Study Guide for

Today's Medical Assistant

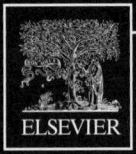

ELSEVIER

evolve

∴ *To access your Resources, visit:*

http://evolve.elsevier.com/Bonewit/today/

Evolve® Student Learning Resources for *Today's Medical Assistant: Clinical & Administrative Procedures* offers the following features:

Learning Resources

- **Apply Your Knowledge**
  Interactive Review Questions that serve as a valuable study tool.

- **Content Updates**
  Continually updated information to provide the latest updates on relevant issues for medical assistants.

- **Prepare for Certification**
  Interactive activities that help prepare for your certification.

Study Guide for

Today's Medical Assistant: Clinical & Administrative Procedures

Kathy Bonewit-West, BS, MEd
Coordinator and Instructor
Medical Assistant Technology
Hocking College
Nelsonville, Ohio

Former Member, Curriculum Review Board
 of the American Association of Medical Assistants

Sue A. Hunt, MA, RN, CMA (AAMA)
Former Professor and Coordinator
Medical Assisting Program
Middlesex Community College
Lowell, Massachusetts

Edith Applegate, MS
Professor of Biological Sciences
Kettering College of Medical Arts
Kettering, Ohio

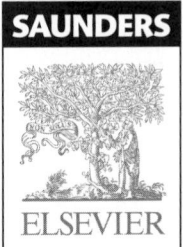

SAUNDERS

ELSEVIER

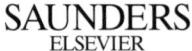

11830 Westline Industrial Drive
St. Louis, Missouri 63146

Notice

Knowledge and best practice in this field are constantly changing. As new research and experience broaden our knowledge, changes in practice, treatment and drug therapy may become necessary or appropriate. Readers are advised to check the most current information provided (i) on procedures featured or (ii) by the manufacturer of each product to be administered, to verify the recommended dose or formula, the method and duration of administration, and contraindications. It is the responsibility of the practitioner, relying on their own experience and knowledge of the patient, to make diagnoses, to determine dosages and the best treatment for each individual patient, and to take all appropriate safety precautions. To the fullest extent of the law, neither the Publisher nor the Authors assume any liability for any injury and/or damage to persons or property arising out or related to any use of the material contained in this book.

The Publisher

ISBN: 978-1-4160-4431-4

Publisher: Michael S. Ledbetter
Associate Developmental Editor: Jennifer Bertucci
Publishing Services Manager: Patricia Tannian
Senior Project Manager: Kristine Feeherty
Design Direction: Charlie Seibel

Printed in the United States of America

Last digit is the print number: 9 8 7 6 5 4 3 2

Preface

Outcome-based education is education directed toward preparing individuals to perform the prespecified tasks of an occupation under "real world" conditions at a level of accuracy and speed required of the entry-level practitioner of that profession. Outcome-based education plays an important role in medical assisting programs to assist in preparing qualified individuals for careers in medical offices, clinics, and related health care facilities. *Study Guide for Today's Medical Assistant: Clinical & Administrative Procedures* has been developed using a complete and thorough outcome-based approach. It meets the criteria stipulated by the CAAHEP Standards and Guidelines for the Medical Assisting Educational Programs (2003) and the ABHES entry-level competencies for medical assistants. The 2008 CAAHEP Standards and Guidelines will be effective in January 2009, and a grid to cross-reference the 2003 standards will be available on the Evolve website at that time. This Study Guide will be a valuable teaching aid for preparing well-trained students who are able to think critically and perform competently in the clinical setting.

Each study guide chapter is organized into the following eight sections:

1. **ASSIGNMENT SHEETS:** The textbook and Study Guide Assignment Sheets indicate the assignments required for each chapter along with a space for the student to document the following: (a) the date each assignment is due, (b) completion of the assignment, and (c) points earned for each assignment. The Laboratory Assignment Sheet presents the procedures required for each chapter along with the textbook and Study Guide reference pages, the number of practices required to attain competency, and a space for documenting the score earned on the Performance Evaluation Checklist.

2. **PRETEST AND POSTTEST:** A Pretest and Posttest have been included for each chapter using true/false questions that allow the student to test his/her acquisition of knowledge for each chapter before and after completing the chapter. These tests can be used as a study guide to prepare for chapter tests.

3. **KEY TERM ASSESSMENT:** The Key Term Assessment section provides the student with an assessment of his/her knowledge of the medical terms relating to each chapter.

4. **EVALUATION OF LEARNING:** The Evaluation of Learning questions help the student evaluate his/her progress throughout each chapter. Once the student has completed these questions and checked them for accuracy, they will serve as an ongoing review of the cognitive knowledge presented in the textbook. Individuals preparing for a national certification examination will find the completed Evaluation of Learning sections a useful study aid for the clinical aspect of the examination.

5. **CRITICAL THINKING ACTIVITIES:** In the Critical Thinking Activities section, the student performs activities that enhance his/her ability to think critically. Some situations require that the student become involved in a game or role-playing situation; others require that the student use independent study in order to answer questions posed by a patient. Independent study helps the student become familiar with resources available to acquire additional knowledge and skills outside the classroom. By learning techniques of self-development, the medical assisting student may become aware of the necessity for continuing education after graduation and entrance into the medical assisting profession.

6. **PRACTICE FOR COMPETENCY:** The Practice for Competency section consists of worksheets that provide the student with a guide for the practice of each clinical skill presented in the textbook.

7. **EVALUATION OF COMPETENCY:** The Evaluation of Competency section is divided into two parts. The first part is the Performance Objective. Its purpose is to provide an exact description of what the learner must be able to demonstrate to attain competency. A performance objective consists of the following three components: (1) the outcome, (2) conditions, and (3) standards. Each Performance Objective in this Study Guide has been developed to correspond with the procedures presented in the textbook.

The second part of the Evaluation of Competency section is the Performance Evaluation Checklist. The Performance Evaluation Checklist provides quality control by comparing the student's performance against an established set of performance standards.

8. **SUPPLEMENTAL EDUCATION:** Due to the nature of the material, several medical assisting content areas are more difficult than others for the student to comprehend and perform. In particular, students have difficulty in taking patient symptoms and in calculating drug dosage. Because of this, two supplemental education sections have been incorporated into this manual. The section "Taking Patient Symptoms" provides supplemental education for Chapter 36 (The Medical Record) in the textbook; the section "Drug Dosage Calculation" provides supplemental education for Chapter 26 (Administration of Medication). In these two sections, a step-by-step, self-directed approach has been used, beginning with basic concepts and advancing to more difficult ones. The student should find that this type of approach facilitates the process of becoming proficient in these areas.

We would like to thank the staff at Elsevier for their assistance and support in preparing this Study Guide. We would also like to express my appreciation to the following individuals who provided encouragement and friendship throughout this endeavor: Dave Brennan, Marlene Donovan, Dawn Bennett, Deborah Murray, Rob Bonewit, Hollie Bonewit, Tristen West, Caitlin Brennan, and Melissa Spencer.

Kathy Bonewit-West, BS, MEd
Sue A. Hunt, MA, RN, CMA (AAMA)
Edith Applegate, MS

CAAHEP competencies used on the "Evaluation of Competency" checklists with permission from the American Association of Medical Assistants, Chicago, Illinois, and the Commission on Accreditation of Allied Health Education Programs, Clearwater, Florida.
ABHES competencies used on the "Evaluation of Competency" checklists with permision from the Accrediting Bureau of Health Education Schools, Falls Church, Virginia.

Message to the Student

This Study Guide has been designed to facilitate the attainment of competency in the clinical theory and procedures in your textbook. Each chapter of the manual has been organized into the eight components outlined below. By completing each component, it is hoped that your ability to assimilate the theory and perform the clinical skills will be greatly enhanced.

1. TEXTBOOK AND STUDY GUIDE ASSIGNMENT SHEETS

    A. Each time your instructor makes an assignment from the textbook, Study Guide, or Companion CD, document the date due in the appropriate space on the Textbook or Study Guide Assignment Sheet.
    B. Complete each assignment by the due date. Place a checkmark in the appropriate space on the Textbook or Study Guide Assignment Sheet after completing each assignment.
    C. Grade your assignment according to the directions stipulated by your instructor.
    D. Record your points earned in the appropriate space on the Textbook or Study Guide Assignment sheet.

2. LABORATORY ASSIGNMENT SHEET

    A. Your instructor will assign the procedure (or procedures) to be completed for each laboratory practice session. Check which procedures are assigned in the appropriate space on the Laboratory Assignment Sheet.
    B. Refer to the page numbers on the Laboratory Assignment Sheet for the Practice for Competency and Evaluation of Competency worksheets required for each procedure your instructor assigned.
    C. Locate and tear out the worksheets required for each procedure to be performed and bring them to your laboratory practice session.
    D. Record the score you earned on the Evaluation of Competency Performance Evaluation Checklist in the appropriate space on the Laboratory Assignment Sheet. This will provide you with an ongoing record of your progress on your clinical procedures.

3. PRETEST AND POSTTEST

    A. Complete the Pretest before beginning a study of each chapter. Complete the Posttest after completing the study of the chapter. Place a checkmark in the appropriate space on the Study Guide Assignment Sheet after completing each test.
    B. Check your work for accuracy with the textbook and correct any errors.
    C. Grade your Pretest and Posttest according to the directions stipulated by your instructor.
    D. Record the points you earned in the appropriate space on the Study Guide Assignment Sheet.
    E. Review the Pretest and Posttest before taking your chapter test.

4. KEY TERM ASSESSMENT

    A. Study the Terminology Review section located at the end of each chapter in the textbook.
    B. Match the medical terms with the definitions. Place a checkmark in the appropriate space on the Study Guide Assignment Sheet after completing.
    C. Check your work for accuracy, using your textbook, and correct any errors.
    D. Grade your Key Term Assessment according to the directions stipulated by your instructor.
    E. Record the points you earned in the appropriate space on the Study Guide Assignment Sheet.
    F. Review the Key Term Assessment before taking your chapter test.

5. EVALUATION OF LEARNING QUESTIONS

    A. Read the textbook chapter.
    B. Complete the Evaluation of Learning questions. Place a checkmark in the appropriate space on the Study Guide Assignment Sheet after completing the questions.
    C. Check your work for accuracy, using the textbook, and correct any errors.
    D. Grade your Evaluation of Learning questions according to the directions stipulated by your instructor.
    E. Record the points you earned in the appropriate space on the Textbook Assignment Sheet.
    F. Review the Evaluation of Learning questions before taking your chapter test.

6. CRITICAL THINKING ACTIVITIES

    A. Review the information required to complete the Critical Thinking Activities.
    B. Obtain any additional materials or resources required.
    C. Complete each Critical Thinking Activity. Place a checkmark in the appropriate space on the Study Guide Assignment Sheet after completing each assigned activity.
    D. Grade each Critical Thinking Activity according to the directions stipulated by your instructor.
    E. Record the points you earned in the appropriate space on the Textbook Assignment Sheet.

7. COMPANION CD ACTIVITIES

    A. Review the information required to complete the companion CD activities.
    B. Using the companion CD, complete the activities.
    C. Place a checkmark in the appropriate space on the Study Guide Assignment Sheet after completing each companion CD activity.
    D. Record the points you earned in the appropriate space on the Study Guide Assignment Sheet.

8. PRACTICE FOR COMPETENCY

    A. Your instructor will assign the procedure (or procedures) to be completed for each laboratory practice session. For each procedure assigned, place a checkmark in the appropriate space on the Laboratory Assignment Sheet.
    B. Refer to the page numbers on the Laboratory Assignment Sheet for the Practice for Competency and Evaluation of Competency sheets required for each procedure your instructor assigned. Locate and tear out the sheets required for each procedure to be performed and bring them to your laboratory practice session.
    C. Practice each assigned procedure the required number of times indicated on the Laboratory Assignment Sheet or as designated by your instructor. Use the following as a guide when practicing the procedure to attain competency over each procedure:
        (1) Information indicated on the Practice for Competency sheet
            • Record your practices in the chart provided on the Practice for Competency sheet.
        (2) Procedure as presented in your textbook
        (3) Video of the procedure (located on the Companion DVDs accompanying your textbook)
            • It is often helpful to view the procedure on the Companion DVD several times to make sure you understand the correct technique and theory for each procedure.
        (4) Evaluation of Competency Performance Checklist
            • Make sure that you are able to perform each procedure according to the criteria stipulated under conditions and standards.
        (5) Peer Evaluation
            • If directed by your instructor, obtain a peer evaluation using the Evaluation of Competency Performance Evaluation Checklist.
    D. Bring the completed Practice for Competency sheet to your laboratory testing session and present it to your instructor for his/her review before testing over the procedure.

9. EVALUATION OF COMPETENCY PERFORMANCE CHECKLIST

    A. Write your name and date in the space indicated on the Evaluation of Competency Performance Evaluation Checklist.
    Important Note: Do not chart the procedure (in advance) on the Evaluation of Competency sheet. You will do this after you have tested over the procedure.

B. For each procedure you are being evaluated over, bring the following to your laboratory testing session and present them to your instructor:
    (1) Completed Practice for Competency sheet
    (2) Evaluation of Competency Performance Checklist
    (3) Outcome Assessment Record
C. Demonstrate the proper procedure for performing the clinical skill for your instructor.
D. Record results (if required) in the chart provided on the Evaluation of Competency Checklist.
E. Obtain your instructor's initials on your Outcome Assessment Record indicating you have performed the procedure with competency.
F. Record the score you earned in the appropriate space on your Laboratory Assignment Sheet.

Once you have completed each chapter in this Study Guide, it is suggested that you place the perforated sheet into a three-ring notebook. This will provide you with an ongoing record of your academic progress. In addition, the notebook will be useful both as a classroom reference and as a certification examination review resource. The author hopes that this Study Guide will assist your attainment of competency in clinical medical assisting procedures, and in turn, facilitate your transition from the classroom to the workplace.

Kathy Bonewit West, BS, MEd
Sue A. Hunt, MA, RN, CMA (AAMA)
Edith Applegate, MS

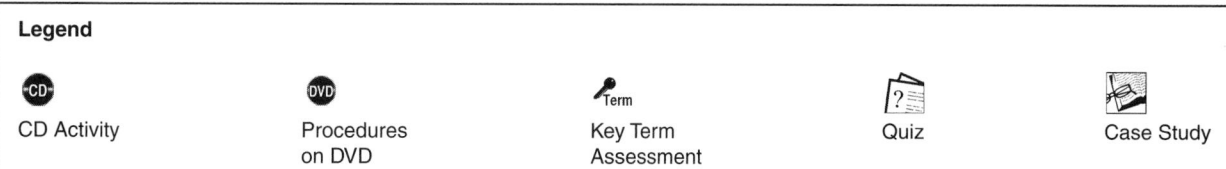

Legend				
CD Activity	Procedures on DVD	Key Term Assessment	Quiz	Case Study

Outcome Assessment Record

Guidelines: This list of outcomes is used to maintain an ongoing record of classroom and practicum outcome assessment. Your instructor should initial each outcome when you have performed it with competency in the classroom. When you have performed the outcome with competency at your practicum facility, it should be initialed by your practicum supervisor. (*Note:* Space is provided for three practicum experiences in the event that you extern at more than one practicum site.)

Name _____	Classroom Performance	Practicum	Practicum	Practicum
MEDICAL ASEPSIS AND THE OSHA STANDARD				
Wash hands.				
Apply an alcohol-based hand rub.				
Apply and remove clean disposable gloves.				
Adhere to the OSHA Standard.				
STERILIZATION AND DISINFECTION				
Sanitize instruments.				
Wrap and label an article for autoclaving.				
Sterilize articles in the autoclave.				
VITAL SIGNS				
Measure oral body temperature.				
Measure axillary body temperature.				
Measure rectal body temperature.				
Measure aural body temperature.				
Measure temporal artery body temperature.				
Measure radial pulse.				
Measure apical pulse.				
Perform pulse oximetry.				
Measure blood pressure.				

Name _____	Classroom Performance	Practicum	Practicum	Practicum
THE PHYSICAL EXAMINATION				
Prepare the examining room.				
Prepare the patient for a physical examination.				
Measure weight and height.				
Position and drape an individual.				
Assist the physician with a physical examination.				
EYE AND EAR PROCEDURES				
Assess distance visual acuity.				
Assess color vision.				
Perform an eye irrigation.				
Perform an eye instillation.				
Perform an ear irrigation.				
Perform an ear instillation.				
PHYSICAL AGENTS TO PROMOTE TISSUE HEALING				
Apply a heating pad.				
Apply a hot soak.				
Apply a hot compress.				
Apply an ice bag.				
Apply a cold compress.				
Apply a chemical cold and hot pack.				
Measure an individual for axillary crutches.				
Instruct an individual in mastering crutch gaits.				
Instruct an individual in the use of a cane.				
Instruct an individual in the use of a walker.				
THE GYNECOLOGIC EXAMINATION AND PRENATAL CARE				
Provide instructions for a breast self-examination.				
Prepare the patient for a gynecologic examination.				
Assist with a gynecologic examination.				
Prepare the patient for a prenatal examination.				
Assist the physician with a prenatal examination.				

Name _____	Classroom Performance	Practicum	Practicum	Practicum
THE PEDIATRIC EXAMINATION				
Carry an infant in the following positions: cradle and upright.				
Measure the weight and length of an infant.				
Measure the head circumference of an infant.				
Measure the chest circumference of an infant.				
Plot pediatric measurements on a growth chart.				
Apply a pediatric urine collector.				
MINOR OFFICE SURGERY				
Apply and remove sterile gloves.				
Open a sterile package.				
Add a sterile article to a sterile filed using a peel-apart package.				
Pour a sterile solution into a container on a sterile field.				
Change a sterile dressing.				
Remove sutures.				
Remove staples.				
Apply and remove adhesive skin closures.				
Set up a surgical tray for minor office surgery.				
Assist the physician with minor office surgery.				
Apply the following bandage turns: circular, spiral, spiral-reverse, figure-eight, and recurrent.				
ADMINISTRATION OF MEDICATION AND INTRAVENOUS THERAPY				
Administer oral medication.				
Prepare an injection from a vial.				
Prepare an injection from an ampule.				
Reconstitute a powdered drug.				
Administer a subcutaneous injection.				
Locate the following intramuscular injection sites: dorsogluteal, deltoid, vastus lateralis, and ventrogluteal.				
Administer an intramuscular injection.				
Administer an injection using the Z-track method.				
Administer an intradermal injection.				
Administer a Mantoux test.				
Read and interpret Mantoux test results.				

Name _____	Classroom Performance	Practicum	Practicum	Practicum
CARDIOPULMONARY PROCEDURES				
Record a 12-lead ECG.				
Perform spirometry testing.				
COLON PROCEDURES AND MALE REPRODUCTIVE HEALTH				
Provide instructions for a fecal occult blood test.				
Develop a fecal occult blood test.				
Provide instructions for a testicular self-examination.				
RADIOLOGY AND DIAGNOSTIC IMAGING				
Instruct a patient in the proper preparation required for each of the following x-ray examinations: mammogram, upper GI, lower GI, and intravenous pyelogram.				
Instruct a patient in the proper preparation required for each of the following: ultrasonography, computed tomography, magnetic resonance imaging, and nuclear medicine.				
INTRODUCTION TO THE CLINICAL LABORATORY				
Use a laboratory directory.				
Complete a laboratory request form.				
Prepare a laboratory report for review by the physician.				
Instruct the patient in advance preparation for a specimen collection.				
Collect a specimen.				
Properly handle and store a specimen.				
Review a laboratory report.				
URINALYSIS				
Instruct a patient in clean-catch midstream urine specimen collection.				
Assess the color and appearance of a urine specimen.				
Perform a chemical assessment of a urine specimen.				
Prepare a urine specimen for microscopic analysis.				
Perform a urine pregnancy test.				

Name _____	Classroom Performance	Practicum	Practicum	Practicum
PHLEBOTOMY				
Perform a venipuncture using the vacuum tube method.				
Perform a venipuncture using the butterfly method.				
Obtain a capillary blood specimen.				
HEMATOLOGY				
Perform a hemoglobin determination.				
Perform a hematocrit determination.				
Prepare a blood smear.				
BLOOD CHEMISTRY AND SEROLOGY				
Perform blood chemistry testing.				
Perform a fasting blood sugar using a glucose meter.				
Perform a rapid mononucleosis test.				
MEDICAL MICROBIOLOGY				
Use a microscope.				
Collect a specimen for a throat culture.				
Obtain a specimen using a collection and transport system.				
Perform a rapid strep test.				
THE MEDICAL RECORD				
Prepare a medical record for a new patient.				
Obtain patient consent for treatment.				
Assist a patient in the completion of a consent to release medical information form.				
Release information according to a completed release of medical information form.				
Complete or assist the patient in completing a health history form.				
Obtain and record patient symptoms.				
PATIENT RECEPTION				
Open the medical office.				
Close the medical office.				
Obtain new patient information.				
Explain office policies and procedures.				

Name _____	Classroom Performance	Practicum	Practicum	Practicum
TELEPHONE TECHNIQUES				
Perform a telephone screening.				
Take a telephone message.				
Take requests for medication or prescription refills.				
Telephone a patient for follow-up.				
SCHEDULING APPOINTMENTS				
Set up the appointment matrix.				
Make an appointment.				
Manage the appointment schedule.				
Complete a referral for managed care.				
Schedule inpatient or outpatient diagnostic testing.				
Schedule inpatient or outpaient admissions.				
MEDICAL RECORDS MANAGEMENT				
File patient records alphabetically.				
File patient records numerically.				
File reports.				
WRITTEN COMMUNICATIONS				
Compose a business letter.				
Respond to written communication.				
Transcribe a dictated letter or report.				
Send a fax.				
Prepare copies of multiple-page documents.				
MAIL				
Process incoming mail.				
Look up a ZIP code.				
Prepare envelopes for mailing.				
MANAGING PRACTICE FINANCES				
Complete a patient charge slip.				
Post charges to the patient ledger.				
Post payments and/or adjustments.				
Record a patient's visit on the day sheet.				
Balance the day sheet.				
Write a check.				
Prepare a bank deposit.				
Reconcile a bank deposit.				

Name _____	Classroom Performance	Practicum	Practicum	Practicum
MEDICAL CODING				
Look up a CPT code.				
Look up a HCPCS code.				
Look up an ICD-9-CM code.				
MEDICAL INSURANCE				
Complete/review the CMS-1500 form.				
BILLING AND COLLECTIONS				
Process patient bills.				
Post an NSF check.				
Post an overpayment.				
Process a refund.				
Create an accounts receivable aging record.				
Write a collection letter.				
Post a collection agency payment.				
THE MEDICAL ASSISTANT AS OFFICE MANAGER				
Perform routine maintenance of equipment.				
Take a supply or equipment inventory.				
Locate community resources.				
ADDITIONAL OUTCOMES (List)				

Contents

Study Guide for

Today's Medical Assistant

1

The Health Care System

CHAPTER ASSIGNMENTS

√ After Completing	Date Due	Textbook Page(s)	TEXTBOOK ASSIGNMENTS	Possible Points	Points You Earned
		1-20	Read Chapter 1: The Health Care System		
		11 18	📖 Read Case Study 1 Case Study questions	5	
		13 18-19	📖 Read Case Study 2 Case Study questions	5	
		18 19	📖 Read Case Study 3 Case Study questions	5	
			TOTAL POINTS		

√ After Completing	Date Due	Study Guide Page(s)	STUDY GUIDE ASSIGNMENTS (CTA: Critical Thinking Activity)	Possible Points	Points You Earned
		3	📝 Pretest	10	
		4	🔑 Key Term Assessment	12	
		5-7	📋 Evaluation of Learning questions	24	
		7	CTA A: Allied Health Professionals	10	
		8	CTA B: The Medical Office	10	
		8	CTA C: Medical Specialties	10	
			💿 CD Activity: Chapter 1 Flashcards: Historical Figures in Medicine (Record points earned)		
			💿 CD Activity: Chapter 1 Apply Your Knowledge questions (Record points earned)		
		3	📝 Posttest	10	

√ After Completing	Date Due	Study Guide Page(s)	STUDY GUIDE ASSIGNMENTS (CTA: Critical Thinking Activity)	Possible Points	Points You Earned
			ADDITIONAL ASSIGNMENTS		
			TOTAL POINTS		

Name _____   Date _____

? PRETEST

True or False

_____   1. Palliative treatment attempts to reduce symptoms but does not cure disease.

_____   2. In the past 30 years there has been a trend to avoid admitting patients to the hospital if possible.

_____   3. The first health insurance plans in the United States were provided by the federal government.

_____   4. The managed care movement has put pressure on physicians to limit time spent with individual patients.

_____   5. After graduating from medical school, a physician spends 2 to 5 years in postgraduate training called an *internship*.

_____   6. If laboratory tests are done in the medical office, there is a specific room or area set aside for this.

_____   7. Some medical offices use paper medical records, but other offices store patient records electronically.

_____   8. The physician who provides general medical care to an adult is usually an internist or a family practitioner.

_____   9. A group practice often consists of three or four physicians in the same specialty.

_____ 10. In addition to standard medical treatment, only a few patients also receive treatments that can be called *complementary medicine*.

? POSTTEST

True or False

_____   1. In order to be hospitalized, a patient's condition must be very unstable or require regulation of therapy.

_____   2. Managed care insurance is another name for fee-for-service insurance.

_____   3. A nurse practitioner manages routine patient care and can write prescriptions in most states.

_____   4. When a patient enters the office, he or she is immediately taken to a treatment room.

_____   5. The government agency that provides for health and safety in the workplace is CLIA.

_____   6. Medical records for all patients who have been seen in the past 10 years are kept in the medical office.

_____   7. The medical office may have a special room just for treatments or procedures.

_____   8. An osteopathic physician (DO) provides primary care and has the same legal status as a physician with an MD degree.

_____   9. The physician who specializes in diseases of the nervous system is a neurologist.

_____ 10. Acupuncture is considered to be a standard medical treatment.

⚷Term KEY TERM ASSESSMENT

Directions: Match each medical term with its definition.

_____ 1. Ambulatory care

_____ 2. Capitation

_____ 3. Empirically

_____ 4. Fee-for-service

_____ 5. Formulary

_____ 6. Health insurance

_____ 7. Holistic

_____ 8. Managed care

_____ 9. Palliative treatment

_____ 10. Residency

_____ 11. Symptomatic treatment

_____ 12. Utilization review

A. A system that manages the delivery of health care with the intention of controlling costs

B. A set payment provided by managed care insurance per patient per month regardless of the amount of service the patient receives

C. Considering the whole; in medicine, considering the entire person when providing health care

D. Therapy that reduces the effects of disease or condition but does not remove the disease itself

E. A program to provide training in a medical specialty to a physician who has finished medical school

F. Medical care that is provided on an outpatient basis

G. Therapy for symptoms of a disease or condition that does not remove the disease itself

H. Purchase of protection for covered services related to health care

I. Assessing medical services to determine whether they are appropriate, necessary, and of high quality

J. A means of payment for health care in which each service provided is reimbursed in full or in part

K. Learned from observation or experiment

L. A list of prescription drugs covered or preferred by a managed care insurance company

EVALUATION OF LEARNING

Directions: Fill in each blank with the correct answer.

1. What is the World Health Organization's definition of health?

   _____

   _____

   _____

2. What historical figure is considered to be the first to see illness as a result of physical and environmental factors? When did he live?

   _____

3. What three trends in modern medicine have increased the importance of ambulatory care?

   _____

   _____

   _____

4. What is fee-for-service health insurance?

   _____

   _____

5. List and give a short description of three government insurance plans that were introduced starting in the 1960s.

   _____

   _____

   _____

6. Briefly describe what managed care is.

   _____

   _____

   _____

7. If a managed care insurance plan uses capitation to pay for health care, what does this mean?

   _____

   _____

   _____

8. How do managed care plans attempt to reduce the cost of prescription medications?

   _____

   _____

   _____

9. List the six steps of an ordinary patient visit to a medical office.

   _____

   _____

   _____

10. Identify at least six other health professionals besides the physician and the medical assistant who may work in the medical office.

_____

_____

_____

11. Describe briefly how physicians are educated.

_____

_____

_____

12. What examination does a physician take to obtain a state license to practice medicine? How does a physician become "board certified"?

_____

_____

_____

13. Describe the education and training of a physician assistant (PA) and a nurse practitioner (NP).

_____

_____

_____

_____

14. What is teamwork? Identify at least four components of effective teamwork.

_____

_____

_____

15. Identify the major areas of a typical medical office and their functions.

_____

_____

_____

_____

16. Identify four other areas that can be found in larger offices.

_____

_____

_____

17. Identify three types of primary care physicians.

_____

_____

18. Describe osteopathy. Are osteopaths licensed to practice medicine?

_____

_____

19. What is podiatry, and what kinds of patients might be referred to a podiatrist?

_____

20. What is chiropractic, and what kinds of patients seek care from a chiropractor?

_____

21. What is the difference between a solo practice and a group practice?

_____

_____

22. What type of medical facility was traditionally called a *clinic?*

_____

_____

23. Describe at least five types of complementary medicine.

_____

_____

_____

24. What is the role of complementary medicine in the United States today?

_____

_____

CRITICAL THINKING ACTIVITIES

A. ALLIED HEALTH PROFESSIONALS

Refer to Table 1-3 and select the allied health professionals, other than a medical assistant, who are most qualified to perform each of the following tasks.

1. Take an x-ray of the lower leg: _____

2. Create a meal plan for a patient with a gastrointestinal disease: _____

3. Supervise laboratory operations: _____

4. Pass instruments during surgery to repair a hernia: _____

5. Plan an exercise program for a patient after replacement of a hip: _____

6. Help a patient learn how to get dressed after a stroke: _____

7. Provide respiratory treatments to a patient with pneumonia: _____

8. Perform an ultrasound of the gallbladder: _____

9. Assign codes to office surgical procedures for billing: _____

10. Set up a medical record filing system: _____

B. THE MEDICAL OFFICE

Where in the medical office shown in Figure 1-4 would the following activities probably take place?

1. Put a patient's medical record after use: _____

2. Physical examination by the physician: _____

3. Patient telephones for an appointment: _____

4. Patient is weighed: _____

5. Test urine specimens: _____

6. Physician meeting with patient and family: _____

7. Prepare patient bills for mailing: _____

8. Suture a laceration: _____

9. Patient checks in: _____

10. Patient charges posted to patient accounts: _____

C. MEDICAL SPECIALTIES

Look up each of the following conditions as needed and refer to Box 1-1 in the textbook to identify which medical specialist would treat an adult patient with the following problems:

1. Recurrent urinary tract infections: _____

2. Tumor of the colon: _____

3. Acne: _____

4. Brain tumor: _____

5. Ovarian cyst: _____

6. Cataract: _____

7. Hip fracture: _____

8. Growth on the vocal cords: _____

9. Stroke with paralysis: _____

10. Repair of fractured cheek bone: _____

2

The Professional Medical Assistant

CHAPTER ASSIGNMENTS

√After Completing	Date Due	Textbook Page(s)	TEXTBOOK ASSIGNMENTS	Possible Points	Points You Earned
		21-33	Read Chapter 2: The Professional Medical Assistant		
		24 32	📖 Read Case Study 1 Case Study questions	5	
		26 32-33	📖 Read Case Study 2 Case Study questions	5	
		27 33	📖 Read Case Study 3 Case Study questions	5	
			TOTAL POINTS		

√After Completing	Date Due	Study Guide Page(s)	STUDY GUIDE ASSIGNMENTS (CTA: Critical Thinking Activity)	Possible Points	Points You Earned
		11	📝 Pretest	10	
		12	🔑 Key Term Assessment	6	
		13-15	📋 Evaluation of Learning questions	25	
		15	CTA A: Professional Appearance	30	
		15	CTA B: Professional Behavior for Physicians	6	
		16	CTA C: Professional Organizations	6	
		16	CTA D: Scope of Practice	5	
			💿 CD Activity: Chapter 2 Apply Your Knowledge questions (Record points earned)		
		11	📝 Posttest	10	

√After Completing	Date Due	Study Guide Page(s)	STUDY GUIDE ASSIGNMENTS (CTA: Critical Thinking Activity)	Possible Points	Points You Earned
			ADDITIONAL ASSIGNMENTS		
			TOTAL POINTS		

Name _____   Date _____

⌷ PRETEST

True or False

_____ 1. The American Medical Technologists was the first professional organization for medical assistants.

_____ 2. A medical assistant who accepts that patients often have different beliefs is displaying dependability.

_____ 3. Being well organized helps the medical assistant respond to sudden changes in schedule or plans.

_____ 4. A medical assistant should always wait for instructions before beginning a new task.

_____ 5. Professionalism is based on both scientific knowledge and a code of ethical behavior.

_____ 6. If a physician engages in unprofessional behavior, the state may suspend or revoke his or her license to practice medicine.

_____ 7. A registered medical assistant has passed a national examination given by the American Association of Medical Assistants (AAMA).

_____ 8. Continuing education is required if a medical assistant wants to maintain certification as a certified medical assistant (CMA [AAMA]) or registered medical assistant (RMA).

_____ 9. Professional organizations for medical assistants publish journals to help medical assistants stay current.

_____ 10. Billing is performed by a specialist in the medical office, not the medical assistant.

⌷ POSTTEST

True or False

_____ 1. Medical assisting programs seek accreditation from the American Association of Medical Assistants or the American Medical Technologists.

_____ 2. To be suited for the profession of medical assisting, an individual must be able to put the needs of a patient first.

_____ 3. In almost all offices, the medical assistant wears professional street clothes for both clinical and administrative tasks.

_____ 4. A medical assistant can demonstrate initiative by restocking examination rooms without having to be told to do so.

_____ 5. A professional medical assistant may have to report a colleague who breaks patient confidentiality.

_____ 6. If a medical assistant is certified, he or she has a state license to be a medical assistant.

_____ 7. In order to become a certified medical assistant, an individual must have graduated from an accredited medical assisting program.

_____ 8. Professional organizations provide programs that carry continuing education credit so that medical assistants can maintain certification.

_____ 9. State, local, and national meetings are held by professional organizations to help medical assistants meet their professional needs.

_____ 10. Risk management is a term used specifically for measures to prevent the spread of infection in a health care setting.

Term KEY TERM ASSESSMENT

Directions: Match each medical term with its definition.

_____ 1. Accreditation

_____ 2. Continuing education unit (CEU)

_____ 3. Externship

_____ 4. Fee splitting

_____ 5. Initiative

_____ 6. Risk management

A. A work experience that is required in an educational program and usually unpaid

B. Processes to protect a health care facility from the risk of legal action

C. The ability to begin or carry through on a plan of action independently

D. Credit or recognition for maintaining certain standards by a regional or national organization

E. The practice of sharing fees with colleagues, especially for making referrals

F. A standard unit of measure on continuing education for professionals, defined as 10 contact hours of participation

EVALUATION OF LEARNING

Directions: Fill in each blank with the correct answer.

1. Identify five changes in medical care over the past 25 years that have affected the profession of medical assisting.

   _____

   _____

2. List two organizations that have worked to define professionalism for medical assistants.

   _____

3. What are four important character traits of a professional medical assistant?

   _____

4. How is caring expressed by a medical assistant?

   _____

5. Identify three reasons why neatness and good grooming are important for the medical assistant.

   _____

   _____

   _____

6. What does the medical assistant usually wear when performing clinical tasks? Administrative tasks?

   _____

7. Give two specific examples of how the medical assistant can demonstrate initiative.

   _____

8. Identify four sources of information about professional practice for physicians.

   _____

   _____

9. What is considered to be the first statement of guidelines for professionalism for physicians?

   _____

10. What are five ethical responsibilities of a professional medical assistant?

    _____

    _____

    _____

11. Identify two written sets of standards that provide guidance for professional medical assistants.

    _____

    _____

12. What is the difference between certification and licensure?

    _____

    _____

13. Describe how an individual becomes a certified medical assistant.

_____

_____

14. Describe how an individual becomes a registered medical assistant.

_____

_____

15. Describe three credentials other than certification that a medical assistant may need to obtain.

_____

_____

_____

16. What are the continuing education requirements for a certified medical assistant to recertify?

_____

_____

17. What are the continuing education requirements for a registered medical assistant to recertify?

_____

_____

18. Describe the medical assistant's role in making appointments.

_____

_____

19. Describe the medical assistant's role in maintaining and filing medical records.

_____

_____

20. Describe the medical assistant's role in billing, accepting payments, and recording payments.

_____

_____

21. Describe six areas of clinical responsibility for the medical assistant.

_____

_____

_____

22. Describe the medical assistant's responsibility if an emergency occurs in the medical office.

_____

23. Explain the medical assistant's responsibility related to supplies and equipment.

_____

_____

24. Give examples of three different types of instruction that a medical assistant might give to patients.

    _____

    _____

25. Discuss three common types of health care facilities where medical assistants often find employment.

    _____

    _____

CRITICAL THINKING ACTIVITIES

A. PROFESSIONAL APPEARANCE

Create a poster with pictures and comments to show the proper clothing, hairstyle, and jewelry (if any) for a medical assistant assigned to various areas in the medical office. If you are female, illustrate female attire. If you are male, illustrate male attire.

1. Using items cut from a magazine (such as a uniform supply company) and items printed from the Internet, colored pencils, and markers, illustrate professional attire for the clinical or laboratory area on one half of your poster. Illustrate both short-sleeve and long-sleeve options. Write comments on the poster to describe appropriate hairstyle, jewelry, fingernail appearance, and footwear as needed.

2. Using items cut from a magazine and items printed from the Internet, colored pencils, and markers, illustrate professional attire for the administrative area of the medical office if street clothes are worn. Write comments on the poster to describe appropriate hairstyle, jewelry, fingernail appearance, and footwear as needed.

3. In the classroom, choose a partner and trade sheets. Discuss the reasons for your choices.

B. PROFESSIONAL BEHAVIOR FOR PHYSICIANS

Give reasons why each of the following behaviors by a physician would be considered professional or unprofessional.

1. Requiring a payment from any physician to whom a patient is referred

    _____

    _____

2. Sending prescriptions automatically to a pharmacy in which the physician owns stock without asking the patient if that is his or her preferred pharmacy

    _____

    _____

3. Meeting with pharmacy representatives during the lunch hour and accepting samples of new medications

    _____

    _____

4. Allowing the medical assistant to obtain blood specimens and perform blood tests

    _____

    _____

5. Dating a former patient who now obtains care from another primary care physician

    _____

    _____

6. Treating a patient outside his or her specialty (e.g., a gynecologist treating a patient for diabetes mellitus)

    _____

    _____

C. PROFESSIONAL ORGANIZATIONS

Find information about local/state/regional chapters of the American Association of Medical Assistants and the American Medical Technologists. The websites of the national organizations have links to state associations.

1. What is the location of the nearest chapter of the AAMA to your school? _____

2. What is the location of the nearest chapter of the AMT to your school? _____

3. Is your medical assisting program accredited? _____ If so, by whom? _____

4. When is the next state meeting of the AAMA in your state? _____ AMT? _____

5. Are students and nonmembers welcome to attend state meetings? _____

6. From your research, identify five reasons to attend the state meeting of one or more of these organizations:

   _____

   _____

   _____

   _____

   _____

D. SCOPE OF PRACTICE

Based on the description of the medical assistant's role in Chapter 2, investigate and discuss whether each of the following is within the medical assistant's scope of practice in your state.

1. The medical assistant obtains and tests urine specimens

   _____

   _____

2. The medical assistant performs routine physical examinations on children and adults

   _____

   _____

3. The medical assistant administers immunizations to infants, children and adults

   _____

   _____

4. The medical assistant authorizes prescription refills for patients on long-term medication therapy

   _____

   _____

5. The medical assistant obtains specimens of venous blood by finger stick and phlebotomy and performs diagnostic tests using the blood specimens

   _____

   _____

3

Ethics and Law for the Medical Office

CHAPTER ASSIGNMENTS

√ After Completing	Date Due	Textbook Page(s)	TEXTBOOK ASSIGNMENTS	Possible Points	Points You Earned
		34-57	Read Chapter 3: Ethics and Law for the Medical Office		
		38 55	Read Case Study 1 Case Study questions	5	
		46 55	Read Case Study 2 Case Study questions	5	
		49 55	Read Case Study 3 Case Study questions	5	
			TOTAL POINTS		
√ After Completing	Date Due	Study Guide Page(s)	STUDY GUIDE ASSIGNMENTS (CTA: Critical Thinking Activity)	Possible Points	Points You Earned
		19	Pretest	10	
		20	Key Term Assessment: Ethics	15	
		20-21	Key Term Assessment: Law	35	
		22-26	Evaluation of Learning questions	50	
		26	CTA A: Ethical Issues	30	
		26-27	CTA B: Making Ethical Decisions	4	
		27	CTA C: Advance Directives	3	
		27	CTA D: Intentional Torts	4	
		28	CTA E: Negligence	4	
			CD Activity: Chapter 3 Apply Your Knowledge questions (Record points earned)		

√ After Completing	Date Due	Study Guide Page(s)	STUDY GUIDE ASSIGNMENTS (CTA: Critical Thinking Activity)	Possible Points	Points You Earned
			CD CD Activity: Chapter 3 Quiz Show (Record points earned)		
		19	? Posttest	10	
			ADDITIONAL ASSIGNMENTS		
			TOTAL POINTS		

Name _____   Date _____

PRETEST

True or False

_____ 1. Patients have the right to autonomy, which includes the right to refuse treatment.

_____ 2. Legal abortions and confidentiality are manifestations of the individual's right to privacy.

_____ 3. The branch of law that regulates interactions between individuals and groups is called *criminal law*.

_____ 4. In order to be enforceable, a contract must be written.

_____ 5. A physician cannot refuse to accept patients who seek treatment.

_____ 6. Written consent forms are usually used for surgery and other invasive procedures.

_____ 7. A wound infection after surgery is caused by negligence on the part of the physician.

_____ 8. If a patient is injured through the negligence of a medical assistant, a patient can sue the medical assistant as well as her physician employer.

_____ 9. If a trial is held for malpractice, it is only necessary to provide photocopies of the medical record.

_____ 10. A patient must begin a lawsuit for malpractice within 10 years of the time the injury occurred.

POSTTEST

True or False

_____ 1. Physician-assisted suicide is illegal in all states because a federal law prohibits it.

_____ 2. Health professionals are considered to have a duty to be faithful to reasonable expectations of patients.

_____ 3. A serious crime, committed with the intent to cause harm, is called a *felony*.

_____ 4. In order for a contract to be valid, there must be a mutual agreement between the parties.

_____ 5. A physician can end a relationship with a patient, provided that the patient is notified in writing.

_____ 6. To give informed consent, a patient must understand the risks and benefits of a procedure.

_____ 7. When a physician fails to care for his patient correctly, causing injury to the patient, it is called *professional negligence* or *malpractice*.

_____ 8. Professional liability insurance only covers a physician for his or her own actions.

_____ 9. Most malpractice lawsuits are settled out of court, and no trial occurs.

_____ 10. The physician is not liable for injury to a patient if the patient refuses to follow medical advice.

🔑 KEY TERM ASSESSMENT: ETHICS

Directions: Match each term with its definition.

_____ 1. Autonomy

_____ 2. Beneficence

_____ 3. Cloning

_____ 4. DNR (do not resuscitate)

_____ 5. Duty

_____ 6. Etiquette

_____ 7. Fidelity

_____ 8. Gene therapy

_____ 9. Genetic engineering

_____ 10. Health care proxy

_____ 11. Living will

_____ 12. Nonmalfeasance

_____ 13. Stem cells

_____ 14. Right

_____ 15. Veracity

A. Making, altering, or repairing genetic material
B. Cells that have the capacity to develop into various types of body tissue
C. Ability to make independent decisions without constraint or coercion from others
D. Truthfulness
E. Faithfulness
F. Ethical concept requiring that an action do no harm, or do less harm than good
G. Giving patients new genes or parts of genes to treat a disease or condition
H. A legal document that names an agent to make decisions about a person's medical care if he or she becomes unable to make wishes known
I. Rules of socially acceptable behavior; manners
J. Commitment to act in a certain way
K. Acting in the best possible way; performing good deeds
L. Producing genetically identical cells or individuals artificially
M. A legal document that specifies the kind of medical treatment a patient wants or does not want if he or she becomes incapacitated
N. A medical order signed by a physician that relieves health care personnel from the obligation to resuscitate a patient who stops breathing or whose heart stops
O. A claim that is expected to be honored

🔑 KEY TERM ASSESSMENT: LAW

Directions: Match each term with its definition.

_____ 1. Abandonment

_____ 2. Act

_____ 3. Arbitration

_____ 4. Assumption of risk

_____ 5. Case law

_____ 6. Common law

_____ 7. Contingency

_____ 8. Controlled substance

_____ 9. Defendant

_____ 10. Drug Enforcement Administration (DEA)

A. A formal process in which the parties to a dispute agree to submit to the decision of a neutral party
B. Law established by decisions of previous court cases
C. Law enacted by a legislative body
D. Agreement to a medical procedure based on understanding of the procedure and its possible consequences and effects
E. Unwritten body of law based on general custom
F. Stealing another person's property or money without violence
G. Intentional deception resulting in injury or loss
H. A legal doctrine making an employer liable for the negligent acts of employees
I. The person or group against whom an action is brought in a court of law
J. Failing to perform on act that should have been performed

_____ 11 Embezzlement

_____ 12. Felony

_____ 13. Fraud

_____ 14. Informed consent

_____ 15. Larceny

_____ 16. Liability

_____ 17. License

_____ 18. Litigation

_____ 19. Malfeasance

_____ 20. Malpractice

_____ 21. Mediation

_____ 22. Misdemeanor

_____ 23. Misfeasance

_____ 24. Negligence

_____ 25. Nonfeasance

_____ 26. Plaintiff

_____ 27. Prescription

_____ 28. Privilege

_____ 29. Prudent

_____ 30. Reciprocity

_____ 31. _Respondeat superior_

_____ 32. Standard of care

_____ 33. Statute of limitations

_____ 34. Statutory law

_____ 35. Subpoena _duces tecum_

K. The person or group that makes the complaint in a lawsuit

L. Failure to continue to provide medical care to a patient without proper notification

M. Fraudulent appropriation of funds or property of an employer or client

N. Failure to act (or refrain from acting) as a reasonably prudent person would in similar circumstances

O. Performing a legal act in an improper way

P. A law limiting the time period for beginning a lawsuit

Q. A person under the age of 18 with the rights of an adult including the ability to consent to medical care

R. The federal agency that enforces the Controlled Substances Act of 1970

S. A defense to a lawsuit that establishes the plaintiff assumed the risk of whatever caused the injury

T. A less serious crime, punishable by a fine or imprisonment for less than 1 year

U. A court order to produce documents or records

V. A drug that has the potential for addiction or abuse

W. A bill or measure that has become law, often referring to legislation with several parts

X. Negotiation by a third party to help two parties resolve a dispute

Y. The process of taking a lawsuit through the courts

Z. A special immunity that protects against legal liability

AA. Using care or common sense

BB. Automatic issuing of a license in one state to the holder of a license in another state

CC. A crime or wrongdoing that is illegal or contrary to official obligation

DD. Legal responsibility

EE. A condition that must be met before a contract is binding

FF. Level of appropriate care required of a health professional

GG. Official permission to perform an activity or practice a profession

HH. A serious crime punishable by death or imprisonment

II. Negligence by a professional

JJ. An order to a pharmacist to dispense a supply of a medication

EVALUATION OF LEARNING

Directions: Fill in each blank with the correct answer.

1. Identify four reasons that medical assisting students can benefit from studying about ethics and bioethics.

   _____

   _____

2. Identify three sources of beliefs about the rights and duties of individuals and society as a whole.

   _____

   _____

   _____

3. Describe briefly what is included in each of the following ethical rights:

   a. Right to life _____

   b. Right to privacy _____

   c. Right to autonomy _____

   d. Right to the means to sustain life _____

4. Identify five duties of a health professional.

   _____

5. When does ethical conflict arise?

   _____

6. What are two issues that create conflict within society related to reproductive issues?

   _____

7. What is the current legal position with respect to stem cell research related to federal legislation?

   _____

   _____

8. Define the following terms:

   a. Stem cell research _____

   b. Genetic engineering _____

   c. Cloning _____

   d. Gene therapy _____

9. What are the general provisions of the Patient Self-Determination Act of 1990?

   _____

10. What is the difference between physician-assisted suicide and euthanasia? Is either legal in the United States?

   _____

   _____

11. What are five recommended steps to make ethical decisions?

_____

_____

12. Describe the medical assistant's ethical responsibility related to patient care in the medical office.

_____

13. What is a DNR order?

_____

14. What is the difference between a living will and a health care proxy? Which is preferable?

_____

_____

15. What is the relationship between law and ethics?

_____

16. Briefly describe the following three types of law:

    a. Criminal law _____

    b. Civil law _____

    c. Contract law _____

17. Explain how an injury can result in both civil and criminal lawsuits.

_____

18. Describe two classifications of crimes.

_____

19. Describe each of the following crimes and identify how each might occur in a medical office:

    a. Manslaughter or criminal negligence _____

    b. Embezzlement _____

    c. Fraud _____

20. What three elements are necessary for a legal contract?

_____

_____

21. Differentiate between an intentional tort and an unintentional tort.

_____

22. Differentiate among a malfeasance, a misfeasance, and a nonfeasance.

_____

_____

23. Identify how the physician-patient relationship meets the definition of a contract.

_____

_____

_____

24. Give examples of each of the following types of contracts:

    a. Implied _____

_____

b. Verbal _____

_____

c. Written _____

_____

25. Identify four groups of people who cannot legally be party to a contract or give informed consent.

_____

_____

26. When can an individual who is not yet 18 consent to medical treatment?

_____

27. When can a physician terminate care to a patient?

_____

_____

28. How should the physician notify the patient that he or she is terminating care? Why?

_____

_____

29. What does the term *standard of care* mean?

_____

30. Why is informed consent usually verified by having the patient sign a consent form?

_____

_____

31. What is the medical assistant's role in obtaining a signature on a consent form?

_____

32. What four elements must be proved in order to prove liability for professional negligence (malpractice)?

_____

_____

33. What does the doctrine of *res ipsa loquitur* refer to?

_____

34. What are two reasons for physicians to purchase professional liability insurance?

_____

35. If a physician believes that a patient is going to initiate a lawsuit, how should he or she respond?

_____

36. What is a subpoena and a subpoena *duces tecum*?

_____

37. Differentiate between mediation and arbitration.

_____

38. Describe the following tort defenses:

    a. Privilege _____

    b. Consent _____

    c. Self-defense _____

    d. Expiration of the statute of limitations _____

    e. Contributory negligence _____

    f. Comparative negligence _____

    g. Assumption of risk _____

39. What are controlled substances, and what law regulates their use?

    _____

    _____

40. What are five measures to prevent misuse of prescription forms and tampering with prescriptions?

    _____

    _____

41. What organization was created by the Health and Safety Act of 1970 to protect employees in the workplace?

    _____

42. What are two examples of measures to protect the health of employees in the medical office?

    _____

    _____

43. What employee rights are protected by the following laws?

    a. Equal Opportunity Employment laws

    _____

    b. Americans with Disabilities Act

    _____

    c. Family and Medical Leave Act

    _____

    d. Fair Labor Standards Act

    _____

    e. Employee Retirement Income Security Act

    _____

44. What is the purpose of the Privacy Rule of the Health Insurance Portability and Accountability Act (HIPAA) of 1996?

    _____

45. What are four other rules included in HIPAA?

    _____

    _____

46. Describe what a mandated report is and give five examples of mandatory reporting for physicians.

    _____

    _____

47. What are the four basic requirements for a physician to be licensed in most states?

_____

_____

_____

48. What are grounds for suspending or revoking a license to practice medicine?

_____

49. Which types of health care facilities usually require a state license?

_____

50. Name two organizations that provide voluntary accreditation for physician's offices.

_____

CRITICAL THINKING ACTIVITIES

A. ETHICAL ISSUES

Select one of the following topics for investigation. Do research about the topic to obtain information. Write a short paper giving information to describe the topic and demonstrate why it is controversial. Be sure to give credit for ideas and/or statistics that you have obtained from a book, journal article, or Internet article.

1. Genetically modified food products

2. Partial birth abortion

3. Federal funding for stem cell research

4. Physician-assisted suicide

5. Gene therapy

B. MAKING ETHICAL DECISIONS

Identify the conflicting values in each of the following situations, choose an action, and justify your action.

1. You find your brother, who is 12 years old, smoking a cigarette in the backyard.

_____

_____

_____

_____

2. A patient tells you that she thinks she may be dependent on the narcotic analgesics she has been taking. Then she asks you not to tell the physician, because she still wants to get a refill for the prescription.

_____

_____

_____

_____

3. An elderly relative that you are extremely close to has a chronic condition causing muscle weakness. She begs you to help her "end everything."

_____

_____

_____

_____

4. An expensive medication has been prescribed for a relative by his personal physician. You mention that there are samples of that medication in your office. The relative asks you if you can get some for him.

_____

_____

_____

_____

C. ADVANCE DIRECTIVES

Answer the following questions that might be included in a health care proxy or living will. Discuss your answers with a classmate.

1. If you have a terminal illness or very serious injury and become unable to make your wishes known, whom do you want to make health care decisions on your behalf?

_____

2. If you have an irreversible condition and in the judgment of your physician you cannot care for yourself or make decisions for yourself, which would you request?

_____ I request that all treatments other than those needed to keep me comfortable be discontinued or withheld.

_____ I request that I be kept alive in this condition using available life-sustaining treatment.

3. Are there specific treatments that you would request to be withheld (e.g., ventilator, feeding tube, intravenous therapy, antibiotics for secondary infections)?

_____

_____

D. INTENTIONAL TORTS

Decide whether the following situations would most likely be examples of invasion of privacy, defamation, assault and battery, misrepresentation, or false imprisonment. Discuss with your classmates what the legal consequences may be.

1. In a casual conversation, an acquaintance says, "That dentist is totally incompetent. He can't even put in a filling that won't fall out."

_____

_____

2. An employee of a medical laboratory mentions to a friend that a well-known person in the community has received a positive result on an HIV test.

_____

_____

3. A patient is taken to an emergency room by ambulance with a leg injury. When he arrives, the physician tells the nurse to cut off his pants so that his leg can be examined. The patient says, "Do not cut my clothes. I don't want to be treated here. I will call my wife to come get me." The nurse gets help to hold him down and begins to cut off his pants.

_____

_____

4. A candidate for employment writes on a job application that she is a registered nurse. After being hired, her employer finds out that she completed nursing school but did not pass state boards and does not have a state license as a registered nurse.

_____

_____

E. NEGLIGENCE

Discuss with your classmates what a "reasonably prudent person" would be expected to do in the following situations.

1. Your elderly neighbor slips and falls on a patch of ice in your driveway. She appears unable to get up and complains of pain in her left hip.

   _____

   _____

2. You are in the washroom at work and you notice that the handle on the hot water tap is not working properly so that very hot water is constantly dripping into the sink.

   _____

   _____

3. You spill some coffee on a tile floor at your school.

   _____

   _____

4. You are in a restaurant, and you see another patron who appears to be starting to choke. The person is not making any coughing audibly, but he is clutching his throat and trying to cough.

   _____

   _____

4

Interacting with Patients

CHAPTER ASSIGNMENTS

√ After Completing	Date Due	Textbook Page(s)	TEXTBOOK ASSIGNMENTS	Possible Points	Points You Earned
		58-73	Read Chapter 4: Interacting with Patients		
		62 72	Read Case Study 1 Case Study questions	5	
		65 72	Read Case Study 2 Case Study questions	5	
		69 72	Read Case Study 3 Case Study questions	5	
			TOTAL POINTS		

√ After Completing	Date Due	Study Guide Page(s)	STUDY GUIDE ASSIGNMENTS (CTA: Critical Thinking Activity)	Possible Points	Points You Earned
		31	Pretest	10	
		32	Key Term Assessment	23	
		33-35	Evaluation of Learning questions	30	
		36-38	CTA A: Nonverbal Cues	4	
		38-39	CTA B: Using Effective Communication Techniques	6	
		39	CTA C: Responses That Inhibit Communication	6	
		39	CTA D: Defense Mechanisms	8	
			CD Activity: Chapter 4 Apply Your Knowledge questions (Record points earned)		
		31	Posttest	10	

√ After Completing	Date Due	Study Guide Page(s)	STUDY GUIDE ASSIGNMENTS (CTA: Critical Thinking Activity)	Possible Points	Points You Earned
			ADDITIONAL ASSIGNMENTS		
			TOTAL POINTS		

Name _____   Date _____

PRETEST

True or False

_____ 1. The medical assistant communicates nonverbally using tone of voice and facial gestures.

_____ 2. A closed question expects a yes/no or very short answer.

_____ 3. Silence is an effective technique to encourage a patient to continue speaking.

_____ 4. A patient who is legally blind will be unable to distinguish light and shadow.

_____ 5. If a patient is not comfortable, translation must be done by a native speaker in person.

_____ 6. In Maslow's hierarchy of needs, the needs for safety and security are lower than needs for esteem and recognition.

_____ 7. A patient experiencing moderate anxiety will have difficulty learning new information.

_____ 8. The patient is aware when he or she is relying on ego defense mechanisms like denial.

_____ 9. The medical assistant should remember that anger is often displaced from the true cause to another target.

_____ 10. If a patient believes that disease has a supernatural cause, the medical assistant should tell the patient tactfully that this is impossible.

POSTTEST

True or False

_____ 1. Internal factors that interfere with communication include excessive noise and lack of privacy.

_____ 2. Open questions encourage a patient to explain symptoms in his or her own way.

_____ 3. Paraphrasing is giving a short summary of a verbal communication.

_____ 4. The medical assistant uses both touch and words to guide a patient who is totally blind.

_____ 5. Both telephone and video translation services are available when patients are uncomfortable with English.

_____ 6. The needs depicted on the highest level of Maslow's hierarchy of needs include oxygen, sleep, and adequate nutrition.

_____ 7. Hyperventilation may be a symptom of a full-blown anxiety attack.

_____ 8. Projection is an unconscious ego defense mechanism where an individual ascribes his or her own feelings to another.

_____ 9. If a patient is using denial as an ego defense mechanism, it is important to correct the patient as soon as possible.

_____ 10. A patient from a different culture may believe that changes in diet will help treat certain diseases.

Term KEY TERM ASSESSMENT

Directions: Match each medical term with its definition.

_____ 1. Acting out

_____ 2. Active listening

_____ 3. Anxiety

_____ 4. Body language

_____ 5. Chronic

_____ 6. Closed questions

_____ 7. Denial

_____ 8. Ego defense mechanism

_____ 9. Empathy

_____ 10. Hierarchy

_____ 11. Judgmental

_____ 12. Nonverbal

_____ 13. Open questions

_____ 14. Oral

_____ 15. Paraphrasing

_____ 16. Physiologic

_____ 17. Projection

_____ 18. Reflecting

_____ 19. Self-actualization

_____ 20. Summarizing

_____ 21. Sympathy

_____ 22. Verbal

_____ 23. Webcam

A. Existing over a long period of time
B. Expressing the meaning and emotion of another's words back to the person
C. Spoken; pertaining to the mouth
D. Unconscious mental process that offers psychological protection
E. The fulfillment of each individual's potential
F. Feeling the same emotions as another
G. Failure to acknowledge the reality of a situation
H. Making judgments about what is good or bad based on personal opinion
I. Using words to communicate
J. Translating unconscious emotions into inappropriate behavior
K. Objective awareness and sensitivity to the feelings and emotions of others
L. Questions that anticipate a yes/no or short answer
M. Pertaining to body processes
N. Small video camera attached to a computer that allows video to be transmitted on the Internet
O. Communication that occurs without words, such as through body posture or facial expression
P. Paying close attention to a speaker without thinking of anything else
Q. Classified according to rank or importance
R. Expressing the most important points of a conversation or written document
S. Communication that is expressed through facial expressions, body position, muscle activity, and other nonverbal means
T. Experiencing one's own emotions as those of another
U. A vague, unpleasant emotion of fear or dread often accompanied by restlessness or nervousness
V. A restatement of the words of another, often to clarify meaning
W. Questions that could have a variety of answers and encourage a personal response

EVALUATION OF LEARNING

Directions: Fill in each blank with the correct answer.

1. Give four examples of different types of verbal communication.

   _____

2. Give four examples of nonverbal communication.

   _____

   _____

3. Identify and describe three examples of outside interference with effective communication.

   _____

   _____

4. Identify and describe three examples of inside interference with communication.

   _____

   _____

5. Describe active listening.

   _____

   _____

6. What are four listening techniques that facilitate good communication between medical assistants and patients?

   _____

   _____

7. How can the medical assistant use eye contact and body posture to facilitate communication?

   _____

   _____

8. Give two examples of how nonverbal communication is different in different cultures.

   _____

   _____

9. When is it appropriate to use closed questions during an interview?

   _____

10. When are open-ended questions more useful than closed questions?

    _____

    _____

11. Identify and describe six communication techniques that draw patients out and encourage them to keep talking.

    a. _____

    b. _____

    c. _____

    d. _____

e. _____

f. _____

12. What are three types of responses that inhibit communication or make the patient defensive?

    _____

    _____

13. How can the medical assistant improve communication with a patient whose understanding is impaired?

    _____

    _____

14. Differentiate between a patient who is totally blind and one who is legally blind.

    _____

15. How do patients who are totally blind usually prefer to be assisted in an unknown setting?

    _____

    _____

16. Differentiate between a patient who is deaf and a patient who is hearing impaired.

    _____

17. What measures will improve communication with a patient who is hearing impaired?

    _____

    _____

18. What measures should be implemented to communicate with a deaf patient?

    _____

    _____

19. What are three ways to provide translation service for a patient who is not comfortable communicating in English?

    _____

    _____

20. What are three things that patients often expect when they seek health care?

    _____

    _____

21. Identify the needs on each level of Maslow's hierarchy of needs.

    a. Level 1 (lowest level): _____

    b. Level 2: _____

    c. Level 3: _____

    d. Level 4: _____

    e. Level 5: _____

22. How do unmet needs affect a patient during illness?

    _____

23. Why is it important for medical assistants to identify the unmet needs of patients?

_____

_____

24. Differentiate between empathy and sympathy.

_____

_____

25. How can a medical assistant communicate caring to a patient?

_____

_____

26. Identify and describe four common reactions that patients experience when confronted with a serious medical condition.

_____

_____

_____

27. How do people use ego defense mechanisms?

_____

_____

28. What do individuals from other cultures sometimes believe is a cause of illness other than physiologic factors?

_____

_____

29. What is a general rule about accepting traditional medical practices that patients may use?

_____

_____

30. Identify and discuss two different cultural practices related to behavioral requirements for women and men.

_____

_____

CRITICAL THINKING ACTIVITIES

A. NONVERBAL CUES

In any interaction, a significant part of communication is nonverbal and includes individual interpretation of nonverbal cues. Examine each of the following photographs and summarize your assumptions about each person in the photograph: Who is each person? What is he or she feeling? What might be happening between the two people in the photograph? What is the location pictured in the photograph? Distinguish between assumptions that you are sure of and those you would need more information to confirm.

1.

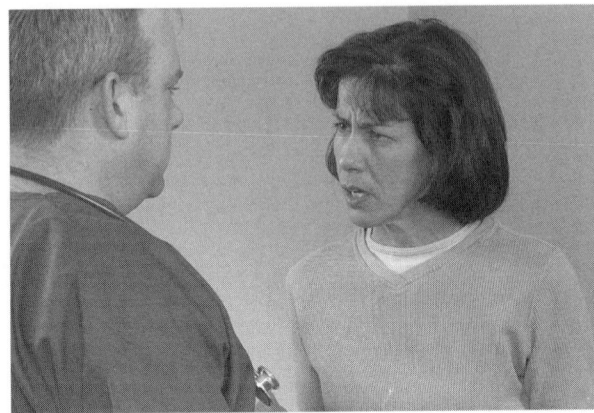

(From Hunt SA: *Student mastery manual for Saunders fundamentals of medical assisting,* Philadelphia, 2002, Saunders.)

_____

_____

_____

_____

2.

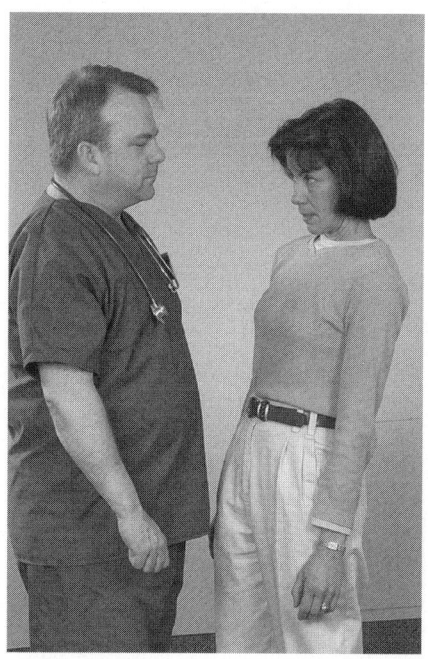

(From Hunt SA: *Student mastery manual for Saunders fundamentals of medical assisting,* Philadelphia, 2002, Saunders.)

_____

_____

_____

_____

3.

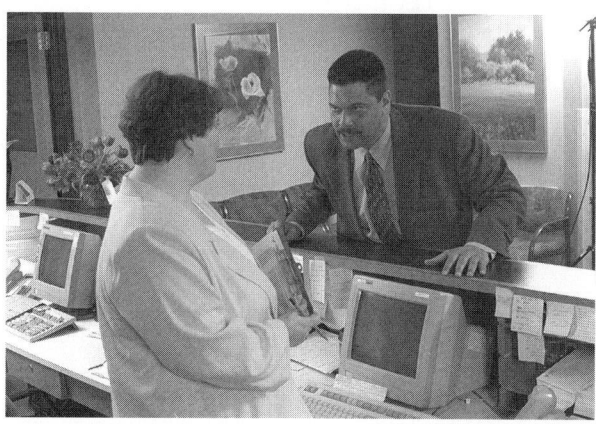

(From Hunt SA: *Student mastery manual for Saunders fundamentals of medical assisting,* Philadelphia, 2002, Saunders.)

_____

_____

_____

_____

4.

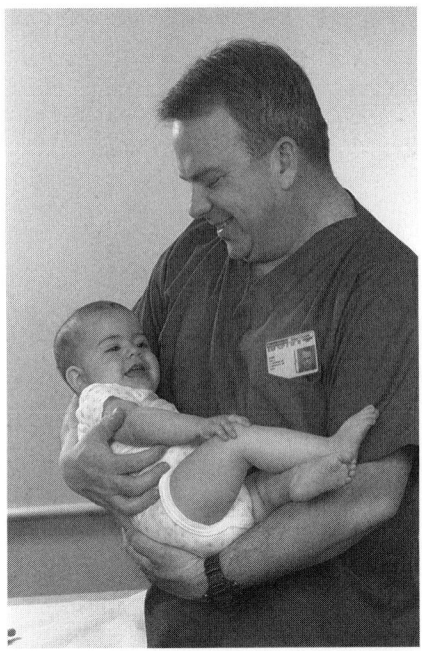

(From Hunt SA: *Student mastery manual for Saunders fundamentals of medical assisting,* Philadelphia, 2002, Saunders.)

_____
_____
_____
_____

B. USING EFFECTIVE COMMUNICATION TECHNIQUES

After you've taken the vital signs of Valerie Hoffman, a 34-year-old teacher, she says, " I don't know if I'm sick or not. I mean, I hope that Dr. Hughes finds something wrong with me to explain why I feel so bad. I don't have any energy, you know. I get up in the morning, when I can finally get myself up, and in about 10 minutes I'm ready to go back to bed for a nap. Everything just seems like it takes so much effort."

Give an example of a response you could make that demonstrates each of the following communication techniques:

1. Paraphrasing

_____
_____

2. Translating a nonverbal message into words

_____
_____

3. Reflecting

_____
_____

4. Summarizing

_____
_____

5. Repeating or restating

_____

_____

6. Asking for clarification

_____

_____

C. RESPONSES THAT INHIBIT COMMUNICATION

Refer to Table 4-2 in your textbook and identify which of the following type of response each of the following examples is. These are responses that inhibit communication.

1. How do you know that bad spirits cause disease? Have you ever seen one?

_____

2. The physician is very busy, you know, because some patients are very ill.

_____

3. You are making a big fuss over a very small problem.

_____

4. After your chemotherapy, you will feel fine in a few hours.

_____

5. Why didn't you take your blood pressure medication?

_____

6. You shouldn't forget to test your blood sugar. That's why it is so high.

_____

D. DEFENSE MECHANISMS

Name the defense mechanism that is illustrated in each of the following examples.

1. A patient says, "The reason I don't use seatbelts is because I am always late." _____

2. A woman has forgotten sexual abuse that occurred during childhood. _____

3. A girl with a facial scar from an accident studies very hard and is always at the top of her class in school. _____

4. An unfaithful husband accuses his wife of having an affair. _____

5. A school-age child starts sucking her thumb and wetting the bed when a new baby is born in the family. _____

6. A man has an unpleasant conversation with his boss at work. When he gets home, he kicks the family dog. _____

7. A woman says to her friend, "No offense, but your hair looks terrible. But I love your outfit, and your skin is perfect." _____

8. After extensive testing and a diagnosis of diabetes mellitus, a patient says, "I know that I don't have diabetes. I am going to get a second opinion." _____

5

Introduction to Anatomy and Physiology

CHAPTER ASSIGNMENTS

√ After Completing	Date Due	Textbook Page(s)	TEXTBOOK ASSIGNMENT	Possible Points	Points You Earned
		74-102	Read Chapter 5: Introduction to Anatomy and Physiology		
√ After Completing	Date Due	Study Guide Page(s)	STUDY GUIDE ASSIGNMENTS (CTA: Critical Thinking Activity)		
		43	📋 Pretest	10	
		44	✎Term Key Term Assessment	26	
		45-56	🗹 Evaluation of Learning questions: The Human Body Cell Structure and Function Tissue and Membranes	19 32 68	
		56	CTA A: Planes of the Body	3	
		57	CTA B: Cavities of the Body	8	
		57	CTA C: Abdominopelvic Quadrants	4	
		58	CTA D: Abdominopelvic Regions	9	
		58	•CD• CTA E: Road to Recovery CD Activity: Body Area Terms (Record points earned)		
		58	•CD• CTA F: Body Spectrum CD Activity: General Human Cell	10	
		59	CTA G: Cell Structure and Function	40	
		60	•CD• CTA H: Chapter 5 Animations CD Activity	32	
		61	CTA I: Crossword Puzzle	25	
		43	📋 Posttest	10	

√ After Completing	Date Due	Study Guide Page(s)	STUDY GUIDE ASSIGNMENTS (CTA: Critical Thinking Activity)		
			ADDITIONAL ASSIGNMENTS		
			TOTAL POINTS		

Name_____ Date_____

PRETEST

True or False

_____ 1. The study of the shape and structure of the human body is known as *human anatomy*.

_____ 2. The integumentary system protects underlying tissue from injury.

_____ 3. The lungs are located in the pelvic cavity.

_____ 4. The nucleolus is the control center that directs the activities of the cell.

_____ 5. The function of lysosomes is to destroy cellular debris and foreign particles.

_____ 6. A human cell has 23 pairs of chromosomes.

_____ 7. Cytology is the microscopic study of tissues.

_____ 8. Fibroblasts secrete mucus.

_____ 9. Adipose tissue protects the body from invasion by pathogens.

_____ 10. Platelets initiate the blood clotting mechanism.

POSTTEST

True or False

_____ 1. An organ is made up of a group of tissues with a similar structure and function.

_____ 2. A frontal plane divides the body into right and left portions.

_____ 3. The plasma membrane determines what can enter or leave a cell.

_____ 4. Ribosomes are responsible for protein synthesis.

_____ 5. Microvilli are hairlike processes that move substances across the surface of a cell.

_____ 6. A red blood cell will hemolyze if it is placed in a hypertonic solution.

_____ 7. Capillary walls are made up of simple squamous epithelial tissue.

_____ 8. An endocrine gland secretes its product onto a free surface through a duct.

_____ 9. Skeletal muscle tissue is under involuntary control.

_____ 10. A mucous membrane lines a body cavity that opens to the outside.

KEY TERM ASSESSMENT

Directions: Match each medical term with its definition.

_____ 1. Active transport

_____ 2. Anatomic position

_____ 3. Chondrocyte

_____ 4. Collagenous fibers

_____ 5. Cytokinesis

_____ 6. Diffusion

_____ 7. Elastic fibers

_____ 8. Fibroblast

_____ 9. Histology

_____ 10. Homeostasis

_____ 11. Human anatomy

_____ 12. Human physiology

_____ 13. Macrophage

_____ 14. Mast cell

_____ 15. Meiosis

_____ 16. Metabolism

_____ 17. Mitosis

_____ 18. Negative feedback

_____ 19. Neuroglia

_____ 20. Neuron

_____ 21. Osmosis

_____ 22. Osteocyte

_____ 23. Passive transport

_____ 24. Phagocytosis

_____ 25. Pinocytosis

_____ 26. Tissue

A. Division of the cytoplasm

B. Connective tissue cell that produces fibers

C. The type of nuclear division in which the number of chromosomes is reduced to half the number found in a body cell; results in the formation of an egg or sperm

D. A response mechanism of the body in which a stimulus initiates a reaction that reduces the stimulus

E. The diffusion of water through a selectively permeable membrane

F. The standard reference position for the body

G. The movement of substances from a region of high concentration to a region of low concentration

H. Fibers composed of elastin that have a stretching quality

I. The study of the shape and structure of the human body and its parts

J. Cells located in nervous tissue that provide support for neurons

K. A group of cells with a similar structure that are specialized to form a certain function

L. Fibers made of collagen that are strong and flexible

M. A membrane transport process in which substances are moved uphill from an area of lower concentration to an area of higher concentration

N. The microscopic study of tissues

O. The engulfing and destruction of foreign particles such as bacteria

P. The scientific study of the functions of the human body and its parts

Q. A nerve cell

R. The formation of vesicles to transfer fluid droplets into a cell; cell drinking

S. The state in which body systems are functioning normally and the internal environment of the body is in equilibrium; the body is in a healthy state

T. A cartilage cell

U. A large phagocytic cell that cleans up cellular debris and foreign particles from the tissues

V. A connective tissue cell that produces heparin and histamine

W. The process by which the nucleus of a body cell divides to form two new (daughter) cells, each identical to the parent cell

X. A mature bone cell

Y. The total of all biochemical reactions that take place in the body

Z. Membrane transport process that does not require cellular energy

EVALUATION OF LEARNING

Directions: Fill in each blank with the correct answer.

The Human Body

1. What is the difference between gross human anatomy and microscopic human anatomy?

   _____

   _____

2. What is the relationship between human anatomy and physiology?

   _____

   _____

3. What are the six levels of organization of the body?

   _____

   _____

4. What are the four main types of tissue found in the body?

   _____

   _____

5. What makes up an organ? List examples of organs.

   _____

   _____

6. What makes up a body system? List examples of body systems.

   _____

   _____

7. What makes up a total human organism?

   _____

8 What is the function of the following systems?

   a. Integumentary: _____

   _____

   b. Skeletal: _____

   _____

   c. Muscular: _____

   _____

   d. Nervous: _____

   _____

   e. Endocrine: _____

   _____

   f. Cardiovascular: _____

   _____

g. Lymphatic: _____

_____

h. Digestive: _____

_____

i. Respiratory: _____

_____

j. Urinary: _____

_____

k. Reproductive: _____

_____

9. What is homeostasis? Why is it important to the body?

_____

_____

_____

10. How does the body maintain normal blood pressure using a negative feedback mechanism?

_____

_____

_____

11. Describe the body in anatomic position.

_____

_____

12. Define the following body directions, and provide an example of each:

a. Superior: _____

_____

b. Inferior: _____

_____

c. Anterior: _____

_____

d. Posterior: _____

_____

e. Medial: _____

_____

f. Lateral: _____

_____

g. Proximal: _____

_____

h. Distal: _____

_____

i. Superficial: _____

_____

j. Deep: _____

_____

k. Visceral: _____

_____

l. Parietal: _____

_____

13. Define the following planes and sections of the body:

a. Sagittal plane: _____

_____

b. Midsagittal plane: _____

_____

c. Transverse plane: _____

_____

d. Frontal plane: _____

_____

14. What are the subdivisions of the dorsal cavity? _____

_____

15. What are the subdivisions of the ventral cavity? _____

_____

16. What structures are located in the thoracic cavity? _____

_____

17. What structures are located in the abdominal cavity? _____

_____

18. What structures are located in the pelvic cavity? _____

_____

19. What structures are located in the following regions of the body?

a. Axial: _____

b. Appendicular: _____

Cell Structure and Function

1. What is the function of the plasma membrane?

_____

_____

2. What is cytoplasm?

_____

3. What are organelles?

_____

4. What substances are dissolved in the intracellular fluid of the cytoplasm?

_____

_____

5. What is the function of the nucleus?

_____

_____

6. Where is the nucleolus located?

_____

7. What is the function of the nucleolus?

_____

_____

8. What is the function of mitochondria?

_____

_____

9. What is the function of ribosomes?

_____

10. What is the function of the endoplasmic reticulum?

_____

_____

11. What is the function of the Golgi apparatus?

_____

_____

12. What is the function of lysosomes?

_____

_____

13. What are cilia, and what is their function?

_____

_____

14. What is simple diffusion?

_____

_____

15. How does diffusion result in the exchange of oxygen and carbon dioxide in the lungs?

_____

_____

_____

16. What is osmosis?

_____

_____

17. What occurs when a red blood cell is placed in an isotonic solution?

_____

_____

18. What occurs when a red blood cell is placed in a hypertonic solution? Explain the reason for your answer.

_____

_____

19. What occurs when a red blood cell is placed in a hypotonic solution? Explain the reason for your answer.

_____

_____

20. What process in the body relies on filtration?

_____

21. What is active transport?

_____

_____

22. What process in the body relies on active transport?

_____

_____

23. What is endocytosis?

_____

_____

24. What occurs during phagocytosis?

_____

_____

25. What is exocytosis?

_____

_____

26. List two examples of exocytosis.

_____

_____

27. What is a somatic cell?

_____

28. What is a gamete?

_____

29. How many pairs of chromosomes are present in a human cell? _____

30. What are the two methods the body uses to reproduce cells?

_____

_____

31. What occurs during the following stages of mitosis?

a. Interphase: _____

_____

b. Prophase: _____

_____

c. Metaphase: _____

_____

d. Anaphase: _____

_____

e. Telophase: _____

_____

32. What is meiosis?

_____

_____

_____

Tissues and Membranes

1. What is histology?

_____

2. What is the intercellular matrix?

_____

_____

3. What are the four main tissues of the body?

_____

4. Where is epithelial tissue located?

_____

_____

5. What is the name of the structure that attaches epithelial cells to underlying connective tissue? _____

_____

6. Describe the shape of the cell and its nucleus for each of the following types of epithelial cells:

a. Squamous: _____

_____

b. Cuboidal: _____

_____

c. Columnar: _____

_____

7. What is the difference between simple epithelium and stratified epithelium?

_____

_____

8. Describe the appearance of simple squamous epithelium. In the margin of this page, draw a sketch of simple squamous epithelium.

_____

_____

9. Where is simple squamous epithelium located in the body?

_____

_____

10. Describe the appearance of simple cuboidal epithelium. In the margin of this page, draw a sketch of simple cuboidal epithelium.

_____

11. Where is simple cuboidal epithelium located in the body?

_____

_____

12. Describe the appearance of simple columnar epithelium. In the margin of this page, draw a sketch of simple columnar epithelium.

_____

_____

13. Where is simple columnar epithelium located in the body?

_____

14. What are microvilli? What is their purpose?

_____

_____

15. What is the purpose of goblet cells?

_____

16. What is the appearance of pseudostratified columnar epithelium? In the margin of this page, draw a sketch of pseudostratified columnar epithelium.

_____

_____

17. Where is pseudostratified columnar epithelium located in the body?

_____

_____

18. What is the appearance of stratified squamous epithelium? In the margin of this page, draw a sketch of stratified squamous epithelium.

_____

_____

19. Where is stratified squamous epithelium located in the body?

_____

_____

20. What special quality is present with transitional epithelium?

_____

_____

21. Where is transitional epithelium located in the body?

_____

22. What is glandular epithelium?

_____

_____

23. What is the difference between an exocrine gland and an endocrine gland?

_____

_____

24. What are examples of exocrine glands?

_____

25. What is the function of connective tissue?

_____

_____

26. What are the characteristics of collagenous fibers?

_____

_____

27. What structures are composed of collagenous fibers?

_____

28. What are the characteristics of elastic fibers?

_____

29. What three cells are most commonly found in connective tissue? List the function of each of these cells.

Cell	**Function**

30. What is the function of loose connective tissue?

_____

_____

31. What is the function of adipose tissue?

_____

_____

32. Describe the characteristics of dense fibrous connective tissue.

_____

_____

33. What is the function of tendons?

_____

_____

34. What is the function of ligaments?

_____

_____

35. What body structures are composed of elastic connective tissue?

_____

_____

36. What is the function of cartilage?

_____

_____

37. Describe the following components of cartilage:
    a. Chondrocyte: _____
    b. Perichondrium: _____

38. Where is hyaline cartilage located?

_____

_____

39. Where is fibrocartilage located in the body?

_____

_____

40. Where is elastic cartilage located in the body?

_____

41. What is the function of bone?

_____

_____

42. Describe the following components of bone:

    a. Osteons (haversian systems): _____

    b. Osteonic canal (haversian canal): _____

    c. Osteocyte: _____

    d. Canaliculi: _____

43. What qualities do the following give to bone?

    a. Collagenous fibers: _____

    b. Calcium: _____

44. What is the function of the following blood components?

    a. Erythrocytes: _____

    _____

    b. Leukocytes: _____

    _____

    c. Thrombocytes: _____

    _____

    d. Plasma: _____

    _____

45. What is the function of muscle tissue?

    _____

    _____

46. Describe the appearance of skeletal muscle cells. In the margin of this page, draw a sketch of skeletal muscle cells.

    _____

    _____

47. What is the function of skeletal muscle in the body?

    _____

48. Describe the appearance of smooth muscle cells. In the margin of this page, draw a sketch of smooth muscle cells.

    _____

    _____

49. Where is smooth muscle located in the body?

    _____

50. What is the function of smooth muscle?

    _____

    _____

51. Describe the appearance of cardiac muscle cells. In the margin of this page, draw a sketch of cardiac muscle cells.

    _____

52. Where is cardiac muscle located in the body?

    _____

53. What is the function of cardiac muscle?

    _____

    _____

54. Where is nervous tissue located in the body?

    _____

55. What is the function of nervous tissue?

    _____

    _____

56. Describe the following components of nervous tissue:

    a. Neuron: _____

    b. Nerve cell body: _____

    c. Dendrites: _____

    d. Axons: _____

    e. Neuroglia: _____

57. What is a mucous membrane?

    _____

    _____

58. Where are mucous membranes located in the body?

    _____

    _____

59. What is the function of the mucus secreted by a mucous membrane?

    _____

60. What is a serous membrane?

    _____

    _____

61. What is the function of serous fluid?

    _____

    _____

62. Where are serous membranes located in the body?

    _____

    _____

63. What are synovial membranes?

    _____

    _____

64. Where are synovial membranes located in the body?

    _____

65. What is the function of synovial fluid?

_____

_____

66. What are the meninges?

_____

_____

67. What is the function of the meninges?

_____

_____

68. List and describe the three layers that make up the meninges.

Name	**Description**
_____	_____
_____	_____
_____	_____

CRITICAL THINKING ACTIVITIES

A. PLANES OF THE BODY
Using Figure 5-3 in your textbook as a reference, label each of the planes of the body on the following diagram.

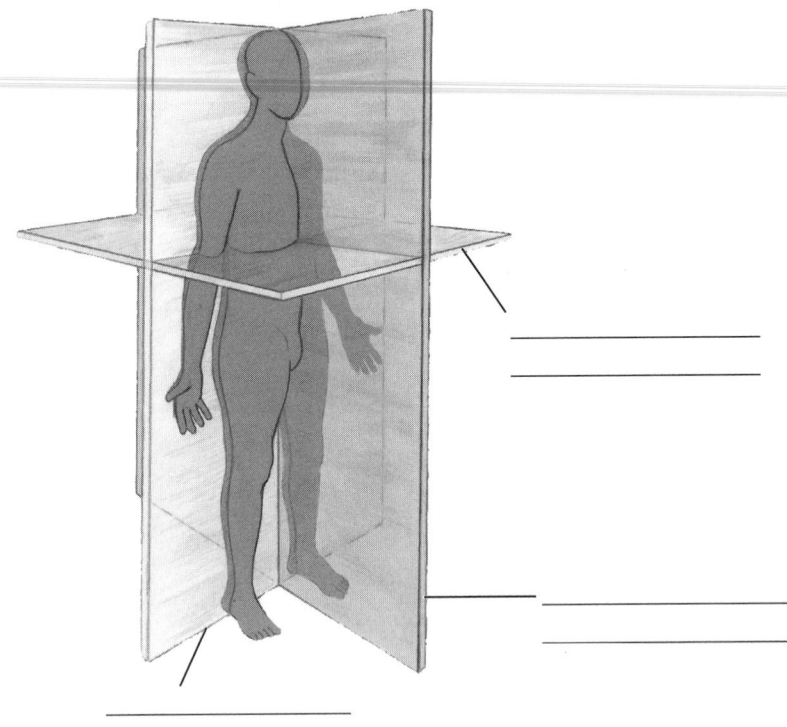

(Modified from Applegate E: *The anatomy and physiology learning system,* ed 3, St. Louis, 2006, Saunders.)

B. CAVITIES OF THE BODY
   Using Figure 5-4 in your textbook as a reference, label each of the cavities of the body on the following diagram.

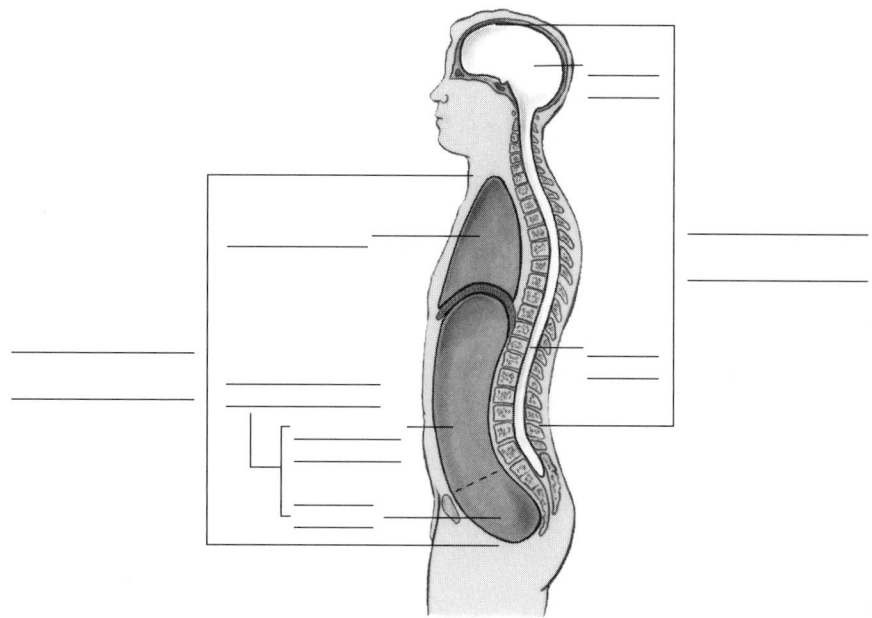

(Modified from Applegate E: *The anatomy and physiology learning system,* ed 3, St. Louis, 2006, Saunders.)

C. ABDOMINOPELVIC QUADRANTS
   Using Figure 5-5 in your textbook as a reference, label each of the quadrants of the body on the following diagram.

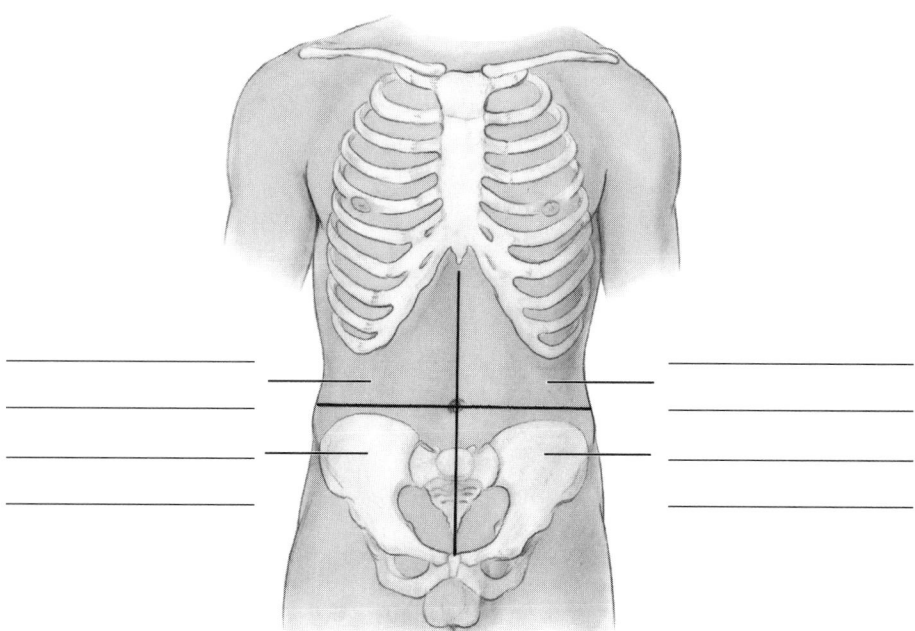

(Modified from Applegate E: *The anatomy and physiology learning system,* ed 3, St. Louis, 2006, Saunders.)

D. ABDOMINOPELVIC REGIONS
Using Figure 5-6 in your textbook as a reference, label each of the planes of the body on the following diagram.

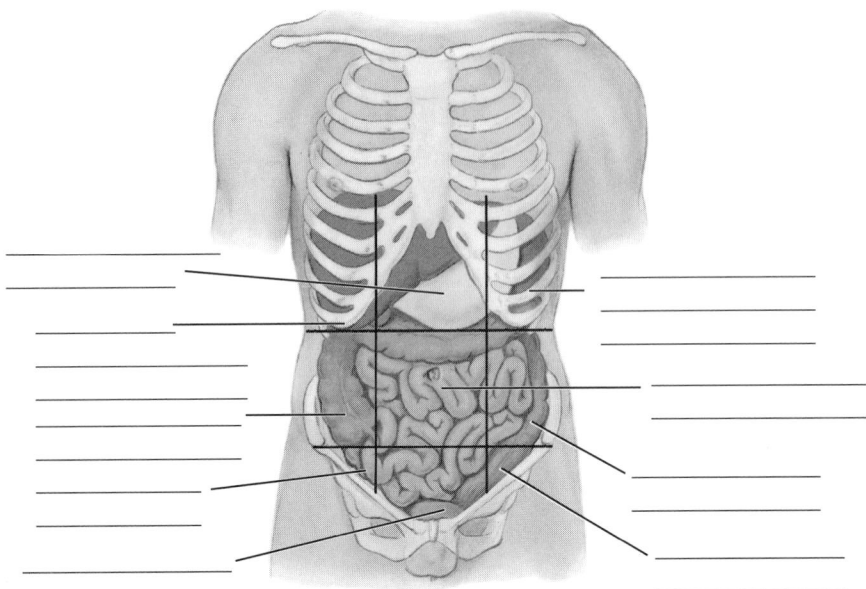

(Modified from Applegate E: *The anatomy and physiology learning system,* ed 3, St. Louis, 2006, Saunders.)

E. ROAD TO RECOVERY CD ACTIVITY
Body Area Terms
Directions:
1. Review the body area terms presented in Table 5-2 of your textbook.
2. Access your Companion CD (accompanying the textbook).
3. Play the Road to Recovery Game presented under Chapter 5.
4. Record your points on your assignment sheet.

F. BODY SPECTRUM CD ACTIVITY
Cell Structure: General Human Cell
Body Spectrum Directions:
1. Access your Body Spectrum program (CD included with your textbook).
2. Go to the Contents screen.
3. Access the HELP screen for directions on using the Body Spectrum program.
4. Select the following category from the Contents screen:
   Cell Structure
5. Select the following anatomic diagram:
   General Human Cell
6. Identify the structures on the diagram.
7. Print out the diagram.

G. CELL STRUCTURE AND FUNCTION

You are an oxygen molecule that has just entered a body cell. In the space provided below, describe all of the structures you see in the cell. Also describe what function each structure is performing in the cell. Each of the following structures should be included in your discussion:

a. Plasma membrane
b. Cytoplasm
c. Nucleus
d. Nuclear membrane
e. Nucleolus
f. Mitochondria
g. Ribosomes
h. Rough endoplasmic reticulum
i. Smooth endoplasmic reticulum
j. Golgi apparatus
k. Lysosomes
l. Centrioles
m. Chromatin
n. Secretory vesicle

_____

_____

_____

_____

_____

_____

_____

_____

_____

_____

_____

_____

_____

_____

_____

_____

_____

_____

_____

_____

_____

_____

_____

_____

_____

_____

H. CHAPTER 5 ANIMATIONS CD ACTIVITY

Directions:

1. View the Chapter 5 Animations on your Companion CD (included with your textbook).
2. For each animation, write two true/false questions in the space provided below.
3. In the classroom, find a partner.
4. For each animation, read your two questions to your partner.
5. For each correct answer, your partner is awarded two points.
6. Next, have your partner read his/her two questions to you. Award yourself two points for each question answered correctly.
7. Continue in this manner until all the questions have been answered.
8. Record your points on your Study Guide Assignment sheet.

True/False Questions

a. Directions of the Body

1. _____

2. _____

b. Parts of the Cell

1. _____

2. _____

c. Cells

1. _____

2. _____

d. Cell Reproduction

1. _____

2. _____

e. Hereditary Traits

1. _____

2. _____

f. Mucous Membrane

1. _____

2. _____

g. Serous Membrane

1. _____

2. _____

h. Synovial Membrane

1. _____

2. _____

I. CROSSWORD PUZZLE
Introduction to Anatomy and Physiology
Directions: Complete the crossword puzzle using the clues presented below.

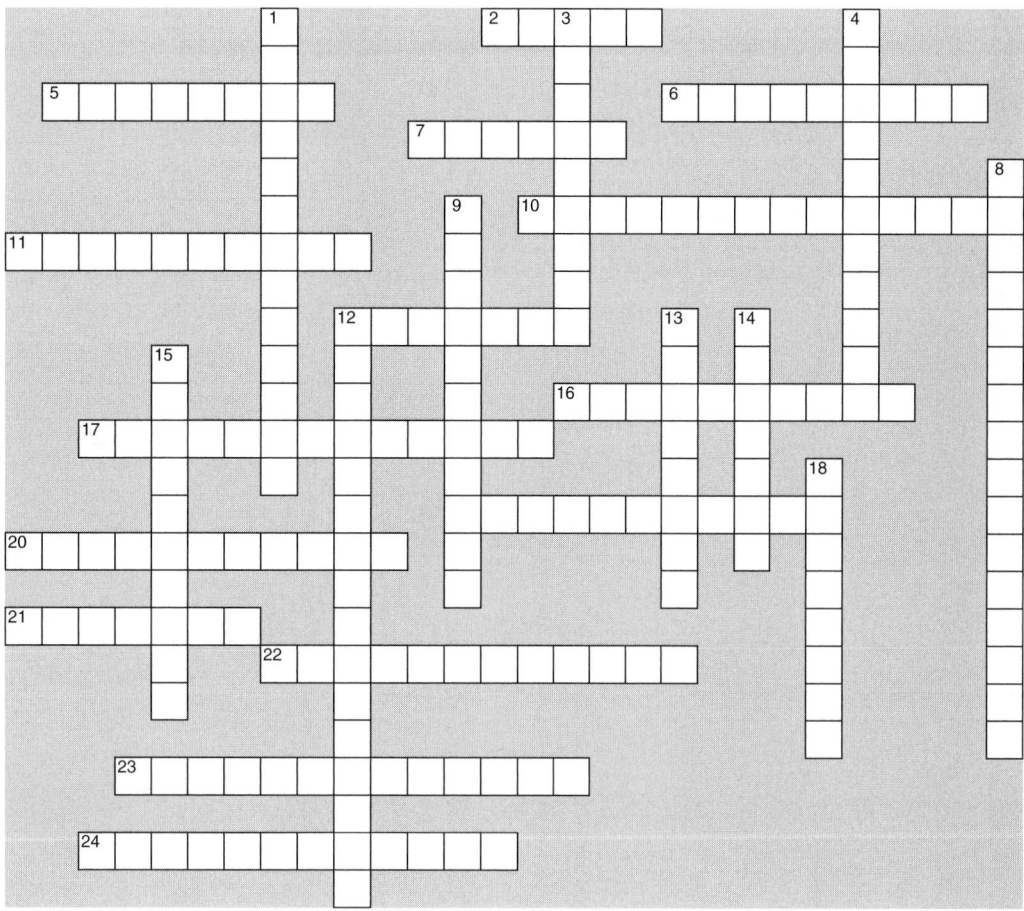

ACROSS
2 Little hairs on cell membrane
5 Number of chromosomes in human cell
6 Synthesizes proteins
7 Connects muscle to bone
10 Packaging and shipping plant
11 Secretes mucus
12 Produces two daughter cells
16 Helps distribute chromosomes to daughter cells
17 Brain, spinal cord, and nerves
19 On or near the surface
20 Everything is A-OK
21 Cell's control center
22 Cell eating
23 Houses the brain
24 Power plant of cell

DOWN
1 Contains fat cells
3 Destroys cellular debris
4 Cartilage cell
8 Has same concentration as RBCs
9 Cell drinking
12 Divides body into right and left halves
13 Toward the front
14 Cell division that produces eggs and sperm
15 Lines abdominopelvic cavity
18 Sperm tail

6

Integumentary System

CHAPTER ASSIGNMENTS

√ After Completing	Date Due	Textbook Page(s)	TEXTBOOK ASSIGNMENT	Possible Points	Points You Earned
		103-110	Read Chapter 6: Integumentary System		
√ After Completing	Date Due	Study Guide Page(s)	STUDY GUIDE ASSIGNMENTS (CTA: Critical Thinking Activity)		
		65	📄 Pretest	10	
		66	🔑Term Key Term Assessment	9	
		67-70	📝 Evaluation of Learning questions	50	
		70	💿 CTA A: Body Spectrum CD Activity: Skin Structure	10	
		70-71	💿 CTA B: Body Spectrum CD Activity: Glands of the Skin	10	
		71	💿 CTA C: Body Spectrum CD Activity: Skin and Hypodermis	10	
		71	💿 CTA D: Body Spectrum CD Activity: Hair Follicle	10	
		71	💿 CTA E: Body Spectrum CD Activity: Hair Follicle Enlarged	10	
		71-72	CTA F: Inquiring Patients Want to Know	20	
		73	CTA G: Crossword Puzzle	24	
		65	📄 Posttest	10	

√ After Completing	Date Due	Study Guide Page(s)	STUDY GUIDE ASSIGNMENTS (CTA: Critical Thinking Activity)		
			ADDITIONAL ASSIGNMENTS		
			TOTAL POINTS		

Name _____   Date _____

PRETEST

True or False

_____ 1. The nails are part of the integumentary system.

_____ 2. The thickest layer of the epidermis is the stratum corneum.

_____ 3. Cerumen provides waterproofing for the skin.

_____ 4. Sensory receptors allow the body to detect changes in the environment.

_____ 5. The subcutaneous layer cushions underlying organs.

_____ 6. The ultraviolet rays of the sun increase melanocyte activity.

_____ 7. The face does not contain hair.

_____ 8. Hair is produced by hair follicles.

_____ 9. The neck and chest have the most sweat glands.

_____ 10. Vitamin A is necessary for the absorption of calcium in the body.

POSTTEST

True or False

_____ 1. The epidermis consists of simple squamous epithelial tissue.

_____ 2. Skin cells grow and multiply in the stratum basale layer of the epidermis.

_____ 3. Melanocytes produce a yellow pigment.

_____ 4. Sebaceous glands are embedded in the dermis.

_____ 5. An individual with a large number of melanin granules in their skin will have dry skin.

_____ 6. The part of the hair that is visible is known as the *shaft*.

_____ 7. The central core of the hair is known as the *cuticle*.

_____ 8. Shivering is caused by contraction of the arrector pili muscles.

_____ 9. Sebum keeps hair and skin soft and pliable.

_____ 10. Merocrine glands are responsible for body odor.

✏Term KEY TERM ASSESSMENT

Directions: Match each medical term with its definition.

_____ 1. Arrector pili

_____ 2. Ceruminous gland

_____ 3. Dermis

_____ 4. Epidermis

_____ 5. Keratinization

_____ 6. Melanin

_____ 7. Sebaceous gland

_____ 8. Subcutaneous layer

_____ 9. Sudoriferous gland

A. A dark brown or black pigment found in parts of the body, especially skin and hair
B. A gland in the ear canal that produces cerumen or earwax
C. A gland in the skin that produces perspiration; also called *sweat gland*
D. An oil gland of the skin that produces sebum or body oil
E. Below the skin; a sheet of areolar connective tissue and adipose tissue beneath the dermis of the skin; also called *hypodermis* or *superficial fascia*
F. Inner layer of the skin that contains the blood vessels, nerves, glands, and hair follicles; also called *stratum corneum*
G. Muscle associated with hair follicles
H. Outermost layer of the skin
I. Process by which the cells of the epidermis become filled with keratin and move to the surface, where they are sloughed off

EVALUATION OF LEARNING

Directions: Fill in each blank with the correct answer.

1. What structures make up the integumentary system?

    _____

2. What is another name for the skin?

    _____

3. What occurs during keratinization?

    _____

    _____

4. Why do cells in the epidermis flatten out and die as they reach the surface of the skin?

    _____

    _____

5. What areas of the body are covered by skin that consists of five strata?

    _____

6. What occurs in the stratum basale?

    _____

    _____

7. What are melanocytes?

    _____

    _____

8. What makes up the stratum germinativum?

    _____

9. What occurs in the stratum granulosum?

    _____

10. What is the appearance of the stratum lucidum?

    _____

    _____

11. What makes up the stratum corneum?

    _____

    _____

12. What is the function of keratin?

    _____

    _____

13. What is another name for the dermis?

    _____

14. What structures are embedded in the dermis?

_____

15. What happens if the dermis is overstretched?

_____

_____

16. What is the function of sensory receptors?

_____

_____

17. What two layers make up the dermis?

_____

18. What causes fingerprints and footprints?

_____

_____

19. What are two other terms for the subcutaneous layer?

_____

20. What type of tissue is located in the subcutaneous layer?

_____

21. What is the function of subcutaneous tissue?

_____

22. Explain the role of melanin in determining skin color.

_____

_____

23. What is the name of the pigment that results in a yellow tint to the skin?

_____

24. What effect does ultraviolet light have on melanocyte activity?

_____

25. What parts of the body do not grow hair?

_____

26. What is the name given to the part of the hair that is visible?

_____

27. Where is the root of the hair located?

_____

28. What is the medulla of a hair?

_____

29. What is the name of the outer covering of a hair? What makes up this covering?

_____

_____

30. What is the function of a hair follicle?

_____

31. How is hair color determined?

_____

_____

32. What occurs when the arrector pili muscles contract?

_____

_____

33. What can cause the arrector pili muscles to contract?

_____

34. What makes up a nail?

_____

_____

35. What is the name given to the visible portion of a nail?

_____

36. What is another name for the cuticle of a nail?

_____

37. What is the function of the nail matrix?

_____

38. Why do nails appear pink?

_____

_____

39. What is the function of sebum?

_____

_____

40. What parts of the body have the most sweat glands?

_____

41. What parts of the body do not have sweat glands?

_____

42. What causes a merocrine gland to secrete sweat?

_____

43. Where are apocrine sweat glands located?

_____

44. When do apocrine sweat glands become active?

_____

45. What causes an apocrine gland to secrete sweat?

_____

46. List four ways in which the skin protects the body.

_____

_____

47. How does the skin regulate body temperature?

_____

48. Vitamin D assists in the absorption of what minerals?

_____

49. What are the functions of calcium and phosphorus in the body?

_____

50. How does the skin produce vitamin D?

_____

_____

CRITICAL THINKING ACTIVITIES

A. BODY SPECTRUM CD ACTIVITY
   Integumentary: Skin Structure
   Body Spectrum Directions:

   1. Access your Body Spectrum program (CD included with your textbook).

   2. Go to the Contents screen.

   3. Access the HELP screen for directions on using the Body Spectrum program.

   4. Select the following category from the Contents screen:

      Integumentary

   5. Select the following anatomic diagram:

      Skin Structure

   6. Identify the structures on the diagram.

   7. Print out the diagram.

B. BODY SPECTRUM CD ACTIVITY
   Integumentary: Glands of the Skin
   Directions: Identify the structures on this diagram following the Body Spectrum Directions outlined under CTA A.

C. BODY SPECTRUM CD ACTIVITY
Integumentary: Skin and Hypodermis
Directions: Identify the structures on this diagram following the Body Spectrum Directions outlined under CTA A.

D. BODY SPECTRUM CD ACTIVITY
Integumentary: Hair Follicle
Directions: Identify the structures on this diagram following the Body Spectrum Directions outlined under CTA A.

E. BODY SPECTRUM CD ACTIVITY
Integumentary: Hair Follicle Enlarged
Directions: Identify the structures on this diagram following the Body Spectrum Directions outlined under CTA A.

F. INQUIRING PATIENTS WANT TO KNOW
You are working in a general practice medical office. Your patients ask you the following questions. In the space provided, indicate how you would respond to each question in terms the patient would understand.

1. What makes skin waterproof?

2. What causes a blister?

3. What causes blushing?

4. What causes curly hair?

5. Why doesn't it hurt when my hair is cut?

6. What causes split ends?

7. How does hair grow?

8. What causes freckles?

9. Why do I have red hair?

10. Why does my skinny friend get cold all the time?

11. What causes age spots?

_____

_____

12. What causes wrinkles?

_____

_____

13. What causes a person to tan?

_____

_____

14. What causes "goose bumps"?

_____

_____

15. What causes pimples?

_____

_____

16. What causes baldness?

_____

_____

17. What causes warts?

_____

_____

18. What causes itching?

_____

_____

19. What causes hair to turn white?

_____

_____

20. How does sunshine cause the body to produce vitamin D?

_____

_____

G. CROSSWORD PUZZLE

Directions: Complete the crossword puzzle using the clues presented below.

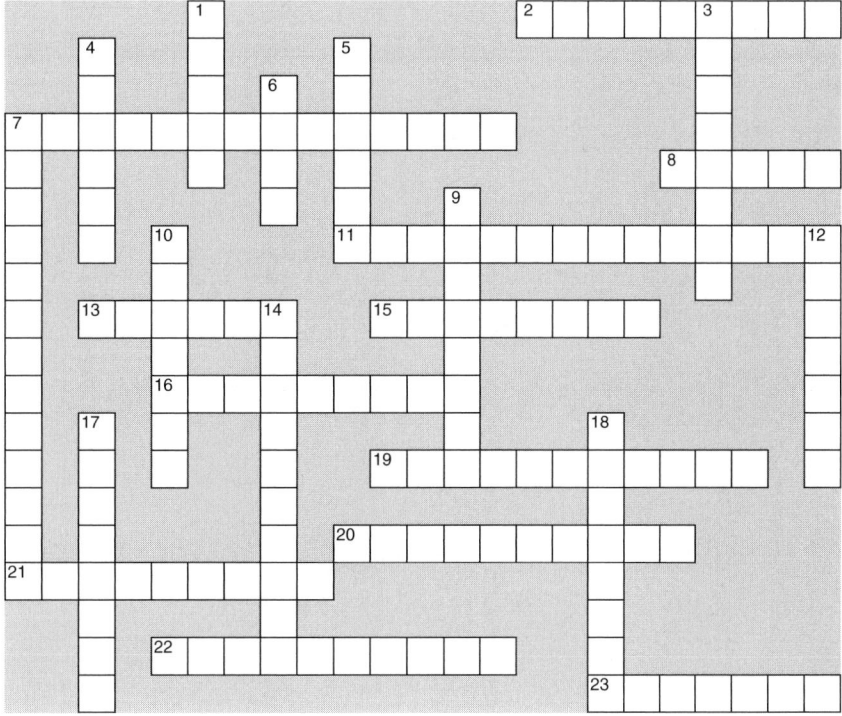

ACROSS

2 Hives
7 Outermost layer of epidermis
8 Mole
11 Present in thick skin
13 Stretch marks
15 Sweat gland in axilla
16 Sweat gland that opens on surface of skin
19 Most numerous on palms and soles
20 Function of skin
21 Outer skin layer
22 Inflammation of the skin
23 Central core of hair

DOWN

1 Oily secretion
3 Baldness
4 Converts precursor in skin to vitamin D
5 Inner skin layer
6 Teenager skin problem
7 Melanocytes live here
9 Yellowish pigment
10 Earwax
12 Responsible for skin color
14 Cuticle
17 Itching
18 Cannot produce melanin

7

Skeletal System

CHAPTER ASSIGNMENTS

√ After Completing	Date Due	Textbook Page(s)	TEXTBOOK ASSIGNMENT	Possible Points	Points You Earned
		111-128	Read Chapter 7: Skeletal System		

√ After Completing	Date Due	Study Guide Page(s)	STUDY GUIDE ASSIGNMENTS (CTA: Critical Thinking Activity)	Possible Points	Points You Earned
		77	Pretest	10	
		78	Key Term Assessment	10	
		79-84	Evaluation of Learning questions	64	
		84	CTA A: Body Spectrum CD Activity: Structure of Bone	10	
		85	CTA B: Long Bone	12	
		85	CTA C: Body Spectrum CD Activity: Skeleton Anterior	10	
		85	CTA D: Body Spectrum CD Activity: Skeleton Posterior	10	
		85	CTA E: Body Spectrum CD Activity: Skull Anterior	10	
		85	CTA F: Body Spectrum CD Activity: Skull Right Lateral	10	
		85	CTA G: Body Spectrum CD Activity: Paranasal Sinuses	40	
		85	CTA H: Body Spectrum CD Activity: Cranial Vault	10	
		86	CTA I: Body Spectrum CD Activity: Skull Inferior	10	
		86	CTA J: Body Spectrum CD Activity: Vertebral Column	10	

√ After Completing	Date Due	Study Guide Page(s)	STUDY GUIDE ASSIGNMENTS (CTA: Critical Thinking Activity)		
		86	CTA K: Body Spectrum CD Activity: Individual Vertebrae	10	
		86	CTA L: Body Spectrum CD Activity: Thorax and Ribs	10	
		86	CTA M: Body Spectrum CD Activity: Right Wrist and Hand	10	
		86	CTA N: Body Spectrum CD Activity: Male Pelvis	10	
		86	CTA O: Body Spectrum CD Activity: Female Pelvis	10	
		86	CTA P: Body Spectrum CD Activity: Right Foot	10	
		86	CTA Q: Synovial Joint	5	
		87	CTA R: Inquiring Patients Want to Know	10	
		88	CTA S: Crossword Puzzle	25	
		77	Posttest	10	
			ADDITIONAL ASSIGNMENTS		
			TOTAL POINTS		

Name _____   Date _____

PRETEST

True or False

_____ 1. The skeletal system provides a rigid framework for the body.

_____ 2. Blood cell formation takes place in the spleen.

_____ 3. Vertebrae are made up of flat bones.

_____ 4. Articular cartilage covers the ends of long bones.

_____ 5. Long bones grow in length at the epiphyseal line.

_____ 6. The maxillary bones form the upper jaw.

_____ 7. The sacrum makes up the small of the back.

_____ 8. The shoulder is an example of a hinge joint.

_____ 9. The patella is the kneecap.

_____ 10. The humerus makes up the thigh.

POSTTEST

True or False

_____ 1. The formation of blood cells is known as *hemogenesis*.

_____ 2. Osteons are the microscopic units of compact bone.

_____ 3. Calcium is located in an osteonic canal.

_____ 4. The shaft of a long bone is the diaphysis.

_____ 5. The endosteum is the tough fibrous connective tissue that covers a long bone.

_____ 6. A mature bone cell is an osteoblast.

_____ 7. The most inferior part of the sternum is the xiphoid process.

_____ 8. The clavicle and scapula make up the pelvic girdle.

_____ 9. The ileum, ischium, and pubis make up the coxal bones.

_____ 10. The ulna is located on the lateral side of the forearm.

⚷ KEY TERM ASSESSMENT

Directions: Match each medical term with its definition.

_____ 1. Amphiarthrosis

_____ 2. Diaphysis

_____ 3. Diarthrosis

_____ 4. Epiphyseal plate

_____ 5. Epiphysis

_____ 6. Osteoblast

_____ 7. Osteoclast

_____ 8. Osteocyte

_____ 9. Osteon

_____ 10. Synarthrosis

A. A slightly movable joint
B. An immovable joint
C. Bone-forming cell
D. Cell that destroys or resorbs bone tissue
E. Freely movable joint characterized by a joint cavity; also called a *synovial joint*
F. Mature bone cell
G. Structural unit of bone; haversian system
H. The cartilaginous plate between the epiphysis and diaphysis of a bone; responsible for the lengthwise growth of a long bone
I. The end of a long bone
J. The long, straight shaft of a long bone

EVALUATION OF LEARNING

Directions: Fill in each blank with the correct answer.

1. What structures make up the skeletal system?

   _____

   _____

2. What are the five functions of the skeletal system?

   _____

   _____

3. How is the blood calcium level maintained in the body?

   _____

   _____

4. What is the function of red bone marrow?

   _____

5. Where is red bone marrow found in the adult?

   _____

   _____

6. What is an osteon?

   _____

7. Describe the following structures that make up an osteon:

   a. Osteonic canal (haversian canal): _____

   _____

   b. Lamella: _____

   _____

   c. Osteocytes: _____

   d. Lacunae: _____

   _____

   e. Canaliculi: _____

   _____

8. What is the difference between spongy bone and compact bone?

   _____

   _____

9. List examples of each of the following classifications of bone:

   a. Long bones: _____

   b. Short bones: _____

   c. Flat bones: _____

   d. Irregular bones: _____

10. Describe each of the following structures that make up a long bone:

   a. Diaphysis: _____

   b. Medullary cavity: _____

   c. Epiphysis: _____

   d. Articular cartilage: _____

   e. Periosteum: _____

   f. Nutrient foramina: _____

   g. Endosteum: _____

11. What is ossification?

   _____

12. What is the function of each of the following types of bone cells?

   a. Osteoblast: _____

   b. Osteocyte: _____

   c. Osteoclast: _____

13. Where is the epiphyseal plate located in a long bone?

   _____

14. What type of cartilage is found in the epiphyseal plate?

   _____

15. How do long bones grow in length?

   _____

   _____

16. When does an individual stop growing in length?

   _____

17. What happens to the epiphyseal plate when long bones stop growing?

   _____

18. What influences bone growth in the body?

   _____

   _____

19. How many bones make up the skeleton of an adult?

   _____

20. What are the two divisions of the skeleton? What structures are included in each division?

   _____

   _____

21. How many bones make up the skull?

   _____

22. What is the function of the cranium?

_____

23. What are sinuses, and what is their function?

_____

24. What bones make up the cranium?

_____

_____

25. What is the function of the facial bones?

_____

_____

26. What are the names of the three small bones located in the middle ear?

_____

27. What is the function of the hyoid bone?

_____

_____

28. How many vertebrae make up the vertebral column?

_____

29. What are the functions of the intervertebral disks?

_____

_____

30. What structures make up vertebrae?

_____

_____

31. How many vertebrae are included in each of the following divisions of the vertebral column?
    a. Cervical: _____
    b. Thoracic: _____
    c. Lumbar: _____

32. Describe the following:
    a. Sacrum: _____

    _____

    b. Coccyx: _____

    _____

33. What are the functions of the thoracic cage?

_____

_____

34. What are the three parts of the sternum?

_____

35. How many pairs of ribs are present in the human skeleton?

_____

36. What is the difference between true ribs and false ribs?

_____

_____

37. What are floating ribs?

_____

38. What is the function of the appendicular skeleton?

_____

39. What two bones make up the pectoral girdle?

_____

40. What is another name for the clavicle?

_____

41. What bone forms the point of the shoulder?

_____

42. What bone is located in the upper arm?

_____

43. What bones are located in the forearm?

_____

44. State the location of the following bones making up the hand:
    a. Carpal bones: _____
    b. Metacarpal bones: _____
    c. Phalanges: _____

45. What are the functions of the pelvic girdle?

_____

_____

46. What three bones fuse to form a coxal bone?

_____

47. What is the symphysis pubis?

_____

48. What bone is located in the thigh?

_____

49. What is the patella?

_____

50. What is the function of the patella?

_____

51. What bones are located in the leg?

_____

52. What does the lateral malleolus do?

_____

53. Describe the location of the following bones making up the foot:

    a. Tarsal bones: _____

    b. Calcaneus bone: _____

    c. Metatarsal bones: _____

    d. Phalanges: _____

54. What is an articulation?

_____

55. What is a synarthrosis?

_____

56. What is an example of a synarthrosis?

_____

57. What is an amphiarthrosis?

_____

58. What is an example of an amphiarthrosis?

_____

59. What is a diarthrosis?

_____

60. Describe the following parts of a diarthrosis:

    a. Articular cartilage: _____

    b. Joint cavity: _____

    c. Joint capsule: _____

    d. Synovial membrane: _____

    e. Synovial fluid: _____

61. What is the function of fibrocartilaginous pads located in the knee?

_____

_____

62. What are bursae?

_____

63. What are the functions of bursae?

_____

_____

64. List examples of the following types of joints. What range of movement is possible with each of the following joints?

Joint	Examples	Range of Movement
a. Ball-and-Socket _____		_____
b. Condyloid _____		_____
c. Saddle _____		_____
d. Pivot _____		_____
e. Hinge _____		_____
f. Gliding _____		_____

CRITICAL THINKING ACTIVITIES

A. BODY SPECTRUM CD ACTIVITY
   Skeletal: Structure of Bone
   Body Spectrum Directions:
   1. Access your Body Spectrum program (CD included with your textbook).
   2. Go to the Contents screen.
   3. Access the HELP screen for directions on using the Body Spectrum program.
   4. Select the following category from the Contents screen:
      Skeletal
   5. Select the following anatomic diagram:
      Structure of Bone
   6. Identify the structures on the diagram.
   7. Print out the diagram.

B. LONG BONE
   Using Figure 7-2 in your textbook as a reference, label each of the parts of a long bone on the following diagram.

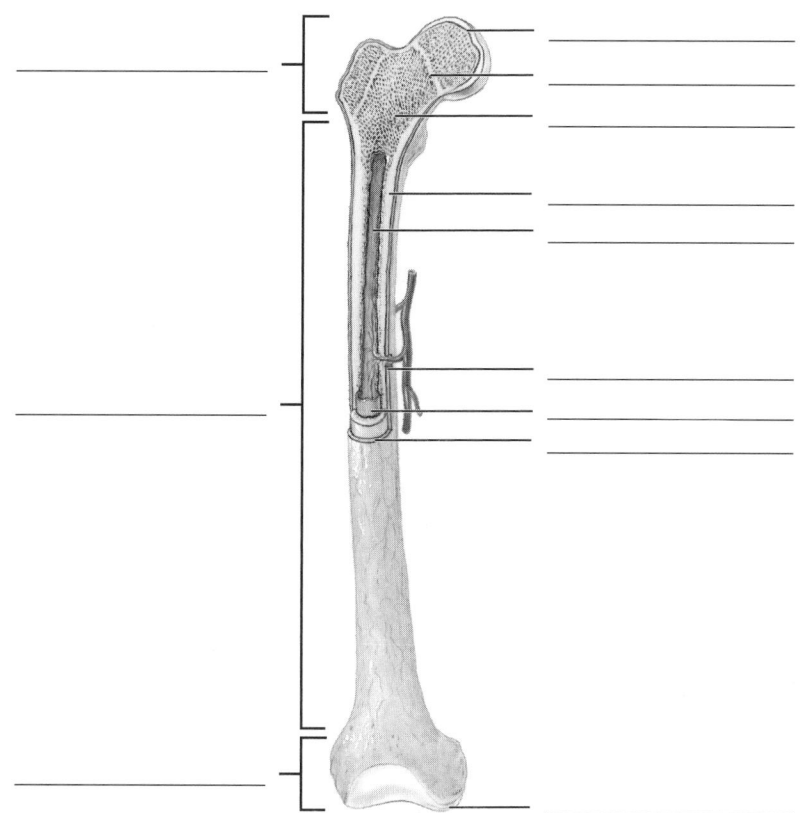

(Modified from Applegate E: *The anatomy and physiology learning system,* ed 3, St. Louis, 2006, Saunders.)

C. BODY SPECTRUM CD ACTIVITY
   Skeletal: Skeleton Anterior
   Directions: Identify the structures on this diagram following the Body Spectrum Directions outlined under CTA A.

D. BODY SPECTRUM CD ACTIVITY
   Skeletal: Skeleton Posterior
   Directions: Identify the structures on this diagram following the Body Spectrum Directions outlined under CTA A.

E. BODY SPECTRUM CD ACTIVITY
   Skeletal: Skull Anterior
   Directions: Identify the structures on this diagram following the Body Spectrum Directions outlined under CTA A.

F. BODY SPECTRUM CD ACTIVITY
   Skeletal: Skull Right Lateral
   Directions: Identify the structures on this diagram following the Body Spectrum Directions outlined under CTA A.

G. BODY SPECTRUM CD ACTIVITY
   Skeletal: Paranasal Sinuses
   Directions: Identify the structures on this diagram following the Body Spectrum Directions outlined under CTA A.

H. BODY SPECTRUM CD ACTIVITY
   Skeletal: Cranial Vault
   Directions: Identify the structures on this diagram following the Body Spectrum Directions outlined under CTA A.

I. BODY SPECTRUM CD ACTIVITY
   Skeletal: Skull Inferior
   Directions: Identify the structures on this diagram following the Body Spectrum Directions outlined under CTA A.

J. BODY SPECTRUM CD ACTIVITY
   Skeletal: Vertebral Column
   Directions: Identify the structures on this diagram following the Body Spectrum Directions outlined under CTA A.

K. BODY SPECTRUM CD ACTIVITY
   Skeletal: Individual Vertebrae
   Directions: Identify the structures on this diagram following the Body Spectrum Directions outlined under CTA A.

L. BODY SPECTRUM CD ACTIVITY
   Skeletal: Thorax and Ribs
   Directions: Identify the structures on this diagram following the Body Spectrum Directions outlined under CTA A.

M. BODY SPECTRUM CD ACTIVITY
   Skeletal: Right Wrist and Hand
   Directions: Identify the structures on this diagram following the Body Spectrum Directions outlined under CTA A.

N. BODY SPECTRUM CD ACTIVITY
   Skeletal: Male Pelvis
   Directions: Identify the structures on this diagram following the Body Spectrum Directions outlined under CTA A.

O. BODY SPECTRUM CD ACTIVITY
   Skeletal: Female Pelvis
   Directions: Identify the structures on this diagram following the Body Spectrum Directions outlined under CTA A.

P. BODY SPECTRUM CD ACTIVITY
   Skeletal: Right Foot
   Directions: Identify the structures on this diagram following the Body Spectrum Directions outlined under CTA A.

Q. SYNOVIAL JOINT
   Using Figure 7-19 in your textbook as a reference, label each of the parts of a synovial joint on the following diagram.

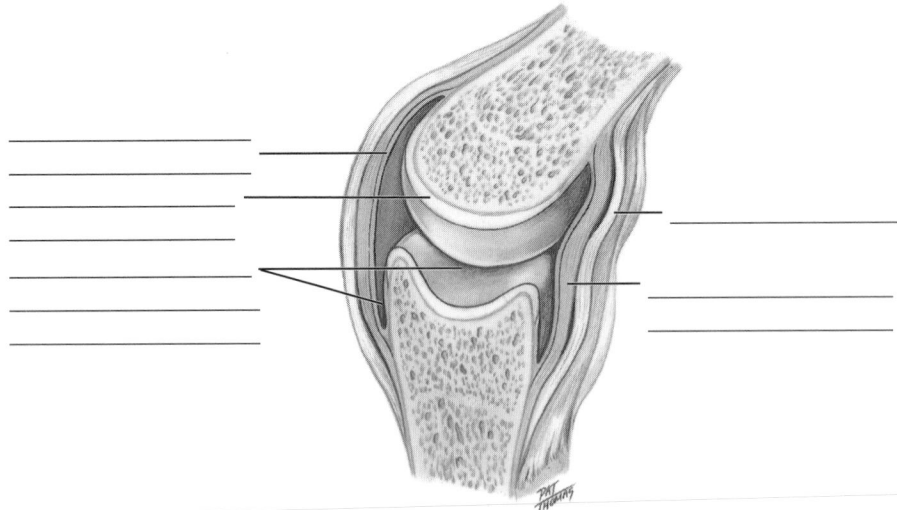

(Modified from Applegate E: *The anatomy and physiology learning system,* ed 3, St. Louis, 2006, Saunders.)

R. INQUIRING PATIENTS WANT TO KNOW

You are working in a general practice medical office. Your patients ask you the following questions. In the space provided, indicate how you would respond to each question in terms the patient would understand. Use your textbook and Internet resources to develop your responses.

1. What causes osteoporosis?

   _____

   _____

2. What causes my sinus headaches?

   _____

   _____

3. How does a baby get through the bones of the pelvis during childbirth?

   _____

   _____

4. What causes older people to break their hips?

   _____

   _____

5. What causes gout?

   _____

   _____

6. Why do people get shorter when they get older?

   _____

   _____

7. Why do babies have "soft spots" on their heads?

   _____

   _____

8. What is the difference between osteoarthritis and rheumatoid arthritis?

   _____

   _____

9. What happens when someone cracks their knuckles?

   _____

   _____

10. What is the difference between a strain and a sprain?

    _____

    _____

S. CROSSWORD PUZZLE
Skeletal System
Directions: Complete the crossword puzzle using the clues presented below.

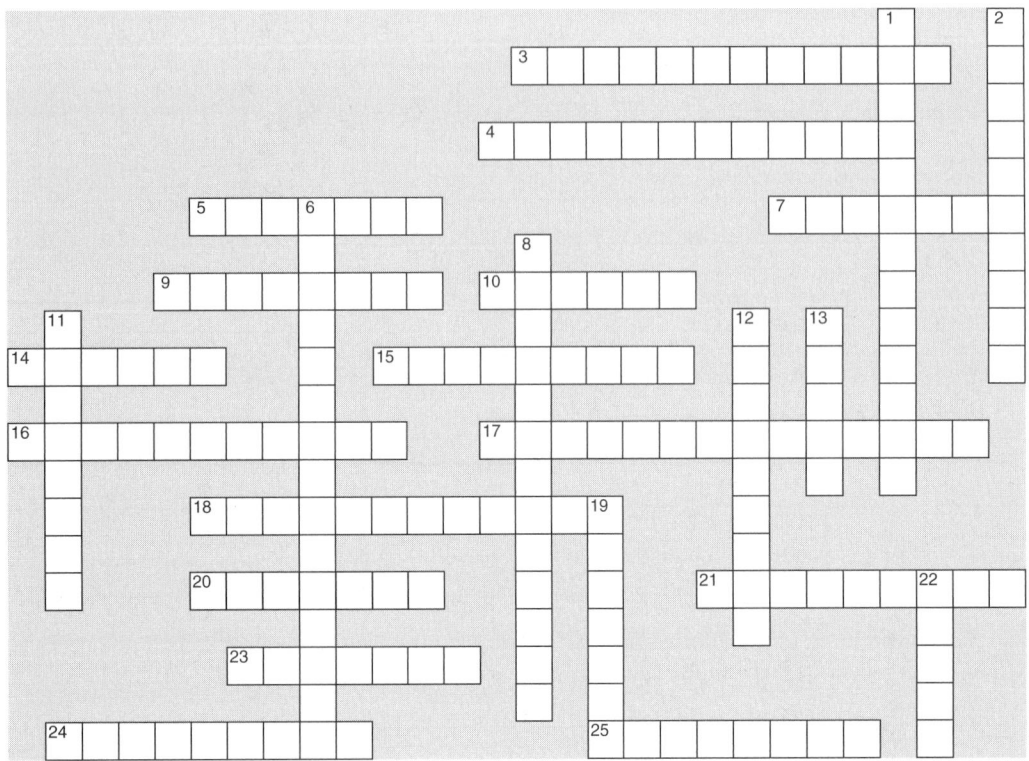

ACROSS
3 Process of bone formation
4 Softening of bones
5 Kneecap
7 Upper arm bone
9 Collarbone
10 Tailbone
14 Ankle
15 Bone cell
16 Freely movable joint
17 Where parietal bones meet
18 Immovable joint
20 Shoulder blade
21 Shaft of a long bone
23 Bones that protect brain
24 Finger bones
25 Lower jaw bones

DOWN
1 Spinal cord passes through this part of skull
2 Outer surface of a long bone
6 Where bones grow in length
8 Where frontal bone meets parietal bones
11 Bones of the upper jaw
12 Abnormal side-to-side spinal curvature
13 Thigh bone
19 Breastbone
22 Air-filled cavity in the skull

8

Muscular System

CHAPTER ASSIGNMENTS

√ After Completing	Date Due	Textbook Page(s)	TEXTBOOK ASSIGNMENT	Possible Points	Points You Earned
		129-146	Read Chapter 8: Muscular System		
√ After Completing	Date Due	Study Guide Page(s)	STUDY GUIDE ASSIGNMENTS (CTA: Critical Thinking Activity)		
		91	Pretest	10	
		92	Key Term Assessment	8	
		93-97	Evaluation of Learning questions	43	
		97	CTA A: Body Spectrum CD Activity: Face—Lateral	10	
		97	CTA B: Body Spectrum CD Activity: Face—Anterior	10	
		97	CTA C: Body Spectrum CD Activity: Anterior Abdominal	10	
		97	CTA D: Body Spectrum CD Activity: Musculature—Anterior	10	
		97	CTA E: Body Spectrum CD Activity: Upper Chest—Superficial	10	
		97	CTA F: Body Spectrum CD Activity: Right Arm—Lateral	10	
		97	CTA G: Body Spectrum CD Activity: Musculature—Posterior	10	
		98	CTA H: Inquiring Patients Want to Know	10	
		98-99	CTA I: Chapter 8 Animations CD Activity	20	
		100	CTA J: Crossword Puzzle	27	

√ After Completing	Date Due	Study Guide Page(s)	STUDY GUIDE ASSIGNMENTS (CTA: Critical Thinking Activity)		
		91	Posttest	10	
			ADDITIONAL ASSIGNMENTS		
			TOTAL POINTS		

Name _____   Date _____

True or False

_____   1. Skeletal muscle is under involuntary control.

_____   2. A ligament indirectly attaches skeletal muscle to bone.

_____   3. The cytoplasm of a muscle fiber is the sarcolemma.

_____   4. Calcium is a neurotransmitter responsible for muscle contractions.

_____   5. Oxygen must be present for aerobic respiration to occur.

_____   6. Bending the elbow is an example of flexion.

_____   7. The orbicularis oculus is used to wink, blink, and squint.

_____   8. The diaphragm forms a partition between the thorax and abdomen.

_____   9. The deltoid muscle moves the shoulder and upper arm.

_____   10. Another name for the calcaneal tendon is the *ankle*.

? POSTTEST

True or False

_____   1. Most of the heat produced in the body is through visceral muscle contractions.

_____   2. The epimysium is a connective tissue sheath that surrounds a muscle.

_____   3. The insertion is the end of a muscle that is attached to a relatively movable part.

_____   4. An axon terminal meets a muscle fiber at the neuromuscular junction.

_____   5. The products of anaerobic respiration are amino acids and carbon dioxide.

_____   6. Moving the arm away from the body is an example of adduction.

_____   7. The sternocleidomastoid muscle is located in the neck.

_____   8. The internal intercostal muscles assist with inspiration.

_____   9. The gluteus maximus muscle is used to administer an intramuscular injection.

_____   10. The quadriceps femoris muscle is used to extend the leg.

𝒯erm KEY TERM ASSESSMENT

Directions: Match each medical term with its definition.

_____ 1. Antagonist

_____ 2. Insertion

_____ 3. Motor unit

_____ 4. Neuromuscular junction

_____ 5. Neurotransmitter

_____ 6. Origin

_____ 7. Prime mover

_____ 8. Synergist

A. A chemical substance that is released at the axon terminals to stimulate a muscle fiber contraction or an impulse in another neuron

B. A muscle that assists a prime mover but is not capable of producing the movement by itself

C. A muscle that has an action opposite to the prime mover

D. A single neuron and all the muscle fibers it stimulates

E. The area of communication between the axon terminal of a motor neuron and the sarcolemma of a muscle fiber; also called a *myoneural junction*

F. The end of a muscle that is attached to a relatively immovable part; the end opposite the insertion

G. The end of a muscle that is attached to a relatively movable part; the end opposite the origin

H. The muscle that is mainly responsible for a particular body movement; also called *agonist*

EVALUATION OF LEARNING

Directions: Fill in each blank with the correct answer.

1. What are the three types of muscle tissue?

   _____

   _____

2. How many skeletal muscles are found in the human body?

   _____

3. List and describe the four characteristics of skeletal muscle.

   _____

   _____

4. What four functions are provided to the body by muscle contractions?

   _____

   _____

5. Describe each of the following parts of a skeletal muscle:
   a. Epimysium: _____
   b. Fascia: _____
   c. Fasciculus: _____
   d. Perimysium: _____
   e. Muscle fiber: _____
   f. Endomysium: _____

6. List and describe the two ways in which skeletal muscle is attached to bone.
   a. _____

   _____
   b. _____

   _____

7. Describe the following parts of a muscle cell:
   a. Sarcolemma: _____

   _____
   b. Sarcoplasm: _____

   _____
   c. Sarcoplasmic reticulum: _____

   _____
   d. T tubules: _____

   _____

8. Why does a muscle cell have numerous mitochondria?

_____

_____

9. What is the name of the nerve cell that stimulates a skeletal muscle to contract?

_____

10. What is a motor unit?

_____

_____

11. What is the neuromuscular junction?

_____

_____

12. What is a synaptic cleft?

_____

_____

13. What is the name of the neurotransmitter responsible for muscle contractions? Where is this neurotransmitter housed before being released?

_____

_____

14. Draw and label a diagram to illustrate what happens when a nerve impulse reaches its axon terminal.

15. What inactivates acetylcholine?

_____

16. What is the function of ATP?

_____

17. What is creatine phosphate?

_____

18. Where are glucose and fatty acids found in the body?

_____

19. What must be available for aerobic respiration to occur?

_____

20. What are the products of aerobic respiration?

_____

21. Where is myoglobin located, and what is its function?

_____

_____

_____

22. How does the body produce energy when it runs out of oxygen?

_____

23. What happens when there is a buildup of lactic acid in the muscles?

_____

24. What is oxygen debt? How is oxygen debt paid back?

_____

_____

_____

25. Describe each of the following types of body movements, and give an example of each:

Type	Definition	Example
Flexion		
Extension		
Hyperextension		
Dorsiflexion		
Plantar flexion		
Abduction		
Adduction		
Rotation		
Supination		
Pronation		
Circumduction		
Inversion		
Eversion		

26. State the function of each of the following muscles involved with facial expressions:

    a. Frontalis: _____

    b. Orbicularis oris: _____

    c. Orbicularis oculi: _____

    d. Buccinator: _____

    e. Zygomaticus: _____

27. What are the names of the muscles responsible for chewing?

    _____

28. What is the function of the following neck muscles?

    a. Sternocleidomastoid: _____

    b. Trapezius: _____

29. What muscles located in the trunk are responsible for maintaining posture?

    _____

30. What is the function of the intercostal muscles?

    _____

31. Where is the diaphragm located?

    _____

32. What is the function of the diaphragm?

    _____

33. What are the four muscle pairs that make up the wall of the abdomen?

    _____

    _____

34. What muscles allow an individual to shrug his or her shoulders?

    _____

35. What is the function of the rotator cuff muscles?

    _____

36. What muscle is responsible for extending the forearm?

    _____

37. What muscles are responsible for flexing the forearm?

    _____

38. What thigh muscle is used to administer an intramuscular injection?

    _____

39. What muscles make up the quadriceps femoris?

    _____

    _____

40. What is the function of the quadriceps femoris?

   _____

41. What muscles are used to flex the leg?

   _____

42. What muscles allow an individual to stand on tiptoe?

   _____

43. What is another name for the calcaneal tendon?

   _____

CRITICAL THINKING ACTIVITIES

A. BODY SPECTRUM CD ACTIVITY
   Muscular: Face—Lateral
   Body Spectrum Directions:
   1. Access your Body Spectrum program (CD included with your textbook).
   2. Go to the Contents screen.
   3. Access the HELP screen for directions on using the Body Spectrum program.
   4. Select the following category from the Contents screen:

      Muscular
   5. Select the following anatomic diagram:

      Face—Lateral
   6. Identify the structures on the diagram.
   7. Print out the diagram.

B. BODY SPECTRUM CD ACTIVITY
   Muscular: Face—Anterior
   Directions: Identify the structures on this diagram following the Body Spectrum Directions outlined under CTA A.

C. BODY SPECTRUM CD ACTIVITY
   Muscular: Anterior Abdominal
   Directions: Identify the structures on this diagram following the Body Spectrum Directions outlined under CTA A.

D. BODY SPECTRUM CD ACTIVITY
   Muscular: Musculature—Anterior
   Directions: Identify the structures on this diagram following the Body Spectrum Directions outlined under CTA A.

E. BODY SPECTRUM CD ACTIVITY
   Muscular: Upper Chest—Superficial
   Directions: Identify the structures on this diagram following the Body Spectrum Directions outlined under CTA A.

F. BODY SPECTRUM CD ACTIVITY
   Muscular: Right Arm—Lateral
   Directions: Identify the structures on this diagram following the Body Spectrum Directions outlined under CTA A.

G. BODY SPECTRUM CD ACTIVITY
   Muscular: Musculature—Posterior
   Directions: Identify the structures on this diagram following the Body Spectrum Directions outlined under CTA A.

H. INQUIRING PATIENTS WANT TO KNOW

You are working in a general practice medical office. Your patients ask you the following questions. In the space provided, indicate how you would respond to each question in terms the patient would understand. Use your textbook and Internet resources to develop your responses.

1. What causes hiccups?

_____

_____

2. What causes menstrual cramps?

_____

_____

3. Why does someone get stiff and rigid after they die?

_____

_____

4. What causes shin splints?

_____

_____

5. What causes an eye tic?

_____

_____

6. Why do my leg muscles burn when I run a 3-mile race?

_____

_____

7. Why do my muscles ache when I have the flu?

_____

_____

8. How does lifting weights make muscles bigger?

_____

_____

9. What causes shivering?

_____

_____

10. What happens to a muscle when it is torn?

_____

_____

I. CHAPTER 8 ANIMATIONS CD ACTIVITY

Directions:

1. View the Chapter 8 Animations on your Companion CD (included with your textbook).
2. For each animation, write two true/false questions in the space provided below.
3. In the classroom, find a partner.
4. For each animation, read your two questions to your partner.
5. For each correct answer, your partner is awarded two points.

6. Next, have your partner read his/her two questions to you. Award yourself two points for each question answered correctly.

7. Continue in this manner until all the questions have been answered.

8. Record your points on your Study Guide Assignment sheet.

True/False Questions

a. Microscopic Structure of Skeletal Muscle

    1. _____

    2. _____

b. The Motor Unit and Muscle Stimulus

    1. _____

    2. _____

c. Types of Skeletal Muscle Contractions

    1. _____

    2. _____

d. Cellular Respiration

    1. _____

    2. _____

e. Carbohydrate Metabolism: Glycolysis

    1. _____

    2. _____

J. CROSSWORD PUZZLE
Muscular System
Directions: Complete the crossword puzzle using the clues presented below.

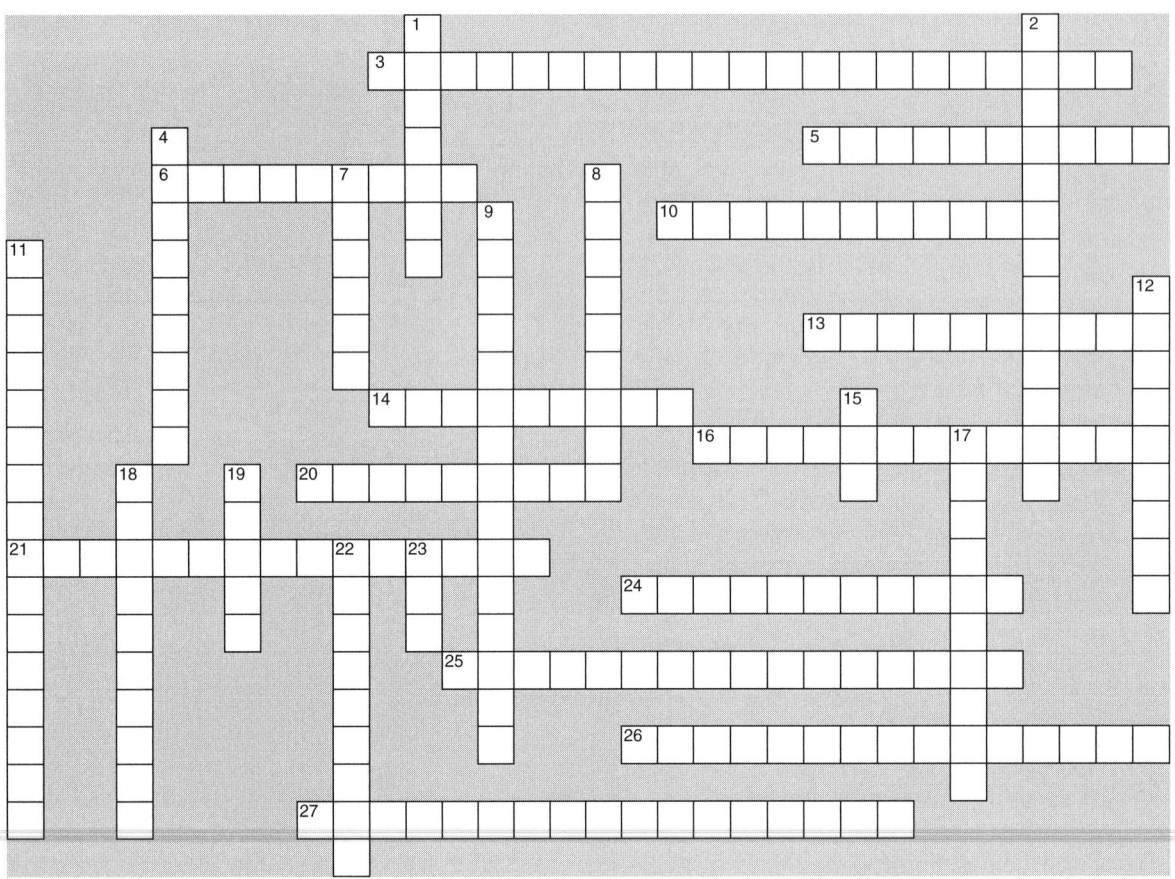

ACROSS	**DOWN**
3 Where an axon meets a muscle fiber	**1** Abducts arm
5 Muscle fiber cell membrane	**2** Flexes forearm
6 Movement away from midline	**4** Bundle of muscle fibers
10 Smiling muscle	**7** Attaches muscle to bone
13 Cheek muscle	**8** Longest muscle in body
14 Movement toward midline	**9** Kissing muscle
16 Extends vertebral column	**11** Where ACh lives
20 Eyebrow-raising muscle	**12** Shrugging shoulders muscle
21 IM injection site for infants	**15** Energy source for muscle contractions
24 Stimulates contraction of skeletal muscle	**17** Muscle fiber cytoplasm
25 Winking muscle	**18** Muscle that opposes a movement
26 Chest muscle	**19** Muscle's fleshy part
27 Muscle group that extends leg	**22** Sheath that surrounds a muscle
	23 Muscle-contraction neurotransmitter

9

Nervous System

CHAPTER ASSIGNMENTS

√ After Completing	Date Due	Textbook Page(s)	TEXTBOOK ASSIGNMENT	Possible Points	Points You Earned
		147-170	Read Chapter 9: Nervous System		
√ After Completing	**Date Due**	**Study Guide Page(s)**	**STUDY GUIDE ASSIGNMENTS (CTA: Critical Thinking Activity)**		
		103	⁇ Pretest	10	
		104	Term Key Term Assessment	10	
		105-110	Evaluation of Learning questions	59	
		110	CD CTA A: Body Spectrum CD Activity: Structure of a Neuron	10	
		111	CTA B: Synapse	7	
		111	CD CTA C: Body Spectrum CD Activity: Brain—Meningeal Coverings	10	
		111	CTA D: Cerebrum	18	
		112	CD CTA E: Body Spectrum CD Activity: Spinal Cord	10	
		112	CTA F: Structure of a Nerve	8	
		112	CD CTA G: Body Spectrum CD Activity: Brain—Inferior	10	
		112-113	CTA H: Inquiring Patients Want to Know	10	
		113-114	CD CTA I: Chapter 9 Animations CD Activity	52	
		115	CTA J: Crossword Puzzle	32	
		103	⁇ Posttest	10	

√ After Completing	Date Due	Study Guide Page(s)	STUDY GUIDE ASSIGNMENTS (CTA: Critical Thinking Activity)		
			ADDITIONAL ASSIGNMENTS		
			TOTAL POINTS		

Name _____   Date _____

? PRETEST

True or False

_____   1. The function of a neuron is to transmit nerve impulses.

_____   2. Neuroglia support and protect neurons.

_____   3. Myelin is a white, fatty substance that surrounds nerve fibers.

_____   4. Sneezing is an example of a reflex.

_____   5. The central sulcus divides the cerebrum into two hemispheres.

_____   6. The hypothalamus functions in the regulation of body temperature.

_____   7. The pons functions in body coordination, posture, and balance.

_____   8. The peripheral nervous system provides a communication network between the central nervous system (CNS) and the body.

_____   9. The endoneurium is a connective tissue sheath that surrounds a nerve.

_____   10. The body has 12 pairs of cranial nerves.

? POSTTEST

True or False

_____   1. An axon transmits impulses toward a neuron cell body.

_____   2. Gray matter is made up of myelinated fibers.

_____   3. A myelin sheath is formed around axons within the CNS by Schwann cells.

_____   4. A synapse is the name of the region of communication between two neurons.

_____   5. The CNS is made up of cranial nerves and spinal nerves.

_____   6. The cerebral cortex consists of gray matter.

_____   7. The spinal cord extends from the base of the skull to the fourth lumbar vertebra.

_____   8. The autonomic nervous system supplies motor impulses to visceral organs.

_____   9. Nerves that carry both sensory and motor fibers are known as *mixed nerves*.

_____   10. The sympathetic division of the autonomic nervous system increases blood flow to skeletal muscle.

Term KEY TERM ASSESSMENT

Directions: Match each medical term with its definition.

_____   1. Action potential

_____   2. Brain stem

_____   3. Cerebellum

_____   4. Cerebrum

_____   5. Diencephalon

_____   6. Myelin

_____   7. Neurilemma

_____   8. Saltatory conduction

_____   9. Synapse

_____   10. Threshold stimulus

A. A nerve impulse; a rapid change in membrane potential that involves depolarization and repolarization

B. Minimum level of stimulation that is required to start a nerve impulse or muscle contraction; also called _liminal stimulus_

C. Part of the brain between the cerebral hemispheres and the midbrain; includes the thalamus, hypothalamus, and epithalamus

D. Process in which a nerve impulse travels along a myelinated nerve fiber by jumping from one node of Ranvier to the next

E. Second largest part of the human brain, located posterior to the pons and medulla oblongata, and involved in the coordination of muscular movements

F. The largest and uppermost part of the human brain; concerned with consciousness, learning, memory, sensations, and voluntary movements

G. The layer of Schwann cells that surrounds a nerve fiber in the peripheral nervous system and, in some cases, produces myelin

H. The portion of the brain, between the diencephalon and spinal cord, that contains the midbrain, pons, and medulla oblongata

I. The region of communication between two neurons

J. White, fatty substance that surrounds many nerve fibers

EVALUATION OF LEARNING

Directions: Fill in each blank with the correct answer.

1. What makes up the nervous system?

   _____

2. Describe the following three general functions of the nervous system:

   a. Sensory functions: _____

   b. Integrative functions: _____

   c. Motor functions: _____

3. What is an effector? What are two types of effectors?

   _____

   _____

4. What are the two main subdivisions of the nervous system?

   _____

5. What is the function of the following subdivisions of the peripheral nervous system?

   a. Afferent (sensory) division: _____

   b. Efferent (motor) division: _____

6. What function is performed by the following subdivisions of the efferent (motor) division?

   a. Somatic nervous system: _____

   b. Autonomic nervous system: _____

7. What are the two subdivisions of the autonomic nervous system?

   _____

8. What are the three basic parts of a neuron?

   _____

9. What is the function of a dendrite?

   _____

10. What is the function of an axon?

   _____

11. What is a myelin sheath?

   _____

12. What makes up the white matter in the central nervous system?

   _____

13. What makes up the gray matter in the central nervous system?

   _____

14. Describe the appearance of a node of Ranvier.

_____

15. What is the neurilemma, and what is its function?

_____

_____

_____

16. What is the function of oligodendrocytes?

_____

17. Why can't nerve fibers in the central nervous system regenerate?

_____

18. Describe the structure and function of the three types of neurons:

   a. Afferent (sensory) neurons: _____

   _____

   b. Efferent (motor) neurons: _____

   _____

   c. Interneurons: _____

   _____

19. What is the function of neuroglia?

_____

20. What is a resting membrane?

_____

21. What happens to sodium ions when a neuron receives a stimulus?

_____

22. Describe how a nerve impulse is propagated along the length of a neuron through an action potential.

_____

_____

_____

_____

23. What is a synapse?

_____

24. How is a nerve impulse transmitted across a synapse?

_____

_____

_____

25. What is a reflex?

_____

_____

26. What are some examples of reflexes that take place in the body?

_____

27. What makes up the central nervous system?

_____

28. What bones surround and protect the brain?

_____

29. What three layers make up the meninges, starting with the outer layer?

_____

30. What are the four parts of the human brain?

_____

31. What is the function of the corpus callosum?

_____

32. What five lobes make up a cerebral hemisphere?

_____

_____

33. Where is the cerebral cortex located? What makes up the cerebral cortex?

_____

_____

34. What functions are controlled by the cerebral cortex?

_____

_____

35. What is the function of the following structures making up the diencephalons?
    a. Thalamus: _____

    _____

    b. Hypothalamus: _____

    _____

    _____

    c. Epithalamus: _____

    _____

36. What structures make up the brain stem?

_____

37. List and explain the function of the three control centers located in the medulla.

      Control Center   **Function**

    a. _____

    b. _____

    c. _____

38. What is the function of the cerebellum?

    _____

    _____

39. What are ventricles?

    _____

40. What is the function of cerebrospinal fluid?

    _____

    _____

    _____

41. What is the starting point and ending point of the spinal cord?

    _____

42. How long is the spinal cord?

    _____

43. What surrounds the spinal cord?

    _____

44. How many pairs of spinal nerves are present in the human body?

    _____

45. What are the functions of the spinal cord?

    _____

    _____

46. What is the difference between ascending tracts and descending tracts of the spinal cord?

    _____

    _____

47. What makes up the peripheral nervous system?

    _____

48. What is the makeup and function of the somatic nervous system?

    _____

    _____

49. What is the makeup and function of the autonomic nervous system?

    _____

50. What type of nerve fibers make up each of the following?

    a. Sensory nerves: _____

    b. Motor nerves: _____

    c. Mixed nerves: _____

51. What is the epineurium?

_____

52. What is a fasciculus?

_____

53. What is the perineurium?

_____

54. What is the endoneurium?

_____

55. What are the names of the 12 cranial nerves, and what is the function of each?

Cranial Nerve	Name	Function
I		
II		
III		
IV		
V		
VI		
VII		
VIII		
IX		
X		
XI		
XII		

56. What are some examples of body functions controlled by the autonomic nervous system?

_____

57. What are the functions of the following two divisions of the autonomic nervous system?

   a. Sympathetic: _____

   _____

   b. Parasympathetic: _____

58. What neurotransmitter is secreted by the postganglionic fibers of the following divisions of the autonomic nervous system?

   a. Sympathetic nervous system: _____

   b. Parasympathetic: _____

59. What effects do the sympathetic and parasympathetic systems have on the following visceral effectors?

Visceral Effector	Sympathetic	Parasympathetic
Pupil of eye		
Heart		
Bronchi		
Digestive glands		
Digestive tract		
Blood vessels to skeletal muscles		
Adrenal medulla		
Urinary bladder		

CRITICAL THINKING ACTIVITES

A. BODY SPECTRUM CD ACTIVITY
   Nervous: Structure of a Neuron
   Body Spectrum Directions:
   1. Access your Body Spectrum program (CD included with your textbook).
   2. Go to the Contents screen.
   3. Access the HELP screen for directions on using the Body Spectrum program.
   4. Select the following category from the Contents screen:
      Nervous
   5. Select the following anatomic diagram:
      Structure of a Neuron
   6. Identify the structures on the diagram.
   7. Print out the diagram.

B. SYNAPSE

Using Figure 9-6 in your textbook as a reference, label each of the components of a synapse on the following diagram.

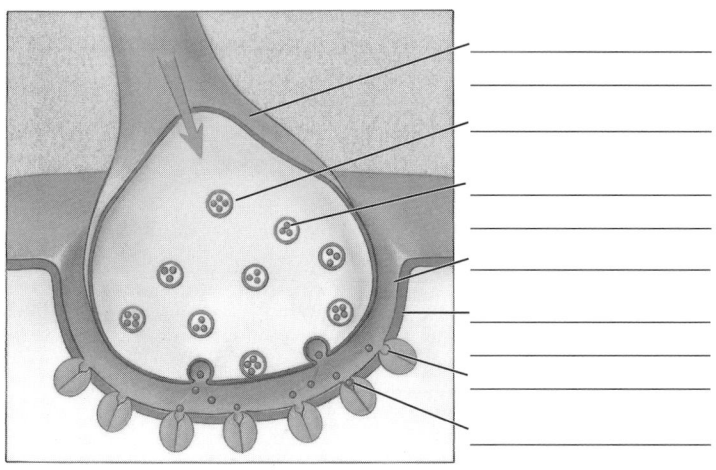

(Modified from Applegate E: *The anatomy and physiology learning system,* ed 3, St. Louis, 2006, Saunders.)

C. BODY SPECTRUM CD ACTIVITY

Nervous: Brain—Meningeal Coverings

Directions: Identify the structures on this diagram following the Body Spectrum Directions outlined under CTA A.

D. CEREBRUM

Using Figure 9-10 in your textbook as a reference, label each of the lobes and functional areas of the cerebrum on the following diagram.

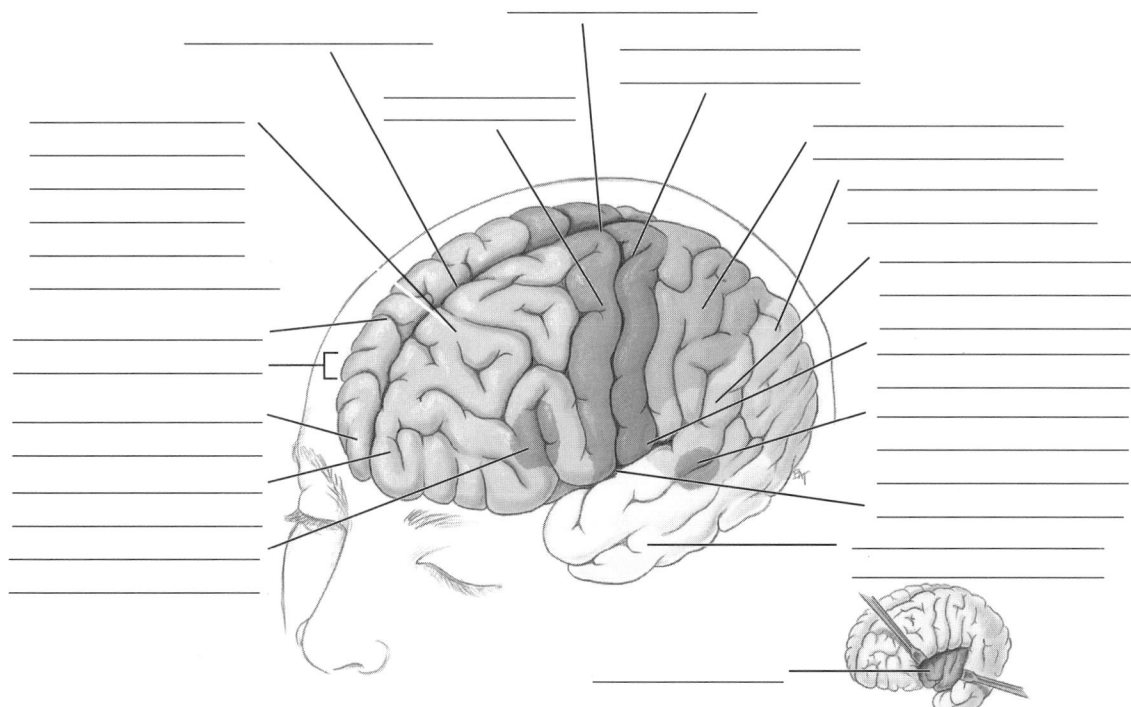

(Modified from Applegate E: *The anatomy and physiology learning system,* ed 3, St. Louis, 2006, Saunders.)

E. BODY SPECTRUM CD ACTIVITY
   Nervous: Spinal Cord
   Directions: Identify the structures on this diagram following the Body Spectrum Directions outlined under CTA A.

F. STRUCTURE OF A NERVE
   Using Figure 9-15 in your textbook as a reference, label each of the structures that make up a nerve on the following diagram.

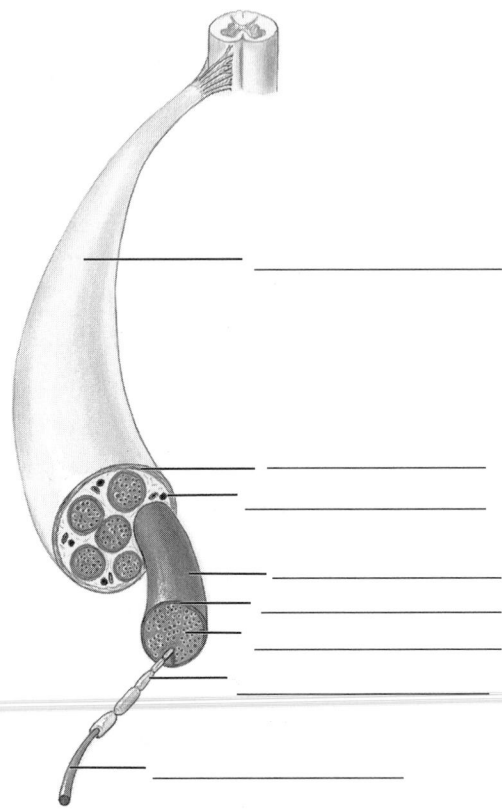

(Modified from Applegate E: *The anatomy and physiology learning system,* ed 3, St. Louis, 2006, Saunders.)

G. BODY SPECTRUM CD ACTIVITY
   Nervous: Brain—Inferior
   Directions: Identify the structures on this diagram following the Body Spectrum Directions outlined under CTA A.

H. INQUIRING PATIENTS WANT TO KNOW
   You are working in a general practice medical office. Your patients ask you the following questions. In the space provided, indicate how you would respond to each question in terms the patient would understand. Use your textbook and Internet resources to develop your responses.

   1. What causes cerebral palsy?

   _____

   _____

   2. What sometimes causes a "brain freeze" when you eat ice cream?

   _____

   _____

3. What does it mean if someone is right-brained or left-brained?

_____

_____

4. What happens in the brain when someone has a migraine headache?

_____

_____

5. Why do you become permanently paralyzed from a spinal cord injury?

_____

_____

6. What makes someone left-handed?

_____

_____

7. How do antidepressants like Prozac work?

_____

_____

8. Is it possible to improve your memory?

_____

_____

9. Why does your knee jerk when the doctor hits it with a rubber hammer?

_____

_____

10. What happens in the brain of a person with Alzheimer's disease?

_____

_____

I. CHAPTER 9 ANIMATIONS CD ACTIVITY
   Directions:
   1. View the Chapter 9 Animations on your Companion CD (included with your textbook).
   2. For each animation, write two true/false questions in the space provided below.
   3. In the classroom, find a partner.
   4. For each animation, read your two questions to your partner.
   5. For each correct answer, your partner is awarded two points.
   6. Next, have your partner read his/her two questions to you. Award yourself two points for each question answered correctly.
   7. Continue in this manner until all the questions have been answered.
   8. Record your points on your Study Guide Assignment sheet.

   True/False Questions
   a. Divisions of the Nervous System

      1. _____
      2. _____
   b. Neurons

      1. _____
      2. _____

c. Nerve Impulses

1. _____

2. _____

d. The Synapse

1. _____

2. _____

e. Reflex Arcs

1. _____

2. _____

f. Physiology of the Brain

1. _____

2. _____

g. Cranial Nerves

1. _____

2. _____

h. Comparison of Anatomic and Somatic Conduction Pathways

1. _____

2. _____

i. The Autonomic Nervous System as a Whole

1. _____

2. _____

j. Sympathetic Nervous System

1. _____

2. _____

k. Parasympathetic Nervous System

1. _____

2. _____

l. Autonomic Neurotransmitters

1. _____

2. _____

m. Spinal Tap

1. _____

2. _____

J. CROSSWORD PUZZLE
Nervous System
Directions: Complete the crossword puzzle using the clues presented below.

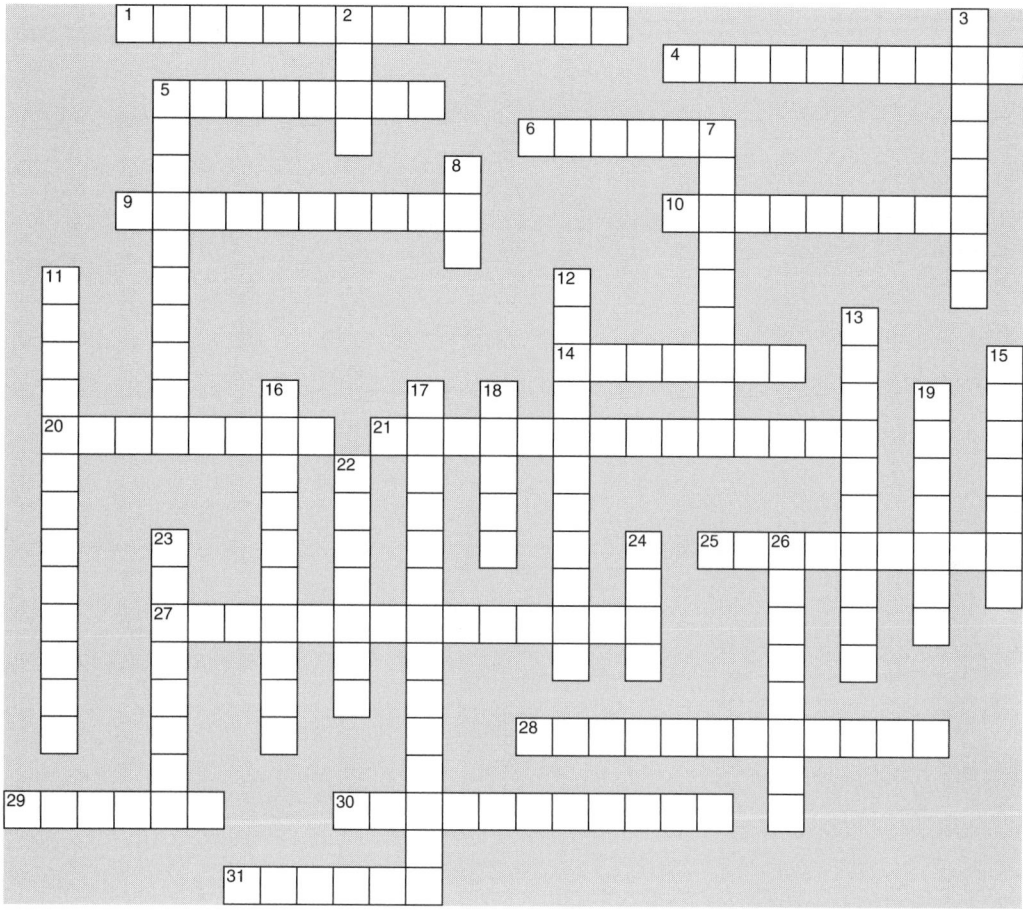

ACROSS
1 Outermost part of cerebrum
4 Cell bodies and unmyelinated fibers
5 Main part of neuron
6 Nerve cell
9 Fluid-filled brain cavities
10 Outer layer of meninges
14 Respiratory center lives here
20 Inner layer of meninges
21 Inside of neuron becomes positive
25 Bundle of nerve fibers
27 Gaps in myelin
28 Regulates body temperature
29 Automatic involuntary response
30 Consists of myelinated nerve fibers
31 White substance surrounding nerve fibers

DOWN
2 Carries impulses away from cell body
3 Largest part of brain
5 In charge of coordination, posture, and balance
7 Support system for neurons
8 Brain and spinal cord fluid
11 Space between neurons
12 "Fight or flight" NS division
13 Protected by vertebral column
15 Communication region between neurons
16 Produces myelin in PNS
17 Restores resting membrane
18 Nerves that carry impulses away from CNS
19 Group of nerve cell bodies outside CNS
22 Nerve that carries impulses toward CNS
23 Transmits impulses to cell body
24 Convolutions on cerebrum
26 Event that alters neuron cell membrane

10

The Senses

CHAPTER ASSIGNMENTS

√ After Completing	Date Due	Textbook Page(s)	TEXTBOOK ASSIGNMENT	Possible Points	Points You Earned
		171-184	Read Chapter 10: The Senses		
√ After Completing	**Date Due**	**Study Guide Page(s)**	**STUDY GUIDE ASSIGNMENTS (CTA: Critical Thinking Activity)**		
		119	☑ Pretest	10	
		120	🖊Term Key Term Assessment	8	
		121-125	☑ Evaluation of Learning questions	65	
		126	CTA A: Taste Locations	4	
		126	💿 CTA B: Body Spectrum CD Activity: Right Eye—Cross Section	10	
		126	💿 CTA C: Body Spectrum CD Activity: Normal Structure of the Eye	10	
		126	💿 CTA D: CD Activity: Eye-Dentify (Record points earned)		
		126-127	CTA E: Light Ray	40	
		127	💿 CTA F: Body Spectrum CD Activity: Ear—Cross Section	10	
		127	💿 CTA G: Body Spectrum CD Activity: Muscles of the Middle Ear	10	
		127	💿 CTA H: CD Activity: Can You Hear Me Now? (Record points earned)		
		128	CTA I: Sound Wave	40	

√ After Completing	Date Due	Study Guide Page(s)	STUDY GUIDE ASSIGNMENTS (CTA: Critical Thinking Activity)		
		128-129	CTA J: Inquiring Patients Want to Know	10	
		129-130	CTA K: Chapter 10 Animations CD Activity	8	
		131	CTA L: Crossword Puzzle	28	
		119	Posttest	10	
			ADDITIONAL ASSIGNMENTS		
			TOTAL POINTS		

Name _____   Date _____

? **PRETEST**

True or False

_____ 1. Special senses have receptors that are localized in a particular area.

_____ 2. Thermoreceptors are located in subcutaneous tissue.

_____ 3. There are more cold receptors in a given area than heat receptors.

_____ 4. The olfactory cortex interprets smell sensations.

_____ 5. The inner layer of the eye that contains rods and cones is the retina.

_____ 6. The region of the retina that produces the sharpest image is the optic disk.

_____ 7. Visual impulses are interpreted in the occipital lobe.

_____ 8. Cerumen helps prevent foreign substances from reaching the eardrum.

_____ 9. The range of frequencies for normal speech is 300 to 4000 vibrations per second.

_____ 10. The cochlea is a coiled structure in the inner ear that functions in hearing.

POSTTEST

True or False

_____ 1. Meissner's corpuscles are stimulated by heavy pressure.

_____ 2. The sense of position or orientation is known as *proprioreception*.

_____ 3. A nociceptor is stimulated by tissue damage.

_____ 4. Taste receptors are stimulated by the pressure of food on the tongue.

_____ 5. The white part of the eye is the choroid.

_____ 6. When the ciliary muscle contracts, the lens bulges for close vision.

_____ 7. Rhodopsin allows the eye to adapt to dim light.

_____ 8. Receptors for hearing are chemoreceptors.

_____ 9. The oval window equalizes the pressure between the outside and the middle ear.

_____ 10. The semicircular canals contain the sense organs for static equilibrium.

KEY TERM ASSESSMENT

Directions: Match each medical term with its definition.

_____ 1. Accommodation

_____ 2. Chemoreceptor

_____ 3. Mechanoreceptor

_____ 4. Nociceptor

_____ 5. Photoreceptor

_____ 6. Proprioception

_____ 7. Sensory adaptation

_____ 8. Thermoreceptor

A. A sensory receptor that detects changes in temperature

B. A sensory receptor that detects light; located in the retina of the eye

C. A sensory receptor that detects the presence of chemicals; responsible for taste, smell, and monitoring the concentration of certain chemicals in body fluids

D. A sensory receptor that responds to a bending or deformation of the cell; examples include receptors for touch, pressure, hearing, and equilibrium

E. A sensory receptor that responds to tissue damage; pain receptor

F. Mechanism that allows the eye to focus at various distances, primarily achieved by changing the curvature of the lens

G. Phenomenon in which some receptors respond when a stimulus is first applied but decrease their response if the stimulus is maintained; receptor sensitivity decreases with prolonged stimulation

H. The sense of body position and movements

EVALUATION OF LEARNING

Directions: Fill in each blank with the correct answer.

1. What is the difference between the general senses and the special senses?

   _____

   _____

2. What are the five types of sense receptors? Provide an example of each.

Type of Receptor	Example

3. What are the steps involved in perceiving sensation?

   _____

   _____

   _____

4. What is sensory adaptation?

   _____

   _____

5. What senses are classified as the general senses?

   _____

   _____

6. What type of stimulus activates a mechanoreceptor?

   _____

7. What is the function of each of the following mechanoreceptors involved with touch and pressure?

   a. Free nerve endings: _____

   b. Meissner's corpuscles: _____

   c. Pacinian corpuscles: _____

8. What is proprioception?

   _____

9. What mechanoreceptors are involved with proprioception?

   _____

10. Where are thermoreceptors located?

    _____

11. In which part of the body are thermoreceptors the most numerous? Where are they the least numerous?

_____

_____

12. How do the number of cold receptors compare to the number of heat receptors?

_____

13. What type of receptors do extreme temperatures stimulate?

_____

14. Describe the sensory adaptation that occurs with thermoreceptors.

_____

_____

15. What stimulates a nociceptor?

_____

16. Where are nociceptors located?

_____

_____

17. How do nociceptors provide a protective function in the body?

_____

_____

18. What senses are classified as special senses?

_____

19. What are the organs of taste?

_____

20. What stimulates the receptors that determine taste?

_____

21. What are the four different taste sensations?

_____

22. What happens when taste hairs are stimulated?

_____

_____

23. What is olfaction?

_____

24. What stimulates the receptors that distinguish smell?

_____

25. What area of the brain interprets smell impulses?

_____

26. What is the function of the following eye structures?

    a. Eyebrows: _____

    b. Eyelids: _____

    c. Eyelashes: _____

    d. Sebaceous glands: _____

27. What eye muscle performs the following?

    a. Closes the eye: _____

    b. Opens the eye: _____

28. Describe the location of the conjunctiva.

    _____

    _____

29. What is the purpose of mucus secreted by the eye?

    _____

30. What is a stye?

    _____

31. What structure produces tears?

    _____

32. What is the function of tears?

    _____

    _____

33. Describe the appearance of the sclera.

    _____

    _____

34. What are two functions of the choroid?

    _____

    _____

35. What effect does contraction of the ciliary muscle have on the lens of the eye?

    _____

    _____

36. How does the iris control the size of the pupil?

    _____

37. Where are the receptor cells of the eye located?

    _____

38. What is the optic disk, and why is it known as the "blind spot" of the eye?

    _____

    _____

39. Describe the location and appearance of the macula lutea.

_____

40. What is the name of the eye structure that produces the sharpest image?

_____

41. Where is the anterior cavity of the eye located?

_____

42. What is the function of aqueous humor?

_____

_____

43. Where is the posterior cavity of the eye located?

_____

44. What is the function of vitreous humor?

_____

45. What is refraction?

_____

46. What four structures of the eye function in refraction?

_____

47. Describe the image that forms when light rays are refracted onto the retina.

_____

48. What occurs in each of these structures during distance and close vision?

Vision	Ciliary Muscle	Suspensory Ligaments	Lens
a. Distance vision			
b. Close vision			

49. What is the function of rods?

_____

50. What is the function of cones?

_____

51. What is the function of rhodopsin?

_____

52. What part of the brain interprets visual impulses?

_____

53. What two functions are performed by the ear?

_____

54. What is the function of the auricle?

_____

_____

55. What is the function of cerumen?

_____

56. What effect do sound waves have on the tympanic membrane?

_____

57. What is the function of the eustachian tube?

_____

_____

58. What are the names of the three auditory ossicles?

_____

59. What structures in the inner ear function in equilibrium?

_____

60. What structure in the inner ear functions in hearing?

_____

61. What structure in the cochlea houses the sound receptors?

_____

62. What is the range of frequencies of normal speech?

_____

63. What nerve carries auditory impulses to the brain?

_____

64. What is static equilibrium?

_____

_____

65. What is dynamic equilibrium?

_____

_____

CRITICAL THINKING ACTIVITIES

A. TASTE LOCATIONS
   Using Figure 10-3 in your textbook, label the taste locations of the tongue on the following diagram:

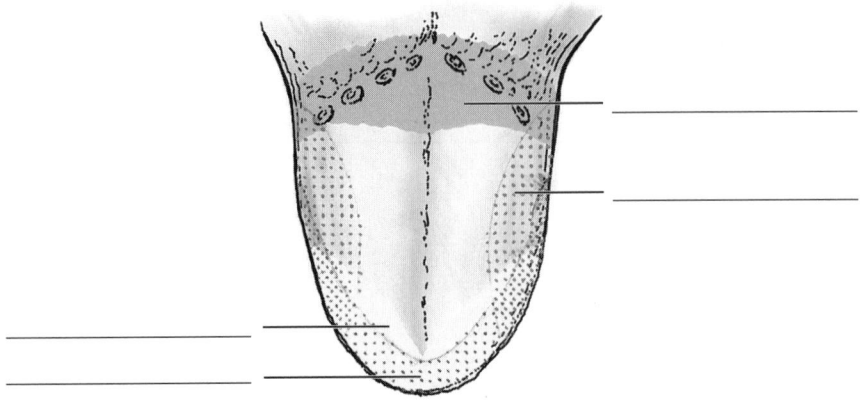

   (Modified from Applegate E: *The anatomy and physiology learning system,* ed 3, St. Louis, 2006, Saunders.)

B. BODY SPECTRUM CD ACTIVITY
   Senses: Right Eye—Cross Section
   Body Spectrum Directions:
   1. Access your Body Spectrum program (CD included with your textbook).
   2. Go to the Contents screen.
   3. Access the HELP screen for directions on using the Body Spectrum program.
   4. Select the following category from the Contents screen:
      Senses
   5. Select the following anatomic diagram:
      Right Eye—Cross Section
   6. Identify the structures on the diagram.
   7. Print out the diagram.

C. BODY SPECTRUM CD ACTIVITY
   Senses: Normal Structure of the Eye
   Directions: Identify the structures on this diagram following the Body Spectrum Directions outlined under CTA A.

D. CD ACTIVITY: EYE-DENTIFY
   Access your Companion CD (included with your textbook) to complete this activity. Record your points earned on your assignment sheet.

E. LIGHT RAY
   You are a ray of light that is getting ready to enter the eye and travel to the brain for interpretation. In the space provided below, describe all of the structures you encounter on your way to the brain. Also describe what function each structure is performing in the eye. Each of the following structures should be included in your discussion:

   a. Lacrimal apparatus
   b. Conjunctiva
   c. Sclera
   d. Iris and pupil
   e. Anterior cavity
   f. Lens and suspensory ligaments
   g. Ciliary muscle
   h. Posterior cavity
   i. Retina

  j. Macula lutea
  k. Rods and cones
  l. Optic nerve
  m. Optic chiasma
  n. Thalamus
  o. Occipital lobe

_____
_____
_____
_____
_____
_____
_____
_____
_____
_____
_____
_____
_____
_____
_____
_____
_____
_____
_____
_____
_____
_____
_____

F. BODY SPECTRUM CD ACTIVITY
    Senses: Ear—Cross Section
    Directions: Identify the structures on this diagram following the Body Spectrum Directions outlined under CTA A.

G. BODY SPECTRUM CD ACTIVITY
    Senses: Muscles of the Middle Ear
    Directions: Identify the structures on this diagram following the Body Spectrum Directions outlined under CTA A.

H. CD ACTIVITY: CAN YOU HEAR ME NOW?
    Access your Companion CD (included with your textbook) to complete this activity. Record your points earned on your assignment sheet.

I. SOUND WAVE

You are a sound wave that is getting ready to enter the ear and travel to the brain for interpretation. In the space provided below, describe all of the structures you encounter on your way to the brain. Also describe what function each structure is performing in the ear. Each of the following structures should be included in your discussion:

a. Auricle
b. External auditory canal
c. Ceruminous glands
d. Tympanic membrane
e. Eustachian tube
f. Auditory ossicles
g. Oval window
h. Cochlea
i. Temporal lobe

_____

_____

_____

_____

_____

_____

_____

_____

_____

_____

_____

_____

_____

_____

_____

_____

_____

_____

_____

_____

_____

_____

_____

J. INQUIRING PATIENTS WANT TO KNOW

You are working in a general practice medical office. Your patients ask you the following questions. In the space provided, indicate how you would respond to each question in terms the patient would understand. Use your textbook and Internet resources to develop your responses.

1. What causes an optical illusion?

_____

_____

2. How does LASIK surgery improve vision?

_____

_____

3. How does loud music damage hearing?

_____

_____

4. What is the reason for putting tubes in the eardrum?

_____

_____

5. What causes eye floaters?

_____

_____

6. Why do my ears get plugged when I'm on an airplane?

_____

_____

7. What can cause an eardrum to rupture?

_____

_____

8. Why does a dog have a better sense of smell than a human?

_____

_____

9. Why can't you taste food when you have a bad cold?

_____

_____

10. Why do you feel dizzy when you spin around?

_____

_____

K. CHAPTER 10 ANIMATIONS CD ACTIVITY
  Directions:
  1. View the Chapter 10 Animations on your Companion CD (included with your textbook).
  2. For each animation, write two true/false questions in the space provided below.
  3. In the classroom, find a partner.
  4. For each animation, read your two questions to your partner.
  5. For each correct answer, your partner is awarded two points.
  6. Next, have your partner read his/her two questions to you. Award yourself two points for each question answered correctly.
  7. Continue in this manner until all the questions have been answered.
  8. Record your points on your Study Guide Assignment sheet.

True/False Questions

a. Smell

    1. _____

    2. _____

b. Pathway of Sound Waves

    1. _____

    2. _____

L. CROSSWORD PUZZLE
  The Senses
  Directions: Complete the crossword puzzle using the clues presented below.

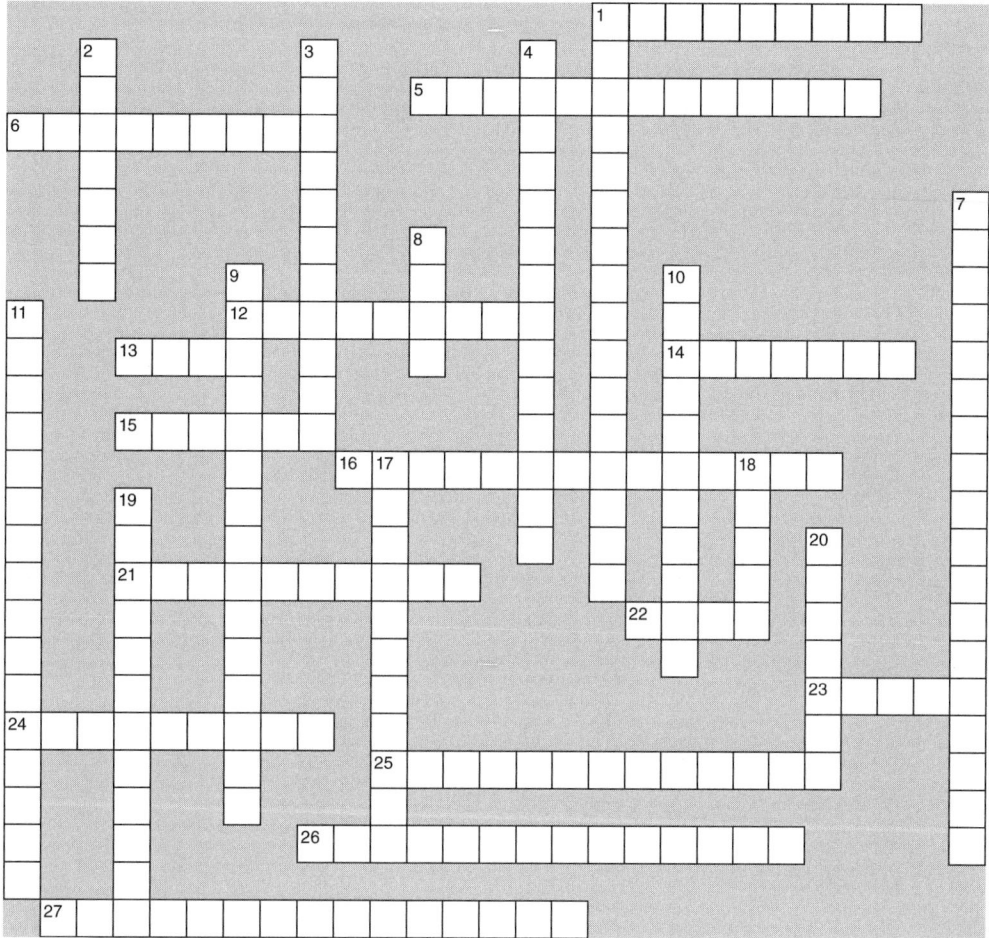

ACROSS
  1 Organs of taste
  5 Produces tears
  6 Visual purple
  12 Blind spot
  13 Colored part of eye
  14 Earwax
  15 White of the eye
  16 Space between cornea and lens
  21 Bending of light rays
  22 This bulges for close vision
  23 Receptors for color vision
  24 Sense of smell
  25 Where visual impulses are interpreted
  26 Connects middle ear with throat
  27 Stimulated by heat and cold

DOWN
  1 Eardrum
  2 Absorbs excess light rays
  3 Covers front of eyeball except for cornea
  4 Sense of position
  7 Stimulated by heavy pressure
  8 Sensitive to dim light
  9 Contains vitreous humor
  10 Yellow spot on retina
  11 Muscle that closes the eye
  17 Pain receptors
  18 Auditory ossicle
  19 Where taste impulses are interpreted
  20 Collects sound waves

11

Endocrine System

CHAPTER ASSIGNMENTS

√ After Completing	Date Due	Textbook Page(s)	TEXTBOOK ASSIGNMENT	Possible Points	Points You Earned
		185-194	Read Chapter 11: Endocrine System		
√ After Completing	Date Due	Study Guide Page(s)	STUDY GUIDE ASSIGNMENTS (CTA: Critical Thinking Activity)		
		135	?≡ Pretest	10	
		136	♪Term Key Term Assessment	6	
		137-140	✓≡ Evaluation of Learning questions	35	
		141	CTA A: Location of Endocrine Glands	20	
		142	CTA B: Pituitary Gland	20	
		142-143	CTA C: Inquiring Patients Want to Know	10	
		143	●CD CTA D: Chapter 11 Animations CD Activity	8	
		144	CTA E: Crossword Puzzle	24	
		135	?≡ Posttest	10	
			ADDITIONAL ASSIGNMENTS		
			TOTAL POINTS		

Notes

Name _____   Date _____

? PRETEST

True or False

_____   1. Endocrine glands have ducts that empty their secretions onto a surface.

_____   2. Sex hormones are made up of proteins.

_____   3. A target tissue is a tissue that has receptor sites for a particular hormone.

_____   4. In an adult, an excess secretion of growth hormone can cause Down syndrome.

_____   5. Oxytocin causes contraction of smooth muscle in the wall of the uterus.

_____   6. Goiter results when there is a lack of iodine in the body.

_____   7. When there is a low blood calcium level, calcium is released from the bones.

_____   8. The adrenal glands are located above the kidneys.

_____   9. Insulin is secreted by the beta cells of the pancreas.

_____   10. Progesterone stimulates the production of milk in the lactating breast.

? POSTTEST

True or False

_____   1. Sebaceous glands are exocrine glands.

_____   2. Luteinizing hormone is produced by the anterior pituitary gland.

_____   3. Follicle-stimulating hormone stimulates development of eggs in the ovaries and sperm in the testes.

_____   4. Diabetes mellitus results when there is not enough antidiuretic hormone secreted by the body.

_____   5. Myxedema is due to a deficiency of thyroid hormone in an adult.

_____   6. Aldosterone reduces the calcium level in the body.

_____   7. Vitamin C is necessary for dietary calcium to be absorbed into the blood from the intestines.

_____   8. Insulin promotes cellular uptake and use of glucose of insulin for energy.

_____   9. Hydrochloric acid stimulates the liver to break down glycogen into glucose.

_____   10. Melatonin is a hormone that regulates the sleep/wake cycle.

✏ Term **KEY TERM ASSESSMENT**

Directions: Match each medical term with its definition.

_____ 1. Adenohypophysis

_____ 2. Endocrine gland

_____ 3. Exocrine gland

_____ 4. Hormone

_____ 5. Neurohypophysis

_____ 6. Target tissue

A. A substance secreted by an endocrine gland
B. A tissue (cells) that responds to a particular hormone because it has receptor sites for that hormone
C. Anterior portion of the pituitary gland
D. Gland that secretes its product directly into the blood
E. Gland that secretes its product to a surface or cavity through ducts
F. Posterior portion of the pituitary gland

EVALUATION OF LEARNING

Directions: Fill in each blank with the correct answer.

1. How do the following systems regulate body activities?

   a. Nervous system: _____

   b. Endocrine system: _____

2. What are exocrine glands?

   _____

   _____

3. What are four examples of exocrine glands?

   _____

   _____

4. How does an endocrine gland function?

   _____

   _____

5. Why must insulin be administered by injection?

   _____

   _____

6. What hormones consist of steroids?

   _____

7. How do hormones exert their action on the body?

   _____

   _____

8. What is the function of the following hormones secreted by the anterior lobe of the pituitary gland?

   a. Growth hormone: _____

   _____

   b. Thyroid stimulating hormone: _____

   _____

   c. ACTH: _____

   _____

   d. Follicle-stimulating hormone (FSH): _____

   _____

   e. Luteinizing hormone:

   Female: _____

   Male: _____

f. Prolactin: _____

_____

9. What is the function of the following hormones secreted by the posterior lobe of the pituitary gland?

a. Antidiuretic hormone: _____

_____

b. Oxytocin: _____

_____

10. What makes up thyroid hormone?

_____

11. Why does the adult thyroid gland enlarge when there is a lack of iodine in the body?

_____

_____

12. What are the causes, symptoms, and treatments of the following conditions?

Condition	Cause	Symptoms	Treatment
a. Cretinism			
b. Myxedema			
c. Hyperthyroidism			

13. How does calcitonin decrease the calcium level in the blood?

_____

_____

14. Where are the parathyroid glands located?

_____

15. What is the function of parathyroid hormone?

_____

_____

16. Where are the adrenal glands located?

_____

17. What is the function of mineralocorticoids secreted by the adrenal glands?

_____

_____

18. What is the name of the principal mineralocorticoid?

_____

19. What is the function of glucocorticoids secreted by the adrenal cortex?

_____

_____

20. What is the principal glucocorticoid?

_____

21. What are the cause and symptoms of Addison's disease?

_____

_____

_____

22. What are the cause and symptoms of Cushing's syndrome?

_____

_____

_____

23. What causes the secretion of epinephrine and norepinephrine by the adrenal medulla?

_____

24. What effect does the secretion of epinephrine and norepinephrine have on the body?

_____

_____

25. What are the names of the cells in the pancreas that secrete the following hormones?
    a. Glucagon: _____
    b. Insulin: _____

26. Why is it important for the body to maintain blood glucose levels within a normal range?

_____

27. How does glucagon work to raise blood glucose levels?

_____

_____

_____

28. How does insulin decrease the blood glucose level?

_____

_____

_____

29. What happens to excess glucose that cannot be stored as glycogen?

_____

30. What are three factors that cause hypoactivity of insulin?

_____

_____

31. What are androgens?

_____

32. What structure secretes testosterone?

_____

33. What is the function of testosterone at the onset of puberty?

_____

_____

_____

34. What is the function of estrogen and progesterone at the onset of puberty?

_____

_____

_____

35. What is the function of melatonin secreted by the pineal gland?

_____

_____

_____

CRITICAL THINKING ACTIVITIES

A. LOCATION OF ENDOCRINE GLANDS

Using Figure 11-2 as a reference, sketch an outline of the human body. Draw, color, and label the major endocrine glands on your sketch.

B. PITUITARY GLAND

You are a pituitary gland and have control over your target tissues. In the chart provided, indicate what hormone you would secrete to stimulate each of the following target tissues. Also indicate what effect each hormone would have on its target tissue.

Target Tissue	What Hormone Would You Secrete to Stimulate This Target Tissue?	What Effect Would This Hormone Have on the Target Tissue?
Thyroid gland		
Adrenal cortex		
Ovarian follicles		
Seminiferous tubules		
Ovaries		
Testes		
Mammary glands		
Kidney		
Uterus and mammary glands		
Most body tissues		

C. INQUIRING PATIENTS WANT TO KNOW

You are working in a general practice medical office. Your patients ask you the following questions. In the space provided, indicate how you would respond to each question in terms the patient would understand. Use your textbook and Internet resources to develop your responses.

1. Why doesn't an adolescent girl with anorexia have a menstrual period?

_____

_____

2. How is the insulin that is used for insulin injections made?

_____

_____

3. Why do some diabetics take medication orally?

_____

_____

4. How does an insulin pump work?

_____

_____

5. What are anabolic steroids, and why are they sometimes abused by athletes?

_____

_____

6. What side effects can occur from taking anabolic steroids?

_____

_____

7. What is an adrenaline rush?

_____

_____

8. Why do I feel so irritable when I am having trouble with hypoglycemia?

_____

_____

9. What is the best diet to follow for hypoglycemia?

_____

_____

10. Can hypoglycemia be cured?

_____

_____

D. CHAPTER 11 ANIMATIONS CD ACTIVITY
Directions:
1. View the Chapter 11 Animations on your Companion CD (included with your textbook).
2. For each animation, write two true/false questions in the space provided below.
3. In the classroom, find a partner.
4. For each animation, read your two questions to your partner.
5. For each correct answer, your partner is awarded two points.
6. Next, have your partner read his/her two questions to you. Award yourself two points for each question answered correctly.
7. Continue in this manner until all the questions have been answered.
8. Record your points on your Study Guide Assignment sheet.

True/False Questions

a. Thyroid Gland

1. _____

2. _____

b. Function of Insulin

1. _____

2. _____

E. CROSSWORD PUZZLE
Endocrine System
Directions: Complete the crossword puzzle using the clues presented below.

ACROSS

2 Responsible for development of male reproductive structures
4 Lethargy, weight gain, loss of hair, low BMR are symptoms of this
7 Stimulates milk production by mammary gland
8 Reduces blood calcium level
10 Fight-or-flight hormone
13 Stimulates growth of bones and muscles
14 Glucocorticoid that counteracts inflammatory response
16 Glands with ducts
18 Causes uterus to contract
21 Sex hormones
22 Regulates circadian rhythms
24 Causes ovulation to occur

DOWN

1 Stimulates development of eggs and sperm
3 Glands that secrete hormones
5 Located on top of kidneys
6 Protruding eyes
9 Causes uterus to thicken
11 Increases blood calcium levels
12 Raises blood glucose level
15 Decreases blood glucose level
17 Mentally retarded dwarf
19 Stimulates adrenal gland to secrete cortisol
20 Promotes reabsorption of water by kidney
23 Stimulates thyroid to secrete thyroid hormone

12

Circulatory System

CHAPTER ASSIGNMENTS

√ After Completing	Date Due	Textbook Page(s)	TEXTBOOK ASSIGNMENT	Possible Points	Points You Earned
		195-215	Read Chapter 12: Circulatory System		

√ After Completing	Date Due	Study Guide Page(s)	STUDY GUIDE ASSIGNMENTS (CTA: Critical Thinking Activity)	Possible Points	Points You Earned
		147	Pretest	10	
		148	Key Term Assessment	15	
		149-155	Evaluation of Learning questions	76	
		155	CTA A: Body Spectrum CD Activity: Heart—Cross Section	10	
		155	CTA B: Body Spectrum CD Activity: Heart Circulation	10	
		155	CTA C: Body Spectrum CD Activity: Coronary Vessels	10	
		155	CTA D: CD Activity: Name That Blood Cell (Record points earned)		
		155-156	CTA E: Blood Clotting	20	
		156	CTA F: Artery	6	
		157	CTA G: Inquiring Patients Want to Know	10	
		157-159	CTA H: Chapter 12 Animations CD Activity	56	
		160	CTA I: Crossword Puzzle	30	
		147	Posttest	10	

√ After Completing	Date Due	Study Guide Page(s)	STUDY GUIDE ASSIGNMENTS (CTA: Critical Thinking Activity)		
			ADDITIONAL ASSIGNMENTS		
			TOTAL POINTS		

Name _____   Date _____

? PRETEST

True or False

_____ 1. The pointed end of the heart is the apex.

_____ 2. The myocardium forms the bulk of the heart wall.

_____ 3. The coronary arteries branch off the aorta to supply the heart with oxygen and nutrients.

_____ 4. The SA node is located in the right atrium.

_____ 5. The adult male has 5 to 6 liters of blood.

_____ 6. Erythrocytes lack a nucleus.

_____ 7. Vitamin K is necessary for the absorption of vitamin B_{12} from the intestines.

_____ 8. Leukocytes defend the body against disease.

_____ 9. Thrombocytes develop from large cells known as *macrophages*.

_____ 10. Veins carry blood toward the heart.

? POSTTEST

True or False

_____ 1. The peritoneum is the loose-fitting sac that encloses the heart.

_____ 2. The superior vena cava returns blood to the heart from the lower extremities.

_____ 3. The mitral valve is located between the right atrium and right ventricle.

_____ 4. When the ventricles are contracting, the AV valves are open.

_____ 5. The buffy coat is made up of white blood cells and platelets.

_____ 6. An immature erythrocyte is a band.

_____ 7. Bile is the yellow pigment that results from the breakdown of hemoglobin.

_____ 8. Acute infections cause an increase in the number of neutrophils.

_____ 9. Thrombin converts fibrinogen to fibrin.

_____ 10. Microscopic arteries are known as *arterioles*.

Term KEY TERM ASSESSMENT

Directions: Match each medical term with its definition.

_____ 1. Atrioventricular valve

_____ 2. Cardiac cycle

_____ 3. Coagulation

_____ 4. Conduction myofibers

_____ 5. Diapedesis

_____ 6. Diastole

_____ 7. Erythrocyte

_____ 8. Erythropoiesis

_____ 9. Erythropoietin

_____ 10. Hemocytoblast

_____ 11. Hematopoiesis

_____ 12. Leukocyte

_____ 13. Semilunar valve

_____ 14. Systole

_____ 15. Thrombocyte

A. A complete heartbeat consisting of contraction and relaxation of both atria and both ventricles

B. A hormone released by the kidneys that stimulates red blood cell production

C. A stem cell in the bone marrow from which the blood cells arise

D. Blood cell production, which occurs in the red bone marrow

E. Cardiac muscle cells specialized for conducting action potentials to the myocardium; part of the conduction system of the heart; also called _Purkinje fibers_

F. Contraction phase of the cardiac cycle

G. One of the formed elements of the blood; functions in blood clotting

H. Red blood cell

I. Relaxation phase of the cardiac cycle

J. The process by which white blood cells squeeze between the cells in a vessel wall to enter the tissue spaces outside the blood vessel

K. The process of blood clotting

L. The process of red blood cell formation

M. Valve between a ventricle of the heart and the vessel that carries blood away from the ventricle

N. Valve between an atrium and a ventricle in the heart

O. White blood cell

EVALUATION OF LEARNING

Directions: Fill in each blank with the correct answer.

1. What is the function of the heart?

   _____

   _____

2. How large is the average human heart?

   _____

3. Describe the following layers of the pericardium:

   a. Fibrous pericardium: _____

   b. Parietal pericardium: _____

   c. Visceral pericardium: _____

   _____

4. What is the function of the epicardium?

   _____

   _____

5. What makes up the myocardium?

   _____

6. Why does the endocardium have a smooth surface?

   _____

7. What type of blood enters the right atrium?

   _____

8. The superior vena cava returns blood to the heart from what parts of the body?

   _____

9. The inferior vena cava returns blood to the heart from what parts of the body?

   _____

10. What is the interarterial septum?

    _____

11. What is the function of the right ventricle?

    _____

12. What is the function of the left ventricle?

    _____

13. Why does the left ventricle have a thicker myocardium than the right ventricle?

    _____

    _____

14. What is the interventricular septum?

_____

_____

15. Describe the location and function of each of the following valves:

Valve	Location	Function
a. Tricuspid valve		
b. Bicuspid valve		
c. Pulmonary semilunar valve		
d. Aortic semilunar valve		

16. Starting with the right atrium, trace the path of the blood through the heart.

_____

_____

_____

_____

17. What are the names of the vessels that supply the heart with oxygen?

_____

18. What is the function of the SA node?

_____

_____

19. What is the function of the AV node?

_____

_____

20. What structures transmit the heart's impulse from the AV node to the ventricles?

_____

21. What occurs with each of the following during atrial systole?

    a. AV valves: _____

    b. Atria: _____

    c. Ventricles: _____

    d. Semilunar valves: _____

22. What are each of the following structures doing during ventricular systole?

    a. AV valves: _____

    b. Atria: _____

    c. Ventricles: _____

    d. Semilunar valves: _____

23. What causes each of the following heart sounds?

    a. Lubb: _____

    b. Dupp: _____

24. What causes a heart murmur?

_____

25. How does blood function in transportation in the body?

_____

_____

_____

26. How does blood function in regulation in the body?

_____

_____

_____

27. How does blood function in protection in the body?

_____

_____

_____

28. What percentage of the blood is made up of the following?

    a. Plasma: _____

    b. Red blood cells: _____

29. What makes up the buffy coat?

_____

30. What is the function of the following plasma proteins?

    a. Albumins: _____

_____

    b. Globulins: _____

_____

    c. Fibrinogen: _____

31. What are the waste products of protein and nucleic acid catabolism? How are these waste products excreted?

_____

32. What simple nutrients are derived from digestion of the following?

    a. Protein: _____

    b. Carbohydrates: _____

    c. Lipids: _____

33. What are four electrolytes found in the plasma of the blood?

_____

34. What seven cells develop from a hemocytoblast?

   _____

   _____

35. What is the normal range for a red blood count for the following?

   a. Adult male: _____

   b. Adult female: _____

36. Describe the appearance of a mature red blood cell.

   _____

37. What is a reticulocyte?

   _____

38. What is the function of erythrocytes?

   _____

39. What is oxyhemoglobin, and what is its color?

   _____

   _____

40. What is deoxyhemoglobin, and what is its color?

   _____

   _____

41. What is the name of the hormone that stimulates the red bone marrow to produce erythrocytes?

   _____

42. What vitamins and minerals are necessary for the production of red blood cells?

   _____

43. What is the function of the intrinsic factor?

   _____

44. What condition results when there is a lack of the intrinsic factor?

   _____

45. What is the lifespan of a red blood cell?

   _____

46. What happens when a red blood cell is worn out?

   _____

   _____

47. What happens to the following components when hemoglobin breaks down?

   a. Protein: _____

   b. Iron: _____

   c. Bilirubin: _____

48. What is the normal range for a white blood count?

_____

49. Where do leukocytes do their work?

_____

50. What is diapedesis?

_____

51. What is the function of neutrophils?

_____

52. What causes an increase in eosinophils?

_____

53. What is the function of the following substances secreted by a basophil?
    a. Histamine: _____
    b. Heparin: _____

54. What are macrophages, and what is their function?

_____

_____

55. What is another name for a thrombocyte?

_____

56. What is a megakaryocyte?

_____

57. What is the normal range for a platelet count?

_____

58. What is the function of thrombocytes?

_____

59. What is the term for the stoppage of bleeding?

_____

60. What is the function of serotonin secreted by platelets when a blood vessel is torn or cut?

_____

_____

61. What is the function of a platelet plug?

_____

62. What are procoagulants?

_____

63. How does blood stay in a liquid form in the blood vessels?

_____

_____

64. What is necessary to convert inactive prothrombin to active thrombin?

_____

65. What is the function of thrombin?

_____

66. Why does a blood clot retract after it forms?

_____

_____

67. What antigens and antibodies occur with each of the following blood types?

Blood Type	Blood Antigens	Blood Antibodies
Type A		
Type B		
Type AB		
Type O		

68. What does it mean if someone is Rh positive? What does it mean if they are Rh negative?

_____

_____

69. What is the function of arteries?

_____

70. What are the three layers that make up the wall of an artery?

_____

71. What makes up the wall of a capillary?

_____

72. What is the function of veins?

_____

73. Why can veins hold more blood than arteries?

_____

74. What is the function of venous valves?

_____

_____

75. What is the function of the pulmonary circuit?

_____

_____

76. What is the function of the systemic circuit?

_____

_____

CRITICAL THINKING ACTIVITIES

A. BODY SPECTRUM CD ACTIVITY
   Circulatory: Heart—Cross Section
   Body Spectrum Directions:
   1. Access your Body Spectrum program (CD included with your textbook).
   2. Go to the Contents screen.
   3. Access the HELP screen for directions on using the Body Spectrum program.
   4. Select the following category from the Contents screen:
      Circulatory
   5. Select the following anatomic diagram:
      Heart—Cross Section
   6. Identify the structures on the diagram.
   7. Print out the diagram.

B. BODY SPECTRUM CD ACTIVITY
   Circulatory: Heart Circulation
   Directions: Identify the structures on this diagram following the Body Spectrum Directions outlined under CTA A.

C. BODY SPECTRUM CD ACTIVITY
   Circulatory: Coronary Vessels
   Directions: Identify the structures on this diagram following the Body Spectrum Directions outlined under CTA A.

D. CD ACTIVITY: NAME THAT BLOOD CELL
   Access your Companion CD (included with your textbook) to complete this activity. Record your points earned on your assignment sheet.

E. BLOOD CLOTTING
   You are a blood vessel located in the finger of a human. Your human is cutting up vegetables and accidentally severs you with a knife. Describe what tasks are performed to heal you during each of the hemostatic processes listed below.

   a. Vascular constriction:

   _____

   _____

   _____

   _____

   _____

   _____

   _____

b. Platelet plug formation:

_____

_____

_____

_____

_____

_____

_____

c. Coagulation:

_____

_____

_____

_____

_____

_____

_____

F. ARTERY

Using Figure 12-15 in your textbook as a reference, label each of the parts of an artery on the following diagram.

ARTERY

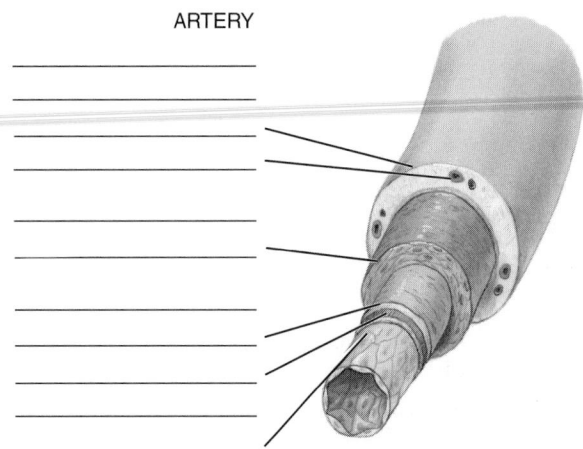

(Modified from Applegate E: *The anatomy and physiology learning system,* ed 3, St. Louis, 2006, Saunders.)

G. INQUIRING PATIENTS WANT TO KNOW

You are working in a general practice medical office. Your patients ask you the following questions. In the space provided, indicate how you would respond to each question in terms the patient would understand. Use your textbook and Internet resources to develop your responses.

1. Why is blood red?

   _____

   _____

2. Why does a bruise eventually turn yellow?

   _____

   _____

3. What causes varicose veins?

   _____

   _____

4. What is the difference between iron-deficiency anemia and pernicious anemia?

   _____

   _____

5. How does a pacemaker work?

   _____

   _____

6. What happens in the body during carbon monoxide poisoning?

   _____

   _____

7. What is done with the plasma that is collected at plasma donor centers?

   _____

   _____

8. What happens to the heart when it is defibrillated?

   _____

   _____

9. How can poor circulation cause gangrene?

   _____

   _____

10. Why does the physician look at the blood vessels in my eye?

   _____

   _____

H. CHAPTER 12 ANIMATIONS CD ACTIVITY

Directions:

1. View the Chapter 12 Animations on your Companion CD (included with your textbook).

2. For each animation, write two true/false questions in the space provided below.

3. In the classroom, find a partner.

4. For each animation, read your two questions to your partner.

5. For each correct answer, your partner is awarded two points.

6. Next, have your partner read his/her two questions to you. Award yourself two points for each question answered correctly.

7. Continue in this manner until all the questions have been answered.

8. Record your points on your Study Guide Assignment sheet.

True/False Questions

a. Location of the Heart

1. _____

2. _____

b. Chambers of the Heart

1. _____

2. _____

c. Heart Valves and Sounds

1. _____

2. _____

d. Conduction of Heart Impulses

1. _____

2. _____

e. The Cardiac Cycle

1. _____

2. _____

f. Red Blood Cells

1. _____

2. _____

g. White Blood Cells

1. _____

2. _____

h. Phagocytes

1. _____

2. _____

i. Platelets and Blood Clotting

1. _____

2. _____

j. Blood Grouping

1. _____

2. _____

k. Rh Compatibility

1. _____

2. _____

l. Pulmonary Circulation

    1. _____

    2. _____

m. Systemic Circulation

    1. _____

    2. _____

n. Physiology of Blood Pressure

    1. _____

    2. _____

I. CROSSWORD PUZZLE
Circulatory System
Directions: Complete the crossword puzzle using the clues presented below.

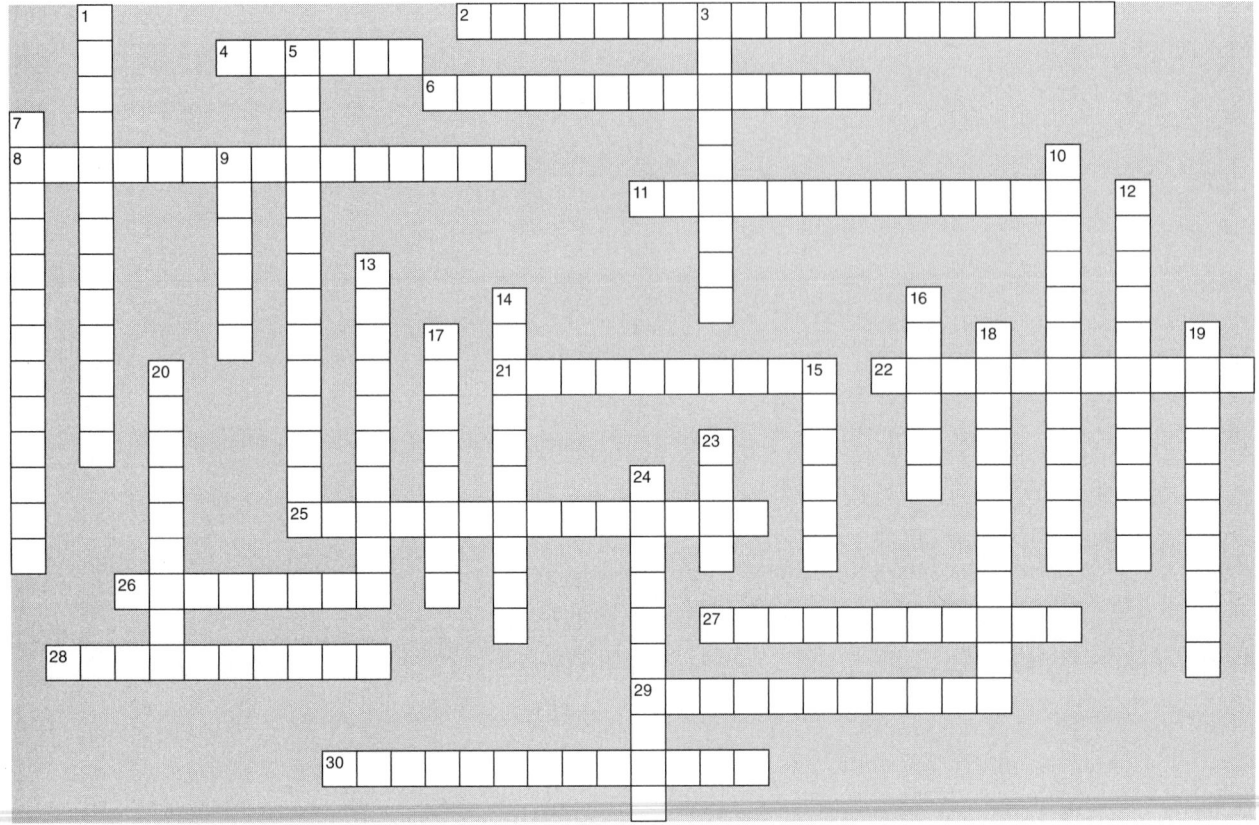

ACROSS
2 Also known as the epicardium
4 Carries blood away from heart
6 Inhibits clotting
8 Needed for absorption of vitamin B_{12}
11 Between left atrium and left ventricle
21 Forms bulk of heart wall
22 Tiny blood vessels
25 Stimulates RBC production
26 Largest WBC
27 Inner lining of heart wall
28 Receives oxygenated blood
29 Sac that encloses the heart
30 Chamber that pumps blood to entire body

DOWN
1 Production of blood cells
3 White blood cell
5 Between right atrium and right ventricle
7 Shape of RBC
9 Pacemaker of the heart
10 Immature erythrocyte
12 Red blood cell
13 Produces antibodies
14 Transports oxygen
15 Abnormal heart sound
16 Liquid part of blood
17 Secretes histamine and heparin
18 Receives deoxygenated blood
19 Stoppage of bleeding
20 Consists of white blood cells and platelets
23 Carries blood toward heart
24 Engulfs bacteria by phagocytosis

13

Respiratory System

CHAPTER ASSIGNMENTS

√ After Completing	Date Due	Textbook Page(s)	TEXTBOOK ASSIGNMENT	Possible Points	Points You Earned
		216-224	Read Chapter 13: Respiratory System		
√ After Completing	Date Due	Study Guide Page(s)	STUDY GUIDE ASSIGNMENTS (CTA: Critical Thinking Activity)		
		163	📄 Pretest	10	
		164	🔑 Key Term Assessment	7	
		165-167	📋 Evaluation of Learning questions	33	
		167	💿 CTA A: Body Spectrum CD Activity: Respiratory System	10	
		168	💿 CTA B: Body Spectrum CD Activity: Nasal Cavity and Pharynx	10	
		168	💿 CTA C: Body Spectrum CD Activity: Larynx and Upper Trachea	10	
		168	CTA D: Inquiring Patients Want to Know	10	
		169	💿 CTA E: Chapter 13 Animations CD Activity	32	
		170	CTA F: Crossword Puzzle	24	
		163	📄 Posttest	10	
			ADDITIONAL ASSIGNMENTS		
			TOTAL POINTS		

Notes

Name _____   Date _____

True or False

_____   1. The lungs are located in the lower respiratory tract.

_____   2. The function of mucus in the respiratory tract is to destroy microorganisms.

_____   3. The nasal septum divides the nose into two parts.

_____   4. The eustachian tubes open into the oropharynx.

_____   5. The uvula is the posterior portion of the soft palate that helps direct food into the oropharynx.

_____   6. The glottis prevents food and water from entering the trachea.

_____   7. The vocal cords are made up of ligaments.

_____   8. The right lung is divided into two lobes.

_____   9. The process of taking air into the lungs is known as *inhalation*.

_____   10. Sneezing is a nonrespiratory air movement.

? POSTTEST

True or False

_____   1. The exchange of gases between the blood and tissue cells is known as *external respiration*.

_____   2. The paranasal sinuses are lined by a serous membrane.

_____   3. Cilia propel mucus toward the pharynx.

_____   4. The nasal conchae separate the nasal cavity from the oral cavity.

_____   5. The oropharynx receives air, food, and water from the oral cavity.

_____   6. The thyroid cartilage located in the larynx is commonly called the *Adam's apple*.

_____   7. The larynx is supported by 15 to 20 C-shaped pieces of hyaline cartilage.

_____   8. The pleura is a double-layered serous membrane that encloses the lungs.

_____   9. The diaphragm consists of muscle.

_____   10. The respiratory center is located in the hypothalamus.

✎Term KEY TERM ASSESSMENT

Directions: Match each medical term with its definition.

_____ 1. Alveoli

_____ 2. Bronchial tree

_____ 3. External respiration

_____ 4. Internal respiration

_____ 5. Respiratory membrane

_____ 6. Surfactant

_____ 7. Ventilation

A. A substance, produced by certain cells in lung tissue, that reduces surface tension between fluid molecules that line the respiratory membrane and helps keep the alveolus from collapsing

B. Any surface in the lungs where diffusion occurs; consists of the layers that the gases must pass through to get into or out of the alveoli

C. Exchange of gases between the blood and tissue cells

D. Exchange of gases between the lungs and the blood

E. Microscopic dilations of terminal bronchioles in the lungs, where diffusion of gases occurs

F. Movement of air into and out of the lungs; breathing

G. The bronchi and all their branches that function as passageways between the trachea and the alveoli

EVALUATION OF LEARNING

Directions: Fill in each blank with the correct answer.

1. What are the functions of the respiratory system?

   _____

   _____

2. What is external respiration?

   _____

3. What is internal respiration?

   _____

4. What structures are located in the upper respiratory tract?

   _____

5. What structures are located in the lower respiratory tract?

   _____

6. Describe the following parts of the nose:

   a. Nasal cavity: _____

   b. Nasal septum: _____

   c. Nostrils: _____

   d. Internal nares: _____

   e. Palate: _____

   f. Uvula: _____

7. What is the difference between the hard palate and soft palate?

   _____

   _____

8. What are the functions of the nasal conchae?

   _____

   _____

9. What are the paranasal sinuses?

   _____

   _____

10. What are three functions of the paranasal sinuses?

   _____

   _____

11. What is the function of the mucus secreted by the mucous membrane of the nose?

   _____

12. What is the function of the cilia in the nasal cavity?

_____

_____

13. What is the nasopharynx?

_____

_____

14. What is the function of the eustachian tubes?

_____

_____

15. What is the oropharynx?

_____

_____

16. What is the laryngopharynx?

_____

17. What is the layman's term for the thyroid cartilage?

_____

18. What is the function of the epiglottis?

_____

_____

19. What are the functions of the following?

    a. False vocal cords: _____

    b. True vocal cords: _____

20. What is the glottis?

_____

21. What holds the trachea open?

_____

22. Describe the components of the bronchial tree.

_____

_____

_____

23. Why do the walls of the alveolar ducts and alveoli consist of simple squamous epithelium?

_____

24. Why are the lungs soft and spongy?

_____

_____

25. How does the right lung differ in appearance from the left lung?

_____

_____

26. What is the pleura?

_____

_____

27. What is another name for breathing?

_____

28. What is the diaphragm?

_____

29. How does air move into the lungs during inhalation?

_____

_____

30. How does air move out of the lungs during exhalation?

_____

_____

31. Where is the respiratory center located?

_____

32. What happens if there is an increase in carbon dioxide in the blood?

_____

_____

33. What are examples of nonrespiratory air movements?

_____

_____

CRITICAL THINKING ACTIVITIES

A. BODY SPECTRUM CD ACTIVITY
   Respiratory: Respiratory System
   Body Spectrum Directions:
   1. Access your Body Spectrum program (CD included with your textbook).
   2. Go to the Contents screen.
   3. Access the HELP screen for directions on using the Body Spectrum program.
   4. Select the following category from the Contents screen:
      Respiratory
   5. Select the following anatomic diagram:
      Respiratory System
   6. Identify the structures on the diagram.
   7. Print out the diagram.

B. BODY SPECTRUM CD ACTIVITY
   Respiratory: Nasal Cavity and Pharynx
   Directions: Identify the structures on this diagram following the Body Spectrum Directions outlined under CTA A.

C. BODY SPECTRUM CD ACTIVITY
   Respiratory: Larynx and Upper Trachea
   Directions: Identify the structures on this diagram following the Body Spectrum Directions outlined under CTA A.

D. INQUIRING PATIENTS WANT TO KNOW
   You are working in a general practice medical office. Your patients ask you the following questions. In the space provided, indicate how you would respond to each question in terms the patient would understand. Use your textbook and Internet resources to develop your responses.

   1. What happens in the body when you sneeze?

      _____

      _____

   2. Why do men have a deeper voice than women?

      _____

      _____

   3. What do your tonsils do?

      _____

      _____

   4. What damage does smoking do to the respiratory tract?

      _____

      _____

   5. What do sinuses do?

      _____

      _____

   6. Can you die from holding your breath?

      _____

      _____

   7. What makes you yawn when someone else yawns?

      _____

      _____

   8. Is it bad for you if you're drinking water and it goes down the wrong tube?

      _____

      _____

   9. Why does your nose run when you have allergies?

      _____

      _____

   10. Can you permanently lose your voice from laryngitis?

      _____

      _____

E. CHAPTER 13 ANIMATIONS CD ACTIVITY
Directions:

1. View the Chapter 13 Animations on your Companion CD (included with your textbook).
2. For each animation, write two true/false questions in the space provided below.
3. In the classroom, find a partner.
4. For each animation, read your two questions to your partner.
5. For each correct answer, your partner is awarded two points.
6. Next, have your partner read his/her two questions to you. Award yourself two points for each question answered correctly.
7. Continue in this manner until all the questions have been answered.
8. Record your points on your Study Guide Assignment sheet.

True/False Questions

a.   Air Distribution through the Upper Respiratory Tract

   1. _____
   2. _____

b.   Air Distribution through the Lower Respiratory Tract

   1. _____
   2. _____

c.   Respiratory Mucosa

   1. _____
   2. _____

d.   Bronchi and Bronchioles

   1. _____
   2. _____

e.   Respiration

   1. _____
   2. _____

f,   External Respiration

   1. _____
   2. _____

g.   Respiratory Membrane

   1. _____
   2. _____

h.   Internal Respiration

   1. _____
   2. _____

F. CROSSWORD PUZZLE
Respiratory System
Directions: Complete the crossword puzzle using the clues presented below.

ACROSS
1 Exchange of gases between tissues and blood
7 Respiratory center
8 Bony ridges that warm air
9 Equalizes air pressure
11 Separates nasal cavity from oral cavity
12 Expelling air from the lungs
14 Windpipe
15 Air-filled cavity in skull
16 Throat
18 Opening between oral cavity and oropharynx
19 Separates thoracic and abdominal cavities
20 Voice box
21 Adam's apple
22 Produces sound
23 Membrane around the lungs

DOWN
2 Prevents food from entering trachea
3 Has three lobes
4 Divides nose into two parts
5 Nonrespiratory air movement
6 Whooping cough
10 Contains serous fluid produced by the pleura
13 Inflammation of the vocal cords
17 Tiny air sacs

14

Digestive System

CHAPTER ASSIGNMENTS

√ After Completing	Date Due	Textbook Page(s)	TEXTBOOK ASSIGNMENT	Possible Points	Points You Earned
		225-241	Read Chapter 14: Digestive System		
√ After Completing	Date Due	Study Guide Page(s)	STUDY GUIDE ASSIGNMENTS (CTA: Critical Thinking Activity)		
		173	🔲 Pretest	10	
		174	🎤 Key Term Assessment	6	
		175-180	📋 Evaluation of Learning questions	66	
		180	•CD• CTA A: Body Spectrum CD Activity: Digestive System	10	
		180	•CD• CTA B: Body Spectrum CD Activity: Teeth	10	
		181	CTA C: Structure of a Tooth	11	
		181	•CD• CTA D: Body Spectrum CD Activity: Salivary Glands	10	
		181	•CD• CTA E: Body Spectrum CD Activity: Anatomy of Large Intestine	10	
		181	•CD• CTA F: Body Spectrum CD Activity: Intestinal Secretion Sources	10	
		181-182	CTA G: Pizza Digestion	20	
		182-183	CTA H: Inquiring Patients Want to Know	10	
		183	•CD• CTA I: Chapter 14 Animations CD Activity	16	
		184	CTA J: Crossword Puzzle	38	

√ After Completing	Date Due	Study Guide Page(s)	STUDY GUIDE ASSIGNMENTS (CTA: Critical Thinking Activity)		
		173	📄 Posttest	10	
			ADDITIONAL ASSIGNMENTS		
			TOTAL POINTS		

Name _____   Date _____

PRETEST

True or False

_____   1. The pancreas is an accessory organ of the digestive system.

_____   2. Peristalsis consists of rhythmic waves of contractions that propel food particles through the digestive tract.

_____   3. The buccinator muscle connects the tongue anteriorly to the floor of the mouth.

_____   4. The total number of primary teeth is 32.

_____   5. Saliva moistens and lubricates the food.

_____   6. The esophagus provides a passageway for food between the pharynx and stomach.

_____   7. The first part of the small intestine is the duodenum.

_____   8. Hepatocytes are liver cells.

_____   9. Iron is stored in the liver.

_____   10. The function of the gallbladder is to produce bile.

POSTTEST

True or False

_____   1. The taking in of food is known as *mastication*.

_____   2. Mechanical digestion breaks down food into smaller particles through the mixing actions of the stomach.

_____   3. The hard palate and uvula direct food away from the nasal cavity and into the oropharynx during swallowing.

_____   4. Cuspids are teeth that have sharp edges used for biting food.

_____   5. The cardiac sphincter acts as a valve between the stomach and small intestine.

_____   6. The intrinsic factor aids in the absorption of vitamin B_{12} from the digestive tract.

_____   7. Chyme is a semifluid that results when food is broken down in the stomach.

_____   8. The large intestine functions in the absorption of nutrients.

_____   9. Bile emulsifies fat into small fat droplets.

_____   10. The end product of protein digestion is glucose.

✎ Term KEY TERM ASSESSMENT

Directions: Match each medical term with its definition.

_____ 1. Absorption

_____ 2. Chyme

_____ 3. Mesentery

_____ 4. Peristalsis

_____ 5. Plicae circulares

_____ 6. Rugae

A. Circular folds in the mucosa and submucosa of the small intestine
B. Extensions of peritoneum that are associated with the intestine
C. Longitudinal folds in the mucosa of the stomach
D. Rhythmic contractions of the intestine that move food along the digestive tract
E. The passage of digestive end products from the gastrointestinal tract into the blood or lymph
F. The semifluid mixture of food and gastric juice that leaves the stomach through the pyloric sphincter

EVALUATION OF LEARNING

Directions: Fill in each blank with the correct answer.

1. What are two other names for the digestive tract?

   _____

2. What structures make up the digestive tract?

   _____

   _____

3. What are the accessory organs of digestion?

   _____

   _____

4. What is ingestion?

   _____

5. What occurs during mechanical digestion?

   _____

   _____

6. What occurs during chemical digestion?

   _____

   _____

7. What is deglutition?

   _____

8. What is peristalsis?

   _____

   _____

9. What are the four layers of the digestive tract?

   _____

10. What tissues make up the lips?

   _____

11. What muscle makes up the cheeks?

   _____

12. Describe the difference between the hard palate and soft palate.

   _____

   _____

   _____

13. What is the function of the uvula?

_____

_____

14. What is the frenulum linguae?

_____

15. What are two functions of the papillae located on the tongue?

_____

_____

16. What is the function of the lingual tonsils?

_____

17. What is the function of the tongue?

_____

_____

18. How many teeth make up the following?

    a. Primary teeth: _____

    b. Secondary teeth: _____

19. What are the functions of the following teeth?

    a. Incisors: _____

    b. Cuspids: _____

    c. Bicuspids and molars: _____

20. Describe the following three main parts of a tooth:

    a. Crown: _____

    b. Root: _____

    c. Neck: _____

21. Describe the following structures that make up a tooth:

    a. Pulp cavity: _____

    b. Pulp: _____

    c. Root canal: _____

    d. Apical foramen: _____

    e. Dentin: _____

    f. Cementum: _____

    g. Periodontal ligaments: _____

    h. Enamel: _____

22. What are the names and locations of the three salivary glands?

Name	Location

23. What is the function of saliva?

_____

_____

_____

24. What are the three regions of the pharynx?

_____

25. What is the function of the esophagus?

_____

26. What is the function of the esophageal sphincter?

_____

27. Describe the following structures that make up the stomach:

    a. Cardiac region: _____

    b. Fundus: _____

    c. Body: _____

    d. Lesser curvature: _____

    e. Greater curvature: _____

    f. Pyloric region: _____

    g. Pyloric sphincter: _____

28. What are rugae, and what is their function?

_____

_____

29. Indicate the type of gastric gland cells that produce the following gastric secretions and the function of each secretion.

Gastric Gland Secretion	Secreted by	Function
a. Thick and alkaline mucus		
b. Thin and watery mucus		
c. Hydrochloric acid		
d. Intrinsic factor		
e. Pepsinogen		

30. What is the function of pepsin?

   _____

31. How is inactive pepsinogen converted to active pepsin?

   _____

32. What is chyme?

   _____

33. What causes gastric juice to be released during the cephalic phase?

   _____

34. What causes gastric juice to be released during the gastric phase?

   _____

35. What triggers the intestinal phase of gastric secretion regulation?

   _____

36. What is the function of the small intestine?

   _____

   _____

37. What is the function of the plicae circulares?

   _____

38. Describe the appearance of the villi. What is the function of villi?

   _____

   _____

39. What are the three regions of the small intestine?

   _____

40. What is the function of the mesentery?

   _____

41. What are the functions of the following enzymes?
   a. Peptidase: _____
   b. Maltase, sucrose, and lactase: _____
   c. Intestinal lipase: _____

42. What is the ileocecal junction?

   _____

43. What are the four regions of the large intestine?

   _____

44. What are the four parts of the colon?

   _____

   _____

45. What is the function of the large intestine?

_____

_____

46. What is the function of the mucus secreted by the large intestine?

_____

_____

47. What is the function of the falciform ligament of the liver?

_____

_____

48. What are hepatocytes?

_____

49. What substances are stored in the liver?

_____

_____

50. What is the function of Kupffer cells?

_____

_____

51. What makes up bile?

_____

52. What are the functions of bile salts?

_____

_____

53. How are bile pigments produced?

_____

_____

54. What is the name of the principal bile pigment?

_____

55. What is the function of the gallbladder?

_____

56. What causes the release of cholecystokinin?

_____

57. What is the function of cholecystokinin?

_____

_____

58. What is the function of the islets of Langerhans?

_____

59. What is the function of pancreatic acinar cells?

_____

_____

60. What is the function of the pancreatic duct?

_____

_____

61. What digestive enzymes are found in pancreatic juice?

_____

62. What effect does cholecystokinin have on the pancreas?

_____

_____

63. What are the end products of carbohydrate digestion?

_____

64. What are the end products of protein digestion?

_____

65. What are the end products of lipid digestion?

_____

66. In what part of the small intestine does most absorption take place?

_____

CRITICAL THINKING ACTIVITES

A. BODY SPECTRUM CD ACTIVITY
   Digestive: Digestive System
   Body Spectrum Directions:
   1. Access your Body Spectrum program (CD included with your textbook).
   2. Go to the Contents screen.
   3. Access the HELP screen for directions on using the Body Spectrum program.
   4. Select the following category from the Contents screen:
      Digestive
   5. Select the following anatomic diagram:
      Digestive System
   6. Identify the structures on the diagram.
   7. Print out the diagram.

B. BODY SPECTRUM CD ACTIVITY
   Digestive: Teeth
   Directions: Identify the structures on this diagram following the Body Spectrum Directions outlined under CTA A.

C. STRUCTURE OF A TOOTH

Using Figure 14-5 in your textbook as a reference, label each of the structures of a tooth on the following diagram.

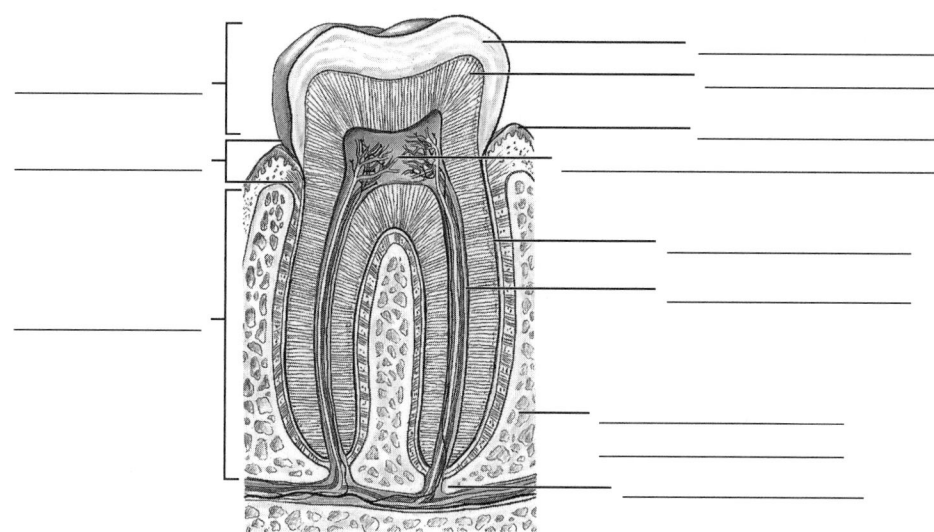

(Modified from Applegate E: *The anatomy and physiology learning system,* ed 3, St. Louis, 2006, Saunders.)

D. BODY SPECTRUM CD ACTIVITY
Digestive: Salivary Glands
Directions: Identify the structures on this diagram following the Body Spectrum Directions outlined under CTA A.

E. BODY SPECTRUM CD ACTIVITY
Digestive: Anatomy of Large Intestine
Directions: Identify the structures on this diagram following the Body Spectrum Directions outlined under CTA A.

F. BODY SPECTRUM CD ACTIVITY
Digestive: Intestinal Secretion Sources
Directions: Identify the structures on this diagram following the Body Spectrum Directions outlined under CTA A.

G. PIZZA DIGESTION

You are a slice of pizza that has just been eaten by a human. Starting at the mouth, describe what you will go through during the digestive process.

_____

_____

_____

_____

_____

_____

_____

_____

_____

_____

_____

_____

_____

_____

_____

_____

_____

_____

_____

_____

_____

_____

_____

H. INQUIRING PATIENTS WANT TO KNOW

You are working in a general practice medical office. Your patients ask you the following questions. In the space provided, indicate how you would respond to each question in terms the patient would understand. Use your textbook and Internet resources to develop your responses.

1. What is a cleft palate?

   _____

   _____

2. What causes cavities?

   _____

   _____

3. How does fluoride make your teeth stronger?

   _____

   _____

4. What causes heartburn?

   _____

   _____

5. What causes vomiting?

   _____

   _____

6. What causes someone to be lactose intolerant?

   _____

   _____

7. What is an ulcer?

   _____

   _____

8. What causes a hiatal hernia?

   _____

   _____

9. What causes gallstones?

   _____

   _____

10. How does drinking cause cirrhosis of the liver?

_____

_____

I. CHAPTER 14 ANIMATIONS CD ACTIVITY
   Directions:
   1. View the Chapter 14 Animations on your Companion CD (included with your textbook).
   2. For each animation, write two true/false questions in the space provided below.
   3. In the classroom, find a partner.
   4. For each animation, read your two questions to your partner.
   5. For each correct answer, your partner is awarded two points.
   6. Next, have your partner read his/her two questions to you. Award yourself two points for each question answered correctly.
   7. Continue in this manner until all the questions have been answered.
   8. Record your points on your Study Guide Assignment sheet.

   True/False Questions
   a. Esophagus

      1. _____

      2. _____

   b. Stomach

      1. _____

      2. _____

   c. Small Intestine

      1. _____

      2. _____

   d. Large Intestine

      1. _____

      2. _____

J. CROSSWORD PUZZLE
Digestive System
Directions: Complete the crossword puzzle using the clues presented below.

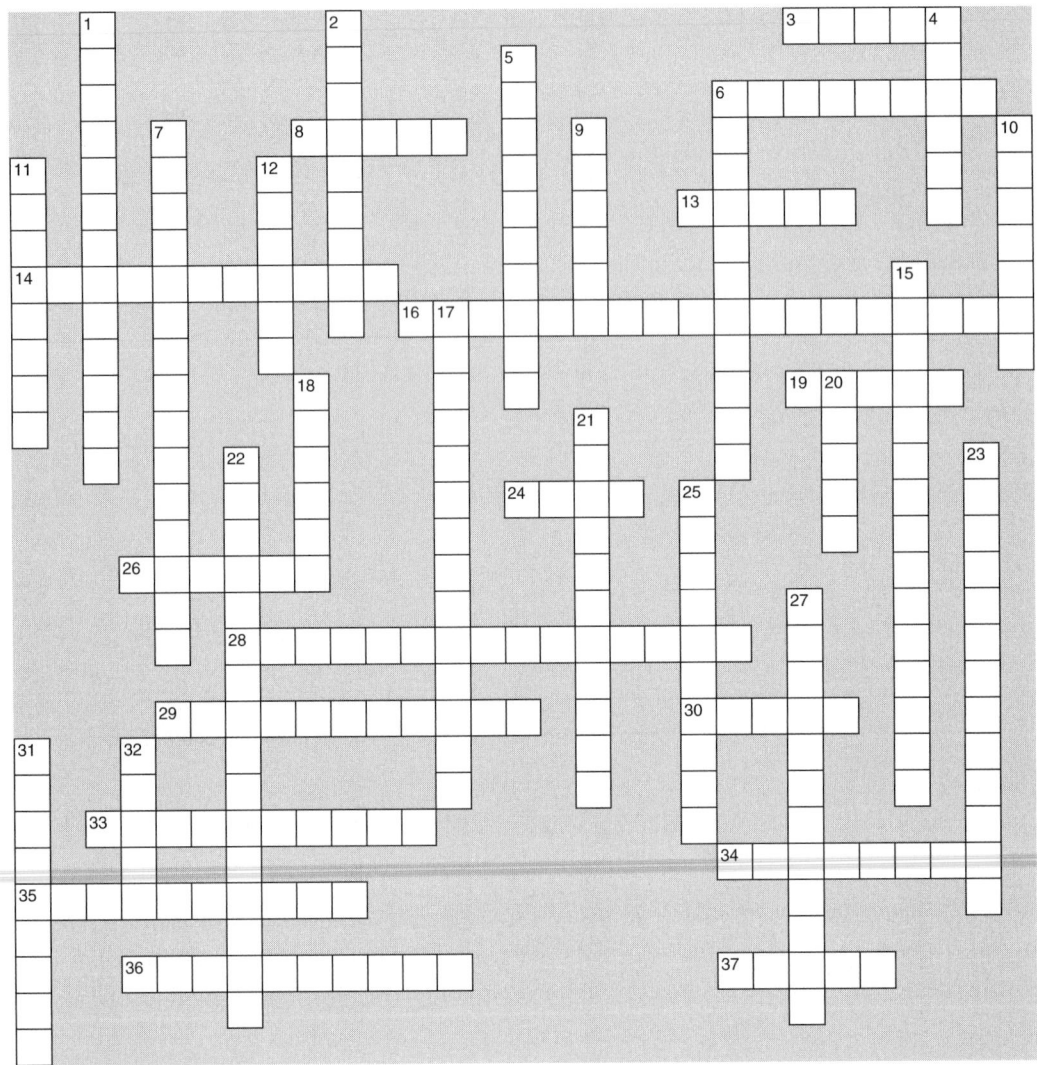

ACROSS

3 Allow stomach to expand
6 Tongue projections that contain taste buds
8 Blind pouch in large intestine
13 Produces and secretes bile
14 Swallowing
16 Secrete insulin and glucagon
19 Increase surface area for food absorption
24 Part of tooth that contains nerves and blood vessels
26 Innermost layer of GI tract
28 Aids in absorption of vitamin B_{12}
29 Chewing
30 Semifluid mixture of food and gastric juice
33 Cheek muscle
34 Teeth used to bite food
35 Liver cell
36 Removal of wastes through anus
37 Visible part of the tooth

DOWN

1 Largest salivary glands
2 Taking in of food
4 Hardest substance in the body
5 Length of GI tract
6 Propels food through GI tract
7 Connects tongue to floor of mouth
9 Teeth used to crush and grind food
10 End product of carbohydrate digestion
11 First part of small intestine
12 Forms bulk of tooth
15 Causes gallbladder to contract
17 Most food absorption occurs here
18 Moistens and lubricates food
20 Last part of small intestine
21 Stores bile
22 Valve between stomach and small intestine
23 Triggered by seeing and smelling food
25 End products of protein digestion
27 S-shaped curve of large intestine
31 Food tube
32 Soft palate projection

15

Urinary System

CHAPTER ASSIGNMENTS

√ After Completing	Date Due	Textbook Page(s)	TEXTBOOK ASSIGNMENT	Possible Points	Points You Earned
		245-250	Read Chapter 15: Urinary System		
√ After Completing	Date Due	Study Guide Page(s)	STUDY GUIDE ASSIGNMENTS (CTA: Critical Thinking Activity)		
		187	📝 Pretest	10	
		188	🔑 Key Term Assessment	4	
		189-191	📋 Evaluation of Learning questions	40	
		192	💿 CTA A: Body Spectrum CD Activity: Urinary Tract	10	
		192	💿 CTA B: Body Spectrum CD Activity: Kidney	10	
		192	CTA C: Nephron	9	
		193	CTA D: Inquiring Patients Want to Know	10	
		193-194	💿 CTA E: Chapter 15 Animations CD Activity	8	
		195	CTA F: Crossword Puzzle	31	
		187	📝 Posttest	10	
			ADDITIONAL ASSIGNMENTS		
			TOTAL POINTS		

Notes

Name _____   Date _____

? PRETEST

True or False

_____   1. The functional unit of the kidney is the nephron.

_____   2. The outer portion of the kidney is known as the *renal medulla*.

_____   3. The indentation in the kidney is known as the *hilum*.

_____   4. The glomerulus is made up of loose connective tissue.

_____   5. The double-layered epithelial cup that surrounds the glomerulus is Bowman's capsule.

_____   6. The ureters transport urine from the urinary bladder to the outside.

_____   7. Rugae located in the wall of the urinary bladder allow the bladder to expand.

_____   8. The urethra in a male functions only in the transport of urine.

_____   9. Glucose is reabsorbed into the body in the renal tubule.

_____ 10. Micturition is the act of expelling urine.

? POSTTEST

True or False

_____   1. The urinary system helps to regulate the blood pressure.

_____   2. The renal pelvis collects urine as it is produced.

_____   3. The nephron is made up of the glomerulus and Bowman's capsule.

_____   4. Blood enters the glomerulus through the efferent arteriole.

_____   5. The renal tubule carries fluid away from the glomerular capsule toward a collecting duct.

_____   6. Urine is expelled from the urinary bladder through contraction of the detrusor muscle.

_____   7. The calyx is made up of three openings and is located in the floor of the urinary bladder.

_____   8. The urethral orifice controls the passage of urine through the urethra.

_____   9. Erythropoietin increases reabsorption of sodium and reduces urine output.

_____ 10. In the absence of ADH, the urine is more dilute.

KEY TERM ASSESSMENT

Directions: Match each medical term with its definition.

_____ 1. Glomerular capsule

_____ 2. Juxtaglomerular apparatus

_____ 3. Nephron

_____ 4. Renal tubule

A. Complex of modified cells in the afferent arteriole and the ascending limb/distal tubule in the kidney; helps regulate blood pressure by secreting renin; consists of the macula densa and juxtaglomerular cells

B. Double-layered epithelial cup that surrounds the glomerulus in a nephron; also called *Bowman's capsule*

C. Functional unit of the kidney consisting of a renal corpuscle and a renal tubule

D. Tubular portion of the nephron that carries the filtrate away from the glomerular capsule; site where tubular reabsorption and secretion occur

EVALUATION OF LEARNING

Directions: Fill in each blank with the correct answer.

1. What are the functions of the urinary system?

   _____

   _____

2. What are the functions of the kidneys?

   _____

   _____

3. What is renal fascia, and what is its function?

   _____

   _____

4. What is the renal capsule, and what is its function?

   _____

   _____

5. Describe each of the following parts of the kidney:

   a. Hilum: _____

   b. Renal sinus: _____

   c. Renal cortex: _____

6. What makes up the renal medulla?

   _____

7. What do renal pyramids contain?

   _____

8. What are renal columns?

   _____

   _____

9. What is the function of the renal pelvis?

   _____

10. What is the function of a minor calyx?

    _____

11. What is a nephron?

    _____

12. What are the two parts of a nephron?

    _____

13. What makes up the glomerulus?

_____

14. Describe Bowman's capsule.

_____

15. What is the name of the vessel that delivers blood to the glomerulus?

_____

16. What vessel carries blood away from the glomerulus?

_____

17. What is the function of the renal tubule?

_____

18. What are the three regions of a renal tubule?

_____

_____

19. What is the function of the ureters?

_____

20. Where do the ureters enter the urinary bladder?

_____

21. What is the function of the muscular layer of the ureter?

_____

22. What is the function of the urinary bladder?

_____

23. What is the function of the rugae located in the wall of the urinary bladder?

_____

24. What is the function of the detrusor muscle?

_____

25. What three openings are located in the trigone of the urinary bladder?

_____

_____

26. Where is the trigone located?

_____

27. What is the function of the urethra?

_____

28. What are the names of the sphincters that control the flow of urine through the urethra?

_____

29. What is the external urethral orifice?

   _____

30. What two functions are served by the urethra in the male?

   _____ _____

31. What are the three parts of the male urethra?

   _____

32. What are the three steps involved in the formation of urine?

   _____

   _____

33. What occurs during glomerular filtration?

   _____

   _____

34. What is tubular reabsorption?

   _____

   _____

35. What are examples of substances that are reabsorbed into the blood?

   _____

36. What is tubular secretion?

   _____

   _____

37. How do the following hormones influence urine concentration and volume?
   a. Aldosterone: _____

   _____

   b. Presence of antidiuretic hormone: _____

   _____

   c. Absence of antidiuretic hormone: _____

   _____

   d. Atrial natriuretic hormone: _____

   _____

38. What is the function of renin?

   _____

39. What is micturition?

   _____

40. What stimulates the micturition reflex?

   _____

   _____

CRITICAL THINKING ACTIVITIES

A. BODY SPECTRUM CD ACTIVITY
Urinary: Urinary Tract
Body Spectrum Directions:
1. Access your Body Spectrum program (CD included with your textbook).

2. Go to the Contents screen.

3. Access the HELP screen for directions on using the Body Spectrum program.

4. Select the following category from the Contents screen:

   Urinary

5. Select the following anatomic diagram:

   Urinary Tract

6. Identify the structures on the diagram.

7. Print out the diagram.

B. BODY SPECTRUM CD ACTIVITY
Urinary: Kidney
Directions: Identify the structures on this diagram following the Body Spectrum Directions outlined under CTA A.

C. NEPHRON
Using Figure 15-4 in your textbook as a reference, label each of the structures making up a nephron.

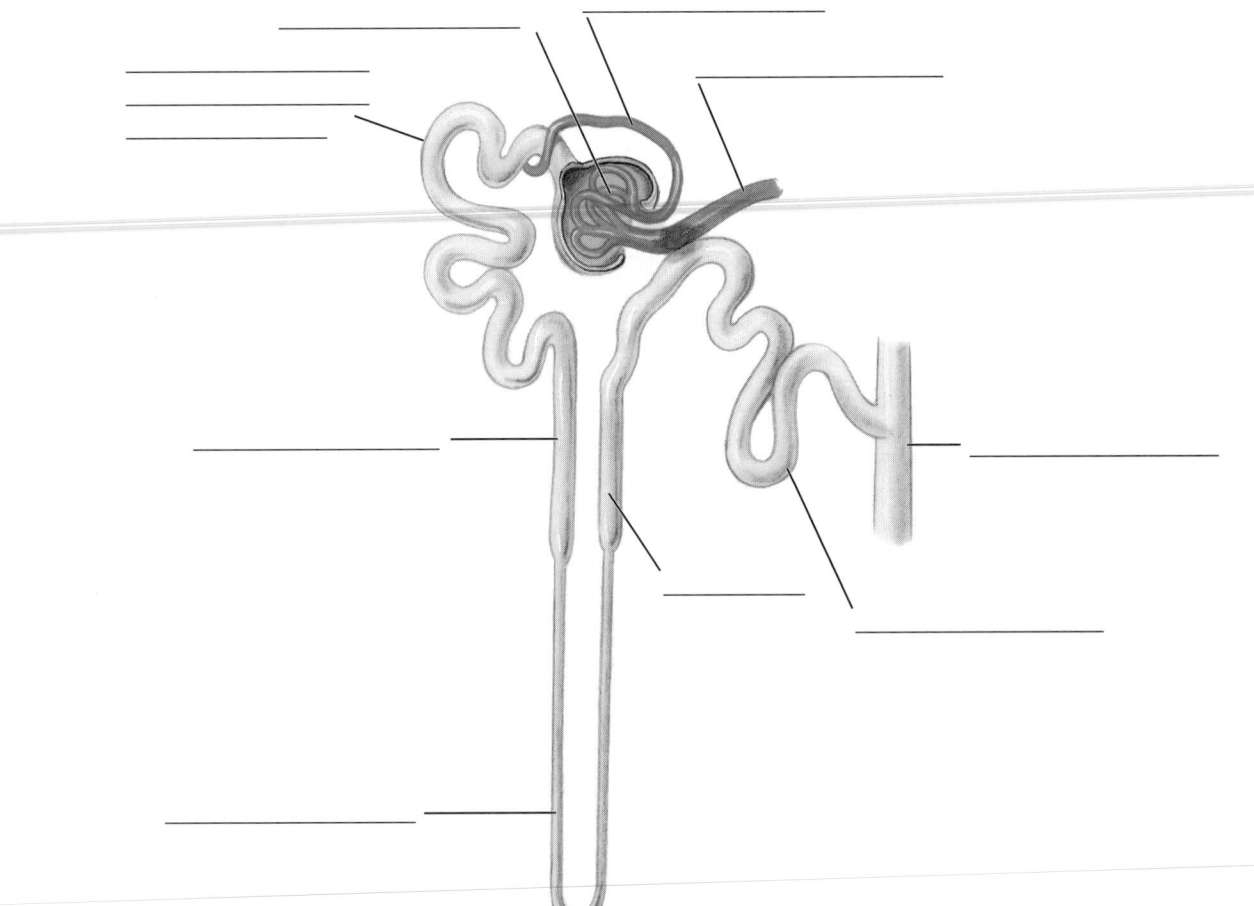

(Modified from Applegate E: *The anatomy and physiology learning system, ed 3,* St. Louis, 2006, Saunders.)

D. INQUIRING PATIENTS WANT TO KNOW

You are working in a general practice medical office. Your patients ask you the following questions. In the space provided, indicate how you would respond to each question in terms the patient would understand. Use your textbook and Internet resources to develop your responses.

1. Why is urine yellow?

    _____

    _____

2. Why do women have more urinary tract infections than men?

    _____

    _____

3. Is it safer to drink bottled water than tap water?

    _____

    _____

4. What causes kidney stones?

    _____

    _____

5. How are kidney stones removed?

    _____

    _____

6. Why is urine a darker yellow color in the morning?

    _____

    _____

7. What causes some older people to be incontinent?

    _____

    _____

8. Why should someone with a UTI drink cranberry juice?

    _____

    _____

9. What happens during kidney dialysis?

    _____

    _____

10. Do dialysis patients still urinate?

    _____

    _____

E. CHAPTER 15 ANIMATIONS CD ACTIVITY

Directions:

1. View the Chapter 15 Animations on your Companion CD (included with your textbook).
2. For each animation, write two true/false questions in the space provided below.
3. In the classroom, find a partner.
4. For each animation, read your two questions to your partner.
5. For each correct answer, your partner is awarded two points.

6. Next, have your partner read his/her two questions to you. Award yourself two points for each question answered correctly.

7. Continue in this manner until all the questions have been answered.

8. Record your points on your Study Guide Assignment sheet.

True/False Questions

a. The Kidneys

    1. _____

    2. _____

b. Aldosterone Regulation Mechanism

    1. _____

    2. _____

F. CROSSWORD PUZZLE
Urinary System
Directions: Complete the crossword puzzle using the clues presented below.

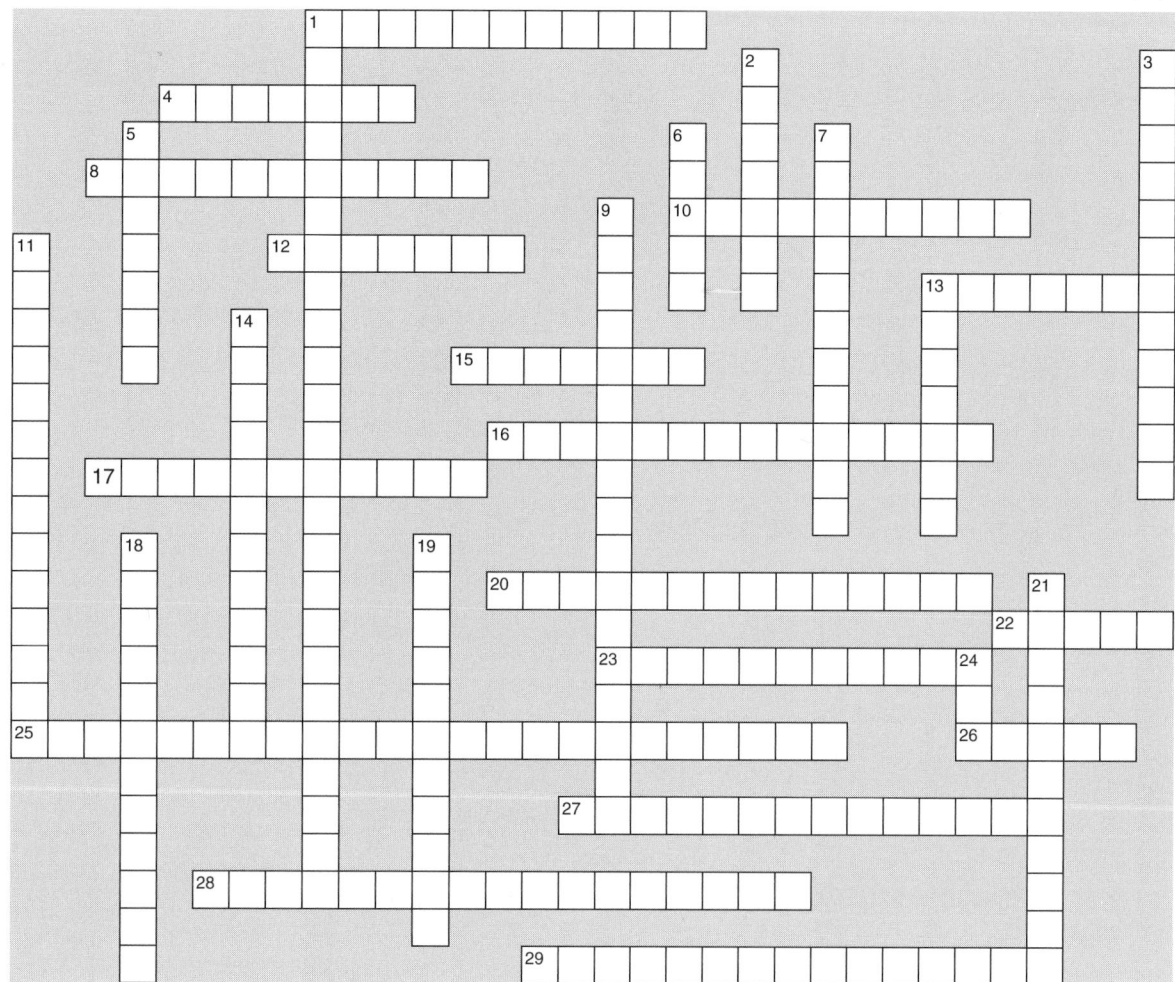

ACROSS

1 How urine moves through ureter
4 Formed by three openings in urinary bladder
8 Act of expelling urine
10 Cluster of capillaries in nephron
12 Cuplike projections of renal pelvis
13 Transports urine from urinary bladder to outside
15 Functional unit of kidney
16 Stores urine
17 Outer region of kidney
20 Controls RBC production
22 Helps maintain normal BP
23 Hold kidney in place
25 Opening of urethra
26 Kidney indentation
27 Expels urine from bladder by contracting
28 Takes blood to glomerulus
29 Transports urine from nephron to minor calyces

DOWN

1 Where most of tubular reabsorption occurs
2 Substance that is reabsorbed by kidney
3 Connective tissue that encases kidney
5 Filters blood and removes wastes
6 Allows bladder to expand
7 Urinary bladder capacity in milliliters
9 Takes blood away from glomerulus
11 Epithelial cup that surrounds glomerulus
13 Transports urine from renal pelvis to urinary bladder
14 Inner region of kidney
18 Adipose tissue surrounding kidney
19 Hormone that increases reabsorption of sodium
21 Collects urine
24 Hormone that increases reabsorption of water

16

Reproductive System

CHAPTER ASSIGNMENTS

√ After Completing	Date Due	Textbook Page(s)	TEXTBOOK ASSIGNMENT	Possible Points	Points You Earned
		251-265	Read Chapter 16: Reproductive System		
√ After Completing	Date Due	Study Guide Page(s)	STUDY GUIDE ASSIGNMENTS (CTA: Critical Thinking Activity)		
		199	📋 Pretest	10	
		200	✒Term Key Term Assessment	8	
		201-204 204-207	🗒 Evaluation of Learning questions: Male Reproductive System Female Reproductive System	44 38	
		207	💿 CTA A: Body Spectrum CD Activity: Male Reproductive System	10	
		207	💿 CTA B: Body Spectrum CD Activity: Female Reproductive System	10	
		207	💿 CTA C: Body Spectrum CD Activity: Fertilization to Implantation	10	
		208	CTA D: Inquiring Patients Want to Know	10	
		208-210	💿 CTA E: Chapter 16 Animations CD Activity	64	
		211	CTA F: Crossword Puzzle	35	
		199	📋 Posttest	10	

√ After Completing	Date Due	Study Guide Page(s)	STUDY GUIDE ASSIGNMENTS (CTA: Critical Thinking Activity)		
			ADDITIONAL ASSIGNMENTS		
			TOTAL POINTS		

Name _____   Date _____

[?] **PRETEST**

True or False

_____ 1. The gonads include egg and sperm cells.

_____ 2. The head of a sperm contains 46 chromosomes.

_____ 3. Sperm are propelled through the ductus deferens by peristalsis.

_____ 4. The prostate gland encircles the urethra.

_____ 5. The scrotum is a pouch of skin and subcutaneous tissue that contains the testes.

_____ 6. The process of egg formation is known as *oogenesis*.

_____ 7. Fertilization usually takes place in the uterus.

_____ 8. The bulk of the uterine wall is made up of the myometrium.

_____ 9. The endometrium is shed from the uterine wall during the secretory phase of the uterine cycle.

_____ 10. The cessation of the female reproductive cycle is known as *menarche*.

[?] **POSTTEST**

True or False

_____ 1. The interstitial cells in the testes produce male sex hormones.

_____ 2. Spermatogonia divide by mitosis.

_____ 3. The epididymis secretes a fluid containing fructose to provide an energy source for sperm.

_____ 4. Ejaculation is the forceful discharge of semen into the urethra.

_____ 5. The epididymis is a tightly coiled tube in which sperm complete the maturation process.

_____ 6. If fertilization does not take place, the corpus luteum continues to grow and enlarge.

_____ 7. Fimbriae help propel sperm through the uterus.

_____ 8. The growth of the ovarian follicle occurs during the follicular phase of the ovarian cycle.

_____ 9. In the female, LH is responsible for stimulating the growth and thickening of the endometrium.

_____ 10. The upper bulging surface of the uterus is the fundus.

⚷ Term KEY TERM ASSESSMENT

Directions: Match each medical term with its definition.

_____ 1. Gametes

_____ 2. Gonads

_____ 3. Oogenesis

_____ 4. Ovarian cycle

_____ 5. Ovarian follicle

_____ 6. Spermatogenesis

_____ 7. Spermiogenesis

_____ 8. Uterine cycle

A. An oocyte surrounded by one or more layers of cells within the ovaries

B. Monthly cycle of events that occur in the ovary from puberty to menopause; occurs concurrently with the uterine cycle

C. Monthly cycle of events that occur in the uterus from puberty to menopause; also called the _menstrual cycle;_ occurs concurrently with the ovarian cycle

D. Morphologic changes that transform a spermatid into a mature sperm

E. Primary reproductive organs; organs that produce the gametes: testes in the male and ovaries in the female

F. Process of meiosis in the female in which one ovum and three polar bodies are produced from one primary oocyte

G. Process of meiosis in the male in which four spermatids are produced from one primary spermatocyte

H. Sex cells: sperm and ova

EVALUATION OF LEARNING

Directions: Fill in each blank with the correct answer.

Male Reproductive System

1. What are the four functions of the reproductive system?

   _____

   _____

2. What is another name for the primary reproductive organs?

   _____

3. What is another name for egg and sperm cells?

   _____

4. What is the function of the secondary reproductive organs?

   _____

   _____

5. Why are the testes located outside of the abdominal cavity?

   _____

   _____

6. What makes up the scrotum?

   _____

7. Describe the characteristics of the following:

   a. Tunica albuginea: _____

   b. Septa: _____

   c. Seminiferous tubules: _____

   d. Rete testis: _____

8. What is the function of the interstitial cells (cells of Leydig)?

   _____

9. Where in the testes does spermatogenesis take place?

   _____

10. What are spermatogonia?

    _____

11. What happens to spermatogonia at puberty? How many chromosomes do they have?

    _____

    _____

12. What occurs during meiosis I of spermatogenesis?

    _____

    _____

13. What occurs during meiosis II of spermatogenesis?

_____

_____

14. How many spermatids are eventually produced by each primary spermatocyte?

_____

15. What occurs during spermiogenesis?

_____

16. How many chromosomes are contained in the head of a sperm?

_____

17. Where is the acrosome located, and what is its function?

_____

_____

18. What are the functions of the following parts of a mature sperm cell?

a. Midpiece: _____

b. Tail: _____

19. How long does it take for a mature sperm to be produced (starting with a primary spermatocyte)?

_____

20. How long can sperm live in the female reproductive tract?

_____

21. List the series of ducts that a sperm passes through to reach the outside of the body from the testes.

_____

_____

22. What occurs to sperm in the epididymis?

_____

23. How are sperm moved through the ductus deferens?

_____

24. What two ducts combine to form the ejaculatory duct?

_____

25. Describe the location of each of the following parts of the male urethra:

a. Prostatic: _____

b. Membranous: _____

c. Penile (spongy): _____

26. What is the name of the opening of the penis to the outside?

_____

27. What is contained in the fluid secreted by the seminal vesicles, and what is its function?

_____

28. What structure does the prostate gland encircle?

_____

29. What is the function of the fluid secreted by the prostate gland?

_____

30. What are the three functions of the fluid secreted by the bulbourethral glands?

_____

_____

31. What is semen?

_____

_____

32. What is the usual number of sperm contained in each milliliter of semen?

_____

33. What are the names and location of the columns of erectile tissue located in the penis?

_____

_____

34. What are the three parts of the penis?

_____

35. What is the prepuce (foreskin)?

_____

36. What causes an erection of the penis?

_____

_____

37. What occurs during emission?

_____

_____

38. What occurs during ejaculation?

_____

_____

39. Why do the sphincters of the urinary bladder constrict during emission and ejaculation?

_____

40. When does puberty usually begin in males? When does it usually end?

_____

41. What hormone causes the pituitary gland to secrete LH and FSH?

_____

42. What is the function of luteinizing hormone in the male?

_____

_____

43. What two hormones are responsible for stimulating spermatogenesis?

_____

44. What effect does testosterone have on the human male at puberty?

_____

_____

Female Reproductive System

1. What is the function of the female reproductive organs?

_____

_____

_____

2. Where are the ovaries located?

_____

3. What is the tunica albuginea?

_____

4. What is located in the cortex of the ovary?

_____

5. What is the name for a female germ cell?

_____

6. What structures are located in the medulla of the ovary?

_____

7. What is oogenesis?

_____

8. When do primitive germ cells in the female develop into primary oocytes?

_____

9. How many chromosomes are present in a primary oocyte?

_____

10. How many primary oocytes are present when a female infant is born?

_____

11. What occurs during meiosis I of oogenesis?

_____

_____

12. What occurs during meiosis II of oogenesis?

_____

_____

_____

13. What makes up an ovarian follicle?

_____

_____

14. What occurs during ovulation?

_____

_____

15. What happens to the secondary oocyte if it is not fertilized?

_____

16. What happens to the secondary oocyte if it is fertilized?

_____

_____

17. What is the corpus luteum?

_____

18. What hormones are secreted by the corpus luteum?

_____

19. What happens to the corpus luteum if fertilization does not take place?

_____

_____

20. What happens to the corpus luteum if fertilization takes place?

_____

_____

21. Describe how an oocyte moves from the ovary and into the fallopian tube.

_____

_____

_____

22. How long does it take an oocyte to move through a fallopian tube?

_____

23. Where does fertilization usually occur?

_____

24. Describe the following parts of the uterus:

    a. Fundus: _____

    b. Body: _____

   c. Cervix: _____

   d. Internal os: _____

   e. External os: _____

25. What are the characteristics of the three layers that make up the wall of the uterus?

Wall of the Uterus	Characteristics
Perimetrium	
Myometrium	
Endometrium	

26. What is the function of the vagina?

_____

_____

27. Describe the characteristics of the following structures that make up the external female genitalia.

Structure	Characteristics
Labia majora	
Mons pubis	
Labia minora	
Vestibule	
Clitoris	
Prepuce	
Paraurethral glands	
Greater vestibular glands	

28. What happens to the follicle during each of the phases of the ovarian cycle?

   a. Follicular phase: _____

   b. Ovulatory phase: _____

   c. Luteal phase: _____

29. What hormones are responsible for the following?

   a. Growth of the ovarian follicle: _____

   b. Estrogen production by the ovaries: _____

   c. Rupture of the mature follicle out of the ovary: _____

   d. Stimulation of the corpus luteum to secrete estrogen and progesterone: _____

30. What is the menstrual cycle?

_____

_____

31. What happens to the endometrium of the uterus during the following phases of the menstrual cycle?

    a. Menstrual phase: _____

    b. Proliferative phase: _____

    c. Secretory phase: _____

32. What is menopause?

    _____

33. What is the function of the mammary glands?

    _____

34. What is the areola?

    _____

35. How many lobes of glandular tissue does each breast contain?

    _____

36. What determines the size and shape of the breasts?

    _____

37. What is the function of lactiferous ducts?

    _____

38. What effect do the following hormones have on the breasts?

    a. Prolactin: _____

    b. Oxytocin: _____

CRITICAL THINKING ACTIVITIES

A. BODY SPECTRUM CD ACTIVITY
   Reproductive: Male Reproductive System
   Body Spectrum Directions:
   1. Access your Body Spectrum program (CD included with your textbook).
   2. Go to the Contents screen.
   3. Access the HELP screen for directions on using the Body Spectrum program.
   4. Select the following category from the Contents screen:
      Reproductive
   5. Select the following anatomic diagram:
      Male Reproductive System
   6. Identify the structures on the diagram.
   7. Print out the diagram.

B. BODY SPECTRUM CD ACTIVITY
   Reproductive: Female Reproductive System
   Directions: Identify the structures on this diagram following the Body Spectrum Directions outlined under CTA A.

C. BODY SPECTRUM CD ACTIVITY
   Reproductive: Fertilization to Implantation
   Directions: Identify the structures on this diagram following the Body Spectrum Directions outlined under CTA A.

D. INQUIRING PATIENTS WANT TO KNOW

You are working in a general practice medical office. Your patients ask you the following questions. In the space provided, indicate how you would respond to each question in terms the patient would understand. Use your textbook and Internet resources to develop your responses.

1. How do birth control pills work?

    _____

    _____

2. What happens in the body during a hot flash?

    _____

    _____

3. Can you get pregnant during your menstrual period?

    _____

    _____

4. How does an erectile dysfunction drug work?

    _____

    _____

5. Is a vasectomy reversible?

    _____

    _____

6. Is it a good idea to douche?

    _____

    _____

7. How are embryos frozen?

    _____

    _____

8. What is a hymen?

    _____

    _____

9. What is the success rate for in vitro fertilization?

    _____

    _____

10. What causes PMS?

    _____

    _____

E. CHAPTER 16 ANIMATIONS CD ACTIVITY

Directions:

1. View the Chapter 16 Animations on your Companion CD (included with your textbook).

2. For each animation, write two true/false questions in the space provided below.

3. In the classroom, find a partner.

4. For each animation, read your two questions to your partner.

5. For each correct answer, your partner is awarded two points.

6. Next, have your partner read his/her two questions to you. Award yourself two points for each question answered correctly.

7. Continue in this manner until all the questions have been answered.

8. Record your points on your Study Guide Assignment sheet.

True/False Questions

a. Testes

    1. _____

    2. _____

b. Spermatogenesis

    1. _____

    2. _____

c. Spermatozoa

    1 _____

    2. _____

d. Male Reproductive Ducts

    1. _____

    2. _____

e. Accessory or Supportive Sex Glands (Male)

    1. _____

    2. _____

f. Male External Genitalia

    1. _____

    2. _____

g. Pathway of Sperm

    1. _____

    2. _____

h. Ovaries

    1. _____

    2. _____

i. Oogenesis

    1. _____

    2. _____

j. Female External Genitalia

    1. _____

    2. _____

k. Accessory or Supportive Sex Glands (Female)

    1. _____

    2. _____

l. Ovarian Cycle

   1. _____

   2. _____

m. Menstrual Cycle: Uterine

   1. _____

   2. _____

n. Pathway of Ovum

   1. _____

   2. _____

o. Fertilization to Implantation

   1. _____

   2. _____

p. Breasts

   1. _____

   2. _____

F. CROSSWORD PUZZLE
Reproductive System
Directions: Complete the crossword puzzle using the clues presented below.

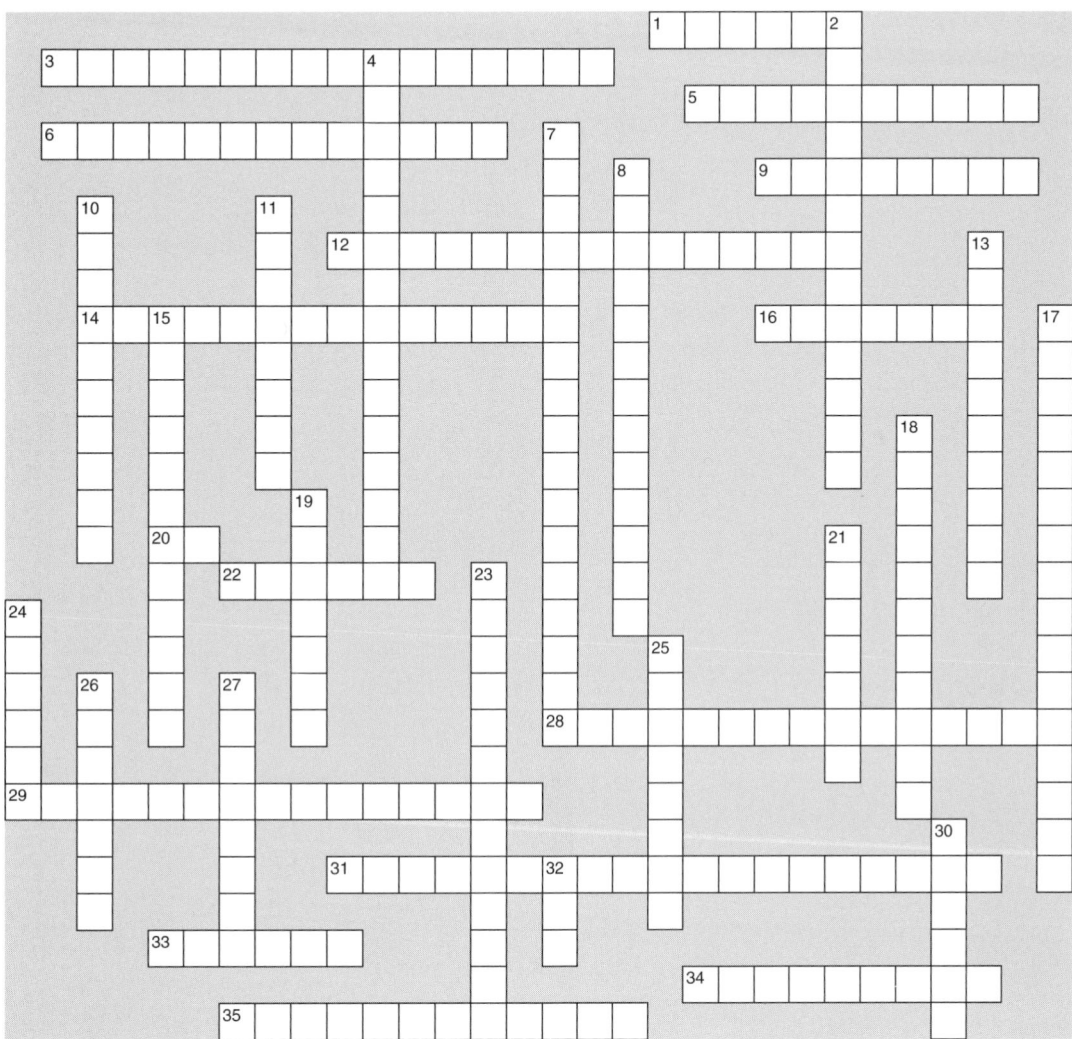

ACROSS	DOWN
1 Primary male reproductive organ	**2** Immature male germ cells
3 Mature follicle	**4** Contains a developing oocyte
5 Muscle layer of uterus	**7** Produce male sex hormones
6 Milk production organs	**8** Holds uterus in place
9 Finger-like extensions of a fallopian tube	**10** Where sperm mature
12 Carries milk from lobule to nipple	**11** Gland that encircles male urethra
14 Transports sperm from epididymis to ejaculatory duct	**13** Distal end of penis
16 Immature female germ cells	**15** Name of follicle after ovulation
20 Stimulates ovulation to occur	**17** Milk reservoir
22 Outer area of ovary	**18** Outer layer of uterus
28 Secrete fructose fluid to provide energy source	**19** Contains the testes
for sperm	**21** Primary female reproductive organs
29 Process of sperm formation	**23** Tube that transports oocyte to uterus
31 Produce sperm	**24** Provides growth environment for a fertilized egg
33 Upper bulging surface of uterus	**25** Discharge of semen into urethra
34 Hormone that stimulates milk production	**26** Egg and sperm cells
35 Hormone responsible for male secondary	**27** Hormone that causes ejection of milk from
sex characteristics	mammary glands
	30 Part of uterus that projects into vagina
	32 Stimulates growth of ovarian follicle

17

Medical Asepsis and the OSHA Standard

CHAPTER ASSIGNMENTS

√ After Completing	Date Due	Textbook Page(s)	TEXTBOOK ASSIGNMENTS	Possible Points	Points You Earned
		266-294	Read Chapter 17: Medical Asepsis and the OSHA Standard		
		277 292	📖 Read Case Study 1 Case Study 1 questions	5	
		282 293	📖 Read Case Study 2 Case Study 2 questions	5	
		286 293	📖 Read Case Study 3 Case Study 3 questions	5	
			TOTAL POINTS		

√ After Completing	Date Due	Study Guide Page(s)	STUDY GUIDE ASSIGNMENTS (CTA: Critical Thinking Activity)	Possible Points	Points You Earned
		217	❓ Pretest	10	
		218	🖊 Key Term Assessment	23	
		219-222	📝 Evaluation of Learning questions	40	
		223	CTA A: Infection Process Cycle	5	
		223	CTA B: Handwashing	8	
		224	CTA C: Personal Protective Equipment: Gloves	8	
		224	CTA D: Personal Protective Equipment	30	
		224-225	CTA E: Discarding Medical Waste	20	
			💿 CD Activity: Chapter 17 Discard It! (Record points earned)		
		225	CTA F: Dear Gabby	10	

√ After Completing	Date Due	Study Guide Page(s)	STUDY GUIDE ASSIGNMENTS (CTA: Critical Thinking Activity)	Possible Points	Points You Earned
		226	CTA G: Crossword Puzzle	25	
		227	CTA H: Road to Recovery Game: OSHA Bloodborne Pathogens Standard (Record points earned)		
			⊙ CD Activity: Chapter 17 Quiz Show (Record points earned)		
			⊙ CD Activity: Chapter 17 Apply Your Knowledge questions (Record points earned)		
		217	📄 Posttest	10	
			ADDITIONAL ASSIGNMENTS		
			TOTAL POINTS		

√ When Assigned by Your Instructor	Study Guide Page(s)	Practices Required	LABORATORY ASSIGNMENTS (Procedure Number and Name)	*Score
	235	5	**DVD** **Practice for Competency** 17-1: Handwashing Textbook reference: pp. 271-273	
	237-238		**Evaluation of Competency** 17-1: Handwashing	*
	235	4	**DVD** **Practice for Competency** 17-2: Applying an Alcohol-Based Hand Rub Textbook reference: pp. 274-275	
	239-240		**Evaluation of Competency** 17-2: Applying an Alcohol-Based Hand Rub	*
	235	5	**DVD** **Practice for Competency** 17-3: Application and Removal of Clean Disposable Gloves Textbook reference: pp. 275-276	
	241-242		**Evaluation of Competency** 17-3: Application and Removal of Clean Disposable Gloves	*
			ADDITIONAL ASSIGNMENTS	

Notes

_____ 10. An empty urine container

_____ 11. Sutures caked with blood

_____ 12. Thermometer probe cover

_____ 13. Patient gown

_____ 14. Disposable diaper

_____ 15. Dressing saturated with a purulent discharge

_____ 16. Clean disposable gloves

_____ 17. Disposable vaginal speculum

_____ 18. An outdated vaccine

_____ 19. Syringe and needle

_____ 20. Examining-table paper

F. DEAR GABBY

Gabby is away on vacation and wants you to fill in for her. In the space provided, respond to the following letter using the knowledge you have acquired in this chapter.

Dear Gabby:

I am writing to you because I am very concerned about my younger sister "Tuesday." For the past 2 weeks, Tuesday has been extremely tired and does not feel like eating. She also vomits several times a day and says that her joints ache. Tuesday is 26 years old and a single mother with two small children. Tuesday has been dating "Alex" for the past 4 months. It is well-known around town that Alex sometimes injects himself with illegal drugs, and I think there's a chance that Tuesday is also using drugs. I told Tuesday that she needs to see her doctor right away, but she will not listen to me. She says it just seems like a prolonged case of the flu, and it will probably go away soon. I did an Internet search of her symptoms, and it sounds to me like she has hepatitis C. Gabby, am I just being overprotective of my sister, or should I insist that she see her doctor?

Wanting to Know in Wyoming

_____
_____
_____
_____
_____
_____
_____
_____
_____
_____

G. CROSSWORD PUZZLE
Medical Asepsis and the OSHA Standard
Directions: Complete the crossword puzzle using the clues provided below.

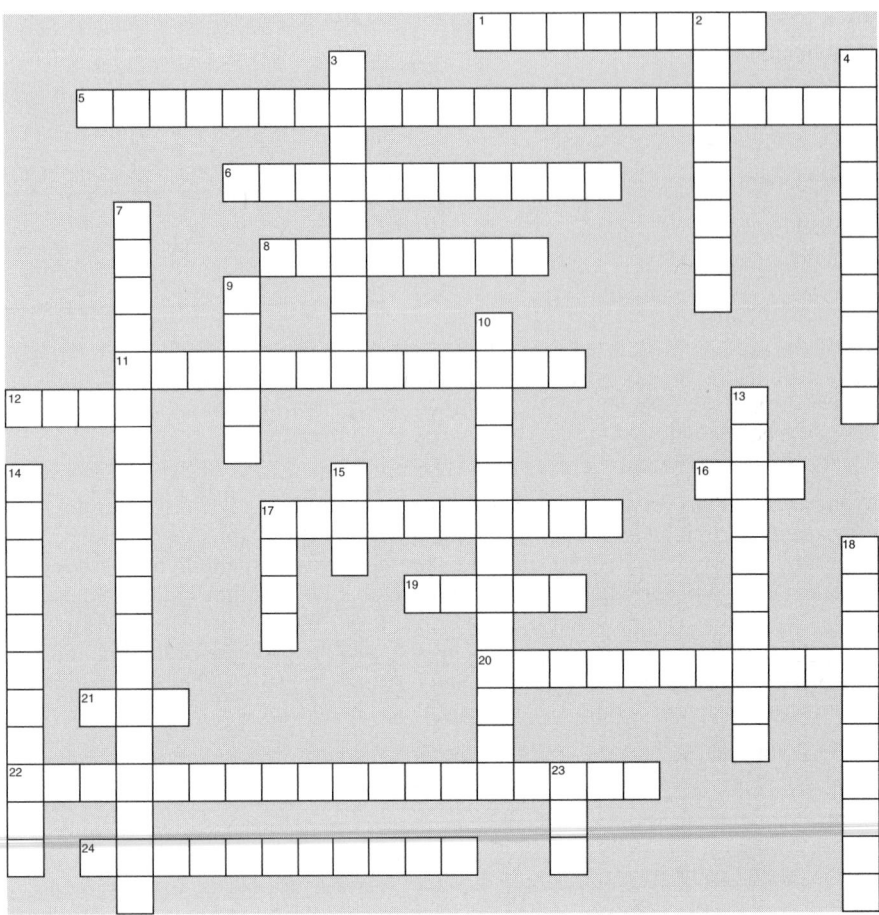

ACROSS
1 Grows best without oxygen
5 Infection resulting from a defective immune system
6 HBV serious complication
8 Microorganism that causes disease
11 Normally live on the skin
12 Vaginal secretions (example)
16 Protector of public health
17 Can live dry for 1 week
19 Traps microorganisms
20 Lacking resistance
21 After exposure: may prevent disease
22 Health hazard eliminator
24 Eats "live stuff"

DOWN
2 Example of a microorganism
3 Body invasion by a pathogen
4 Found in antimicrobial soap
7 Way to prevent a needlestick injury
9 HIV screening test
10 Broken skin
13 #1 chronic viral disease in United States
14 #1 aseptic practice
15 Scrubs are not this
17 Hepatitis B passive immunizing agent
18 Piercing of the skin barrier
23 Discard in a biohazard container

H. ROAD TO RECOVERY GAME: OSHA BLOODBORNE PATHOGENS STANDARD

Object: To lead your "patient" to recovery by correctly determining if an action taken to a situation in the medical office meets the OSHA Bloodborne Pathogens Standard or violates the OSHA standard

Needed: **Road to Recovery** game board (located at the end of your study guide)
                     A token for each player (e.g., a button or coin)
                     Dice (1)
                     Game cards
                     Score card

Directions:
1. Cut out the situation game cards on the following pages.
2. On the reverse of each card, respond to the situation by indicating an action that could be taken. For approximately half of your cards, state an action that would **meet** the OSHA standard, and for the other half, state an action that would **violate** the OSHA standard.
3. Get into a group of two.
4. Get into your playing groups, and trade your cards with a player from another group.
5. Place one complete set of cards on the game board with the Situations facing up (and the Actions facing down).
6. Play **Road to Recovery** following the directions on the reverse side of the game board. A player should pick up a card and read the Situation and the Action and respond by indicating whether the action **meets** the OSHA standard or **violates** the OSHA standard. If the rest of the players agree with your response, award yourself 5 points. If a question arises as to the correct answer, consult your instructor for assistance.
7. Keep track of your points using the score card provided.
8. After completing one set of cards on the game board, place a second set on the board and continue playing the game. Continue playing until all the sets of cards have been used.

ROAD TO RECOVERY
SCORE CARD

Name: _____

Recording Points:
Using the Game Card Points box, cross off a number each time you answer a game card correctly (starting with 5 and continuing in sequence). Your Total Game Card Points will be equal to the last number you crossed off. Record this number in the space provided (1). Record any extra points you were awarded during the game (2) and any points that were deducted (3). To determine your total points, add (1) and (2) together and deduct (3). Record this number in the Total Points Earned space provided. Compare your score with the other player and determine where you placed. Place a check mark next to the level of recovery your patient attained.

Game Card Points:		
5	75	145
10	80	150
15	85	155
20	90	160
25	95	165
30	100	170
35	105	175
40	110	180
45	115	185
50	120	190
55	125	195
60	130	200
65	135	205
70	140	210

Calculation of Points:

(1) Total Game Card Points: _____

(2) Additional Points Awarded: _____

(3) Deducted Points: _____

TOTAL POINTS EARNED: _____

LEVEL OF RECOVERY:

Patient's Name: _____

☐ First Place: **Fully Recovered**
☐ Second Place: **Almost Recovered**

Notes

SITUATION: You go into an examining room and notice that the biohazard sharps container in that room is completely full.

SITUATION: You are performing laboratory testing and accidentally drop a blood tube, and it breaks.

SITUATION: You are wearing a protective laboratory coat over your scrubs, and you are getting ready to leave for the day.

SITUATION: A part-time clinical medical assistant was just hired. She is not immunized against hepatitis B.

SITUATION: A clinical medical assistant who has worked at the office for 5 years changes her mind and decides she wants the hepatitis B vaccine.

SITUATION: You are wearing a protective lab coat over your scrubs. While performing a laboratory test, some blood splashes onto your lab coat but does not penetrate through to your scrubs.

SITUATION: You just gave an injection to a patient and after withdrawing the needle, you notice that there is no sharps container in the room.

SITUATION: You are getting ready to apply gloves and notice that you have a cut on your finger.

SITUATION: You accidentally get some blood on your bare hands while removing your gloves.

ACTION:

ACTION:

ACTION:

ACTION:

ACTION:

ACTION:

ACTION:

ACTION:

ACTION:

SITUATION: During an office meeting, a coworker suggests an idea to save money by emptying full sharps containers into a biohazard bag so that the containers can be reused.

SITUATION: A new employee wants to know where she should eat her lunch.

SITUATION: You are applying a pair of disposable gloves, and one of the gloves tears while you are pulling it on.

SITUATION: A new clinical medical assistant was just hired at the medical office, and she is allergic to latex gloves.

SITUATION: You have just drawn blood from a patient, and you accidentally stick yourself with the needle.

SITUATION: Your office only has one refrigerator and blood tubes need to be stored in it, but the staff would like to put their lunches in it.

SITUATION: You remove your gloves after giving an injection to a patient and accidentally drop them into the biohazard sharps container.

SITUATION: You are separating serum from whole blood, and you accidentally spill some of the serum on the countertop.

SITUATION: By mistake, you throw a reusable tourniquet into the sharps container after drawing a patient's blood.

ACTION:

ACTION:

ACTION:

ACTION:

ACTION:

ACTION:

ACTION:

ACTION:

ACTION:

SITUATION: A technician is coming to your office today to repair your blood chemistry analyzer.

SITUATION: Your office has run out of biohazard bags used to transport specimens to the laboratory, and you notice that an employee is using plastic bags as a substitute.

SITUATION: You notice that after an externship student performs a finger puncture, she lays the used, exposed lancet on the counter. She then discards it in the sharps container after applying a Band-Aid to the patient's finger.

SITUATION: You have just been assigned the responsibility of performing all required venipunctures in your office. You notice that the sharps container is located on the side of the room opposite the blood drawing chair.

SITUATION: Utility gloves are used and reused in your office for the sanitization of medical instruments.

SITUATION: You accidentally close (and lock in place) the lid of a sharps container that is only half full.

SITUATION: You are removing a stopper from a tube of blood so that you can transfer the serum to another tube. A small amount of serum accidentally spatters into your eye.

SITUATION: A new employee has been hired who says she has already had the hepatitis B vaccination series.

SITUATION: A medical assisting externship student does not wear gloves to recap a needle after drawing medication into a syringe to give an injection to a patient.

ACTION:

ACTION:

ACTION:

ACTION:

ACTION:

ACTION:

ACTION:

ACTION:

ACTION:

PRACTICE FOR COMPETENCY

Medical Asepsis

Procedure 17-1: Handwashing. Perform the handwashing procedure. List five medically aseptic steps that must be followed during this procedure.

Medically Aseptic Steps to Follow during Handwashing

1. _____
   _____

2. _____
   _____

3. _____
   _____

4. _____
   _____

5. _____
   _____

Procedure 17-2: Alcohol-Based Hand Rub. Apply an alcohol-based hand rub. Practice applying both a gel and a foam hand rub. List the brand name(s) of the hand rubs you applied, and list the ingredients contained in them.

_____

_____

Procedure 17-3: Clean Disposable Gloves. Apply and remove clean disposable gloves. What size gloves fit you the best?

_____

_____

Notes

EVALUATION OF COMPETENCY

Procedure 17-1: Handwashing

Name: _____   Date: _____

Evaluated By: _____   Score: _____

Performance Objective

Outcome:	Perform handwashing.
Conditions:	Using a sink.
	Given liquid soap or bar soap and paper towels.
Standards:	Time: 5 minutes. Student completed procedure in _____ minutes.
	Accuracy: Satisfactory score on the Performance Evaluation Checklist.

Performance Evaluation Checklist

Trial 1	Trial 2	Point Value	Performance Standards
		•	Removed watch or pushed it up on the forearm.
		•	Removed rings.
		▷	Stated the reason for removing rings.
		•	Stood at sink with clothing away from edge of sink.
		•	Turned on faucets with paper towel.
		▷	Explained the reason for turning on faucets with paper towel.
		•	Adjusted the water to a warm temperature.
		•	Discarded towel into trash can.
		•	Wet hands and forearms with water.
		•	Held hands lower than elbows at all times.
		▷	Explained why the hands should be held lower than elbows.
		•	Did not touch the inside of sink with hands.
		•	Applied soap to hands.
		•	Washed palms and backs of hands with 10 circular motions and friction.
		▷	Explained why circular motions and friction are needed to wash hands.
		•	Washed fingers with 10 circular motions.
		•	Washed fingers while interlaced using friction and circular motions.
		•	Rinsed well (keeping hands lower than elbows).
		•	Washed wrists and forearms using friction and circular motions.
		•	Cleaned fingernails using manicure stick.

Trial 1	Trial 2	Point Value	Performance Standards
		•	Rinsed arms and hands.
		•	Repeated handwashing procedure (if necessary).
		•	Dried hands gently and thoroughly.
		▷	Stated the reason for drying hands gently and completely.
		•	Turned off faucets using paper towel.
		•	Did not touch sink area with bare hands.
		▷	Explained the reason for not touching sink area with bare hands.
		✻	Completed the procedure within 5 minutes.
			TOTALS

Evaluation of Student Performance

EVALUATION CRITERIA			COMMENTS
Symbol	Category	Point Value	
✻	Critical Step	16 points	
•	Essential Step	6 points	
▷	Theory Question	2 points	

Score calculation: 100 points

− _____ points missed

_____ Score

Satisfactory score: 85 or above

CAAHEP Competencies Achieved:

Psychomotor (Skills)
☑ III. 2. Practice Standard Precautions.
☑ III. 4. Perform handwashing.
☑ IX. 8. Apply local, state, and federal health care legislation and regulation appropriate to the medical assisting practice setting.

Affective (Behavior)
☑ IX. 3. Recognize the importance of local, state, and federal legislation and regulations in the practice setting.

ABHES Competencies Achieved:

☑ 4. f. Comply with federal, state, and local health laws and regulations.
☑ 9. b. Apply principles of aseptic techniques and infection control.
☑ 9. i. Use standard precautions.

EVALUATION OF COMPETENCY

Procedure 17-2: Applying an Alcohol-Based Hand Rub

Name: _____   Date: _____

Evaluated By: _____   Score: _____

Performance Objective

Outcome:	Perform handwashing.
Conditions:	Given liquid soap or bar soap and paper towels.
Standards:	Time: 2 minutes. Student completed procedure in _____ minutes.
	Accuracy: Satisfactory score on the Performance Evaluation Checklist.

Performance Evaluation Checklist

Trial 1	Trial 2	Point Value	Performance Standards
		●	Inspected the hands to make sure they are not visibly soiled.
		▷	Stated the procedure to follow if the hands are visibly soiled.
		●	Removed watch or pushed it up on the forearm.
		●	Removed rings.
			Applied the alcohol-based hand rub to the palm of one hand as follows:
		●	*Gel or lotion:* Applied an amount of gel or lotion approximately equal to the size of a dime.
		●	*Foam:* Applied an amount of foam approximately equal to the size of a walnut.
		▷	Explained why it is important not to use more than the recommended amount of hand rub.
		●	Thoroughly spread the hand rub over the surface of both hands up to ½ inch above the wrist.
		●	Spread the hand rub around and under the fingernails.
		▷	Explained why it is important to cover the entire surface of the hands.
		●	Rubbed the hands together until they are dry.
		●	Did not touch anything until the hands were dry.
		＊	Completed the procedure within 2 minutes.
			TOTALS

Evaluation of Student Performance

EVALUATION CRITERIA			COMMENTS
Symbol	Category	Point Value	
✳	Critical Step	16 points	
●	Essential Step	6 points	
▷	Theory Question	2 points	

Score calculation: 100 points

−_____ points missed

_____ Score

Satisfactory score: 85 or above

CAAHEP Competencies Achieved:

Psychomotor (Skills)
☑ III. 2. Practice Standard Precautions.
☑ IX.8. Apply local, state, and federal health care legislation and regulation appropriate to the medical assisting practice setting.

Affective (Behavior)
☑ IX. 3. Recognize the importance of local, state, and federal legislation and regulations in the practice setting.

ABHES Competencies Achieved:

☑ 4. f. Comply with federal, state, and local health laws and regulations.
☑ 9. b. Apply principles of aseptic techniques and infection control.
☑ 9. i. Use standard precautions.

EVALUATION OF COMPETENCY

DVD Procedure 17-3: Application and Removal of Clean Disposable Gloves

Name: _____   Date: _____

Evaluated By: _____   Score: _____

Performance Objective

Outcome:	Apply and remove clean disposable gloves.
Conditions:	Given the appropriate size clean disposable gloves.
Standards:	Time: 5 minutes. Student completed procedure in _____ minutes.
	Accuracy: Satisfactory score on the Performance Evaluation Checklist.

Performance Evaluation Checklist

Trial 1	Trial 2	Point Value	Performance Standards
			Application of Clean Gloves
		•	Removed all rings.
		▷	Stated why rings should be removed.
		•	Sanitized the hands.
		•	Chose the appropriate size gloves.
		▷	Explained what can happen if the gloves are too small or too large.
		•	Applied the gloves.
		•	Adjusted the gloves so that they fit comfortably.
		•	Inspected the gloves for tears.
		▷	Stated the procedure to follow if a glove is torn.
			Removal of Clean Gloves
		•	Grasped the outside of the left glove 1 to 2 inches from the top with the gloved right hand.
		•	Slowly pulled left glove off the hand.
		•	Pulled the left glove free and scrunched it into a ball with the gloved right hand.
		•	Placed the index and middle fingers of the left hand on the inside of the right glove.
		•	Did not allow the clean hand to touch outside of the glove.
		•	Pulled the glove off the right hand enclosing the balled-up left glove.
		•	Discarded both gloves in an appropriate waste container.

		▷	Stated when gloves should be discarded in a biohazardous waste container.
		●	Sanitized the hands.
		✳	Completed the procedure in 5 minutes.
			TOTALS

Evaluation of Student Performance

EVALUATION CRITERIA			COMMENTS
Symbol	Category	Point Value	
✳	Critical Step	16 points	
●	Essential Step	6 points	
▷	Theory Question	2 points	

Score calculation: 100 points

−_____ points missed

_____ Score

Satisfactory score: 85 or above

CAAHEP Competencies Achieved:

Psychomotor (Skills)
☑ III. 2. Practice Standard Precautions.
☑ IX.8. Apply local, state, and federal health care legislation and regulation appropriate to the medical assisting practice setting.

Affective (Behavior)
☑ IX. 3. Recognize the importance of local, state, and federal legislation and regulations in the practice setting.

ABHES Competencies Achieved:

☑ 4. f. Comply with federal, state, and local health laws and regulations.
☑ 9. b. Apply principles of aseptic techniques and infection control.
☑ 9. i. Use standard precautions.

18

Sterilization and Disinfection

CHAPTER ASSIGNMENTS

√ After Completing	Date Due	Textbook Page(s)	TEXTBOOK ASSIGNMENTS	Possible Points	Points You Earned
		295-324	Read Chapter 18: Sterilization and Disinfection		
		298 323	Read Case Study 1 Case Study 1 questions	5	
		308 323	Read Case Study 2 Case Study 2 questions	5	
		310 323	Read Case Study 3 Case Study 3 questions	5	
			TOTAL POINTS		

√ After Completing	Date Due	Study Guide Page(s)	STUDY GUIDE ASSIGNMENTS (CTA: Critical Thinking Activity)	Possible Points	Points You Earned
		247	Pretest	10	
		248	Key Term Assessment	17	
		249-251	Evaluation of Learning questions	28	
		251-253	CTA A: Material Safety Data Sheet	17	
		253-254	CTA B: Obtaining a Material Safety Data Sheet	10	
		254	CTA C: Sanitization	8	
		255	CTA D: Sterilization	10	
		256	CTA E: What Comes Next? Game (Record points earned)		
			CD Activity: Chapter 18 What Happens Now? (Record points earned)		

√ After Completing	Date Due	Study Guide Page(s)	STUDY GUIDE ASSIGNMENTS (CTA: Critical Thinking Activity)	Possible Points	Points You Earned
			CD Activity: Chapter 18 Quiz Show (Record points earned)		
			CD Activity: Chapter 18 Apply Your Knowledge questions (Record points earned)		
		247	Posttest	10	
			ADDITIONAL ASSIGNMENTS		
			TOTAL POINTS		

√ When Assigned by Your Instructor	Study Guide Page(s)	Practices Required	LABORATORY ASSIGNMENTS (Procedure Number and Name)	*Score
	259	3	**DVD Practice for Competency** 18-1: Sanitization of Instruments Textbook reference: pp. 303-307	
	261-263		**Evaluation of Competency** 18-1: Sanitization of Instruments	*
	259	Paper: 3 Muslin: 3	**DVD Practice for Competency** 18-2: Wrapping Instruments Using Paper or Muslin Textbook reference: pp. 313-315	
	265-266		**Evaluation of Competency** 18-2: Wrapping Instruments Using Paper or Muslin	*
	259	3	**DVD Practice for Competency** 18-3: Wrapping Instruments Using a Pouch Textbook reference: pp. 315-316	
	267-268		**Evaluation of Competency** 18-3: Wrapping Instruments Using a Pouch	*
	259	3	**DVD Practice for Competency** 18-4: Sterilizing Articles in the Autoclave Textbook reference: pp. 320-322	
	269-270		**Evaluation of Competency** 18-4: Sterilizing Articles in the Autoclave	*
			ADDITIONAL ASSIGNMENTS	

Notes

Name _____   Date _____

PRETEST

True or False

_____ 1. A bacterial spore consists of a hard, thick-walled capsule that can resist adverse conditions.

_____ 2. The purpose of sanitization is to remove all microorganisms and spores from a contaminated article.

_____ 3. According to OSHA, gloves do not need to be worn during the sanitization process.

_____ 4. Glutaraldehyde (Cidex) is a high-level disinfectant.

_____ 5. High-level disinfection kills all microorganisms but not spores.

_____ 6. Sterilization is the process of destroying all forms of microbial life except for bacterial spores.

_____ 7. Autoclave tape indicates whether or not an autoclaved item is sterile.

_____ 8. The wrapper used to autoclave articles should prevent contaminants from getting in during handling and storage.

_____ 9. Tap water should be used in the autoclave.

_____ 10. The inside of the autoclave should be wiped every day with a damp cloth.

POSTTEST

True or False

_____ 1. The agent used to destroy microorganisms on an article depends on the size of the article.

_____ 2. The purpose of the Hazard Communications Standard is to make sure that employees do not use hazardous chemicals in the workplace.

_____ 3. The Hazard Communications Standard requires that the label of a hazardous chemical include information on how to store and handle the chemical.

_____ 4. Stethoscopes must be decontaminated using a high-level disinfectant.

_____ 5. The most common temperature and pressure for autoclaving is 212°F at 15 lb of pressure/square inch.

_____ 6. A sterilization strip should be positioned in the center of a wrapped pack.

_____ 7. The best means of determining the effectivness of the sterilization process are biologic indicators.

_____ 8. The proper time for sterilizing an article in the autoclave depends on what is being autoclaved.

_____ 9. A pack that has been in the storage cupboard for 4 weeks should be resterilized.

_____ 10. Ethylene oxide gas is used by medical manufacturers to sterilize disposable items.

Term KEY TERM ASSESSMENT

Directions: Match each medical term with its definition.

D   1. Antiseptic

H   2. Autoclave

B   3. Contaminate

G   4. Critical item

P   5. Decontamination

I   6. Detergent

L   7. Disinfectant

Q   8. Hazardous chemical

A   9. Incubate

K   10. Load

M   11. Material safety data sheet

E   12. Noncritical item

N   13. Sanitization

J   14. Semicritical item

F   15. Spore

O   16. Sterilization

C   17. Thermolabile

A. To provide proper conditions for growth and development

B. To soil, stain, or pollute; to make impure

C. Easily affected or changed by heat

D. A substance that inhibits disease-producing microorganisms but not their spores (usually applied to living tissues)

E. An item that comes in contact with intact skin but not mucous membranes

F. A hard, thick-walled capsule formed by some bacteria that contains only the essential parts of the protoplasm of the bacterial cell

G. An item that comes in contact with sterile tissue or the vascular system

H. An apparatus for the sterilization of materials, using steam under pressure

I. An agent that cleanses by emulsifying dirt and oil

J. An item that comes in contact with nonintact skin or intact mucous membranes

K. The articles that are being sterilized

L. An agent used to destroy pathogenic microorganisms but not necessarily their spores (usually applied to inanimate objects)

M. A sheet that provides information regarding a chemical and its hazards, and measures to take to avoid injury and illness when handling the chemical

N. A process to remove organic matter from an article and to lower the number of microorganisms to a safe level as determined by public health requirements

O. The process of destroying all forms of microbial life, including bacterial spores

P. The use of physical or chemical means to destroy bloodborne pathogens on an item so that it is no longer capable of transmitting disease, making it safe to handle

Q. Any chemical that presents a threat to the health and safety of an individual coming into contact with it

Spore : Harder to kill
Drying
Sunlight
Heat
Disinfectan

Sanitization - process
Disinfection - Agent
Sterilization - Sterile
process

EVALUATION OF LEARNING

Directions: Fill in each blank with the correct answer.

1. How does one determine what type of physical or chemical agent to use to destroy microorganisms on an article?

   Depends on the level of disinfection desired

2. List two diseases that are caused by bacteria that produce spores.

   Clostridium botulinum
   Clostridium tetani

3. What is the purpose of the Hazard Communications Standard?

   to ensure employees are informed of hazardous chemicals in the workplace

4. List four examples of hazardous chemicals that may be used in the medical office.

   disinfectants, developing solutions, anesthetics, toner

5. What information must be included on a hazardous chemical label as required by the Hazard Communications Standard?

   manufacturer label with warning to alert chemical dangers

6. List and describe the information that must be included in an MSDS.

   Identification
   Composition of ingredents
   Physical and chemical properties
   fire and explosion hazard data
   Reactivity DATA

7. What are the purposes of sanitizing an article?

   to reduce number of microorganisms to a safe level

8. What is the advantage of using the ultrasound method to clean instruments?

   Safety advantage, dont have to handle during cleaning process

9. Why should gloves be worn during the sanitization procedure?

   protects employee from infectious disease,

10. What is the definition of high-level disinfection?

process that destroys all micro-organisms with the exception of spores.

11. List one example of an item that requires high-level disinfection. List one example of a high-level disinfectant.

2% glutaraldehyde

12. List two examples of items that can be disinfected through intermediate-level disinfection. List one example of an intermediate-level disinfectant.

Stethoscopes, bP cuff
Alcohol wipes

13. List two examples of items that are disinfected by low-level disinfection.

exam tables, Counter tops

14. What is the purpose of the pressure used in the autoclaving process?

to produce steam and heat to kill microorganisms

15. Why is it important that all air be removed from the autoclave during the sterilization process?

Certain bacteria can survive

16. What are the most common temperature and pressure used to sterilize materials with the autoclave?

250° at 15lbs of pressure for 15 min or more

17. What information does the Centers for Disease Control and Prevention recommend be recorded in an autoclave log regarding each cycle?

Date, time, Description of load, Exposure time, temp, initials of operator

18. What is the function of a sterilization indicator?

to determine effectiveness of the sterilization procedure

19. What is the purpose of wrapping articles to be autoclaved?

to help protect and maintain Sterility of instruments

20. List two properties of a good wrapper for use in autoclaving.

Sterilization paper, pouches and muslin

21. List three examples of wrapping material used for the autoclave, and identify an advantage of each type.

Sterilization paper, pouches and Muslin

22. Why is more time necessary to autoclave a large minor office surgery pack?

Larger amount of instruments to be sterilized

23. What is "event-related sterility"?

if the article is comprimised, it must be resterilized.

24. Describe the care an autoclave should receive on a daily basis.

Wipe inside/outside - clean and Inspect rubber gasket

25. Why is a longer exposure time necessary to ensure sterilization when using the dry heat oven?

Microorganisms and spores are more resistant to dry heat alone

26. What effect does moist heat have on instruments with sharp cutting edges?

More corrosive and can errode edges

27. How does the medical manufacturing industry use ethylene oxide gas sterilization?

producing prepacked sterile disposable items

28. What guidelines must be followed when using cold sterilization?

precise guidelines according to manufacture instructions

CRITICAL THINKING ACTIVITIES

A. MATERIAL SAFETY DATA SHEET

Refer to the MSDS in the text (Figure 18-2), and answer the following questions.

1. When was this MSDS last revised?

8/8/09

2. Is glutaraldehyde soluble in water?

yes

3. Describe the appearance and odor of glutaraldehyde.

Sharp Odor - bluis green liquid

4. What is the pH of glutaraldehyde?

   7.5 – 8.5

5. Is glutaraldehyde flammable?

   No

6. Is glutaraldehyde stable?

   Under recommended Storage

7. What conditions should be avoided with glutaraldehyde?

   direct Sunlight / temp above 104°F

8. How can glutaraldehyde enter the body?

   Skin, eyes, inhalation, ingestion

9. What types of symptoms occur if glutaraldehyde does the following?

   a. Comes in contact with the skin: moderate irratation, dermatitis

   b. Is splashed into the eyes: flush 15 min

   c. Is inhaled: remove to fresh air

   d. Is ingested: Do not induce vomiting - medical attention

10. What preexisting conditions can an individual possess that can be aggravated by glutaraldehyde?

    Asthma

11. Does glutaraldehyde cause cancer?

    No

12. What are the emergency and first aid procedures for glutaraldehyde for the following?

    a. Skin: WASh for 15 min

    b. Eyes: flush water for 15min

    c. Inhalation: Fresh Air move to

    d. Ingestion: Do not induce Vomiting

13. What should be done if glutaraldehyde is spilled?

    Ventilate area, wear PPE, wipe Sponge, flush with large amount of water

14. What is the disposal method for glutaraldehyde?

    in accordance wit State and federal guidelines

15. How should glutaraldehyde be stored?

Cool dry place (59-86°F) away from heat in container.

16. What type of ventilation is necessary when working with glutaraldehyde?

Ensure adequate ventilation

17. What skin and eye protection should be taken with glutaraldehyde?

Chemical resistant gloves and eye goggles

B. OBTAINING A MATERIAL SAFETY DATA SHEET

Obtain an MSDS for one of the following hazardous chemicals, and answer the questions below. Internet sites for obtaining an MSDS are listed below:

www.msdssearch.com
www.hazard.com/msds

- Cidex
- MetriCide
- Cidex OPA
- Cavicide
- Wavicide
- Biozide
- Sporox II
- Vesphene
- Envirocide
- Clorox bleach

1. What is the chemical name of this hazardous chemical?

Sodium Hypochlorite

2. What is the trade or brand name of this chemical?

Bleach

3. Who manufactures this chemical?

Great Value (Wal-Mart)

4. What number would you call if an emergency occurred with this chemical?

911 - poision control

5. What types of symptoms occur if this chemical does the following?

   a. Comes in contact with the skin: _Chemical burns to broken Skin_

   b. Is splashed into the eyes: _Causes eye damage_

   c. Is inhaled: _Avoid breathing vapors_

   d. Is ingested: _Mucosal damage_

6. What are the emergency and first aid procedures for this chemical?

Flush with water 15-20 min, Do not induce vomiting

7. What should be done if this chemical is spilled?

dilute with water, mop up, do not mix with other chemicals

8. What is the disposal method for this chemical?

Cool dry area away from heat and sunlight

9. How should this chemical be stored?

dilute with water before disposal in sewer

10. What type of protection should be taken when working with this chemical?

Wear safety goggles and rubber gloves.

C. SANITIZATION

For each of the following situations involving sanitization, write *C* if the technique is correct and *I* if the technique is incorrect. If the situation is correct, state the principle underlying the technique. If the situation is incorrect, explain what might happen if the technique were performed in the incorrect manner.

I 1. A contaminated surgical instrument is left in the examination room.

Should be taken out to be cleaned and sanitized.

I 2. The MA does not wear gloves when sanitizing surgical instruments.

DuH! Protect yourself.

I 3. The MA piles instruments in a heap while preparing them for sanitization.

Cannot be propely Sanitized.

I 4. The MA forgets to read the MSDS before decontaminating some surgical instruments in Cidex.

Read the MSDS.

I 5. The MA uses laundry detergent to sanitize surgical instruments.

must use proper chemicals to Sanitize.

I 6. Dried blood is not completely cleansed from hemostatic forceps before they are sterilized in the autoclave.

All visible material must be Scrubbed.

C 7. The MA checks all instruments for proper working condition before sterilizing them.

Correct

C *I* 8. The MA lubricates hemostatic forceps with a steam-penetrable lubricant before sterilizing them.

After Correct

D. STERILIZATION

For each of the following situations involving sterilization of articles in the autoclave, write *C* if the technique is correct and *I* if the technique is incorrect. If the situation is correct, state the principle underlying the technique. If the situation is incorrect, explain what might happen if the technique were performed in the incorrect manner.

_I_ 1. The MA opens a hemostat before placing it in a sterilization pouch.

never open prior

_I_ 2. Tap water is used to fill the water reservoir of the autoclave.

must use distilled water

_C_ 3. When loading the autoclave, the MA places glass jars in an upright position.

_I_ 4. The MA places four sterilization pouches on top of each other in the autoclave.

must never place on top of each other

_C_ 5. The MA places small packs to be sterilized approximately 1 to 3 inches apart in the autoclave.

Ensures proper sanitation

_I_ 6. Spore strips are placed in the autoclave, where steam would penetrate them most easily.

Spore strips should be placed in the wraps

_C_ 7. The MA begins timing the load in the autoclave after the proper temperature of 250°F has been reached.

_I_ 8. The MA removes the load from the autoclave while it is still wet.

must go through a dry cycle

_C_ 9. The MA notices a tear in one of the wrappers while removing articles from the autoclave. She rewraps and resterilizes the article.

_I_ 10. The MA notices that a sterilized wrapped article has unwrapped. She retapes the pack and places it back on the storage shelf.

must resterilize

E. WHAT COMES NEXT? GAME

Object: To achieve sterilization of an article by determining the correct sequence of events in the sanitization and sterilization procedure

Directions:

1. Cut out the game cards on the following page.
2. Make your cards unique by coloring and decorating them.
3. Review the sequence of steps in the sanitization and sterilization procedures.
4. Get into a group of three students.
5. Hold your game cards with the steps facing you.
6. Each player places the first step in the sanitization/sterilization procedure face down on the table.
7. When all players have placed a card on the table, turn the cards over.
8. Award yourself 5 points if you have correctly determined the proper step in the sequence. If you have a question regarding the correct answer, consult your instructor.
9. In turn, each player can earn an additional 5 points by stating a fact about that step in the procedure. For example, if the step is "Apply Gloves," a fact about this step would be that both clean gloves and utility gloves must be worn during the sanitization procedure.
10. Keep track of your points on the score card provided.
11. Keep the cards in their proper sequence on the table, and continue the game until all of the game cards have been used.

WHAT COMES NEXT?
SCORE CARD

Name: _____

Recording Points:

Cross off a number each time you properly sequence a game card (starting with 5 and continuing in sequence). Cross off another number if you are able to state a fact about the step in the procedure. Your total points will be equal to the last number you crossed off. Record this number in the space provided and check the level that you achieved.

Game Card Points:	
5	75
10	80
15	85
20	90
25	95
30	100
35	105
40	110
45	115
50	120
55	125
60	130
65	135
70	140

TOTAL POINTS: _____

LEVEL:

☐ 100 to 120 points: **Sterile**—You got rid of all MOs and spores!
☐ 80 to 100 points: **Aseptic**—You got rid of the pathogenic MOs.
☐ 60 to 80 points: **Contaminated**—Your article is still contaminated.

PRACTICE FOR COMPETENCY

Sterilization and Disinfection

Procedure 18-1: Sanitization of Instruments. Sanitize instruments. In the space provided, indicate the following:

A. Name of the disinfectant _____

B. Name of the instrument cleaner _____

C. Names of instruments sanitized _____

_____

_____

Procedures 18-2 and 18-3: Wrapping Articles for the Autoclave. Wrap articles for autoclaving. In the space provided, list the information you indicated on the label of each pack, which includes the contents of the pack, the date, and your initials.
Information indicated on the label of the wrapped article:

_____

_____

_____

_____

_____

_____

_____

Procedure 18-4: Sterilizing Articles in the Autoclave. Sterilize articles in the autoclave. In the space provided, indicate the articles you sterilized.

_____

_____

_____

_____

Notes

EVALUATION OF COMPETENCY

Procedure 18-1: Sanitization of Instruments

Name: _____   Date: _____

Evaluated By: _____   Score: _____

Performance Objective

Outcome:	Sanitize instruments.
Conditions:	Given the following: disposable gloves, utility gloves, contaminated instruments, chemical disinfectant and MSDS, disinfectant container, cleaning solution and MSDS, basin, nylon brush, wire brush, paper towels, cloth towel, and instrument lubricant.
Standards:	Time: 10 minutes. Student completed procedure in ____ minutes.
	Accuracy: Satisfactory score on the Performance Evaluation Checklist.

Performance Evaluation Checklist

Trial 1	Trial 2	Point Value	Performance Standards
		●	Reviewed the MSDS for hazardous chemicals being used.
		●	Applied gloves.
		●	Transported the contaminated instruments to the cleaning area.
		●	Applied heavy-duty utility gloves over the disposable gloves.
		▷	Stated the purpose of the utility gloves.
		●	Separated sharp instruments and delicate instruments from other instruments.
		▷	Explained why instruments should be separated.
		●	Immediately rinsed the instruments thoroughly under warm running water.
		▷	Stated why the instruments should be rinsed immediately.
			Decontaminated the Instruments
		●	Checked the expiration date of the chemical disinfectant.
		▷	Explained why an expired disinfectant should not be used.
		●	Observed all personal safety precautions listed on the label.
		●	Followed label directions for proper use and mixing of the disinfectant.
		●	Labeled the disinfecting container with the name of the disinfectant and the reuse expiration date.
		●	Poured the disinfectant into the labeled container.
		●	Completely submerged the articles in the disinfectant.
		●	Covered the disinfectant container.

Trial 1	Trial 2	Point Value	Performance Standards
		▷	Stated the reason for covering the container.
		●	Disinfected the articles for 10 minutes.
		▷	Explained the reason for decontaminating the instruments.
			Cleaned the Instruments: Manual Method
		●	Checked the expiration date of the cleaning agent.
		●	Observed all personal safety precautions.
		●	Followed label directions for proper use and mixing of the cleaning agent.
		●	Removed articles from disinfectant and placed them in the cleaning solution.
		●	Cleaned the surface of the instruments with a nylon brush.
		●	Cleaned grooves, crevices, or serrations with a wire brush.
		●	Removed stains using commercial stain remover.
		●	Scrubbed the instruments until they were visibly clean.
		▷	Explained why all organic matter must be removed.
			Cleaned the Instruments: Ultrasound Method
		●	Prepared the cleaning solution in the ultrasonic cleaner.
		●	Observed all personal safety precautions listed on the label.
		●	Removed the articles from the disinfectant.
		●	Separated instruments of dissimilar metals.
		●	Properly placed the instruments in the ultrasonic cleaner.
		●	Positioned hinged instruments in an open position.
		▷	Stated why hinged instruments must be in an open position.
		●	Ensured that sharp instruments did not touch other instruments.
		●	Checked to see that all instruments were fully submerged.
		●	Placed the lid on the ultrasonic cleaner.
		●	Turned on the ultrasonic cleaner.
		●	Cleaned the instruments for the length of time recommended by the manufacturer.
		●	Removed the instruments from the machine.
		●	Rinsed each instrument thoroughly with warm water for 20 to 30 seconds.
		▷	Explained why instruments should be rinsed thoroughly.
		●	Dried each instrument with a paper towel.
		●	Placed instrument on a towel for additional drying.
		▷	Stated the reason for drying the instruments.
		●	Checked each instrument for defects and proper working condition.
		●	Lubricated hinged instruments in an open position.
		●	Opened and closed the instrument to distribute the lubricant.
		●	Placed the lubricated instrument on a towel to drain.

Trial 1	Trial 2	Point Value	Performance Standards
		▷	Stated the reason for lubricating instruments.
		●	Disposed of the cleaning solution according to the manufacturer's instructions.
		●	Removed both sets of gloves.
		●	Sanitized hands.
		●	Wrapped the instruments.
		●	Sterilized the instruments in the autoclave.
		＊	Completed the procedure within 10 minutes.
			TOTALS

Evaluation of Student Performance

EVALUATION CRITERIA			COMMENTS
Symbol	Category	Point Value	
＊	Critical Step	16 points	
●	Essential Step	6 points	
▷	Theory Question	2 points	
Score calculation: 100 points			
− _____ points missed			
_____ Score			
Satisfactory score: 85 or above			

CAAHEP Competencies Achieved:

Psychomotor (Skills)
☑ III. 5. Prepare items for autoclaving.

ABHES Competencies Achieved:

☑ 9. b. Apply principles of aseptic techniques and infection control.

Notes

EVALUATION OF COMPETENCY

Procedure 18-2: Wrapping Instruments Using Paper or Muslin

Name: _____   Date: _____

Evaluated By: _____   Score: _____

Performance Objective

Outcome:	Wrap an instrument for autoclaving.
Conditions:	Given the following: sanitized instrument, wrapping material, sterilization indicator strip, autoclave tape, and a permanent marker.
Standards:	Time: 5 minutes. Student completed procedure in _____ minutes.
	Accuracy: Satisfactory score on the Performance Evaluation Checklist.

Performance Evaluation Checklist

Trial 1	Trial 2	Point Value	Performance Standards
		●	Sanitized hands.
		●	Assembled equipment.
		●	Selected the appropriate-sized wrapping material.
		●	Checked the expiration date on the sterilization indicator box.
		▷	Stated why outdated strips should not be used.
		●	Placed wrapping material on clean, flat surface.
		●	Turned the wrap in a diagonal position.
		●	Placed instrument in the center of wrapping material.
		●	Placed instruments with movable joints in an open position.
		▷	Stated why instruments with movable joints must be placed in an open position.
		●	Placed a sterilization indicator in the center of the pack.
		●	Folded wrapping material up from the bottom and doubled back a small corner.
		●	Folded over the right edge of wrapping material and doubled back the corner.
		●	Folded over the left edge of wrapping material and doubled back the corner.
		●	Folded the pack up from the bottom and secured with autoclave tape.
		●	Ensured that the pack was firm enough for handling, but loose enough to permit proper circulation of steam.
		▷	Stated why instruments are wrapped for autoclaving.
		●	Labeled and dated the pack. Included your initials.
		▷	Stated the purpose for dating the pack.
		✳	Completed the procedure within 5 minutes.
			TOTALS

Evaluation of Student Performance

EVALUATION CRITERIA			COMMENTS
Symbol	Category	Point Value	
∗	Critical Step	16 points	
●	Essential Step	6 points	
▷	Theory Question	2 points	

Score calculation: 100 points

− _____ points missed

_____ Score

Satisfactory score: 85 or above

CAAHEP Competencies Achieved:

Psychomotor (Skills)

☑ III. 5. Prepare items for autoclaving.

ABHES Competencies Achieved:

☑ 9. h. Wrap items for autoclaving.

EVALUATION OF COMPETENCY

Procedure 18-3: Wrapping Instruments Using a Pouch

Name: _____   Date: _____

Evaluated By: _____   Score: _____

Performance Objective

Outcome:	Wrap an instrument for autoclaving.
Conditions:	Given the following: sanitized instrument, sterilization pouch, and a permanent marker.
Standards:	Time: 5 minutes. Student completed procedure in ____ minutes.
	Accuracy: Satisfactory score on the Performance Evaluation Checklist.

Performance Evaluation Checklist

Trial 1	Trial 2	Point Value	Performance Standards
		●	Sanitized hands.
		●	Assembled equipment.
		●	Selected the appropriate-sized pouch.
		●	Placed the pouch on a clean, flat surface.
		●	Labeled and dated the pack. Included your initials.
		●	Inserted the instrument into the open end of the pouch.
		●	Sealed the pouch.
		●	Sterilized the pack in the autoclave.
		▷	Stated how long the pack is sterile once it has been autoclaved.
		＊	Completed the procedure within 5 minutes.
			TOTALS

Evaluation of Student Performance

EVALUATION CRITERIA			COMMENTS
Symbol	Category	Point Value	
∗	Critical Step	16 points	
●	Essential Step	6 points	
▷	Theory Question	2 points	

Score calculation: 100 points
        −_____ points missed
        _____ Score

Satisfactory score: 85 or above

CAAHEP Competencies Achieved:

Psychomotor (Skills)
☑ III. 5. Prepare items for autoclaving.

ABHES Competencies Achieved:

☑ 9. h. Wrap items for autoclaving.

EVALUATION OF COMPETENCY

Procedure 18-4: Sterilizing Articles in the Autoclave

Name: _____   Date: _____

Evaluated By: _____   Score: _____

Performance Objective

Outcome:	Sterilize a load of contaminated articles in the autoclave.
Conditions:	Using an autoclave.
	Given the following: autoclave operating manual, distilled water, wrapped articles, and heat-resistant gloves.
Standards:	Time: 10 minutes. Student completed procedure in ____ minutes.
	Accuracy: Satisfactory score on the Performance Evaluation Checklist.

Performance Evaluation Checklist

Trial 1	Trial 2	Point Value	Performance Standards
		•	Assembled equipment.
		•	Checked the water level in the autoclave.
		•	Properly loaded the autoclave.
			Manually Operated the Autoclave
		•	Determined the sterilizing time for the type of articles being autoclaved.
		•	Turned on the autoclave.
		•	Filled the chamber with water.
		•	Closed and latched the door.
		•	Set the timing control.
		▷	Stated when the timer should be set.
		•	Vented the chamber of steam.
		•	Dried the load.
		▷	Stated the reason for drying the load.
			Automatically Operated the Autoclave
		•	Closed and latched the door.
		•	Turned on the autoclave.
		•	Determined the sterilization program.
		•	Pressed the appropriate program button.
		•	Pressed the start button.

Trial 1	Trial 2	Point Value	Performance Standards
		▷	Stated the purpose of each control or indicator on the autoclave.
		●	Turned off the autoclave.
		●	Removed the load with heat-resistant gloves.
		▷	Stated the reason for using heat-resistant gloves.
		●	Inspected the packs as they were removed for damage.
		▷	Explained what should be done if a pack is torn.
		●	Checked the sterilization indicators on the outside of the packs.
		●	Recorded information in the autoclave log.
		●	Stored the articles in a clean, dust-proof area.
		●	Placed the most recently sterilized packs behind previously sterilized packs.
		●	Maintained appropriate daily care of the autoclave.
		▷	Described the care the autoclave should receive each day.
		✳	Completed the procedure within 10 minutes.
			TOTALS

Evaluation of Student Performance

EVALUATION CRITERIA			COMMENTS
Symbol	**Category**	**Point Value**	
✳	Critical Step	16 points	
●	Essential Step	6 points	
▷	Theory Question	2 points	

Score calculation: 100 points

− _____ points missed

_____ Score

Satisfactory score: 85 or above

CAAHEP Competencies Achieved:

Psychomotor (Skills)
☑ III. 6. Perform sterilization procedures.

Affective (Behavior)
☑ IX. 3. Recognize the importance of local, state, and federal legislation and regulations in the practice setting.

ABHES Competencies Achieved:

☑ 9. o.(4) Perform sterilization techniques.

19

Vital Signs

CHAPTER ASSIGNMENTS

√ After Completing	Date Due	Textbook Page(s)	TEXTBOOK ASSIGNMENTS	Possible Points	Points You Earned
		325-374	Read Chapter 19: Vital Signs		
		336 372	Read Case Study 1 Case Study 1 questions	5	
		349 372	Read Case Study 2 Case Study 2 questions	5	
		362 372	Read Case Study 3 Case Study 3 questions	5	
			TOTAL POINTS		
√ After Completing	Date Due	Study Guide Page(s)	STUDY GUIDE ASSIGNMENTS (CTA: Critical Thinking Activity)	Possible Points	Points You Earned
		275	Pretest	10	
		276-277	Key Term Assessment	55	
		278-285	Evaluation of Learning questions	88	
		285-287	CTA A: Measurement of Body Temperature	18	
		287	CTA B: Alterations in Body Temperature	5	
		288	CTA C: Pulse Sites	6	
		288	CTA D: Pulse and Respiratory Rates	3	
		288-289	CTA E: Pulse Oximetry	18	
		289-290	CTA F: Blood Pressure Measurement	6	
		290	CTA G: Proper BP Cuff Selection	12	
		291	CTA H: Reading Blood Pressure Values	8	

√ After Completing	Date Due	Study Guide Page(s)	STUDY GUIDE ASSIGNMENTS (CTA: Critical Thinking Activity)	Possible Points	Points You Earned
			CD Activity: Chapter 19 Under Pressure (Record points earned)		
		291	CTA I: Interpreting Blood Pressure Readings	10	
		292	CTA J: Hypertension	20	
		294	CTA K: Crossword Puzzle	30	
		296	CTA L: GO TO! Game (Record points earned)		
			CD Activity: Chapter 19 Road to Recovery Game: Vital Signs Terminology (Record points earned)		
			CD Activity: Chapter 19 Animations	20	
			CD Activity: Chapter 19 Apply Your Knowledge questions (Record points earned)		
		275	Posttest	10	
			ADDITIONAL ASSIGNMENTS		
			TOTAL POINTS		

√ When Assigned by Your Instructor	Study Guide Page(s)	Practices Required	LABORATORY ASSIGNMENTS	*Score
	299	5	**DVD Practice for Competency** 19-1: Measuring Oral Body Temperature: Electronic Thermometer Textbook reference: pp. 336-338	
	305-306		**Evaluation of Competency** 19-1: Measuring Oral Body Temperature: Electronic Thermometer	*
	299	3	**DVD Practice for Competency** 19-2: Measuring Axillary Body Temperature: Electronic Thermometer Textbook reference: pp. 338-339	
	307-308		**Evaluation of Competency** 19-2: Measuring Axillary Body Temperature: Electronic Thermometer	*
	299	3	**DVD Practice for Competency** 19-3: Measuring Rectal Body Temperature: Electronic Thermometer Textbook reference: pp. 340-341	
	309-310		**Evaluation of Competency** 19-3: Measuring Rectal Body Temperature: Electronic Thermometer	*
	299	5	**DVD Practice for Competency** 19-4: Measuring Aural Body Temperature: Tympanic Membrane Thermometer Textbook reference: pp. 341-343	
	311-312		**Evaluation of Competency** 19-4: Measuring Aural Body Temperature: Tympanic Membrane Thermometer	*
	299	5	**DVD Practice for Competency** 19-5: Measuring Temporal Artery Body Temperature Textbook reference: pp. 344-346	
	313-314		**Evaluation of Competency** 19-5: Measuring Temporal Artery Body Temperature	*
	301	10	**DVD Practice for Competency** 19-6: Measuring Pulse and Respiration Textbook reference: pp. 356-357	
	315-316		**Evaluation of Competency** 19-6: Measuring Pulse and Respiration	*
	301	5	**DVD Practice for Competency** 19-7: Measuring Apical Pulse Textbook reference: pp. 357-358	

√ When Assigned by Your Instructor	Study Guide Page(s)	Practices Required	LABORATORY ASSIGNMENTS	*Score
	317-318		▨ **Evaluation of Competency** 19-7: Measuring Apical Pulse	*
	301	5	⊙ **Practice for Competency** 19-8: Performing Pulse Oximetry Textbook reference: pp. 358-360	
	319-321		▨ **Evaluation of Competency** 19-8: Performing Pulse Oximetry	*
	303	10	⊙ **Practice for Competency** 19-9: Measuring Blood Pressure Textbook reference: pp. 368-371	
	323-325		▨ **Evaluation of Competency** 19-9: Measuring Blood Pressure	*
			ADDITIONAL ASSIGNMENTS	

Name _____   Date _____

PRETEST

True or False

_____ 1. The heat-regulating center of the body is the medulla.

_____ 2. A vague sense of body discomfort, weakness, and fatigue that often marks the onset of a disease is known as the *blahs*.

_____ 3. If an axillary temperature of 100°F was taken orally, it would register as 101°F.

_____ 4. If the lens of a tympanic membrane thermometer is dirty, the reading may be falsely low.

_____ 5. Chemical thermometers should be stored in the freezer.

_____ 6. The femoral pulse site can be used to assess circulation to the foot.

_____ 7. The term used to describe an irregularity in the heart's rhythm is dysrhythmia.

_____ 8. Pulse oximetry provides the physician with information on the amount of oxygen being delivered to the tissues.

_____ 9. Blood pressure measures the contraction and relaxation of the heart.

_____ 10. When taking BP, the stethoscope is placed over the brachial artery.

POSTTEST

True or False

_____ 1. A temperature of 100°F is classified as a low-grade fever.

_____ 2. The rectal site should not be used to take the temperature of a newborn.

_____ 3. A tympanic membrane thermometer should not be used to measure temperature on a patient who has a normal amount of cerumen in the ear.

_____ 4. A temporal artery temperature reading is the same as an oral reading.

_____ 5. Excessive pressure should not be applied when measuring pulse because it could obstruct the pulse.

_____ 6. A child has a faster pulse rate than an adult.

_____ 7. The normal respiratory rate of an adult ranges between 10 and 18 respirations per minute.

_____ 8. The term used to describe a bluish discoloration of the skin due to a lack of oxygen is hypoxia.

_____ 9. The oxygen saturation level of a healthy individual falls between 85% and 90%.

_____ 10. When measuring blood pressure, the patient's arm should be positioned above the level of the heart.

KEY TERM ASSESSMENT

Temperature

Directions: Match each medical term with its definition.

_____ 1. Afebrile

_____ 2. Antipyretic

_____ 3. Axilla

_____ 4. Celsius scale

_____ 5. Conduction

_____ 6. Convection

_____ 7. Crisis

_____ 8. Disinfectant

_____ 9. Fahrenheit scale

_____ 10. Febrile

_____ 11. Fever

_____ 12. Frenulum linguae

_____ 13. Hyperpyrexia

_____ 14. Hypothermia

_____ 15. Malaise

_____ 16. Radiation

A. An extremely high fever
B. An agent used to destroy disease-producing microorganisms but not necessarily their spores (usually applied to inanimate objects)
C. A body temperature that is below normal
D. The armpit
E. The transfer of energy, such as heat, through air currents
F. A body temperature that is above normal (pyrexia)
G. An agent that reduces fever
H. A temperature scale on which the freezing point of water is 32° and the boiling point of water is 212°
I. The transfer of energy, such as heat, in the form of waves
J. A temperature scale on which the freezing point of water is 0° and the boiling point is 100°
K. The midline fold that connects the undersurface of the tongue with the floor of the mouth
L. Pertaining to fever
M. The transfer of energy, from one object to another
N. A sudden falling of an elevated body temperature to normal
O. Without fever; the body temperature is normal
P. A vague sense of body discomfort, weakness, and fatigue often marking the onset of a disease and continuing through the course of the illness

Pulse

Directions: Match each medical term with its definition.

_____ 1. Antecubital space

_____ 2. Aorta

_____ 3. Bounding pulse

_____ 4. Bradycardia

_____ 5. Dysrhythmia

_____ 6. Intercostal

_____ 7. Pulse rhythm

_____ 8. Pulse volume

_____ 9. Tachycardia

_____ 10. Thready pulse

A. Between the ribs
B. A pulse with an increased volume that feels very strong and full
C. The strength of the heartbeat
D. The space located at the front of the elbow
E. An abnormally fast heart rate (greater than 100 beats per minute)
F. The major trunk of the arterial system of the body
G. The time interval between heartbeats
H. A pulse with a decreased volume that feels weak and thin
I. An irregular rhythm
J. An abnormally slow heart rate (greater than 60 beats per minute)

Respiration and Pulse Oximetry

Directions: Match each medical term with its definition.

_____ 1. Alveolus

_____ 2. Apnea

_____ 3. Bradypnea

_____ 4. Cyanosis

_____ 5. Dyspnea

_____ 6. Eupnea

_____ 7. Exhalation

_____ 8. Hyperpnea

_____ 9. Hyperventilation

_____ 10. Hypopnea

_____ 11. Hypoxemia

_____ 12. Hypoxia

_____ 13. Inhalation

_____ 14. Orthopnea

_____ 15. Pulse oximeter

_____ 16. Pulse oximetry

_____ 17. SaO_2

_____ 18. SpO_2

_____ 19. Tachypnea

A. The act of breathing out
B. A reduction in the oxygen supply to the tissues of the body
C. A decrease in the oxygen saturation of the blood; may lead to hypoxia
D. The temporary cessation of breathing
E. An abnormal increase in the respiratory rate of more than 20 respirations per minute
F. A computerized device consisting of a probe and monitor used to measure the oxygen saturation of arterial blood
G. An abnormal decrease in the rate and depth of respiration
H. A thin-walled air sac of the lungs in which the exchange of oxygen and carbon dioxide takes place
I. The use of a pulse oximeter to measure the oxygen saturation of arterial blood
J. The act of breathing in
K. A bluish discoloration of the skin and mucous membranes first observed in the nail beds and lips
L. Abbreviation for the percentage of hemoglobin that is saturated with oxygen in arterial blood
M. The condition in which breathing is easier when an individual is in a standing or sitting position
N. Shortness of breath or difficulty in breathing
O. Abbreviation for the percentage of hemoglobin that is saturated with oxygen in arterial blood as measured by a pulse oximeter
P. Normal respiration
Q. An abnormally fast and deep type of breathing usually associated with acute anxiety conditions
R. An abnormal decrease in the respiratory rate of less than 10 respirations per minute
S. An abnormal increase in the rate and depth of respiration

Blood Pressure

Directions: Match each medical term with its definition.

_____ 1. Diastole

_____ 2. Diastolic pressure

_____ 3. Hypertension

_____ 4. Hypotension

_____ 5. Meniscus

_____ 6. Pulse pressure

_____ 7. Sphygmomanometer

_____ 8. Stethoscope

_____ 9. Systole

_____ 10. Systolic pressure

A. The curved surface on a column of liquid in a tube
B. High blood pressure
C. The point of maximum pressure on the arterial walls
D. The phase in the cardiac cycle in which the heart relaxes between contractions
E. An instrument for measuring arterial blood pressure
F. The point of lesser pressure on the arterial walls
G. Low blood pressure
H. The phase in the cardiac cycle in which the ventricles contract, sending blood out of the heart and into the aorta and pulmonary aorta
I. An instrument for amplifying and hearing sounds produced by the body
J. The difference between the systolic and diastolic pressures

EVALUATION OF LEARNING

Temperature

Directions: Fill in each blank with the correct answer.

1. Define a vital sign.

   _____

2. What are the four vital signs?

   _____
   _____
   _____
   _____

3. What general guidelines should be followed when measuring vital signs?

   _____
   _____
   _____
   _____

4. List four ways in which heat is produced in the body.

   _____
   _____
   _____
   _____

5. List four ways in which heat is lost from the body.

   _____
   _____
   _____
   _____

6. What is the normal body temperature range?

   _____

7. What is a fever?

   _____
   _____

8. How do diurnal variations affect body temperature?

   _____
   _____

9. How does vigorous physical exercise affect body temperature?

   _____

10. How do emotional states affect the body temperature?

_____

11. What symptoms occur with a fever?

_____

_____

12. Describe the following fever patterns:

   a. Continuous fever: _____

   _____

   b. Intermittent fever: _____

   _____

   c. Remittent fever: _____

   _____

13. What is the subsiding stage of a fever?

_____

14. What five sites are used for taking body temperature?

_____

15. List three instances in which the axillary site for taking body temperature would be preferred over the oral site.

_____

_____

_____

16. Why does the rectal method for taking body temperature provide an accurate temperature measurement?

_____

_____

_____

17. When might the rectal method be used to take body temperature?

_____

_____

18. When might the aural method be used to take body temperature?

_____

_____

19. How does a temperature taken through the rectal and axillary methods compare (in terms of degrees) with a temperature taken through the oral method?

_____

_____

_____

20. List and describe the four types of thermometers available for taking body temperature.

_____

_____

_____

_____

21. What is the purpose of using a probe cover with an electronic thermometer?

_____

22. Describe the advantages of a tympanic membrane thermometer.

_____

_____

23. Explain how a tympanic membrane thermometer measures body temperature.

_____

_____

_____

24. Explain how to clean the lens of a tympanic membrane thermometer.

_____

_____

25. List two reasons why the temporal artery is a good site to measure body temperature.

_____

_____

26. How does the temperature obtained through the temporal site compare with oral, rectal, and axillary body temperature?

_____

_____

_____

27. List four factors that can result in a falsely low temperature reading when using the temporal artery thermometer.

_____

_____

28. Where should a chemical thermometer be stored? Explain why.

_____

_____

Pulse

Directions: Fill in each blank with the correct answer.

1. What causes the pulse to occur?

_____

_____

2. What measurement unit is used in checking the pulse rate?

_____

3. How does physical activity affect the pulse rate?

_____

4. What is the most common site for taking the pulse?

_____

5. List two reasons for taking the pulse at the apical pulse site.

_____

_____

6. Where is the apex of the heart located?

_____

_____

7. When is the brachial artery used as a pulse site?

_____

8. When is the carotid artery used as a pulse site?

_____

9. When is the femoral artery used as a pulse site?

_____

10. What two pulse sites can be used to assess circulation to the foot?

_____

11. List two reasons for measuring the pulse rate.

_____

_____

12. State the normal range for a pulse rate for an adult.

_____

13. What is the normal pulse range for the following age groups?
    a. Newborn: _____
    b. Toddler: _____
    c. Preschool child: _____
    d. School-age child: _____
    e. Adult older than age 60: _____

14. What is the normal pulse range for a well-trained athlete?

_____

15. What may cause tachycardia?

_____

16. If the rhythm and volume of a patient's pulse are normal, the medical assistant (MA) would record it as:

_____

Respiration

Directions: Fill in each blank with the correct answer.

1. What is the purpose of respiration?

   _____

   _____

2. What is the purpose of inhalation?

   _____

   _____

3. What is the purpose of exhalation?

   _____

   _____

4. What is included in one complete respiration?

   _____

   _____

5. The exchange of oxygen and carbon dioxide between the body cells and blood is known as:

   _____

6. What is the name of the control center for involuntary respiration?

   _____

7. Why must respiration be taken without the patient's awareness?

   _____

8. What is the normal respiratory rate (range) for a normal adult?

   _____

9. List two factors that increase the respiratory rate.

   _____

   _____

10. Describe a normal rhythm for respiration.

    _____

    _____

11. What are two conditions in which hyperventilation may occur?

    _____

12. What type of patient might experience hypopnea?

    _____

13. Where is cyanosis first observed?

    _____

    _____

14. In which kind of patients might cyanosis occur?

    _____

15. What are two conditions in which dyspnea may occur?

_____

_____

16. Describe the character of normal breath sounds.

_____

_____

17. Describe the character of the following abnormal breath sounds:

   a. Crackles: _____

   _____

   b. Rhonchi: _____

   _____

   c. Wheezes: _____

   _____

Pulse Oximetry

Directions: Fill in each blank with the correct answer.

1. What is the purpose of pulse oximetry?

   _____

   _____

2. What is the function of hemoglobin?

   _____

3. What is the oxygen saturation level of a healthy individual?

   _____

4. What might occur if the oxygen saturation level is 85% to 90%?

   _____

   _____

5. List three patient conditions that can cause a decreased SpO_2 value.

   _____

   _____

   _____

6. When might pulse oximetry be used for the short-term continuous monitoring of a patient?

   _____

   _____

7. What is the purpose of the power-on self-test (POST)?

   _____

   _____

8. What type of site must be used for applying a pulse oximeter probe?

   _____

   _____

9. How can dark fingernail polish cause a falsely low SpO$_2$ reading?

_____

_____

10. How can patient movement cause an inaccurate SpO$_2$ reading?

_____

_____

11. What type of patients may make it difficult to align the oximeter probe properly?

_____

_____

12. List three conditions that can cause poor peripheral blood flow.

_____

_____

13. Why must a reusable oximeter probe be free of all dirt and grime before it is used?

_____

_____

Blood Pressure

Directions: Fill in each blank with the correct answer.

1. What does blood pressure measure?

_____

_____

2. Why is the diastolic pressure lower than the systolic pressure?

_____

_____

_____

3. What is considered normal blood pressure for an adult?

_____

4. State the blood pressure range for each of the following:

   a. Prehypertension: _____

   b. Hypertension, stage 1: _____

   c. Hypertension, stage 2: _____

5. Why should blood pressure readings always be interpreted using the patient's baseline blood pressure?

_____

_____

6. How does age affect blood pressure?

_____

7. How do diurnal variations affect the blood pressure?

_____

_____

8. What are the two types of stethoscope chest pieces, and what is the use of each?

_____

_____

_____

_____

9. What are the parts of a sphygmomanometer?

_____

_____

10. Name the two types of sphygmomanometers.

_____

11. List the three different cuff sizes, and give examples of when each would be employed.

_____

_____

_____

12. Explain how to determine the proper cuff size for a patient.

_____

_____

13. What may occur if blood pressure is taken using a cuff that is too small or too large?

_____

_____

14. List the five phases included in the Korotkoff sounds and what type of sound is heard during each phase.

_____

_____

_____

_____

CRITICAL THINKING ACTIVITIES

A. MEASUREMENT OF BODY TEMPERATURE

For each of the following situations involving the measurement of body temperature, write _C_ if the technique is correct and _I_ if the technique is incorrect. If the situation is correct, state the principle underlying the technique. If the situation is incorrect, explain what might happen if the technique were performed in the incorrect manner.

Electronic Thermometer

_____ 1. The MA takes a patient's oral temperature immediately after the patient has consumed a cup of coffee.

_____

_____

_____ 2. The MA instructs the patient not to talk while his or her oral temperature is being measured.

_____

_____

_____ 3. The MA forgets to lubricate the rectal probe before taking a patient's rectal temperature.

_____

_____

_____ 4. An axillary temperature reading is recorded as follows: 102.2°F.

_____

_____

_____ 5. The MA discards a used rectal probe in a regular waste container.

_____

_____

_____ 6. The MA's bare fingers accidentally touch a used oral probe cover while discarding it.

_____

_____

Tympanic Membrane Thermometer

_____ 1. A tympanic membrane thermometer is used to take the temperature of a patient with impacted cerumen.

_____

_____

_____ 2. A thermometer with a dirty probe lens is used to take the patient's temperature.

_____

_____

_____ 3. The MA straightens the ear canal before taking a patient's aural temperature.

_____

_____

_____ 4. The MA does not seal the opening of the ear canal with the probe when taking aural temperature.

_____

_____

_____ 5. The probe is positioned toward the opposite temple when taking aural temperature.

_____

_____

_____ 6. The MA waits 30 seconds before taking the patient's temperature in the same ear.

_____

_____

Temporal Artery Thermometer

_____ 1. The MA checks to ensure the probe lens is clean and intact before using a temporal artery thermometer.

_____

_____

____ 2. The MA brushes hair away from the patient's forehead before measuring the patient's temperature.

_____

_____

____ 3. The MA slides the temporal artery probe across the patient's forehead while continually depressing the scan button.

_____

_____

____ 4. The MA quickly scans the patient's forehead during temporal artery temperature measurement.

_____

_____

____ 5. After scanning the forehead, the MA records the patient's temporal artery temperature reading.

_____

_____

____ 6. The MA cleans the temporal artery thermometer by immersing it in warm sudsy water.

_____

_____

B. ALTERATIONS IN BODY TEMPERATURE
Label the diagram below with the terms that describe the body temperature alteration.

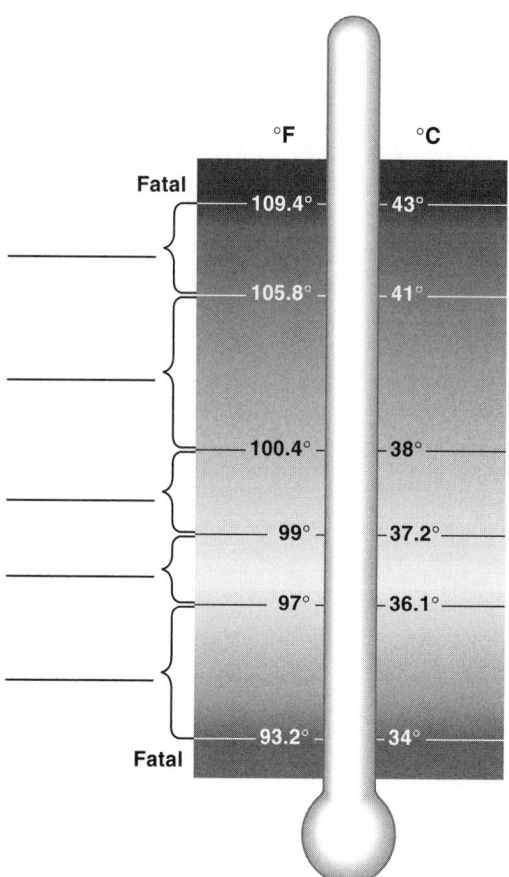

(From Bonewit-West K: _Study guide for clinical procedures for medical assistants_, ed 7, St. Louis, 2008, Saunders.)

C. PULSE SITES
Locate the pulse at the following sites, and record the pulse rates.

1. Brachial pulse: _____

2. Temporal pulse: _____

3. Carotid pulse: _____

4. Femoral pulse: _____

5. Popliteal pulse: _____

6. Dorsalis pedis pulse: _____

D. PULSE AND RESPIRATORY RATES
Measure the pulse and respiration of a person before and after vigorous exercise, and record the results.

1. Before vigorous exercise

   _____

   _____

2. After vigorous exercise

   _____

   _____

3. Compare the results, and explain how exercise affects the pulse and respiratory rates.

   _____

   _____

E. PULSE OXIMETRY
The physician asks you to measure the oxygen saturation level of the following patients. For each situation, answer the following questions:

a. What would you do in each situation to prevent an inaccurate pulse oximetry reading?

b. What occurs with each of these situations, and how does it affect the SpO_2 reading?

1. Kelly Collins, a patient with chronic bronchitis, is wearing navy blue nail polish.

   _____

   _____

2. Melvin Hosey has Parkinson's disease and is having difficulty controlling tremors in his hands.

   _____

   _____

3. Scott Kimes, a patient with emphysema, frequently experiences periods of prolonged coughing.

   _____

   _____

4. Nicole Lowe has returned to the office for a recheck of her pneumonia condition. You are getting ready to measure her oxygen saturation and notice that bright sunlight is coming through the window where she is seated and is shining on her hand.

   _____

   _____

5. Rebecca Bensie, a patient on oxygen therapy, is morbidly obese, and you are having trouble properly aligning the oximeter probe on her finger.

_____

_____

6. Doug Habbershaw, a patient with peripheral vascular disease, has come to the office for a health checkup.

_____

_____

7. Emily Lacey has come to the office because she has been experiencing dyspnea. Her hands are cold, and this is interfering with the pulse oximetry procedure.

_____

_____

8. Susan Boone, a patient with asthma, is wearing artificial fingernails.

_____

_____

9. Frank Stewart, a patient with congestive heart failure, is at the office to have a mole removed from his back. There are bright overhead lights in the room, and they cannot be turned off because the physician needs good lighting to perform the surgery.

_____

_____

10. Wanda Weaver is having a sebaceous cyst removed from her chest and has been sedated for the procedure. You have applied an automatic blood pressure cuff to her right arm. The physician asks you to apply an oximeter probe to monitor her oxygen saturation level continuously during the procedure.

_____

_____

11. Which control, indicator, or display is involved when the following occurs?

a. The oximeter is searching for a pulse: _____

b. The oximeter cannot find a pulse: _____

c. The oximeter is portraying the strength of the pulse: _____

d. You turn up the audible beeping sound of the pulse rate: _____

e. The oximeter displays the oxygen saturation level: _____

f. The oximeter displays the pulse rate: _____

g. The battery is low: _____

h. You turn the oximeter off: _____

F. BLOOD PRESSURE MEASUREMENT

Using the principles outlined in the Procedure for Measuring Blood Pressure, explain what happens under the following circumstances:

1. The BP is taken on a patient who has just undergone vigorous physical exercise.

_____

2. The BP is taken on a patient with tight sleeves.

_____

_____

3. An adult cuff is used to measure BP on a young child.

_____

_____

4. The rubber bladder is not centered over the brachial artery.

_____

_____

5. The cuff is placed ½ inch above the bend in the elbows.

_____

_____

6. The manometer is viewed from a distance of 4 feet.

_____

_____

G. PROPER BP CUFF SELECTION

Listed below are the measurements of the arm circumference (in cm) of different patients. Using Table 19-9, indicate what size blood pressure cuff (child, small adult, adult, large adult, or adult thigh) should be used with each of these patients.

1. 47 cm: _____

2. 20 cm: _____

3. 32 cm: _____

4. 16 cm: _____

5. 38 cm: _____

6. 27 cm: _____

7. 52 cm: _____

8. 24 cm: _____

Measure the arm circumference of four classmates, and record the values. Next to each value, indicate what size blood pressure cuff should be used with each of these individuals.

1. _____

2. _____

3. _____

4. _____

H. READING BLOOD PRESSURE VALUES

Read and record the following blood pressure measurements in the space provided.

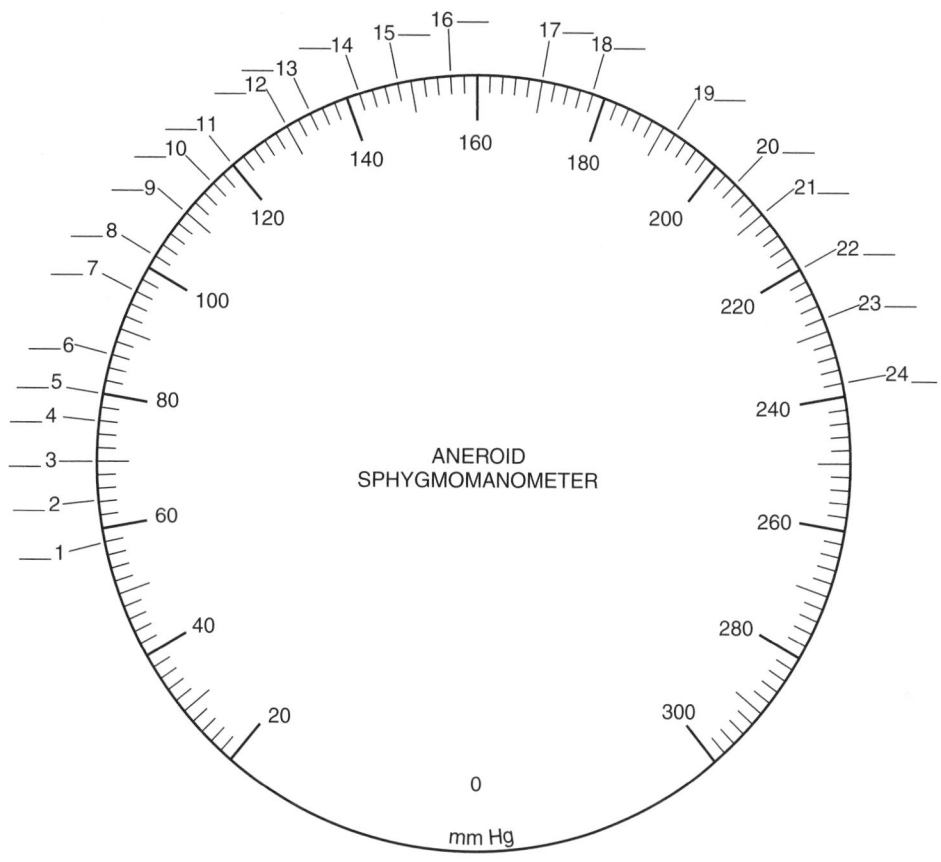

(From Bonewit-West K: *Study guide for clinical procedures for medical assistants*, ed 7, St. Louis, 2008, Saunders.)

I. INTERPRETING BLOOD PRESSURE READINGS

Classify each of the following blood pressure readings into its appropriate category. The readings are based on the average of two or more properly measured, seated blood pressure readings taken at each of two or more visits.

Normal
Prehypertension
Hypertension: stage 1
Hypertension: stage 2

1. 90/66: _____
2. 126/76: _____
3. 146/88: _____
4. 120/88: _____
5. 120/80: _____
6. 158/102: _____
7. 134/82: _____
8. 180/106: _____
9. 104/60: _____
10. 148/94: _____

J. HYPERTENSION

Create a profile of an individual who is at risk for developing hypertension following these guidelines:

1. Using colored pencils, crayons, or markers, draw a figure of an individual exhibiting risk factors for hypertension. Be as creative as possible.

2. Do not use any text in your drawing, other than to label items you have drawn in your picture (e.g., cigarettes). (A picture is worth a thousand words!)

3. Include at least six risk factors for hypertension in your drawing. The Patient Teaching box on hypertension in your textbook can be used as a reference source.

4. In the classroom, choose a partner and trade drawings. Identify the risk factors for hypertension in your partner's drawing. With your partner, discuss what this person could do to lower his or her chances of developing hypertension.

K. CROSSWORD PUZZLE
Vital Signs
Directions: Complete the crossword puzzle using the clues presented below. All of your answers can be found in either a box or a table in your textbook.

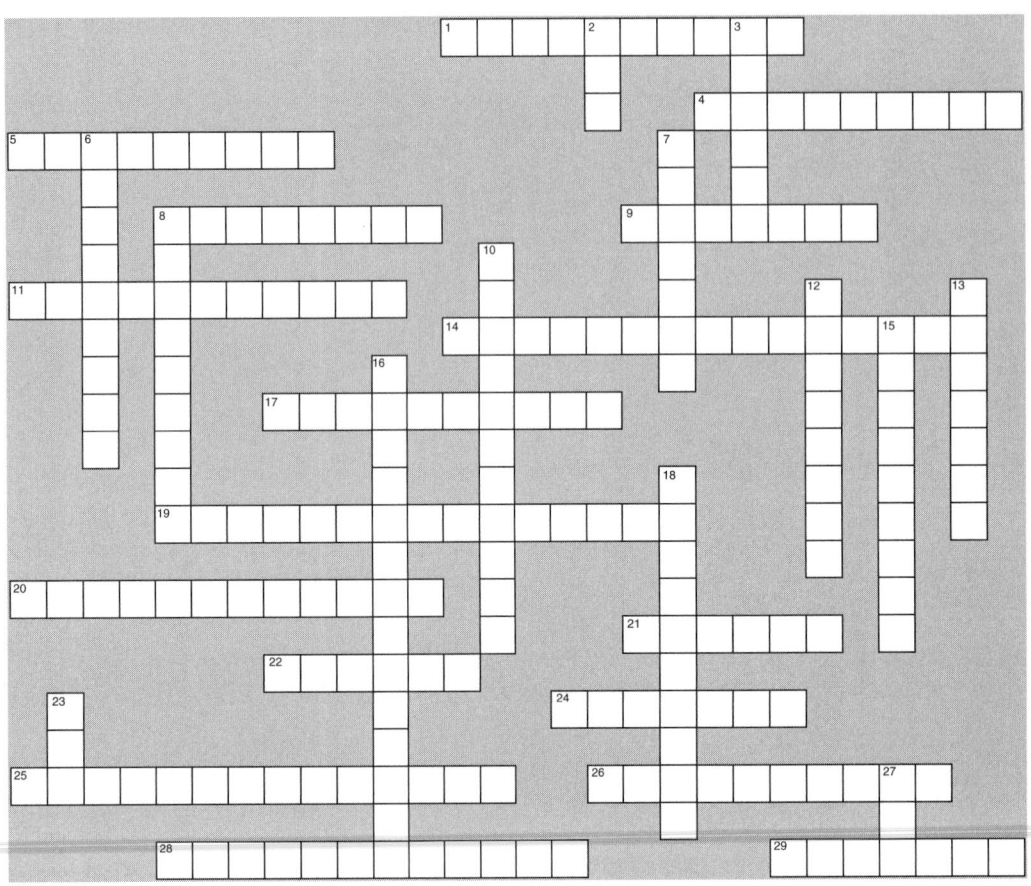

(From Bonewit-West K: *Study guide for clinical procedures for medical assistants*, ed 7, St. Louis, 2008, Saunders.)

ACROSS

1 Diaphragm or bell
4 Angled stethoscope earpieces
5 BP sounds
8 Has an S shape
9 European temperature measurement
11 Fever reducer
14 Fever increases this by 7%
17 U.S. temperature measurement
19 Lowers pulse rate over time
20 Above 140/90
21 High BP might cause this
22 2400 mg or less per day
24 Asthma breath sounds
25 Center BP cuff over this
26 Risk factor for high BP
28 Cools body
29 Cracked earpieces can cause this

DOWN

2 Pulse range for exercising
3 Body temperature increaser
6 Fever that occurs with the flu
7 Invented the stethoscope
8 COPD example
10 Profuse perspiration
12 Do this after aerobic exercise
13 Leading cause of COPD
15 Fever causer
16 Drug to help COPD
18 BP position for patient's arm
23 220 minus your age
27 Good cholesterol

Notes

L. GO TO! GAME

Object:	To demonstrate your knowledge of locating pulse sites and answering questions relating to the vital signs
Needed:	**GO TO!** game board (located in this chapter)
	Completed Evaluation of Learning questions from this chapter
	A small token for each player (e.g., a small button)
	Dice (2)
	Score card

Directions:

1. Complete and review the Vital Signs Evaluation of Learning questions in your Student Study Guide.
2. Get into a group of four players.
3. Each player selects one of the four vital sign question sections (temperature, pulse, respiration, or blood pressure). The player tears that page out of his or her manual.
4. In turn, each player rolls the dice and GOES TO the pulse site indicated on the game board. (If a player rolls an 11, he or she loses a turn and the next player rolls the dice.)
5. If the player:
   a. Goes to the correct pulse site, he or she asks for a question from a vital signs category (other than his or her own category). Example: "Blood pressure."
   b. Does not go to the correct pulse site, the player is not permitted to ask for a question and must wait until his or her next turn to earn points.
6. The player with the category selected reads a question from his or her page of questions.
7. If the player answers the question correctly, he or she is awarded 5 points. If the player does not answer the question correctly, he or she receives no points.
8. If you have any questions regarding the correct pulse site or answer to a question, consult your instructor for assistance.
9. Keep track of your points using the score card provided.
10. When all of the questions from a category have been used, that category is deleted as a possible selection.
11. Continue until all of the Evaluation of Learning questions have been answered.
12. Calculate your points, and determine the knowledge level you attained.

GO TO!
SCORE CARD

Name: _____

Recording Points:
Cross off a number each time you answer a question correctly (starting with 5 and continuing in sequence). Your points will be equal to the last number you crossed off. Record this number in the space provided and determine the Knowledge Level you attained.

Points:	
5	75
10	80
15	85
20	90
25	95
30	100
35	105
40	110
45	115
50	120
55	125
60	130
65	135
70	140

TOTAL POINTS: _____

LEVEL OF KNOWLEDGE:

☐ 75 points and above: **Sheer genius**
☐ 55 to 70 points: **Shows great promise**
☐ 35 to 50 points: **Time to study**
☐ Below 35 points: **Brain freeze**

GO TO!

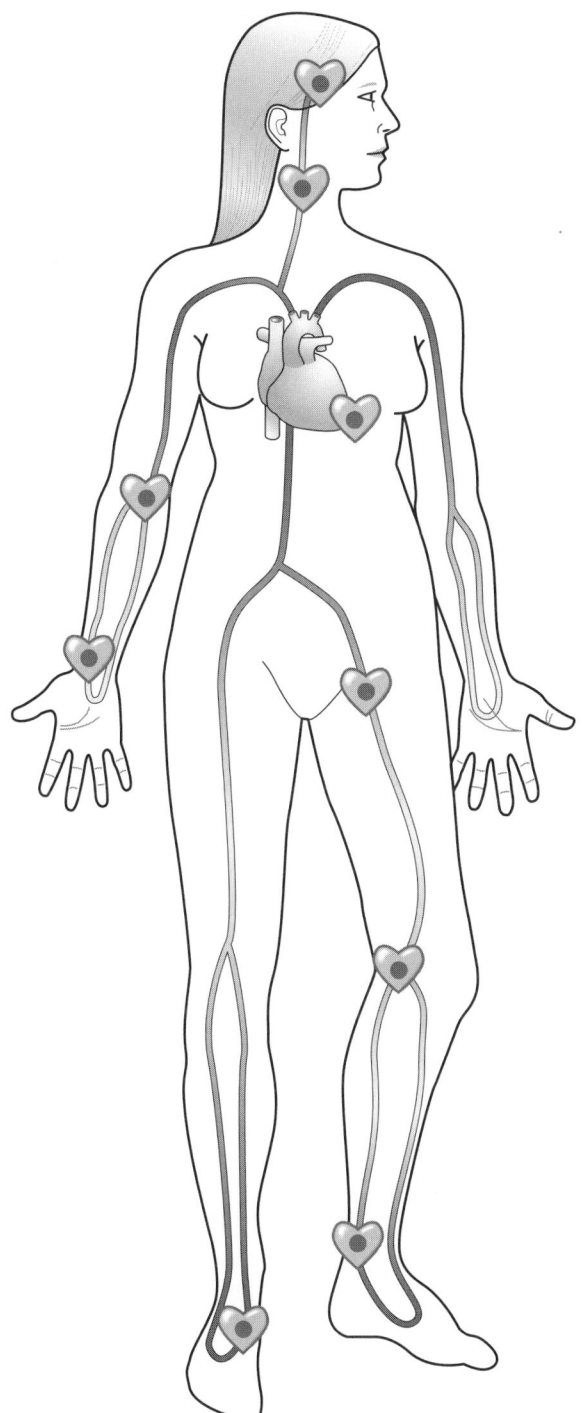

PULSE SITES	
Dice throws:	
Value	Go to
2	Radial
3	Apical
4	Brachial
5	Temporal
6	Carotid
7	Femoral
8	Popliteal
9	Dorsalis pedis
10	Posterior tibial
11	Dysrhythmia detected *Lose this turn*
12	Pulse is regular and strong Go wherever you want *Bonus of 5 points*

(From Bonewit-West K: *Study guide for clinical procedures for medical assistants*, ed 7, St. Louis, 2008, Saunders.)

PRACTICE FOR COMPETENCY

Measuring Body Temperature

Measure body temperature with each of the following types of thermometers, and record results in the chart provided.

Procedures 19-1, 19-2, and 19-3: Electronic Thermometer (Oral, Axillary, and Rectal)

Procedure 19-4: Tympanic Membrane Thermometer (Aural)

Procedure 19-5: Temporal Artery Thermometer

CHART	
Date	

CHART	
Date	

PRACTICE FOR COMPETENCY

Measuring Pulse, Respiration, and Oxygen Saturation

Procedure 19-6: Pulse and Respiration. Measure the radial pulse and respiration. Describe the rhythm and volume of the pulse. Describe the rhythm and depth of the respirations. Record the results in the chart provided.

Procedure 19-7: Apical Pulse. Measure apical pulse. Describe the rhythm and volume of the pulse. Record the results in the chart provided.

Procedure 19-8: Pulse Oximetry. Measure the oxygen saturation level, and record the results in the chart provided.

CHART	
Date	

CHART	
Date	

PRACTICE FOR COMPETENCY

Measuring Blood Pressure

Procedure 19-9: Blood Pressure. Measure blood pressure. Record results in the chart provided.

CHART	
Date	

CHART	
Date	

EVALUATION OF COMPETENCY

Procedure 19-1: Measuring Oral Body Temperature—Electronic Thermometer

Name: _____   Date: _____

Evaluated By: _____   Score: _____

Performance Objective

Outcome:	Measure oral body temperature.
Conditions:	Given the following: electronic thermometer and oral probe, probe cover, and a waste container.
Standards:	Time: 5 minutes. Student completed procedure in ____ minutes.
	Accuracy: Satisfactory score on the Performance Evaluation Checklist.

Performance Evaluation Checklist

Trial 1	Trial 2	Point Value	Performance Standards
		●	Sanitized hands.
		●	Assembled equipment.
		●	Removed thermometer from its base.
		●	Attached oral probe to thermometer unit.
		●	Inserted probe into the thermometer.
		●	Greeted the patient and introduced yourself.
		●	Identified the patient and explained the procedure.
		●	Asked the patient if he/she has ingested hot or cold beverages.
		▷	Explained what to do if the patient has recently ingested a hot or cold beverage.
		●	Removed probe from the thermometer.
		▷	Explained what occurs when probe is removed from the thermometer.
		●	Attached probe cover to probe.
		●	Stated the purpose of the probe cover.
		●	Correctly inserted the probe in patient's mouth.
		●	Instructed the patient to keep the mouth closed.
		▷	Explained why the mouth should be kept closed.
		●	Held probe in place until an audible tone was heard.
		●	Noted patient's temperature reading on display screen.
		●	Removed probe from patient's mouth.
		●	Discarded probe cover in a regular waste container.
		●	Did not allow fingers to come in contact with cover.

Trial 1	Trial 2	Point Value	*Performance Standards*
		●	Returned probe to the thermometer unit.
		▷	Stated what occurs when probe is returned to the thermometer.
		●	Returned the thermometer unit to its storage base.
		●	Sanitized hands.
		●	Charted the results correctly.
		✳	The temperature recording was identical to the reading on the display screen.
		▷	Stated the normal body temperature range for an adult (97°F to 99°F).
		✳	Completed the procedure within 5 minutes.
			TOTALS

CHART		
Date		

Evaluation of Student Performance

EVALUATION CRITERIA			COMMENTS
Symbol	Category	Point Value	
✳	Critical Step	16 points	
●	Essential Step	6 points	
▷	Theory Question	2 points	

Score calculation: 100 points

−_____ points missed

_____ Score

Satisfactory score: 85 or above

CAAHEP Competencies Achieved:

Psychomotor (Skills)
☑ I. 1. Obtain vital signs.

Affective (Behavior)
☑ I. 1. Apply critical thinking skills in performing patient assessment and care.

ABHES Competencies Achieved:

☑ 9. c. Take vital signs.

EVALUATION OF COMPETENCY

DVD   **Procedure 19-2: Measuring Axillary Body Temperature—Electronic Thermometer**

Name: _____ Date: _____

Evaluated By: _____ Score: _____

Performance Objective

Outcome:	Measure axillary body temperature.
Conditions:	Given the following: electronic thermometer and oral probe, probe cover, and a waste container.
Standards:	Time: 5 minutes. Student completed procedure in ____ minutes.
	Accuracy: Satisfactory score on the Performance Evaluation Checklist.

Performance Evaluation Checklist

Trial 1	Trial 2	Point Value	Performance Standards
		●	Sanitized hands.
		●	Assembled equipment.
		●	Removed thermometer from its storage base.
		●	Attached oral probe to thermometer unit.
		●	Inserted probe into the thermometer.
		●	Greeted the patient and introduced yourself.
		●	Identified the patient and explained the procedure.
		●	Removed clothing from patient's shoulder and arm.
		●	Made sure that the axilla was dry.
		●	Removed probe from the thermometer.
		●	Attached probe cover to probe.
		●	Placed probe in the center of the patient's axilla.
		●	Ensured that the arm was held close to the body.
		▷	Explained why the arm must be held close to the body.
		●	Held probe in place until an audible tone was heard.
		●	Removed probe from patient's axilla.
		●	Noted patient's temperature reading on display screen.
		●	Discarded probe cover in a regular waste container.
		●	Did not allow fingers to come in contact with cover.
		●	Returned probe to the thermometer unit.
		●	Returned the thermometer unit to its storage base.

Trial 1	Trial 2	Point Value	Performance Standards
		●	Sanitized hands.
		●	Charted the results correctly.
		✳	The temperature recording was identical to the reading on the display screen.
		✳	Completed the procedure within 5 minutes.
			TOTALS

CHART	
Date	

Evaluation of Student Performance

EVALUATION CRITERIA			COMMENTS
Symbol	Category	Point Value	
✳	Critical Step	16 points	
●	Essential Step	6 points	
▷	Theory Question	2 points	

Score calculation: 100 points

−_____ points missed

_____ Score

Satisfactory score: 85 or above

CAAHEP Competencies Achieved:

Psychomotor (Skills)
☑ I. 1. Obtain vital signs.

Affective (Behavior)
☑ I. 1. Apply critical thinking skills in performing patient assessment and care.

ABHES Competencies Achieved:

☑ 9. c. Take vital signs.

EVALUATION OF COMPETENCY

Procedure 19-3: Measuring Rectal Body Temperature—Electronic Thermometer

Name: _____   Date: _____

Evaluated By: _____   Score: _____

Performance Objective

Outcome:	Measure rectal body temperature.
Conditions:	Given the following: electronic thermometer rectal probe, probe cover, lubricant, disposable gloves, tissues, and a waste container.
Standards:	Time: 5 minutes. Student completed procedure in ____ minutes.
	Accuracy: Satisfactory score on the Performance Evaluation Checklist.

Performance Evaluation Checklist

Trial 1	Trial 2	Point Value	Performance Standards
		●	Sanitized hands.
		●	Assembled equipment.
		●	Removed thermometer from its storage base.
		●	Attached rectal probe to thermometer unit.
		●	Inserted probe into the thermometer.
		●	Greeted the patient and introduced yourself.
		●	Identified the patient and explained the procedure.
		●	Applied gloves.
		▷	Stated the reason for applying gloves.
		●	Positioned and draped the patient.
		▷	Explained how to position an adult and an infant.
		●	Removed probe from the thermometer.
		●	Attached probe cover to probe.
		●	Applied lubricant up to a level of 1 inch.
		▷	Stated the purpose of the lubricant.
		●	Instructed patient to lie still.
		●	Separated the buttocks and properly inserted the thermometer.
		▷	Stated how far the thermometer should be inserted for adults, children, and infants.
		●	Held probe in place until an audible tone was heard.
		●	Removed the probe in the same direction as it was inserted.
		●	Noted patient's temperature reading on display screen.

Trial 1	Trial 2	Point Value	*Performance Standards*
		●	Discarded probe cover in a regular waste container.
		▷	Explained why the cover can be discarded in a regular waste container.
		●	Returned probe to the thermometer unit.
		●	Returned the thermometer unit to its base.
		●	Wiped the anal area with tissues.
		●	Removed gloves and sanitized hands.
		●	Charted the results correctly.
		✳	The temperature recording was identical to the reading on the display screen.
		✳	Completed the procedure within 5 minutes.
			TOTALS

CHART

Date	

Evaluation of Student Performance

EVALUATION CRITERIA			COMMENTS
Symbol	Category	Point Value	
✳	Critical Step	16 points	
●	Essential Step	6 points	
▷	Theory Question	2 points	

Score calculation: 100 points

− _____ points missed

_____ Score

Satisfactory score: 85 or above

CAAHEP Competencies Achieved:

Psychomotor (Skills)
☑ I. 1. Obtain vital signs.

Affective (Behavior)
☑ I. 1. Apply critical thinking skills in performing patient assessment and care.

ABHES Competencies Achieved:

☑ 9. c. Take vital signs.

EVALUATION OF COMPETENCY

Procedure 19-4: Measuring Aural Body Temperature—Tympanic Membrane Thermometer

Name: _____   Date: _____

Evaluated By: _____   Score: _____

Performance Objective

Outcome:	Measure aural body temperature.
Conditions:	Given the following: tympanic membrane thermometer probe cover, and a waste container.
Standards:	Time: 5 minutes. Student completed procedure in _____ minutes.
	Accuracy: Satisfactory score on the Performance Evaluation Checklist.

Performance Evaluation Checklist

Trial 1	Trial 2	Point Value	Performance Standards
		●	Sanitized hands.
		●	Assembled equipment.
		●	Greeted the patient and introduced yourself.
		●	Identified the patient and explained the procedure.
		●	Removed thermometer from its storage base.
		●	Checked to make sure the probe lens was clean and intact.
		▷	Stated what might occur if the lens was dirty.
		●	Placed a cover on the probe.
		▷	Explained the purpose of the probe cover.
		●	Observed the screen to determine if the thermometer was ready to use.
		●	Held the thermometer in the dominant hand.
		●	Straightened the patient's ear canal with the nondominant hand.
		▷	Explained the purpose of straightening the ear canal.
		●	Inserted the probe into the patient's ear canal and sealed the opening without causing the patient discomfort.
		●	Pointed the tip of the probe toward the opposite temple.
		▷	Stated the reason for pointing the probe toward the opposite temple.
		●	Asked the patient to remain still.
		●	Depressed the activation button for 1 full second or until an audible tone was heard.
		●	Removed the thermometer from the ear canal and noted the patient's temperature on the display screen.
		▷	Stated what should be done if the temperature seems too low.

Trial 1	Trial 2	Point Value	Performance Standards
		•	Disposed of the probe cover in a waste container.
		•	Replaced the thermometer in its storage base.
		▷	Explained the reason for storing the thermometer in its storage base.
		•	Sanitized hands.
		•	Charted the results correctly.
		∗	The temperature recording was identical to the reading on the display screen.
		∗	Completed the procedure within 5 minutes.
			TOTALS

CHART	
Date	

Evaluation of Student Performance

EVALUATION CRITERIA			COMMENTS
Symbol	Category	Point Value	
∗	Critical Step	16 points	
•	Essential Step	6 points	
▷	Theory Question	2 points	

Score calculation: 100 points

− _____ points missed

_____ Score

Satisfactory score: 85 or above

CAAHEP Competencies Achieved:

Psychomotor (Skills)
☑ I. 1. Obtain vital signs.

Affective (Behavior)
☑ I. 1. Apply critical thinking skills in performing patient assessment and care.

ABHES Competencies Achieved:

☑ 9. c. Take vital signs.

EVALUATION OF COMPETENCY

DVD **Procedure 19-5: Measuring Temporal Artery Body Temperature**

Name: _____ Date: _____

Evaluated By: _____ Score: _____

Performance Objective

Outcome:	Measure temporal body temperature.
Conditions:	Given the following: temporal artery thermometer, disposal probe cover, antiseptic wipe, waste container.
Standards:	Time: 5 minutes.　　　　　Student completed procedure in ____ minutes.
	Accuracy: Satisfactory score on the Performance Evaluation Checklist.

Performance Evaluation Checklist

Trial 1	Trial 2	Point Value	Performance Standards
		●	Sanitized hands and assembled equipment.
		●	Greeted the patient and introduced yourself.
		●	Identified the patient and explained the procedure.
		●	Checked to make sure the probe lens was clean and intact.
		▷	Stated why the lens should be clean.
		●	Placed a disposable cover onto the probe or cleaned the probe with an antiseptic wipe and allowed it to dry.
		●	Selected an appropriate site.
		●	Brushed away any hair that was covering the scanning sites.
		▷	Explained why hair must be brushed away.
		●	Held the thermometer in the dominant hand with the thumb on the scan button.
		●	Gently positioned the probe of the thermometer on the center of the patient's forehead.
		●	Depressed the scan button and kept it depressed for the entire measurement.
		▷	Stated why the scan button must be continually depressed.
		●	Slowly and gently slid the probe straight across the forehead midway between the eyebrow and the upper hairline.
		●	Continued until the hairline was reached, making sure to keep the probe flush against the forehead.
		●	Keeping the button depressed, lifted the probe from the forehead and placed it behind the earlobe for 1 to 2 seconds.
		▷	Stated why the probe is placed behind the earlobe.
		●	Released the scan button and noted the temperature on the display screen.

Trial 1	Trial 2	Point Value	Performance Standards
		•	Disposed of the probe cover in a regular waste container.
		•	Wiped the probe with an antiseptic wipe and allowed it to dry.
		•	Sanitized hands.
		•	Charted the results correctly.
		✳	The temperature recording was identical to the reading on the display screen.
		•	Stored the thermometer in a clean, dry area.
		✳	Completed the procedure within 5 minutes.
			TOTALS

CHART	
Date	

Evaluation of Student Performance

EVALUATION CRITERIA			COMMENTS
Symbol	Category	Point Value	
✳	Critical Step	16 points	
•	Essential Step	6 points	
▷	Theory Question	2 points	

Score calculation: 100 points

− _____ points missed

_____ Score

Satisfactory score: 85 or above

CAAHEP Competencies Achieved:

Psychomotor (Skills)
☑ I. 1. Obtain vital signs.

Affective (Behavior)
☑ I. 1. Apply critical thinking skills in performing patient assessment and care.

ABHES Competencies Achieved:

☑ 9. c. Take vital signs.

EVALUATION OF COMPETENCY

Procedure 19-6: Measuring Pulse and Respiration

Name: _____   Date: _____

Evaluated By: _____   Score: _____

Performance Objective

Outcome:	Measure radial pulse and respiration.
Conditions:	Using a watch with a second hand.
Standards:	Time: 5 minutes. Student completed procedure in ____ minutes.
	Accuracy: Satisfactory score on the Performance Evaluation Checklist.

Performance Evaluation Checklist

Trial 1	Trial 2	Point Value	Performance Standards
		●	Sanitized hands.
		●	Greeted and introduced yourself.
		●	Identified the patient and explained the procedure.
		●	Observed patient for any signs that might influence the pulse rate or respiratory rate.
		▷	Stated two factors that would increase the pulse rate.
		●	Positioned patient in a comfortable position.
		●	Placed three middle fingertips over the radial pulse site.
		▷	Explained why the pulse should not be taken with the thumb.
		●	Applied moderate, gentle pressure until the pulse was felt.
		▷	Stated what would occur if too much pressure is applied over the radial artery.
		●	Counted the pulse for 30 seconds and made a mental note of the number.
		●	Determined the rhythm and volume of the pulse.
		▷	Stated when the pulse should be measured for a full minute.
		●	Continued to hold the fingers on the patient's wrist.
		▷	Explained why respirations should be taken without the patient's awareness.
		●	Observed the rise and fall of patient's chest.
		●	Counted the number of respirations for 30 seconds and made a mental note of the number.
		▷	Stated what makes up one respiration.
		●	Determined the rhythm and depth of the respirations.
		●	Observed the patient's color.
		●	Sanitized hands.

Trial 1	Trial 2	Point Value	Performance Standards
		●	Multiplied the pulse and respiration values by 2.
		●	Charted the results correctly.
		✳	The pulse rate was within plus or minus 2 beats of the evaluator's reading
		✳	The respiratory rate was within 1 respiration of the evaluator's measurement.
		▷	Stated the normal adult range for the pulse rate (60 to 100 beats per minute).
		▷	Stated the normal adult range for the respiratory rate (12 to 20 respirations per minute).
		✳	Completed the procedure within 5 minutes.
			TOTALS

	CHART
Date	

Evaluation of Student Performance

EVALUATION CRITERIA			COMMENTS
Symbol	Category	Point Value	
✳	Critical Step	16 points	
●	Essential Step	6 points	
▷	Theory Question	2 points	

Score calculation: 100 points

− _____ points missed

_____ Score

Satisfactory score: 85 or above

CAAHEP Competencies Achieved:

Psychomotor (Skills)
☑ I. 1. Obtain vital signs.

Affective (Behavior)
☑ I. 1. Apply critical thinking skills in performing patient assessment and care.

ABHES Competencies Achieved:

☑ 9. c. Take vital signs

EVALUATION OF COMPETENCY

Procedure 19-7: Measuring Apical Pulse

Name: _____   Date: _____

Evaluated By: _____   Score: _____

Performance Objective

Outcome:	Measure apical pulse.
Conditions:	Given the following: stethoscope and antiseptic wipe. Using a watch with a second hand.
Standards:	Time: 5 minutes. Student completed procedure in _____ minutes.
	Accuracy: Satisfactory score on the Performance Evaluation Checklist.

Performance Evaluation Checklist

Trial 1	Trial 2	Point Value	Performance Standards
		•	Sanitized hands.
		•	Greeted the patient and introduced yourself.
		•	Identified the patient and explained the procedure.
		•	Observed the patient for any signs that might affect the pulse rate.
		•	Assembled equipment.
		•	Rotated the chest piece to the bell position.
		•	Cleaned earpieces and chest piece with antiseptic wipe.
		▷	Stated the reason for cleaning stethoscope with an antiseptic.
		•	Positioned patient.
		•	Asked the patient to unbutton or remove his/her shirt.
		•	Warmed chest piece of the stethoscope.
		▷	Explained the reason for warming chest piece.
		•	Inserted earpieces of stethoscope in a forward position in the ears.
		▷	Explained why the earpieces must be directed forward.
		•	Placed the chest piece over the apex of the heart.
		▷	Described the location of the apex of the heart.
		•	Counted the number of heartbeats for 30 seconds and multiplied by 2.
		∗	The reading was within ± 2 beats of the evaluator's reading.
		•	Sanitized hands.
		•	Charted the results correctly.

Trial 1	Trial 2	Point Value	Performance Standards
		●	Cleaned earpieces and chest piece with an antiseptic wipe.
		*	Completed the procedure within 5 minutes.
			TOTALS

CHART	
Date	

Evaluation of Student Performance

EVALUATION CRITERIA			COMMENTS
Symbol	Category	Point Value	
*	Critical Step	16 points	
●	Essential Step	6 points	
▷	Theory Question	2 points	

Score calculation: 100 points

– _____ points missed

_____ Score

Satisfactory score: 85 or above

CAAHEP Competencies Achieved:

Psychomotor (Skills)
☑ I. 1. Obtain vital signs.

Affective (Behavior)
☑ I. 1. Apply critical thinking skills in performing patient assessment and care.

ABHES Competencies Achieved:

☑ 9. c. Take vital signs.

EVALUATION OF COMPETENCY

Procedure 19-8: Performing Pulse Oximetry

Name: _____ Date: _____

Evaluated By: _____ Score: _____

Performance Objective

Outcome:	Perform pulse oximetry.
Conditions:	Given the following: handheld pulse oximeter, reusable finger probe, and an antiseptic wipe.
Standards:	Time: 5 minutes. Student completed procedure in _____ minutes.
	Accuracy: Satisfactory score on the Performance Evaluation Checklist.

Performance Evaluation Checklist

Trial 1	Trial 2	Point Value	Performance Standards
		•	Sanitized hands and assembled equipment.
		•	Ensured the probe opened and closed smoothly and that the windows were clean.
		•	Disinfected the probe windows and platforms and allowed them to dry.
		▷	Stated the purpose of disinfecting the probe windows.
		•	If necessary, connected the probe to the cable.
		•	Connected the cable to the monitor.
		•	Did not lift or carry the monitor by the cable.
		•	Greeted and introduced yourself.
		•	Identified the patient and explained the procedure.
		•	Seated the patient in a chair with the lower arm supported and the palm facing down.
		▷	Explained why the arm should be supported.
		•	Selected an appropriate finger to apply the probe.
		•	Observed the patient's finger to make sure it was free of dark fingernail polish or an artificial nail.
		•	Checked to make sure the patient's finger tip was clean.
		•	Checked to make sure the patient's finger was not cold.
		▷	Explained what to do if the patient's finger is cold.
		•	Made sure that ambient light would not interfere with the measurement.
		▷	Explained why ambient light should be avoided.
		•	Positioned the probe securely on the fingertip.
		•	Allowed the cable to lay across the palm of the hand and parallel to the arm of the patient.

Trial 1	Trial 2	Point Value	Performance Standards
		●	Instructed the patient to remain still and to breathe normally.
		▷	Stated why the patient must remain still.
		●	Turned on the pulse oximeter.
		●	Waited while the oximeter went through its power-on self-test (POST).
		▷	Explained what to do if the oximeter fails the POST.
		●	Allowed several seconds for the oximeter to detect the pulse and calculate the oxygen saturation.
		●	Ensured that the pulse-strength indicator fluctuated with each pulsation and that the pulse signal was strong.
		▷	Stated what should be done if the oximeter is unable to locate a pulse.
		●	Left the probe in place until the oximeter displayed a reading.
		●	Noted the oxygen saturation value and pulse rate.
		✳	The reading was identical to the evaluator's reading.
		▷	Stated the normal oxygen saturation level of a healthy adult (95% to 99%).
		●	Removed the probe from the patient's finger and turned off the oximeter.
		●	Sanitized hands.
		●	Charted the results correctly.
		●	Disconnected the cable from the monitor.
		●	Disinfected the probe with an antiseptic wipe.
		●	Properly stored the monitor in a clean, dry area.
		✳	Completed the procedure within 5 minutes.
			TOTALS
			CHART
Date			

Evaluation of Student Performance

EVALUATION CRITERIA			COMMENTS
Symbol	Category	Point Value	
✳	Critical Step	16 points	
●	Essential Step	6 points	
▷	Theory Question	2 points	

Score calculation: 100 points

−_____ points missed

_____ Score

Satisfactory score: 85 or above

CAAHEP Competencies Achieved:

Psychomotor (Skills)
☑ I. 1. Obtain vital signs.

Affective (Behavior)
☑ I. 1. Apply critical thinking skills in performing patient assessment and care.

ABHES Competencies Achieved:

☑ 9. c. Take vital signs.

Notes

EVALUATION OF COMPETENCY

Procedure 19-9: Measuring Blood Pressure

Name: _____ Date: _____

Evaluated By: _____ Score: _____

Performance Objective

Outcome:	Measure blood pressure.
Conditions:	Given the following: stethoscope, sphygmomanometer, and an antiseptic wipe.
Standards:	Time: 5 minutes. Student completed procedure in _____ minutes.
	Accuracy: Satisfactory score on the Performance Evaluation Checklist.

Performance Evaluation Checklist

Trial 1	Trial 2	Point Value	Performance Standards
		●	Sanitized hands.
		●	Assembled equipment.
		●	Rotated the chest piece to the diaphragm position.
		●	Cleaned earpieces and chest piece of stethoscope with an antiseptic wipe.
		●	Greeted the patient and introduced yourself.
		●	Identified the patient and explained the procedure.
		●	Observed patient for any signs that might influence the blood pressure reading.
		▷	Listed signs that would influence the blood pressure reading.
		●	Determined how high to pump the cuff (palpated systolic pressure or checking the patient's chart).
		●	Positioned patient in a sitting position.
		●	Made sure that the patient's arm was uncovered.
		●	Explained why blood pressure should not be taken over clothing.
		●	Positioned patient's arm at heart level with the palm facing up.
		●	Selected the proper cuff size.
		▷	Explained how to determine the proper cuff size.
		●	Located the brachial pulse with the fingertips.
		▷	Stated the location of the brachial pulse.
		●	Centered bladder over the brachial pulse site.
		▷	Explained why the bladder should be centered over the brachial pulse site.
		●	Placed cuff on patient's arm 1 inch above bend in elbow.

Trial 1	Trial 2	Point Value	Performance Standards
		●	Wrapped cuff smoothly and snugly around patient's arm and secured it.
		●	Positioned self and/or manometer for direct viewing and at a distance of no more than 3 feet.
		●	Inserted earpieces of stethoscope in a forward position in the ears.
		●	Located the brachial pulse again.
		▷	Stated the purpose of locating the brachial pulse again.
		●	Placed diaphragm of the stethoscope over the brachial pulse site to make a tight seal.
		▷	Explained why there should be good contact of the chest piece with the skin.
		●	Made sure chest piece was not touching cuff.
		▷	Explained why the chest piece should not touch the cuff.
		●	Closed valve on bulb by turning thumbscrew to the right.
		●	Rapidly pumped air into cuff up to a level of 20 to 30 mm Hg above the palpated or previously measured systolic pressure.
		●	Released pressure at a moderate, steady rate by turning thumbscrew to the left.
		●	Heard and noted the first clear tapping sound (systolic pressure).
		●	Continued to deflate the cuff for another 10 mm Hg.
		●	Heard and noted the point on the scale at which the sounds ceased (diastolic pressure).
		●	Quickly and completely deflated cuff to zero and removed earpieces from ears.
		▷	Stated how long one should wait before taking the blood pressure again on the same arm.
		●	Carefully removed cuff from patient's arm.
		●	Sanitized hands.
		●	Charted the results correctly.
		✳	The reading was within ±2 mm Hg of the evaluator's reading.
		▷	Stated the normal blood pressure for an adult (less than 120/80).
		●	Cleaned earpieces and chest piece with an antiseptic wipe.
		✳	Completed the procedure within 5 minutes.
			TOTALS
			CHART
Date			

Evaluation of Student Performance

EVALUATION CRITERIA			COMMENTS
Symbol	**Category**	**Point Value**	
∗	Critical Step	16 points	
●	Essential Step	6 points	
▷	Theory Question	2 points	

Score calculation: 100 points

−_____ points missed

____ Score

Satisfactory score: 85 or above

CAAHEP Competencies Achieved:

Psychomotor (Skills)

☑ I. 1. Obtain vital signs.

Affective (Behavior)

☑ I. 1. Apply critical thinking skills in performing patient assessment and care.

ABHES Competencies Achieved:

☑ 9. c. Take vital signs.

Notes

20

The Physical Examination

CHAPTER ASSIGNMENTS

√ After Completing	Date Due	Textbook Page(s)	TEXTBOOK ASSIGNMENTS	Possible Points	Points You Earned
		375-407	Read Chapter 20: The Physical Examination		
		380 406	Read Case Study 1 Case Study 1 questions	5	
		382 406	Read Case Study 2 Case Study 2 questions	5	
		402 406	Read Case Study 3 Case Study 3 questions	5	
			TOTAL POINTS		

√ After Completing	Date Due	Study Guide Page(s)	STUDY GUIDE ASSIGNMENTS (CTA: Critical Thinking Activity)	Possible Points	Points You Earned
		331	Pretest	10	
		332	Key Term Assessment	16	
		333-334	Evaluation of Learning questions	20	
		335	CTA A: Reading Weight Measurements	15	
			CD Activity: Chapter 20 By the Pound (Record points earned)		
		336	CTA B: Reading Height Measurements	11	
			CD Activity: Chapter 20 Feet and Inches (Record points earned)		
		337	CTA C: Calculating BMI	2	
		337	CTA D: Dear Gabby	10	

√ After Completing	Date Due	Study Guide Page(s)	STUDY GUIDE ASSIGNMENTS (CTA: Critical Thinking Activity)	Possible Points	Points You Earned
		337-338	CTA E: Patient Positions	10	
			🔵CD CD Activity: Chapter 20 Let's Get Physical (Record points earned)		
		338	CTA F: Examination Techniques	10	
		338	CTA G: Otoscope	4	
		339	CTA H: Crossword Puzzle	25	
			🔵CD CD Activity: Chapter 20 Animations	10	
			🔵CD CD Activity: Chapter 20 Apply Your Knowledge questions (Record points earned)		
		331	📄 Posttest	10	
			ADDITIONAL ASSIGNMENTS		
			TOTAL POINTS		

√ When Assigned by Your Instructor	Study Guide Page(s)	Practices Required	LABORATORY ASSIGNMENTS (Procedure Number and Name)	*Score
	341	5	📀 **Practice for Competency** 20-1: Measuring Weight and Height Textbook reference: pp. 386-387	
	343-345		📝 **Evaluation of Competency** 20-1: Measuring Weight and Height	*
	341	3	📀 **Practice for Competency** 20-2: Sitting Position Textbook reference: pp. 388-389	
	347-348		📝 **Evaluation of Competency** 20-2: Sitting Position	*
	341	3	📀 **Practice for Competency** 20-3: Supine Position Textbook reference: pp. 389-390	
	349-350		📝 **Evaluation of Competency** 20-3: Supine Position	*
	341	3	📀 **Practice for Competency** 20-4: Prone Position Textbook reference: pp. 390-391	
	351-352		📝 **Evaluation of Competency** 20-4: Prone Position	*
	341	3	📀 **Practice for Competency** 20-5: Dorsal Recumbent Position Textbook reference: pp. 391-392	
	353-354		📝 **Evaluation of Competency** 20-5: Dorsal Recumbent Position	*
	341	3	📀 **Practice for Competency** 20-6: Lithotomy Position Textbook reference: pp. 392-393	
	355-356		📝 **Evaluation of Competency** 20-6: Lithotomy Position	*
	341	3	📀 **Practice for Competency** 20-7: Sims Position Textbook reference: p. 394	
	357-358		📝 **Evaluation of Competency** 20-7: Sims Position	*
	341	3	📀 **Practice for Competency** 20-8: Knee-Chest Position Textbook reference: p. 395	
	359-360		📝 **Evaluation of Competency** 20-8: Knee-Chest Position	*
	341	3	📀 **Practice for Competency** 20-9: Fowler's Position Textbook reference: p. 396	

√ When Assigned by Your Instructor	Study Guide Page(s)	Practices Required	LABORATORY ASSIGNMENTS (Procedure Number and Name)	*Score
	361-362		📖 **Evaluation of Competency** 20-9: Fowler's Position	*
	341	3	📀 **Practice for Competency** 20-10: Assisting with the Physical Examination Textbook reference: pp. 403-405	
	363-365		📖 **Evaluation of Competency** 20-10: Assisting with the Physical Examination	*
			ADDITIONAL ASSIGNMENTS	

Name _____   Date _____

? PRETEST

True or False

_____   1. A complete patient examination consists of a physical examination and laboratory tests.

_____   2. Arthritis is an example of a chronic illness.

_____   3. An otoscope is used to examine the eyes.

_____   4. A patient should be identified by name and date of birth.

_____   5. The reason for weighing a prenatal patient is to determine the baby's due date.

_____   6. The height of an adult is measured during every office visit.

_____   7. The lithotomy position is used to examine the vagina.

_____   8. Inspection involves the observation of the patient for any signs of disease.

_____   9. Measuring blood pressure is an example of auscultation.

_____   10. The supine position is used to examine the back.

? POSTTEST

True or False

_____   1. The prognosis is what is wrong with the patient.

_____   2. A *risk factor* means that a patient will develop a certain disease.

_____   3. A CT scan is an example of a therapeutic procedure.

_____   4. The function of a speculum is to open a body orifice for viewing.

_____   5. The process of measuring the patient is called *mensuration*.

_____   6. A reason for weighing a child is to determine drug dosage.

_____   7. The purpose of draping a patient is to make it easier for the physician to examine the patient.

_____   8. Sims position is used for flexible sigmoidoscopy.

_____   9. Measuring pulse is an example of percussion.

_____   10. BMI is the abbreviation for body mass index.

⚲Term KEY TERM ASSESSMENT

Directions: Match each medical term with its definition.

_____ 1. Audiometer

_____ 2. Auscultation

_____ 3. Bariatrics

_____ 4. Clinical diagnosis

_____ 5. Diagnosis

_____ 6. Differential diagnosis

_____ 7. Inspection

_____ 8. Mensuration

_____ 9. Ophthalmoscope

_____ 10. Otoscope

_____ 11. Palpation

_____ 12. Percussion

_____ 13. Percussion hammer

_____ 14. Prognosis

_____ 15. Speculum

_____ 16. Symptom

A. An instrument for examining the interior of the eye

B. A tentative diagnosis obtained through the evaluation of the health history and the physical examination, without the benefit of laboratory or diagnostic tests

C. An instrument for opening a body orifice or cavity for viewing

D. An instrument used to measure hearing

E. The process of measuring the patient

F. The scientific method for determining and identifying a patient's condition

G. The process of tapping the body to detect disease

H. The process of observing a patient to detect any signs of disease

I. Any change in the body or its functioning that indicates that a disease might be present

J. The process of listening to the sounds produced within the body to detect signs of disease

K. A determination of which of two or more diseases with similar symptoms is producing the patient's symptoms

L. An instrument for examining the external ear canal and tympanic membrane

M. The process of feeling with the hands to detect signs of disease

N. An instrument with a rubber head, used for testing reflexes

O. The probable course and outcome of a patient's condition and the patient's prospects for recovery

P. The branch of medicine that deals with the treatment and control of obesity

EVALUATION OF LEARNING

Directions: Fill in each blank with the correct answer.

1. What are the three parts of a complete patient examination?

   _____

   _____

2. List two functions of the patient examination.

   _____

   _____

3. What is the purpose of establishing a final diagnosis?

   _____

   _____

4. Why is there a space for indicating the clinical diagnosis on the laboratory request form?

   _____

   _____

5. What is a risk factor?

   _____

   _____

6. What is an acute illness? List two examples of acute illnesses.

   _____

   _____

7. What is a chronic illness? List two examples of chronic illnesses.

   _____

   _____

8. What is the difference between a therapeutic procedure and a diagnostic procedure?

   _____

   _____

   _____

9. How can patient apprehension be reduced during a physical examination?

   _____

   _____

10. Why should patients be asked if they need to empty their bladder before the physical examination?

   _____

   _____

11. What is the purpose for measuring weight?

_____

_____

_____

12. What is the purpose of positioning and draping?

_____

_____

_____

13. Indicate three types of examinations for which the supine position is used.

_____

_____

14. Indicate two types of examinations for which the lithotomy position is used.

_____

_____

15. Indicate one type of examination for which the knee-chest position is used.

_____

_____

16. List four types of assessments that can be made through inspection.

_____

_____

17. List four types of assessments that can be made through palpation.

_____

_____

18. Explain what can be assessed through the use of percussion.

_____

_____

19. What type of assessments can be made using auscultation?

_____

_____

20. What type of stethoscope chest piece should be used to assess the heart?

_____

CRITICAL THINKING ACTIVITIES

A. READING WEIGHT MEASUREMENTS

The following diagram is an illustration of a portion of the calibration bar of an upright balance beam scale. In the spaces provided, record the weight measurements indicated on the calibration bar. In all cases, assume that the lower weight is resting in the 100-lb notched groove.

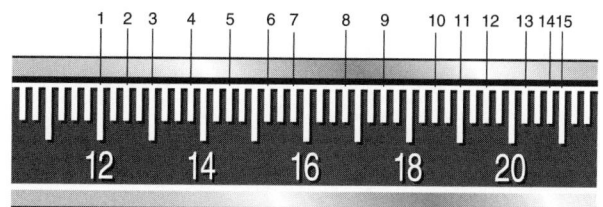

(From Bonewit-West K: *Study guide for clinical procedures for medical assistants,* ed 7, St. Louis, 2008, Saunders.)

1. _____
2. _____
3. _____
4. _____
5. _____
6. _____
7. _____
8. _____
9. _____
10. _____
11. _____
12. _____
13. _____
14. _____
15. _____

B. READING HEIGHT MEASUREMENTS

The following diagram is an illustration of a portion of the calibration rod of an upright balance beam scale. In the spaces provided, indicate the height measurement in feet and inches indicated on the calibration rod.

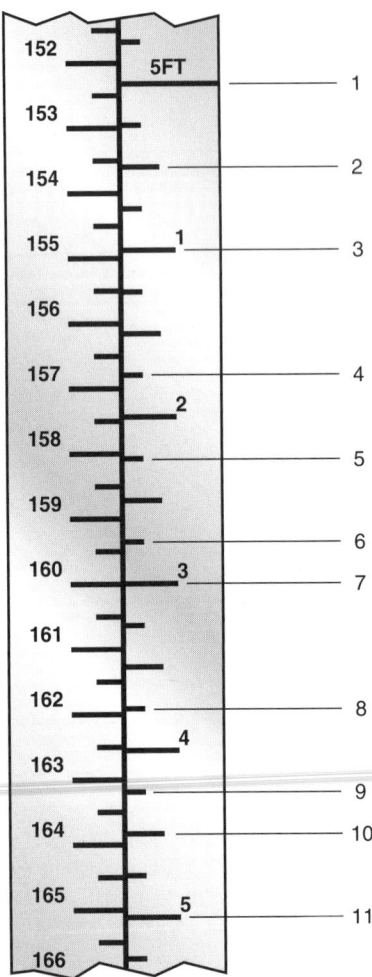

(From Bonewit-West K: *Study guide for clinical procedures for medical assistants,* ed 7, St. Louis, 2008, Saunders.)

1. _____
2. _____
3. _____
4. _____
5. _____
6. _____
7. _____
8. _____
9. _____
10. _____
11. _____

C. CALCULATING BMI

1. Using the *Highlight on Interpreting Body Weight* box on page 385 of your textbook, calculate and interpret your BMI and record the results below.

_____

2. List the diseases that an individual with an above-normal BMI has an increased chance of developing.

_____

_____

_____

_____

D. DEAR GABBY

Gabby is attending a writer's convention and wants you to fill in for her. In the space provided, respond to the following letter using the knowledge you have acquired in this chapter.

Dear Gabby:

I have been reading your column in the local newspaper for many years. I had a problem with this young doctor that I saw recently, and it has me very concerned. I am 67 years "'young'" and am very active. I drink herbal teas, eat lots of fruits and vegetables, and do housework and gardening. I rarely have a cold or get sick, so it has been many years since I have been to see a doctor.

This young doctor did something called a BMI. I know it is probably one of those new-fangled tests they do, and I hope it was covered by my health insurance policy. Anyway, the doctor told me that I have a BMI of 27 and that I should exercise more and eat a little less. His medical assistant came in afterward and gave me some information on a healthy diet and exercising, but I was so upset at that point, I think I threw the information away when I got home!

There used to be an insurance company table that showed whether or not you were within your ideal weight. It seems to me that the last time I checked it, I was not a bit overweight. But now this young doctor and his assistant are trying to tell me that I need to lose weight. Gabby, what should I do?

Signed,

Confused and Concerned in Connecticut

_____

_____

_____

_____

_____

_____

_____

_____

_____

_____

_____

_____

E. PATIENT POSITIONS

In which position would you place the patient for the following examinations or procedures?

1. Measurement of rectal temperature of an adult: _____

2. Examination of the back: _____

3. Measurement of vital signs: _____

4. Pelvic examination: _____

5. Examination of the upper extremities: _____

6. Examination of the eyes, ears, nose, and throat: _____

7. Examination of the breasts: _____

8. Flexible sigmoidoscopy: _____

9. Administration of an enema: _____

10. Examination of the upper body of a patient with emphysema: _____

F. EXAMINATION TECHNIQUES

List the examination technique (inspection, palpation, percussion, auscultation) that is used in each of the following situations.

1. A patient with a stutter: _____

2. Taking the radial pulse: _____

3. Finding the location of the apical pulse: _____

4. Taking the apical pulse: _____

5. Taking respiration (may be two answers, depending on method): _____

6. A patient with cracked lips: _____

7. Checking for lumps in the breast: _____

8. Checking reflexes: _____

9. Obtaining the fetal heart rate: _____

10. A patient with a fever (may be several methods): _____

G. OTOSCOPE

Obtain an otoscope and an ophthalmoscope. Following the manufacturer's instructions, perform the following. Place a check mark next to each after performing it.

_____ 1. Turn the otoscope on and off.

_____ 2. Change the bulb in the otoscope.

_____ 3. Change the batteries or recharge the otoscope.

_____ 4. Change the speculum of the otoscope.

H. CROSSWORD PUZZLE
Assisting with a Physical Examination
Directions: Complete the crossword puzzle using the clues presented below.

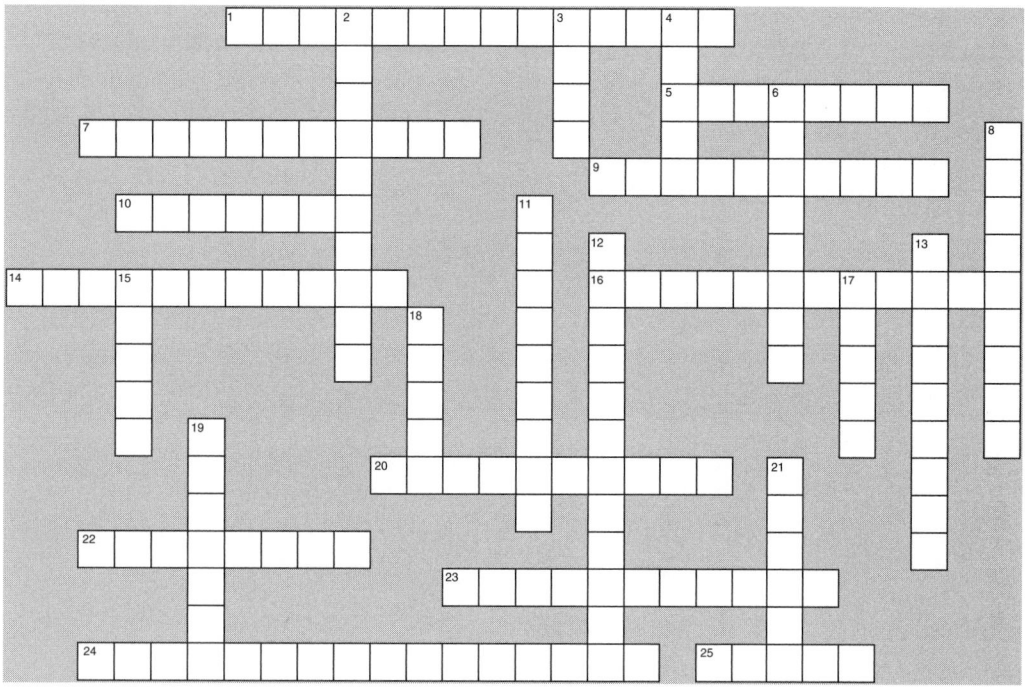

(From Bonewit-West K: *Study guide for clinical procedures for medical assistants,* ed 7, St. Louis, 2008, Saunders.)

ACROSS
1 Eye examiner
5 Ear examiner
7 BMI: less than 18.5
9 BMI: 25 to 29.9
10 "Listen to heart" position
14 Measuring the patient
16 I am listening
20 Metric unit of height
22 Metric unit of weight
23 Curative procedure
24 Reflex tester
25 BMI: 30 or more

DOWN
2 Hearing tester
3 Flex sigmoid position
4 Face-down
6 Orifice opener
8 What is the probable outcome?
11 What is wrong with you?
12 Before you measure weight
13 GYN position
15 Five feet in inches
17 Severe and intense condition
18 Provides warmth and modesty
19 Long-time illness
21 Face-up

Notes

PRACTICE FOR COMPETENCY

Procedure 20-1: Weight and Height. Take weight and height measurements. Record results in the chart provided.

Procedures 20-2 to 20-9: Positioning and Draping. Position and drape an individual in each of the following positions: Sitting, Supine, Prone, Dorsal Recumbent, Lithotomy, Sims, Knee-Chest, and Fowler's.

Procedure 20-10: Assisting with the Physical Examination. Prepare the patient and assist with a physical examination. In the chart provided, record the results of the procedures you performed while assisting with the examination (e.g., vital signs, height, and weight).

CHART	
Date	

CHART	
Date	

⬛ EVALUATION OF COMPETENCY

Procedure 20-1: Measuring Weight and Height

Name: _____   Date: _____

Evaluated By: _____   Score: _____

Performance Objective

Outcome:	Measure weight and height.
Conditions:	Given a paper towel.
	Using an upright balance scale.
Standards:	Time: 5 minutes. Student completed procedure in ____ minutes.
	Accuracy: Satisfactory score on the Performance Evaluation Checklist.

Performance Evaluation Checklist

Trial 1	Trial 2	Point Value	Performance Standards
			WEIGHT
		●	Sanitized hands.
			Checked the balance scale for accuracy
		●	Verified that the upper and lower weights were on zero.
		●	Looked at the indicator point to make sure the scale was balanced.
		▷	Stated what would be observed if the scale is balanced.
		▷	Explained what to do if the indicator point rests below the center.
		▷	Explained what to do if the indicator point rests above the center.
		▷	Stated what occurs if the scale is not balanced.
		●	Greeted the patient and introduced yourself.
		●	Identified the patient and explained the procedure.
		●	Instructed patient to remove shoes and heavy outer clothing.
		●	Placed paper towel on the scale.
		●	Assisted patient onto the scale.
		●	Instructed patient not to move.
			Balanced the scale
		●	Moved the lower weight to the groove that did not cause the indicator point to drop to the bottom of the balance area.
		▷	Stated why the lower weight should be seated firmly in its groove.

Trial 1	Trial 2	Point Value	*Performance Standards*
		●	Slid the upper weight slowly until the indicator point came to a rest at the center of the balance area.
		●	Read the results to the nearest quarter pound. Jotted down this value or made a mental note of it.
		＊	The reading was identical to the evaluator's reading.
		●	Asked the patient to step off the scale.
			HEIGHT
		●	Slid the calibration rod until it was above the patient's height.
		●	Opened the measuring bar to its horizontal position.
		●	Instructed the patient to step onto the scale platform with his/her back to the scale.
		●	Instructed patient to stand erect and to look straight ahead.
		●	Carefully lowered the measuring bar until it rested gently on top of the patient's head.
		●	Verified that the bar was in a horizontal position.
		●	Instructed the patient to step down and put on his/her shoes.
		●	Read the marking to the nearest quarter inch. Jotted down this value or made a mental note of it.
		＊	The reading was identical to the evaluator's reading.
		●	Returned the measuring bar to its vertical position.
		●	Slid the calibration rod to its lowest position.
		●	Returned the weights to zero.
		●	Sanitized hands.
		●	Charted the results correctly.
		＊	Completed the procedure within 5 minutes.
			TOTALS
			CHART
Date			

Evaluation of Student Performance

EVALUATION CRITERIA			COMMENTS
Symbol	Category	Point Value	
✶	Critical Step	16 points	
●	Essential Step	6 points	
▷	Theory Question	2 points	

Score calculation: 100 points

− _____ points missed

_____   Score

Satisfactory score: 85 or above

CAAHEP Competencies Achieved:

Psychomotor (Skills)
☑ IV. 6. Prepare a patient for procedures and/or treatments.

Affective (Behavior)
☑ IV. 1. Demonstrate empathy in communicating with patients, family, and staff.
☑ IV. 9. Recognize and protect personal boundaries in communicating with others.

ABHES Competencies Achieved:

☑ 8. bb. Are impartial and show empathy when dealing with patients.
☑ 9. l. Prepare patient for examinations and treatments.

Notes

EVALUATION OF COMPETENCY

Procedure 20-2: Sitting Position

Name: _____   Date: _____

Evaluated By: _____   Score: _____

Performance Objective

Outcome:	Position and drape an individual in the sitting position.
Conditions:	Using an examining table.
	Given the following: a patient gown and a drape.
Standards:	Time: 5 minutes. Student completed procedure in _____ minutes.
	Accuracy: Satisfactory score on the Performance Evaluation Checklist.

Performance Evaluation Checklist

Trial 1	Trial 2	Point Value	Performance Standards
		●	Sanitized hands.
		●	Greeted the patient and introduced yourself.
		●	Identified the patient.
		●	Explained what type of examination would be performed.
		●	Provided patient with a patient gown.
		●	Instructed patient to remove clothing and to put on a patient gown with the opening in front.
		▷	Stated what qualities the disrobing facility should have.
		●	Pulled out the footrest and assisted the patient into a sitting position.
		●	The patient's buttocks and thighs were firmly supported on the edge of the table.
		●	Placed a drape over the patient's thighs and legs.
		●	Assisted the patient off the table after the examination.
		●	Returned the footrest to its normal position.
		●	Instructed the patient to get dressed.
		●	Discarded the gown and drape in a waste container.
		▷	Stated one use of the sitting position.
		✶	Completed the procedure within 5 minutes.
			TOTALS

Evaluation of Student Performance

EVALUATION CRITERIA			COMMENTS
Symbol	Category	Point Value	
✳	Critical Step	16 points	
●	Essential Step	6 points	
▷	Theory Question	2 points	

Score calculation: 100 points

− _____ points missed

_____ Score

Satisfactory score: 85 or above

CAAHEP Competencies Achieved:

Psychomotor (Skills)

☑ IV. 6. Prepare a patient for procedures and/or treatments.

☑ XI.11. Use proper body mechanics.

Affective (Behavior)

☑ IV.4. Demonstrate awareness of the territorial boundaries of the person with whom communicating.

ABHES Competencies Achieved:

☑ 9. 1. Prepare patient for examinations and treatments.

EVALUATION OF COMPETENCY

Procedure 20-3: Supine Position

Name: _____   Date: _____

Evaluated By: _____   Score: _____

Performance Objective

Outcome:	Position and drape an individual in the sitting position.
Conditions:	Using an examining table.
	Given the following: a patient gown and a drape.
Standards:	Time: 5 minutes. Student completed procedure in _____ minutes.
	Accuracy: Satisfactory score on the Performance Evaluation Checklist.

Performance Evaluation Checklist

Trial 1	Trial 2	Point Value	Performance Standards
		●	Sanitized hands.
		●	Greeted the patient and introduced yourself.
		●	Identified the patient
		●	Explained what type of examination or procedure would be performed.
		●	Provided patient with a patient gown.
		●	Instructed patient to remove clothing and to put on a patient gown with the opening in front.
		●	Pulled out the footrest and assisted the patient into a sitting position.
		●	Placed a drape over the patient's thighs and legs.
		●	Asked the patient to move back on the table.
		●	Pulled out the table extension while supporting the patient's lower legs.
		●	Asked the patient to lie down on his or her back with the legs together.
		●	Placed the patient's arms above the head or alongside the body.
		●	Positioned the drape lengthwise over the patient.
		▷	Stated the purpose of the drape.
		●	Moved the drape according to the body parts being examined.
		●	Assisted the patient back into a sitting position after the examination.
		●	Slid the table extension back into place while supporting the patient's lower legs.
		●	Assisted the patient from the examining table.
		●	Returned the footrest to its normal position.

Trial 1	Trial 2	Point Value	Performance Standards
		●	Instructed the patient to get dressed.
		●	Discarded the gown and drape in a waste container.
		▷	Stated one use of the supine position.
		✱	Completed the procedure within 5 minutes.
			TOTALS

Evaluation of Student Performance

EVALUATION CRITERIA			COMMENTS
Symbol	**Category**	**Point Value**	
✱	Critical Step	16 points	
●	Essential Step	6 points	
▷	Theory Question	2 points	
Score calculation: 100 points			
− _____ points missed			
_____ Score			
Satisfactory score: 85 or above			

CAAHEP Competencies Achieved:

Psychomotor (Skills)
☑ IV. 6. Prepare a patient for procedures and/or treatments.
☑ XI.11. Use proper body mechanics.

Affective (Behavior)
☑ IV.4. Demonstrate awareness of the territorial boundaries of the person with whom communicating.

ABHES Competencies Achieved:

☑ 9. 1. Prepare patient for examinations and treatments.

[✔] EVALUATION OF COMPETENCY

(DVD) Procedure 20-4: Prone Position

Name: _____   Date: _____

Evaluated By: _____   Score: _____

Performance Objective

Outcome:	Position and drape an individual in the prone position.
Conditions:	Using an examining table.
	Given the following: a patient gown and a drape.
Standards:	Time: 5 minutes. Student completed procedure in ____ minutes.
	Accuracy: Satisfactory score on the Performance Evaluation Checklist.

Performance Evaluation Checklist

Trial 1	Trial 2	Point Value	Performance Standards
		●	Sanitized hands.
		●	Greeted the patient and introduced yourself.
		●	Identified the patient.
		●	Explained what type of examination or procedure would be performed.
		●	Provided patient with a patient gown.
		●	Instructed patient to remove clothing and to put on a patient gown with the opening in back.
		●	Pulled out the footrest and assisted the patient into a sitting position.
		●	Placed a drape over the patient's thighs and legs.
		●	Asked the patient to move back on the table.
		●	Pulled out the table extension while supporting the patient's lower legs.
		●	Asked the patient to lie down on his/her back.
		●	Positioned the drape lengthwise over the patient.
		●	Asked the patient to turn onto his or her stomach by rolling toward you.
		●	Provided assistance.
		▷	Stated the reason for providing assistance.
		●	Positioned the patient with his/her legs together and the head turned to one side.
		●	Placed the patient's arms above his/her head or alongside his/her body.
		●	Adjusted the drape as needed.
		●	Moved the drape according to the body parts being examined.

Trial 1	Trial 2	Point Value	Performance Standards
		●	Assisted the patient into the supine position after the examination.
		●	Assisted the patient into a sitting position.
		●	Slid the table extension back into place while supporting the patient's lower legs.
		●	Assisted the patient from the examining table.
		●	Returned the footrest to its normal position.
		●	Instructed the patient to get dressed.
		●	Discarded the gown and drape in a waste container.
		▷	Stated one use of the prone position.
		✳	Completed the procedure within 5 minutes.
			TOTALS

Evaluation of Student Performance

EVALUATION CRITERIA			COMMENTS
Symbol	Category	Point Value	
✳	Critical Step	16 points	
●	Essential Step	6 points	
▷	Theory Question	2 points	

Score calculation: 100 points

− _____ points missed

_____ Score

Satisfactory score: 85 or above

CAAHEP Competencies Achieved:

Psychomotor (Skills)

☑ IV. 6. Prepare a patient for procedures and/or treatments.

☑ XI.11. Use proper body mechanics.

Affective (Behavior)

☑ IV.4. Demonstrate awareness of the territorial boundaries of the person with whom communicating.

ABHES Competencies Achieved:

☑ 9. 1. Prepare patient for examinations and treatments.

EVALUATION OF COMPETENCY

Procedure 20-5: Dorsal Recumbent Position

Name: _____   Date: _____

Evaluated By: _____   Score: _____

Performance Objective

Outcome:	Position and drape an individual in the dorsal recumbent position.
Conditions:	Using an examining table.
	Given the following: a patient gown and a drape.
Standards:	Time: 5 minutes. Student completed procedure in ____ minutes.
	Accuracy: Satisfactory score on the Performance Evaluation Checklist.

Performance Evaluation Checklist

Trial 1	Trial 2	Point Value	Performance Standards
		●	Sanitized hands.
		●	Greeted the patient and introduced yourself.
		●	Identified the patient.
		●	Explained what type of examination would be performed.
		●	Provided patient with a patient gown.
		●	Instructed patient to remove clothing and to put on a patient gown with the opening in front.
		●	Pulled out the footrest and assisted the patient into a sitting position.
		●	Placed a drape over the patient's thighs and legs.
		●	Asked the patient to move back on the table.
		●	Pulled out the table extension while supporting the patient's lower legs.
		●	Asked the patient to lie down on his/her back.
		●	Placed the patient's arms above his/her head or alongside his/her body.
		●	Positioned the drape diagonally over the patient.
		●	Asked the patient to bend his/her knees and place each foot at the edge of the table with the soles of his/her feet flat on the table.
		●	Provided assistance.
		●	Pushed in the table extension and the footrest.
		●	Adjusted the drape as needed.
		●	Folded back the center corner of the drape when the physician was ready to examine the patient.
		●	Pulled out the footrest and the table extension after the examination.

Trial 1	Trial 2	Point Value	Performance Standards
		•	Assisted the patient back into a supine position and then into a sitting position.
		•	Slid the table extension back into place while supporting the patient's lower legs.
		•	Assisted the patient from the examining table.
		•	Returned the footrest to its normal position.
		•	Instructed the patient to get dressed.
		•	Discarded the gown and drape in a waste container.
		▷	Stated one use of the dorsal recumbent position.
		＊	Completed the procedure within 5 minutes.
			TOTALS

Evaluation of Student Performance

EVALUATION CRITERIA			COMMENTS
Symbol	**Category**	**Point Value**	
＊	Critical Step	16 points	
•	Essential Step	6 points	
▷	Theory Question	2 points	
Score calculation: 100 points			
– _____ points missed			
_____ Score			
Satisfactory score: 85 or above			

CAAHEP Competencies Achieved:

Psychomotor (Skills)
☑ IV. 6. Prepare a patient for procedures and/or treatments.
☑ XI.11. Use proper body mechanics.

Affective (Behavior)
☑ IV.4. Demonstrate awareness of the territorial boundaries of the person with whom communicating.

ABHES Competencies Achieved:

☑ 9. 1. Prepare patient for examinations and treatments.

EVALUATION OF COMPETENCY

Procedure 20-6: Lithotomy Position

Name: _____   Date: _____

Evaluated By: _____   Score: _____

Performance Objective

Outcome:	Position and drape an individual in the lithotomy position.
Conditions:	Using an examining table.
	Given the following: a patient gown and a drape.
Standards:	Time: 5 minutes. Student completed procedure in _____ minutes.
	Accuracy: Satisfactory score on the Performance Evaluation Checklist.

Performance Evaluation Checklist

Trial 1	Trial 2	Point Value	Performance Standards
		•	Sanitized hands.
		•	Greeted the patient and introduced yourself.
		•	Identified the patient.
		•	Explained what type of examination would be performed.
		•	Provided patient with a patient gown.
		•	Instructed patient to remove clothing and to put on a patient gown with the opening in front.
		•	Pulled out the footrest and assisted the patient into a sitting position.
		•	Placed a drape over the patient's thighs and legs.
		•	Asked the patient to move back on the table.
		•	Pulled out the table extension while supporting the patient's lower legs.
		•	Asked the patient to lie down on his/her back.
		•	Placed the patient's arms above head or alongside body.
		•	Positioned drape diagonally over the patient.
		•	Pulled out the stirrups and positioned them at an angle.
		•	Positioned the stirrups so that they were level with the examining table and pulled out approximately 1 foot from the edge of the table.
		•	Asked the patient to bend at the knees and place each foot into a stirrup.
		•	Provided assistance.
		•	Pushed in the table extension and the footrest.

Trial 1	Trial 2	Point Value	Performance Standards
		●	Instructed the patient to slide buttocks to the edge of the table and to rotate thighs outward as far as is comfortable.
		●	Repositioned the drape as needed.
		●	Folded back the center corner of the drape when the physician was ready to examine the genital area.
		●	After completion of the examination, pulled out the footrest and the table extension.
		●	Asked the patient to slide the buttocks back from the end of the table.
		●	Lifted the patient's legs out of the stirrups at the same time and placed them on the table extension.
		▷	Stated why both legs should be lifted at the same time.
		●	Returned stirrups to the normal position.
		●	Assisted the patient back into a sitting position.
		●	Slid the table extension back into place while supporting the patient's lower legs.
		●	Assisted the patient from the examining table.
		●	Returned the footrest to its normal position.
		●	Instructed the patient to get dressed.
		●	Discarded the gown and drape in a waste container.
		▷	Stated one use of the lithotomy position.
		✶	Completed the procedure within 5 minutes.
			TOTALS

Evaluation of Student Performance

EVALUATION CRITERIA			COMMENTS
Symbol	Category	Point Value	
✶	Critical Step	16 points	
●	Essential Step	6 points	
▷	Theory Question	2 points	

Score calcu lation: 100 points

−_____ points missed

_____ Score

Satisfactory score: 85 or above

CAAHEP Competencies Achieved:

Psychomotor (Skills)
☑ IV. 6. Prepare a patient for procedures and/or treatments.
☑ XI.11. Use proper body mechanics.

Affective (Behavior)
☑ IV.4. Demonstrate awareness of the territorial boundaries of the person with whom communicating.

ABHES Competencies Achieved:

☑ 9. 1. Prepare patient for examinations and treatments.

EVALUATION OF COMPETENCY

Procedure 20-7: Sims Position

Name: _____   Date: _____

Evaluated By: _____   Score: _____

Performance Objective

Outcome:	Position and drape an individual in the Sims position.
Conditions:	Using an examining table.
	Given the following: a patient gown and a drape.
Standards:	Time: 5 minutes. Student completed procedure in ____ minutes.
	Accuracy: Satisfactory score on the Performance Evaluation Checklist.

Performance Evaluation Checklist

Trial 1	Trial 2	Point Value	Performance Standards
		●	Sanitized hands.
		●	Greeted the patient and introduced yourself.
		●	Identified the patient.
		●	Explained what type of examination or procedure would be performed.
		●	Provided patient with a patient gown.
		●	Instructed patient to remove clothing and to put on a patient gown with the opening in back.
		●	Pulled out the footrest and assisted the patient into a sitting position.
		●	Placed a drape over the patient's thighs and legs.
		●	Asked the patient to move back on the table.
		●	Pulled out the table extension while supporting the patient's lower legs.
		●	Asked the patient to lie down on his/her back.
		●	Positioned the drape lengthwise over the patient.
		●	Asked the patient to turn onto his/her left side.
		●	Provided assistance.
		●	Positioned the left arm behind the body and the right arm forward with the elbow bent.
		●	Assisted the patient in flexing the legs with the right leg flexed sharply and the left leg flexed slightly.
		●	Adjusted the drape by folding back the drape to expose the anal area when the physician was ready to examine the patient.

Trial 1	Trial 2	Point Value	Performance Standards
		•	Assisted the patient into a supine position and then into a sitting position following the examination.
		•	Slid the table extension back into place while supporting the patient's lower legs.
		•	Assisted the patient from the examining table.
		•	Returned the footrest to its normal position.
		•	Instructed the patient to get dressed.
		•	Discarded the gown and drape in a waste container.
		▷	Stated one use of the Sims position.
		∗	Completed the procedure within 5 minutes.
			TOTALS

Evaluation of Student Performance

EVALUATION CRITERIA			COMMENTS
Symbol	Category	Point Value	
∗	Critical Step	16 points	
•	Essential Step	6 points	
▷	Theory Question	2 points	
Score calculation: 100 points			
−_____ points missed			
_____ Score			
Satisfactory score: 85 or above			

CAAHEP Competencies Achieved:

Psychomotor (Skills)
☑ IV. 6. Prepare a patient for procedures and/or treatments.
☑ XI.11. Use proper body mechanics.

Affective (Behavior)
☑ IV.4. Demonstrate awareness of the territorial boundaries of the person with whom communicating.

ABHES Competencies Achieved:

☑ 9. 1. Prepare patient for examinations and treatments.

EVALUATION OF COMPETENCY

Procedure 20-8: Knee-Chest Position

Name: _____ Date: _____

Evaluated By: _____ Score: _____

Performance Objective

Outcome:	Position and drape an individual in the knee-chest position.
Conditions:	Using an examining table.
	Given the following: a patient gown and a drape.
Standards:	Time: 5 minutes. Student completed procedure in _____ minutes.
	Accuracy: Satisfactory score on the Performance Evaluation Checklist.

Performance Evaluation Checklist

Trial 1	Trial 2	Point Value	*Performance Standards*
		●	Sanitized hands.
		●	Greeted the patient and introduced yourself.
		●	Identified the patient.
		●	Explained what type of examination or procedure would be performed.
		●	Provided patient with a patient gown.
		●	Instructed patient to remove clothing and to put on a patient gown with the opening in back.
		●	Pulled out the footrest and assisted the patient into a sitting position.
		●	Placed a drape over the patient's thighs and legs.
		●	Asked the patient to move back on the table.
		●	Pulled out the table extension while supporting the patient's lower legs.
		●	Assisted the patient into the supine position and then into the prone position.
		●	Positioned the drape diagonally over the patient.
		●	Asked the patient to bend his/her arms at the elbows and rest them alongside his/her head.
		●	Asked the patient to elevate the buttocks while keeping his/her back straight.
		●	Turned the patient's head to one side, with the weight of his/her body supported by their chest.
		●	Used a pillow for additional support, if needed.
		●	Separated the knees and lower legs approximately 12 inches.
		●	Adjusted the drape diagonally as needed.

Trial 1	Trial 2	Point Value	Performance Standards
		●	Folded back a small portion of the drape to expose the anal area when the physician was ready to examine the patient.
		●	Assisted the patient into a prone position and then into a supine position after the examination.
		●	Allowed the patient to rest in a supine position before sitting up.
		▷	Stated why the patient should be allowed to rest.
		●	Assisted the patient into a sitting position.
		●	Slid the table extension back into place while supporting the patient's lower legs.
		●	Assisted the patient from the examining table.
		●	Returned the footrest to its normal position.
		●	Instructed the patient to get dressed.
		●	Discarded the gown and drape in a waste container.
		▷	Stated one use of the knee-chest position.
		✳	Completed the procedure within 5 minutes.
			TOTALS

Evaluation of Student Performance

EVALUATION CRITERIA			COMMENTS
Symbol	Category	Point Value	
✳	Critical Step	16 points	
●	Essential Step	6 points	
▷	Theory Question	2 points	

Score calculation: 100 points

−_____ points missed

_____ Score

Satisfactory score: 85 or above

CAAHEP Competencies Achieved:

Psychomotor (Skills)
☑ IV. 6. Prepare a patient for procedures and/or treatments.
☑ XI.11. Use proper body mechanics.

Affective (Behavior)
☑ IV.4. Demonstrate awareness of the territorial boundaries of the person with whom communicating.

ABHES Competencies Achieved:

☑ 9. 1. Prepare patient for examinations and treatments.

EVALUATION OF COMPETENCY

DVD   Procedure 20-9: Fowler's Position

Name: _____   Date: _____

Evaluated By: _____   Score: _____

Performance Objective

Outcome:	Position and drape an individual in the Fowler's position.
Conditions:	Using an examining table.
	Given the following: a patient gown and a drape.
Standards:	Time: 5 minutes. Student completed procedure in _____ minutes.
	Accuracy: Satisfactory score on the Performance Evaluation Checklist.

Performance Evaluation Checklist

Trial 1	Trial 2	Point Value	Performance Standards
		●	Sanitized hands.
		●	Greeted the patient and introduced yourself.
		●	Identified the patient.
		●	Explained what type of examination or procedure would be performed.
		●	Provided patient with a patient gown.
		●	Instructed patient to remove clothing and to put on a patient gown with the opening in front.
		●	Positioned the head of the table at a 45-degree angle for a semi-Fowler's position or at a 90-degree angle for a full Fowler's position.
		●	Pulled out the footrest and assisted the patient into a sitting position.
		●	Placed a drape over the patient's thighs and legs.
		●	Pulled out the table extension while supporting the patient's lower legs.
		●	Asked the patient to lean back against the table head.
		●	Provided assistance.
		●	Positioned a drape over the patient.
		●	Moved the drape according to the body parts being examined.
		●	Assisted the patient into a sitting position after the examination.
		●	Slid the table extension back into place while supporting the patient's lower legs.
		●	Assisted the patient from the examining table.
		●	Instructed the patient to get dressed.

Trial 1	Trial 2	Point Value	Performance Standards
		●	Returned the head of the table and the footrest to their normal positions.
		●	Discarded the gown and drape in a waste container.
		▷	Stated one use of the Fowler's position.
		✳	Completed the procedure within 5 minutes.
			TOTALS

Evaluation of Student Performance

EVALUATION CRITERIA			COMMENTS
Symbol	Category	Point Value	
✳	Critical Step	16 points	
●	Essential Step	6 points	
▷	Theory Question	2 points	

Score calculation: 100 points

− _____ points missed

_____ Score

Satisfactory score: 85 or above

CAAHEP Competencies Achieved:

Psychomotor (Skills)
☑ IV. 6. Prepare a patient for procedures and/or treatments.
☑ XI.11. Use proper body mechanics.

Affective (Behavior)
☑ IV.4. Demonstrate awareness of the territorial boundaries of the person with whom communicating.

ABHES Competencies Achieved:

☑ 9. l. Prepare patient for examinations and treatments.

☑ EVALUATION OF COMPETENCY

DVD **Procedure 20-10: Assisting with the Physical Examination**

Name: _____   Date: _____

Evaluated By: _____   Score: _____

Performance Objective

Outcome:	Prepare the patient and assist with a physical examination.
Conditions:	Using an examining table.
	Given the following: equipment for the type of examination to be performed, patient examination gown, and drapes.
Standards:	Time: 20 minutes. Student completed procedure in _____ minutes.
	Accuracy: Satisfactory score on the Performance Evaluation Checklist.

Performance Evaluation Checklist

Trial 1	Trial 2	Point Value	Performance Standards
		●	Prepared examining room.
		●	Sanitized hands.
		●	Assembled all necessary equipment.
		●	Arranged instruments in a neat and orderly manner.
		●	Obtained the patient's medical record.
		●	Went to the waiting room and asked the patient to come back.
		●	Escorted the patient to the examining room.
		●	Asked the patient to be seated.
		●	Greeted the patient and introduced yourself.
		●	Identified the patient by full name and date of birth.
		▷	Stated why a calm and friendly manner should be used.
		●	Seated yourself facing the patient at a distance of 3 to 4 feet.
		●	Obtained and recorded patient symptoms.
		●	Measured vital signs and charted results.
		▷	State the adult normal range for temperature (97°F-99°F), pulse (60-100 beats/min), respiration (12-20/min), and blood pressure (less than 120/80).
		●	Measured weight and height, and charted results.
		●	Asked patient if he or she needs to void.
		▷	Stated why the patient should be asked to void.
		●	Instructed patient to remove all clothing and put on an examining gown.

Trial 1	Trial 2	Point Value	Performance Standards
		•	Informed the patient that the physician would be in soon.
		•	Left the room to provide patient with privacy.
		•	Made patient's medical record available to the physician.
		•	Checked to make sure patient was ready to be seen.
		•	Informed physician that the patient was ready.
			Assisted the physician
		•	Ensured the patient was in a sitting position on examining table.
		•	Handed the ophthalmoscope to the physician when requested.
		•	Dimmed the lights when the physician was ready to use the ophthalmoscope.
		▷	Stated why the lights are dimmed.
		▷	Stated the proper use of the ophthalmoscope.
		•	Handed the otoscope to the examiner when requested.
		▷	Stated the proper use of the otoscope.
		•	Was able to change the speculum and bulb in the otoscope.
		•	Handed the tongue depressor to the examiner when requested.
		•	Offered reassurance to patient as needed.
		•	Positioned patient as required for examination of the remaining body systems.
			Assisted and instructed patient
		•	Allowed patient to rest in a sitting position before getting off the examining table.
		▷	Stated why the patient should be allowed to rest before getting off the table.
		•	Assisted patient off the examining table.
		•	Instructed patient to get dressed.
		•	Provided patient with any necessary instructions.
		▷	Stated what type of instructions may need to be relayed to the patient.
		•	Sanitized hands and charted any instructions given to the patient.
		•	Escorted the patient to the reception area.
			Cleaned the examining room
		•	Discarded paper on the examining table and unrolled a fresh length.
		•	Discarded all disposable supplies into an appropriate waste container.
		•	Checked to make sure ample supplies were available.
		•	Removed reusable equipment for sanitization, sterilization, or disinfection.
		✶	Completed the procedure within 20 minutes.
			TOTALS

	CHART	
Date		

Evaluation of Student Performance

EVALUATION CRITERIA			COMMENTS
Symbol	Category	Point Value	
∗	Critical Step	16 points	
●	Essential Step	6 points	
▷	Theory Question	2 points	

Score calculation: 100 points

－_____ points missed

_____   Score

Satisfactory score: 85 or above

CAAHEP Competencies Achieved:

Psychomotor (Skills)

☑ I. 10. Assist physician with patient care.

☑ IV. 5. Instruct patients according to their needs to promote health maintenance and disease prevention.

☑ IV. 6. Prepare a patient for procedures and/or treatments.

☑ IV. 12. Develop and maintain a current list of community resources related to patients' health care needs.

☑ V. 9. Perform routine maintenance of office equipment with documentation.

☑ XI.11. Use proper body mechanics.

Affective (Behavior)

☑ I. 3. Demonstrate respect for diversity in approaching patients and families.

☑ IV.2. Apply active listening skills.

☑ IV.3. Use appropriate body language and other nonverbal skills in communicating with patients, family, and staff.

☑ IV.8. Analyze communications in providing appropriate responses/feedback.

☑ IV.10. Demonstrate respect for individual diversity, incorporating awareness of one's own biases in areas including gender, race, religion, age, and economic status.

☑ X. 3. Demonstrate awareness of diversity in providing patient care.

ABHES Competencies Achieved:

☑ 8. y. Perform routine maintenance of administrative and clinical equipment.

☑ 8. z. Maintain inventory equipment and supplies.

☑ 8. aa. Are attentive, listen, and learn.

☑ 8. cc. Communicate on the recipient's level of comprehension.

☑ 8. ii. Recognize and respond to verbal and non-verbal communication.

☑ 8. kk. Adapt to individualized needs.

☑ 9. k. Prepare and maintain examination and treatment area.

☑ 9. l. Prepare patient for examinations and treatments.

☑ 9. m. Assist physician with routine and specialty examinations and treatments.

☑ 9. p. Advise patients of office policies and procedures.

☑ 9. r. Teach patients methods of health promotion and disease prevention.

Notes

21

Eye and Ear Assessment and Procedures

CHAPTER ASSIGNMENTS

√ After Completing	Date Due	Textbook Page(s)	TEXTBOOK ASSIGNMENTS	Possible Points	Points You Earned
		408-432	Read Chapter 21: Eye and Ear Assessment and Procedures		
		413 430	🖾 Read Case Study 1 Case Study 1 questions	5	
		417 430-431	🖾 Read Case Study 2 Case Study 2 questions	5	
		422 431	🖾 Read Case Study 3 Case Study 3 questions	5	
			TOTAL POINTS		

√ After Completing	Date Due	Study Guide Page(s)	STUDY GUIDE ASSIGNMENTS (CTA: Critical Thinking Activity)	Possible Points	Points You Earned
		371	📑 Pretest	10	
		372	🔑 Key Term Assessment	11	
		373-375	📝 Evaluation of Learning questions	21	
		375	CTA A: Measuring Distance Visual Acuity	6	
		375	CTA B: Interpreting Visual Acuity Results	4	
		375-376	CTA C: Charting Visual Acuity Results	4	
		376	CTA D: Ear Procedures	8	
		377	CTA E: Dear Gabby	10	
		378	CTA F: Crossword Puzzle	23	
		380	CTA G: Eye and Ear Conditions	40	

√ After Completing	Date Due	Study Guide Page(s)	STUDY GUIDE ASSIGNMENTS (CTA: Critical Thinking Activity)	Possible Points	Points You Earned
			💿 CD Activity: Chapter 21 Animations	10	
			💿 CD Activity: Chapter 21 Apply Your Knowledge questions (Record points earned)		
		371	Posttest	10	
			ADDITIONAL ASSIGNMENTS		
			TOTAL POINTS		

√ When Assigned by Your Instructor	Study Guide Page(s)	Practices Required	LABORATORY ASSIGNMENTS (Procedure Number and Name)	*Score
	383	5	(DVD) **Practice for Competency** 21-1: Assessing Distance Visual Acuity: Snellen Chart Textbook reference: pp. 415-416	
	385-386		**Evaluation of Competency** 21-1: Assessing Distance Visual Acuity: Snellen Chart	*
	383	3	(DVD) **Practice for Competency** 21-2: Assessing Color Vision: Ishihara Test Textbook reference: pp. 416-417	
	387-389		**Evaluation of Competency** 21-2: Assessing Color Vision: Ishihara Test	*
	383	3	(DVD) **Practice for Competency** 21-3: Performing an Eye Irrigation Textbook reference: pp. 418-420	
	391-393		**Evaluation of Competency** 21-3: Performing an Eye Irrigation	*
	383	3	(DVD) **Practice for Competency** 21-4: Performing an Eye Instillation Textbook reference: pp. 420-421	
	395-396		**Evaluation of Competency** 21-4: Performing an Eye Instillation	*
	383	3	(DVD) **Practice for Competency** 21-5: Performing an Ear Irrigation Textbook reference: pp. 427-428	
	397-399		**Evaluation of Competency** 21-5: Performing an Ear Irrigation	*
	383	3	(DVD) **Practice for Competency** 21-6: Performing an Ear Instillation Textbook reference: pp. 429-430	
	401-402		**Evaluation of Competency** 21-6: Performing an Ear Instillation	*
			ADDITIONAL ASSIGNMENTS	

Notes

Name _____   Date _____

?≡ PRETEST

True or False

_____ 1. *Refraction* refers to the bending of light rays so that they can be focused on the retina.

_____ 2. A person who is farsighted has a condition known as *myopia*.

_____ 3. An optometrist can perform eye surgery.

_____ 4. The Snellen eye test is conducted at a distance of 20 feet.

_____ 5. The Snellen eye chart should be positioned at the patient's eye level.

_____ 6. An eye instillation may be performed to treat an eye infection.

_____ 7. The function of cerumen is to inhibit the growth of pathogens.

_____ 8. The most specific type of hearing test is the tuning fork test.

_____ 9. Serous otitis media can result in a conductive hearing loss.

_____ 10. An ear instillation may be performed to treat an ear infection.

?≡ POSTTEST

True or False

_____ 1. A person who cannot see objects close up has a condition known as *amblyopia*.

_____ 2. *Visual acuity* refers to sharpness of vision.

_____ 3. Presbyopia is a decrease in the elasticity of the lens due to the aging process.

_____ 4. An optician fills prescriptions for eyeglasses.

_____ 5. The Snellen Big E chart is used with school-aged children.

_____ 6. The most common color vision defects are congenital in nature.

_____ 7. The external auditory canal of an adult is straightened by pulling the ear downward and backward.

_____ 8. The range of frequencies for normal speech is 300 to 4000 Hz.

_____ 9. Intense noise can result in a sensorineural hearing loss.

_____ 10. Tympanometry is used to diagnose patients with auditory nerve damage.

Directions: Match each medical term with its definition.

_____ 1. Audiometer

_____ 2. Canthus

_____ 3. Cerumen

_____ 4. Hyperopia

_____ 5. Instillation

_____ 6. Irrigation

_____ 7. Myopia

_____ 8. Otoscope

_____ 9. Presbyopia

_____ 10. Refraction

_____ 11. Tympanic membrane

A. The washing of a body canal with a flowing solution

B. A decrease in the elasticity of the lens that occurs with aging, resulting in a decreased ability to focus on close objects

C. Farsightedness

D. The deflection or bending of light rays by a lens

E. The junction of the eyelids at either corner of the eye

F. Nearsightedness

G. The dropping of a liquid into a body cavity

H. An instrument for examining the external ear canal and tympanic membrane

I. Earwax

J. An instrument used to quantitatively measure hearing acuity for the various frequencies of sound waves

K. A thin, semitransparent membrane located between the external ear canal and the middle ear that receives and transmits sound waves

EVALUATION OF LEARNING

Directions: Fill in each blank with the correct answer.

The Eye

1. What are each of the following eye professionals qualified to perform?

   a. Ophthalmologist

   _____

   _____

   b. Optometrist

   _____

   _____

   c. Optician

   _____

   _____

2. What is visual acuity?

   _____

   _____

3. What condition can be detected by measuring distance visual acuity (DVA)?

   _____

4. What type of patient would warrant use of the Snellen Big E eye chart? (Give two examples.)

   _____

   _____

5. Explain the significance of the top number and bottom number next to each line of letters of the Snellen eye chart.

   _____

   _____

6. List two conditions that can be detected by measuring near visual acuity.

   _____

   _____

7. Explain the difference between congenital and acquired color vision defects.

   _____

   _____

   _____

8. What is a polychromatic plate?

   _____

   _____

   _____

9. List three reasons for performing an eye irrigation.

_____

_____

_____

10. List three reasons for performing an eye instillation.

_____

_____

The Ear

11. What is the range of frequencies for normal speech?

_____

12. List five conditions that may cause a conductive hearing loss.

_____

_____

_____

13. List four conditions that may cause a sensorineural hearing loss.

_____

_____

14. How is hearing acuity tested with the gross screening test?

_____

_____

_____

15. What are the names of the hearing acuity tests that require the use of a tuning fork?

_____

_____

16. What information is obtained through audiometry?

_____

_____

_____

17. What information is obtained through tympanometry?

_____

_____

_____

18. List three reasons for performing an ear irrigation.

_____

_____

19. List three reasons for performing an ear instillation.

_____

_____

20. Explain how impacted cerumen is removed from the ear.

_____

_____

_____

21. Explain how to straighten the external auditory canal in adults and in children 3 years old and younger.

_____

_____

_____

CRITICAL THINKING ACTIVITIES

A. MEASURING DISTANCE VISUAL ACUITY
   For each of the following situations, write *C* if the technique is correct and *I* if the technique is incorrect.

_____ 1. The patient is not given an opportunity to study the Snellen chart before beginning the test.

_____ 2. The Snellen chart is positioned at the MA's eye level.

_____ 3. The patient is instructed to use his or her hand to cover the eye that is not being tested.

_____ 4. The MA instructs the patient to close the eye that is not being tested.

_____ 5. The first line that the MA asks the patient to identify is the 20/20 line.

_____ 6. The MA observes the patient for signs of squinting or leaning forward during the test.

B. INTERPRETING VISUAL ACUITY RESULTS
   1. A patient has a DVA reading of 20/30 in the right eye. Using this information, answer the following questions:

   a. How far was the patient from the eye chart?

   _____

   b. At what distance would a person with normal acuity be able to read this line?

   _____

   2. A patient has a DVA reading of 20/10 in the left eye. Using this information, answer the following questions:

   a. How far was the patient from the eye chart?

   _____

   b. At what distance would a person with normal acuity be able to read this line?

   _____

C. CHARTING VISUAL ACUITY RESULTS
   Properly chart the DVA results in the spaces provided. In all cases, the line indicated is the smallest line the patient could read at a distance of 20 feet.

   1. The patient read the line marked 20/30 with the right eye with two errors and read the line marked 20/30 with the left eye with one error. The patient was wearing corrective lenses.

   _____

   _____

2. The patient read the line marked 20/20 with the right eye with one error and read the line marked 20/20 with the left eye with no errors. The patient was wearing corrective lenses.

_____

_____

3. The patient read the line marked 20/40 with the right eye with two errors and read the line marked 20/30 with the left eye with one error. The patient exhibited squinting and frowning during the test. The patient was not wearing corrective lenses.

_____

_____

4. The patient read the line marked 20/15 with the right eye with no errors and read the line marked 20/20 with the left eye with one error. The patient was not wearing corrective lenses.

_____

_____

D. EAR PROCEDURES
Explain the principle for each of the following:

Ear Irrigation

1. Positioning the patient's head so that it is tilted toward the affected ear

_____

_____

2. Cleansing the outer ear before irrigating

_____

_____

3. Straightening the external auditory canal

_____

_____

4. Injecting the irrigating solution toward the roof of the ear canal

_____

_____

5. Making sure not to obstruct the canal opening

_____

_____

Ear Instillation

6. Positioning the patient's head so that it is tilted toward the unaffected ear

_____

_____

7. Instructing the patient to lie on the unaffected side after the instillation

_____

_____

8. Placing a cotton wick in the patient's ear

_____

_____

E. DEAR GABBY

Gabby has a middle ear infection and is not feeling well. She wants you to fill in for her. In the space provided, respond to the following letter.

Dear Gabby:

I am dating the sweetest and dearest guy. "Mike" has only one flaw. He likes loud music. He had those big boom boxes installed in his car. When we drive somewhere in his car, he blasts the music. Sometimes when we are driving down a street, people even turn around to see where the loud music is coming from. The music hurts my ears and I cannot think straight.

My ears even start ringing when we go on a trip. When I am talking to Mike, he says I mumble, and so I have to speak extra loud around him. I keep telling Mike that the loud music is going to damage our hearing, but he says that we are way too young for that and that only old people have trouble hearing.

Please help me Gabby, because I love going on trips with Mike, but not if my ears hurt afterward.

Signed, Ears Are Ringing

_____

_____

_____

_____

_____

_____

_____

_____

_____

_____

_____

F. CROSSWORD PUZZLE
Eye and Ear
Directions: Complete the crossword puzzle using the clues provided below.

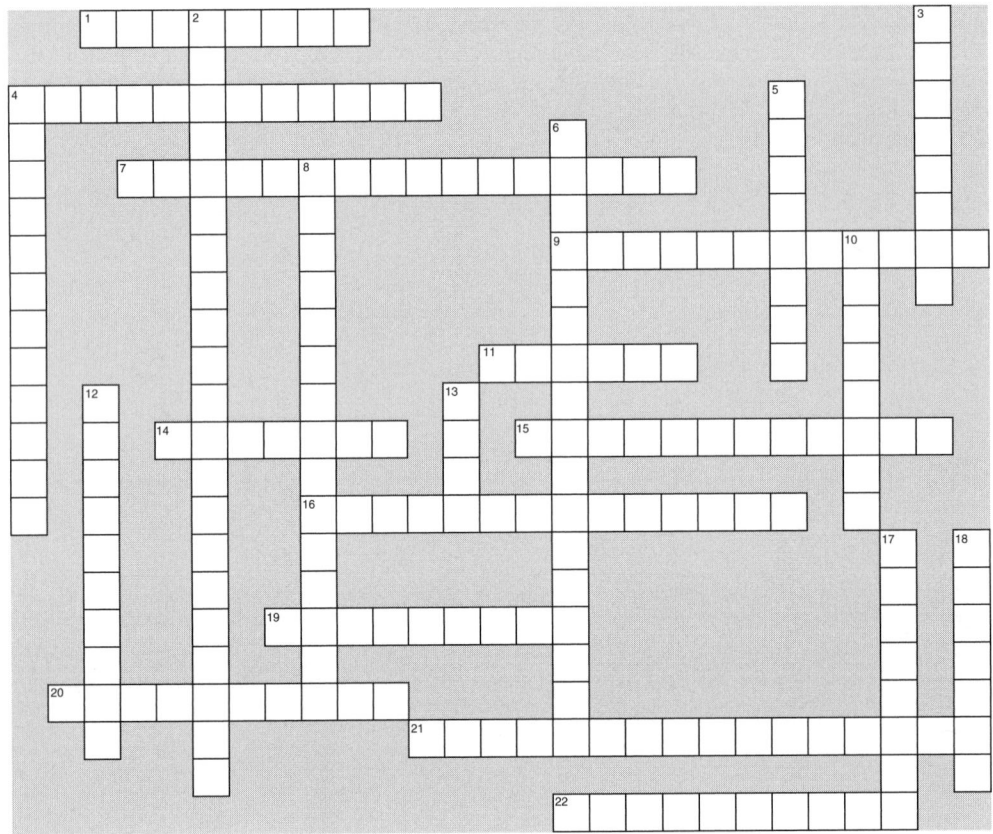

ACROSS
1 Has an S shape
4 Assesses mobility of eardrum
7 Middle ear infection
9 Fixed stapes
11 Cannot see far away
14 Earwax
15 Sharpness of vision
16 20/200 OU c̄c
19 Symptom of pink eye
20 Instrument that measures hearing
21 Drum in your ear
22 Decreased lens elasticity

DOWN
2 Impacted cerumen may cause this
3 A cause of pink eye
4 Normal DVA
5 Risk factor for eye disorders
6 Fluid in middle ear
8 Physician who diagnoses and treats eye disorders
10 Fills eyeglasses prescriptions
12 Caught it!
13 Music that is too loud may cause this
17 Color blind test
18 Measurement for sound

Notes

G. EYE AND EAR CONDITIONS

1. You and your classmates work at a large clinic. It is National Eye and Ear Week. The physicians at your clinic ask you to develop informative, creative, and colorful brochures for patients relating to eye and ear conditions. Choose a condition from the following list, and design a brochure using the blank FAQ (Frequently Asked Questions) brochure provided on the following page. Each student in the class should select a different topic. On a separate sheet of paper, write three true-or-false questions relating to the information in your brochure.

2. Present your brochure to the class. After all the brochures have been presented, each student should ask his or her three questions to the entire class to see how well the class understands eye and ear conditions. (*Note:* You can take notes during the presentations and refer to them when answering the questions.)

Eye

1. Amblyopia (lazy eye)
2. Age-related macular degeneration
3. Astigmatism
4. Blepharitis
5. Cataracts
6. Cytomegalovirus retinitis
7. Corneal ulcer
8. Corneal abrasion
9. Strabismus (cross-eyed)
10. Diabetic retinopathy
11. Drooping eyelids (ptosis)
12. Dry eyes
13. Floaters and spots
14. Glaucoma
15. Keratoconus
16. Ocular hypertension
17. Retinal detachment
18. Retinitis pigmentosa
19. Stye

Ear

1. Acute mastoiditis
2. External otitis
3. Meniere's disease
4. Noise-induced hearing loss
5. Serous otitis media

FAQ
on:

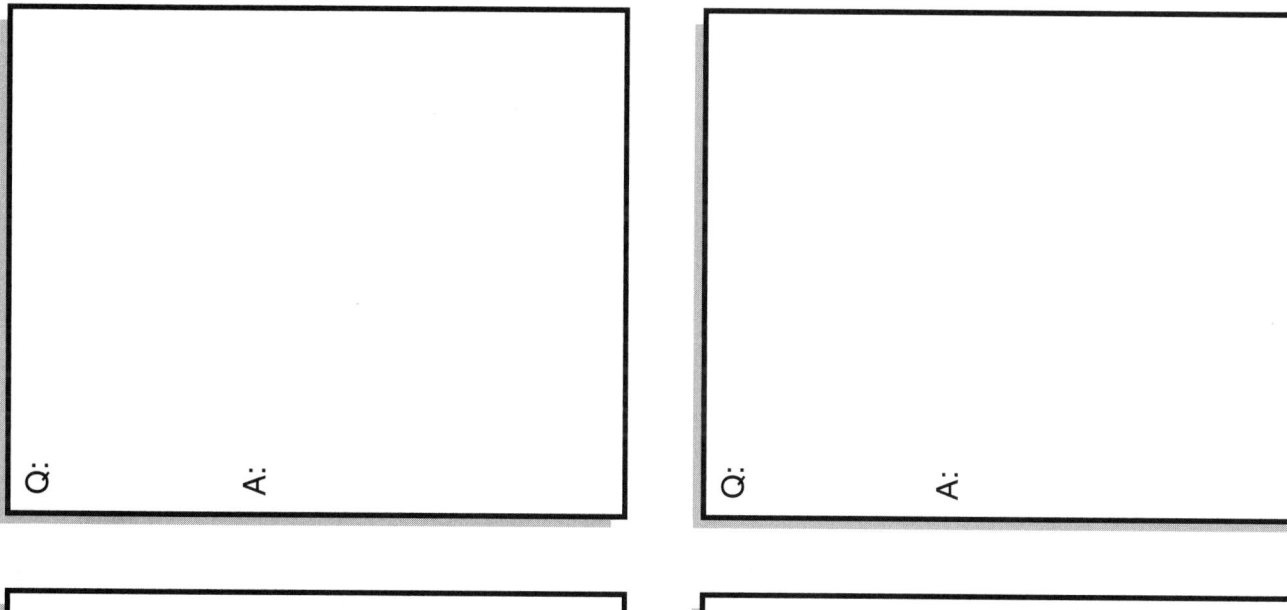

Q: A:

Q: A:

Q: A:

Q: A:

Q:

A:

Q:

A:

Illustration

Q:

A:

Q:

A:

PRACTICE FOR COMPETENCY

Eye Assessment and Procedures

Procedure 21-1: Distance Visual Acuity. Assess distance visual acuity using a Snellen eye chart and record results in the chart provided. Circle any readings that indicate distance visual acuity above or below average.

Procedure 21-2: Color Vision. Assess color vision and record results in the chart provided. Circle any abnormal results.

Procedure 21-3: Eye Irrigation. Perform an eye irrigation and record the procedure in the chart provided.

Procedure 21-4: Eye Instillation. Perform an eye instillation and record the procedure in the chart provided.

Ear Procedures

Procedure 21-5: Ear Irrigation. Perform an ear irrigation and record the procedure in the chart provided.

Procedure 21-6: Ear Instillation. Perform an ear instillation and record the procedure in the chart provided.

CHART	
Date	

CHART	
Date	

EVALUATION OF COMPETENCY

Procedure 21-1: Assessing Distance Visual Acuity—Snellen Chart

Name: _____   Date: _____

Evaluated By: _____   Score: _____

Performance Objective

Outcome:	Assess distance visual acuity.
Conditions:	Given the following: Snellen eye chart, eye occluder, and an antiseptic wipe.
Standards:	Time: 5 minutes. Student completed procedure in _____ minutes.
	Accuracy: Satisfactory score on the Performance Evaluation Checklist.

Performance Evaluation Checklist

Trial 1	Trial 2	Point Value	Performance Standards
		●	Sanitized hands.
		●	Assembled equipment.
		●	Disinfected the eye occluder with an antiseptic wipe.
		●	Greeted the patient and introduced yourself.
		●	Identified the patient and explained the procedure.
		●	Determined if patient wears corrective lenses and instructed patient to leave them on during the test.
		●	Positioned patient 20 feet from the eye chart.
		●	Positioned the center of the eye chart at patient's eye level.
		●	Instructed patient to cover the left eye with the occluder and to keep the left eye open.
		▷	Stated how the occluder should be positioned if the patient wears glasses.
		▷	Explained why the patient's left eye should remain open.
		●	Instructed patient not to squint during the test.
		▷	Explained why patient should not squint during the test.
		●	Asked patient to identify the 20/70 line, using the right eye.
		▷	Stated why the test should begin with a line that is above the 20/20 line.
		●	Proceeded down the chart if the patient identified the 20/70 line or proceeded up the chart if the patient was unable to identify the 20/70 line.
		●	Continued until the smallest line of letters that the patient could read was reached.

Trial 1	Trial 2	Point Value	Performance Standards
		•	Observed patient for any unusual symptoms.
		•	Jotted down the numbers next to the smallest line read by the patient.
		•	Asked patient to cover the right eye and to keep the right eye open.
		•	Measured visual acuity in the left eye.
		•	Jotted down the numbers next to the smallest line read by the patient.
		✳	The visual acuity measurements were identical to the evaluator's measurements.
		•	Charted the results correctly.
		•	Disinfected the occluder with an antiseptic wipe.
		•	Sanitized hands.
		✳	Completed the procedure within 5 minutes.
			TOTALS

CHART

Date	

Evaluation of Student Performance

EVALUATION CRITERIA			COMMENTS
Symbol	**Category**	**Point Value**	
✳	Critical Step	16 points	
•	Essential Step	6 points	
▷	Theory Question	2 points	

Score calculation: 100 points

− _____ points missed

_____ Score

Satisfactory score: 85 or above

CAAHEP Competencies Achieved:

Psychomotor (Skills)
☑ IV. 6. Prepare a patient for procedures and/or treatments.

Affective (Behavior)
☑ I. 2. Use language/verbal skills that enable patients' understanding.
☑ IV. 7. Demonstrate recognition of the patient's level of understanding in communications.

ABHES Competencies Achieved:

☑ 8. cc. Communicate on the recipient's level of comprehension.
☑ 9. l. Prepare patient for examinations and treatments.

EVALUATION OF COMPETENCY

Procedure 21-2: Assessing Color Vision—Ishihara Test

Name: _____   Date: _____

Evaluated By: _____   Score: _____

Performance Objective

Outcome:	Assess color vision.
Conditions:	Given an Ishihara book of color plates and a cotton swab.
Standards:	Time: 10 minutes. Student completed procedure in _____ minutes.
	Accuracy: Satisfactory score on the Performance Evaluation Checklist.

Performance Evaluation Checklist

Trial 1	Trial 2	Point Value	Performance Standards
		●	Sanitized hands.
		●	Assembled equipment.
		●	Conducted the test in a quiet room illuminated by natural daylight.
		▷	Stated why natural daylight should be used.
		●	Greeted the patient and introduced yourself.
		●	Identified the patient.
		●	Explained the procedure using the practice plate.
		▷	Stated the purpose of the practice plate.
		●	Held the first plate 30 inches from the patient at a right angle to the patient's line of vision.
		●	Instructed patient to keep both eyes open.
		●	Told patient that he/she would have 3 seconds to identify each plate.
		●	Asked the patient to identify the number on the plate.
		●	Asked the patient to trace plates with winding lines with a cotton swab.
		▷	Stated why a cotton swab should be used to make the tracing.
		●	Recorded the results after identification of each plate.
		●	Continued until the patient viewed all plates.
		●	Charted the results correctly.
		✻	The results were identical to the evaluator's results.
		●	Returned the Ishihara book to its proper place, storing it in a closed position.
		▷	Explained why the book should be stored in a closed position.
		✻	Completed the procedure within 10 minutes.
			TOTALS

CHART	
Date	

CHART		
Plate No.	Normal Person	Results
1	12	
2	8	
3	5	
4	29	
5	74	
6	7	
7	45	
8	2	
9	X	
10	16	
11	Traceable	
Date :		
Evaluated by :		

(From Bonewit-West K: *Study guide for clinical procedures for medical assistants,* ed 7, St. Louis, 2008, Saunders.)

Evaluation of Student Performance

EVALUATION CRITERIA			COMMENTS
Symbol	Category	Point Value	
∗	Critical Step	16 points	
●	Essential Step	6 points	
▷	Theory Question	2 points	
Score calculation: 100 points			
− _____ points missed			
_____ Score			
Satisfactory score: 85 or above			

CAAHEP Competencies Achieved:

Psychomotor (Skills)

☑ IV. 6. Prepare a patient for procedures and/or treatments.

Affective (Behavior)

☑ I. 2. Use language/verbal skills that enable patients' understanding.
☑ IV. 7. Demonstrate recognition of the patient's level of understanding in communications.

ABHES Competencies Achieved:

☑ 8. cc. Communicate on the recipient's level of comprehension.
☑ 9. l. Prepare patient for examinations and treatments.

Notes

EVALUATION OF COMPETENCY

Procedure 21-3: Performing an Eye Irrigation

Name: _____   Date: _____

Evaluated By: _____   Score: _____

Performance Objective

Outcome:	Perform an eye irrigation.
Conditions:	Given the following: disposable gloves (nonpowdered), irrigating solution, solution container, disposable rubber bulb syringe, basin, moisture-resistant towel, and sterile gauze pads.
Standards:	Time: 5 minutes. Student completed procedure in ____ minutes.
	Accuracy: Satisfactory score on the Performance Evaluation Checklist.

Performance Evaluation Checklist

Trial 1	Trial 2	Point Value	Performance Standards
		•	Sanitized hands.
		•	Assembled equipment.
		•	Checked the solution label with the physician's instructions.
		•	Checked expiration date of the solution.
		▷	Stated the reason for checking the expiration date.
		•	Warmed the irrigating solution to body temperature.
		▷	Explained why the solution should be at body temperature.
		•	Checked the label a second time and poured the solution into a basin.
		•	Checked the label a third time before returning the container to storage.
		•	Greeted the patient and introduced yourself.
		•	Identified the patient and explained the procedure.
		•	Asked patient to remove glasses or contact lenses.
		•	Positioned patient in a lying or sitting position.
		•	Placed a moisture-resistant towel on the patient's shoulder.
		•	Positioned a basin tightly against the patient's cheek.
		•	Asked the patient to tilt head in the direction of the affected eye and hold the basin in place.
		▷	Explained why patient's head is turned in the direction of the affected eye.
		•	Applied nonpowdered gloves.
		▷	Stated why nonpowdered gloves should be used.
		•	Cleanse the eyelids from inner to outer canthus.

Trial 1	Trial 2	Point Value	Performance Standards
		▷	Stated why eyelids are cleansed.
		●	Filled irrigating syringe.
		●	Instructed patient to keep both eyes open and to look at a focal point.
		▷	Stated the reason for looking at a focal point.
		●	Separated eyelids.
		●	Held tip of syringe 1 inch above the eye at the inner canthus.
		●	Allowed solution to flow over the eye at a moderate rate from the inner canthus to the outer canthus and directed solution to the lower conjunctiva.
		▷	Explained why the syringe should be directed toward the lower conjunctiva.
		●	Did not allow syringe to touch the eye.
		●	Refilled the syringe and continued irrigating until the desired results were obtained or all the solution was used.
		●	Dried eyelids with gauze pad from inner to outer canthus.
		●	Removed gloves and sanitized hands.
		●	Charted the procedure correctly.
		▷	Stated the abbreviation for both eyes (OU), the right eye (OD), and the left eye (OS).
		●	Returned equipment.
		✶	Completed the procedure within 5 minutes.
			TOTALS

	CHART
Date	

Evaluation of Student Performance

EVALUATION CRITERIA			COMMENTS
Symbol	**Category**	**Point Value**	
✶	Critical Step	16 points	
●	Essential Step	6 points	
▷	Theory Question	2 points	

Score calculation: 100 points

−_____ points missed

_____ Score

Satisfactory score: 85 or above

CAAHEP Competencies Achieved:

Psychomotor (Skills)
☑ II. 1. Prepare proper dosages of medication for administration.
☑ IV. 6. Prepare a patient for procedures and/or treatments.

Affective (Behavior)
☑ II. 1. Verify ordered doses/dosages prior to administration.
☑ IV. 5. Demonstrate sensitivity appropriate to the message being delivered.

ABHES Competencies Achieved:

☑ 8. bb. Are impartial and show empathy when dealing with patients.
☑ 9. d. Recognize and understand various treatment protocols.
☑ 9. l. Prepare patient for examinations and treatments.

Notes

EVALUATION OF COMPETENCY

DVD **Procedure 21-4: Performing an Eye Instillation**

Name: _____ Date: _____

Evaluated By: _____ Score: _____

Performance Objective

Outcome:	Perform an eye instillation.
Conditions:	Given the following: disposable (nonpowdered) gloves, ophthalmic medication, tissues, and gauze pads.
Standards:	Time: 5 minutes. Student completed procedure in _____ minutes.
	Accuracy: Satisfactory score on the Performance Evaluation Checklist.

Performance Evaluation Checklist

Trial 1	Trial 2	Point Value	Performance Standards
		●	Sanitized hands.
		●	Assembled equipment.
		●	Checked the drug label when removing it from storage.
		▷	Stated what word must appear on the medication label.
		●	Checked drug label and dosage against the physician's instructions.
		●	Checked the expiration date of the medication.
		●	Greeted the patient and introduced yourself.
		●	Identified the patient and explained the procedure.
		●	Positioned patient in a sitting or supine position.
		●	Applied nonpowdered gloves.
		●	Prepared the medication.
		●	Checked the drug label and removed the cap.
		●	Asked patient to look up and exposed the lower conjunctival sac.
		▷	Explained the reason for asking patient to look up.
		●	Drew the skin of the cheek downward and exposed the conjunctival sac.
		●	Inserted the medication correctly.
		▷	Explained how to instill eye drops and ointment.
		●	Instructed patient to close eyes gently and move eyeballs.
		▷	Stated the reason for closing the eyes and moving the eyeballs.
		●	Told patient that the instillation may temporarily blur vision.

Trial 1	Trial 2	Point Value	Performance Standards
		●	Dried eyelids with a gauze pad from inner to outer canthus.
		●	Removed gloves and sanitized hands.
		●	Charted the procedure correctly.
		●	Returned equipment.
		✶	Completed the procedure within 5 minutes.
			TOTALS

	CHART
Date	

Evaluation of Student Performance

EVALUATION CRITERIA			COMMENTS
Symbol	**Category**	**Point Value**	
✶	Critical Step	16 points	
●	Essential Step	6 points	
▷	Theory Question	2 points	
Score calculation: 100 points			
− _____ points missed			
_____ Score			
Satisfactory score: 85 or above			

CAAHEP Competencies Achieved:

Psychomotor (Skills)
☑ II. 1. Prepare proper dosages of medication for administration.
☑ IV. 6. Prepare a patient for procedures and/or treatments.

Affective (Behavior)
☑ II. 1. Verify ordered doses/dosages prior to administration.
☑ IV. 5. Demonstrate sensitivity appropriate to the message being delivered.

ABHES Competencies Achieved:

☑ 8. bb. Are impartial and show empathy when dealing with patients.
☑ 9. d. Recognize and understand various treatment protocols.
☑ 9. l. Prepare patient for examinations and treatments.

EVALUATION OF COMPETENCY

Procedure 21-5: Performing an Ear Irrigation

Name: _____   Date: _____

Evaluated By: _____   Score: _____

Performance Objective

Outcome:	Perform an ear irrigation.
Conditions:	Given the following: disposable gloves, irrigating solution, solution container, irrigating syringe, ear basin, moisture-resistant towel, gauze pads, and ear wick.
Standards:	Time: 10 minutes. Student completed procedure in ____ minutes.
	Accuracy: Satisfactory score on the Performance Evaluation Checklist.

Performance Evaluation Checklist

Trial 1	Trial 2	Point Value	Performance Standards
		●	Sanitized hands.
		●	Assembled equipment.
		●	Checked the label of the irrigating solution with the physician's instructions.
		●	Checked expiration date of the solution.
		●	Warmed the irrigating solution to body temperature.
		▷	Stated the reason for warming the irrigating solution.
		●	Check the label a second time and poured the solution into a basin.
		●	Check the label a third time before returning the container to storage.
		●	Greeted the patient and introduced yourself.
		●	Identified the patient and explained procedure.
		●	Positioned patient with the head tilted toward the affected ear.
		▷	Explained why the head should be tilted toward the affected ear.
		●	Placed a towel on patient's shoulder and instructed patient to hold the ear basin under the affected ear.
		●	Applied gloves.
		●	Cleansed the outer ear.
		▷	Explained why the outer ear should be cleansed.
		●	Filled the irrigating syringe.
		●	Expelled air from syringe.
		▷	Explained why air should be expelled from syringe.
		●	Properly straightened the ear canal.
		▷	Stated why the canal must be straightened.

Trial 1	Trial 2	Point Value	Performance Standards
		•	Inserted syringe tip into the ear.
		•	Did not insert the syringe too deeply.
		•	Made sure that tip of syringe did not obstruct the canal opening.
		▷	Stated why the canal should not be obstructed.
		•	Injected the irrigating solution toward the roof of the ear canal.
		▷	Stated why solution should be injected toward roof of the canal.
		•	Refilled the syringe and continued irrigating until the desired results were obtained or all the solution was used.
		•	Observed the returning solution to note the material present and the amount.
		•	Dried outside of the ear with a gauze pad.
		•	Informed patient that the ear will feel sensitive.
		•	Instructed patient to lie on the affected side on treatment table.
		▷	Explained why patient should lie on the affected side.
		•	Inserted a cotton wick loosely in the ear canal for 15 minutes.
		▷	Stated the purpose of the cotton wick.
		•	Removed gloves and sanitized hands.
		•	Charted the procedure correctly.
		▷	Stated the abbreviation for both ears (AU), the right ear (AD), and the left ear (AS).
		•	Returned equipment.
		∗	Completed the procedure within 10 minutes.
			TOTALS
			CHART
	Date		

Evaluation of Student Performance

EVALUATION CRITERIA			COMMENTS
Symbol	Category	Point Value	
＊	Critical Step	16 points	
●	Essential Step	6 points	
▷	Theory Question	2 points	

Score calculation: 100 points

– _____ points missed

_____ Score

Satisfactory score: 85 or above

CAAHEP Competencies Achieved:

Psychomotor (Skills)
☑ II. 1. Prepare proper dosages of medication for administration.
☑ IV. 6. Prepare a patient for procedures and/or treatments.

Affective (Behavior)
☑ II. 1. Verify ordered doses/dosages prior to administration.
☑ IV. 5. Demonstrate sensitivity appropriate to the message being delivered.

ABHES Competencies Achieved:

☑ 8. bb. Are impartial and show empathy when dealing with patients.
☑ 9. d. Recognize and understand various treatment protocols.
☑ 9. l. Prepare patient for examinations and treatments.

Notes

EVALUATION OF COMPETENCY

Procedure 21-6: Performing an Ear Instillation

Name: _____   Date: _____

Evaluated By: _____   Score: _____

Performance Objective

Outcome:	Perform an ear instillation.
Conditions:	Given the following: disposable gloves, otic medication, and gauze pad.
Standards:	Time: 5 minutes. Student completed procedure in _____ minutes.
	Accuracy: Satisfactory score on the Performance Evaluation Checklist.

Performance Evaluation Checklist

Trial 1	Trial 2	Point Value	Performance Standards
		●	Sanitized hands.
		●	Assembled equipment.
		●	Checked the drug label when removing the medication from storage.
		▷	Stated what word must appear on the medication label.
		●	Checked the drug label and dosage against the physician's instructions.
		●	Checked the expiration date of the medication.
		▷	Explained what might occur if the medication is outdated.
		●	Greeted the patient and introduced yourself.
		●	Identified the patient and explained the procedure.
		●	Positioned patient in a sitting position.
		●	Warmed the ear drops with your hands.
		●	Applied gloves.
		●	Mixed medication if required.
		●	Check the drug label and removed the cap.
		●	Asked the patient to tilt the head in the direction of the unaffected ear.
		●	Properly straightened the ear canal.
		▷	Stated the reason for straightening the canal.
		●	Placed tip of dropper at the opening of the ear canal and inserted the proper amount of medication.
		●	Instructed patient to lie on the unaffected side for 2 to 3 minutes.
		▷	Explained why patient should lie on the unaffected side.
		●	Placed a moistened cotton wick loosely in the ear canal for 15 minutes.

Trial 1	Trial 2	Point Value	Performance Standards
		▷	Stated the reason for moistening the wick.
		●	Removed gloves and sanitized hands.
		●	Charted the procedure correctly.
		●	Returned equipment.
		✳	Completed the procedure within 5 minutes.
			TOTALS

CHART

Date	

Evaluation of Student Performance

EVALUATION CRITERIA			COMMENTS
Symbol	Category	Point Value	
✳	Critical Step	16 points	
●	Essential Step	6 points	
▷	Theory Question	2 points	

Score calculation: 100 points

−_____ points missed

_____ Score

Satisfactory score: 85 or above

CAAHEP Competencies Achieved:

Psychomotor (Skills)

☑ II. 1. Prepare proper dosages of medication for administration.
☑ IV. 6. Prepare a patient for procedures and/or treatments.

Affective (Behavior)
☑ II. 1. Verify ordered doses/dosages prior to administration.
☑ IV. 5. Demonstrate sensitivity appropriate to the message being delivered.

ABHES Competencies Achieved:

☑ 8. bb. Are impartial and show empathy when dealing with patients.
☑ 9. d. Recognize and understand various treatment protocols.
☑ 9. l. Prepare patient for examinations and treatments.

22

Physical Agents to Promote Tissue Healing

CHAPTER ASSIGNMENTS

√ After Completing	Date Due	Textbook Page(s)	TEXTBOOK ASSIGNMENTS	Possible Points	Points You Earned
		433-451	Read Chapter 22: Physical Agents to Promote Tissue Healing		
		436 450	Read Case Study 1 Case Study 1 questions	5	
		446 450	Read Case Study 2 Case Study 2 questions	5	
			TOTAL POINTS		

√ After Completing	Date Due	Study Guide Page(s)	STUDY GUIDE ASSIGNMENTS (CTA: Critical Thinking Activity)	Possible Points	Points You Earned
		407	Pretest	10	
		408	Key Term Assessment	9	
		409-410	Evaluation of Learning questions	15	
		411	CTA A: Dear Gabby	10	
		411-412	CTA B: Crutch Guidelines	8	
		412	CTA C: Accessibility for Physical Disabilities	7	
		413	CTA D: Crossword Puzzle	26	
		414	CTA E: Bone and Joint Conditions	40	
			CD Activity: Chapter 22 Animations	20	
			CD Activity: Chapter 22 Quiz Show (Record points earned)		

√ After Completing	Date Due	Study Guide Page(s)	STUDY GUIDE ASSIGNMENTS (CTA: Critical Thinking Activity)	Possible Points	Points You Earned
			CD Activity: Chapter 22 Apply Your Knowledge questions (Record points earned)		
		407	Posttest	10	
			ADDITIONAL ASSIGNMENTS		
			TOTAL POINTS		

√ When Assigned by Your Instructor	Study Guide Page(s)	Practices Required	LABORATORY ASSIGNMENTS (Procedure Number and Name)	*Score
	417	3	**DVD Practice for Competency** 22-1: Applying a Heating Pad Textbook reference: p. 437	
	419-420		**Evaluation of Competency** 22-1: Applying a Heating Pad	*
	417	3	**DVD Practice for Competency** 22-2: Applying a Hot Soak Textbook reference: p. 438	
	421-422		**Evaluation of Competency** 22-2: Applying a Hot Soak	*
	417	3	**DVD Practice for Competency** 22-3: Applying a Hot Compress Textbook reference: p. 439	
	423-424		**Evaluation of Competency** 22-3: Applying a Hot Compress	*
	417	3	**DVD Practice for Competency** 22-4: Applying an Ice Bag Textbook reference: p. 440	
	425-426		**Evaluation of Competency** 22-4: Applying an Ice Bag	*
	417	3	**DVD Practice for Competency** 22-5: Applying a Cold Compress Textbook reference: p. 441	
	427-428		**Evaluation of Competency** 22-5: Applying a Cold Compress	*
	417	3	**DVD Practice for Competency** 22-6: Applying a Chemical Pack Textbook reference: p. 442	
	429-430		**Evaluation of Competency** 22-6: Applying a Chemical Pack	*
	417	3	**DVD Practice for Competency** 22-7: Measuring for Axillary Crutches Textbook reference: p. 446	
	431-432		**Evaluation of Competency** 22-7: Measuring for Axillary Crutches	*
	417	3× for each gait	**DVD Practice for Competency** 22-8: Instructing a Patient in Crutch Gaits Textbook reference: pp. 447-449	
	433-435		**Evaluation of Competency** 22-8: Instructing a Patient in Crutch Gaits	*

√ When Assigned by Your Instructor	Study Guide Page(s)	Practices Required	LABORATORY ASSIGNMENTS (Procedure Number and Name)	*Score
	417	Cane: 3 Walker: 3	(DVD) **Practice for Competency** 22-9 and 22-10: Instructing a Patient in the Use of a Cane and Walker Textbook reference: pp. 449-450	
	437-438		**Evaluation of Competency** 22-9 and 22-10: Instructing a Patient in the Use of a Cane and Walker	*
			ADDITIONAL ASSIGNMENTS	

Name _____   Date _____

? PRETEST

True or False

_____ 1. A hot compress is an example of moist heat.

_____ 2. Erythema is redness of the skin caused by dilation of superficial blood vessels.

_____ 3. The local application of cold may be used to relieve muscle spasms.

_____ 4. Heat is often prescribed by the physician for black eyes.

_____ 5. The medical assistant should instruct the patient to adjust the heating pad to a higher setting if it no longer feels warm.

_____ 6. Chemical cold packs should be stored in the refrigerator.

_____ 7. Forearm crutches are often used by patients with cerebral palsy.

_____ 8. The three-point gait is the most stable and slowest crutch gait.

_____ 9. *Ambulation* refers to the inability to walk.

_____ 10. A patient using crutches should be instructed to support his weight against the axilla.

? POSTTEST

True or False

_____ 1. The recommended time for the application of heat is 15-30 minutes.

_____ 2. The local application of heat results in constriction of blood vessels in the area to which it is applied.

_____ 3. The most frequent cause of low back pain is poor posture.

_____ 4. After immersing a patient's foot in a hot soak, the MA should add crushed ice to the soak.

_____ 5. A patient with diabetes mellitus may have a more than usual sensitivity to the local application of heat.

_____ 6. An ice bag should be filled with large pieces of ice.

_____ 7. If axillary crutches have been fitted properly, the elbow will be flexed at an angle of 30 degrees.

_____ 8. Walkers are primarily used by pediatric patients.

_____ 9. Incorrectly fitted crutches may cause crutch palsy.

_____ 10. A cane should be held on the strong side of the body.

✏️Term KEY TERM ASSESSMENT

Directions: Match each medical term with its definition.

D 1. Ambulation

C 2. Compress

F 3. Edema

G 4. Erythema

A 5. Exudate

E 6. Soak

H 7. Sprain

B 8. Strain

I 9. Suppuration

A. A discharge produced by the body's tissues
B. An overstretching of a muscle caused by trauma
C. A soft, moist, absorbent cloth that is folded in several layers and applied to a part of the body in the local application of heat or cold
D. Walking or moving from one place to another
E. The direct immersion of a body part in water or a medicated solution
F. The retention of fluid in the tissues, resulting in swelling
G. Redness of the skin caused by congestion of capillaries in the lower layers of skin
H. Trauma to a joint that causes injury to the ligaments
I. The process of pus formation

EVALUATION OF LEARNING

Directions: Fill in each blank with the correct answer.

1. State whether the following is an example of dry heat, moist heat, dry cold, or moist cold.

   a. Hot compress

   moist heat

   b. Ice bag

   dry cold

   c. Heating pad

   dry heat

   d. Chemical hot pack

   dry heat

   e. Cold compress

   moist cold

2. List three factors that must be taken into consideration when applying heat or cold.

   Location of application, age of patient, Impairment of circulation

3. How does the local application of heat to an affected area for a short period of time influence the following?

   a. The diameter of the blood vessels in the affected area

   dilated

   b. The blood supply to the affected area

   Increased

   c. Tissue metabolism in the affected area

   increased

4. What happens to the diameter of the blood vessels if heat is applied for a prolonged time (more than 1 hour)?

   Constriction blood supply to area decreases,

5. List three reasons for applying heat locally.

   relieve pain
   Congestion
   muscle Spasms

6. How does the local application of cold for a short time to an affected area influence the following?

   a. The diameter of the blood vessels in the affected area

   Constricted by cold

   b. The blood supply to the affected area

   decreased

c. Tissue metabolism in the affected area

decreases

7. List two reasons for applying cold locally.

prevent edema
prevent pain

8. What factors does the physician take into consideration when prescribing an ambulatory assistive device?

type of disabilty, amount of support required, patient age and coordination

9. Describe one advantage of the forearm crutch.

Can release hand grip for hand use

10. What may occur if axillary crutches are not fitted properly?

Crutch palsy radial nerve damage

11. List eight guidelines that must be followed during crutch use to ensure safety.

Good shoes non-skid
Correct posture
Look ahead when walking, not down
be mindful of where your walking
Extra padding
Inspect crutches for crakes in
rubber sole

12. List one use of each of the following crutch gaits.
    a. Four-point gait: _Weight on both legs_
    b. Three-point gait: _Weight on one leg only_
    c. Swing-to gait: _for disabilities._

13. List and describe the three types of canes.

Standard, tripod cane and
quad cane.

14. List two reasons for prescribing a cane.

Weakness on one side, defects

15. List two reasons for prescribing a walker.

balance problems, knee or hip replacement

CRITICAL THINKING ACTIVITIES

A. DEAR GABBY

Gabby was called out of town unexpectedly and wants you to fill in for her. In the space provided, respond to the following letter.

Dear Gabby:

I am 15 years old and in the 10th grade. I need your help. I have a backpack that my dad weighed, and he said it was 40 pounds. I only weigh 105. My back and neck hurt from lugging it around. I have to walk almost half a mile to the bus stop. I do not have time to use my locker between classes because it is down a flight of stairs and at the end of the hall. Once, when I tried using my locker, my science teacher got mad at me because I was late getting to class. Gabby, what should I do?

Signed,

Pain in the Neck

You should get your parents to buy you a rolling backpack.

B. CRUTCH GUIDELINES

Each of the following patients is wearing a long leg cast because of a broken tibia and is using wooden axillary crutches to ambulate. Evaluate the crutch technique being practiced by each patient. Write *C* if the technique is correct and *I* if the technique is incorrect. If the technique is *correct*, explain why it should be performed this way. If the technique is *incorrect*, indicate what might happen from performing the technique in this manner.

1. Andy Morris wears Nike sports shoes when ambulating with his crutches.

   Correct

2. Juliet Wright does not stand up straight when using her crutches.

   Incorrect

3. Miguel Saldivia puts his weight on the axilla when getting around on his crutches.

   Incorrect

4. Lindy Campbell has a lot of decorative throw rugs in her house and she does not want to remove them.

   Incorrect

5. Andrew Spence likes to make speed on his crutches, so he moves them forward about 20 inches with each step when using the swing-through gait.

   Incorrect

6. Hanna Romes has tingling in her hands but thinks it is just part of what happens when one uses crutches.

Incorrect

7. Tamra Hetrick pads the shoulder rests and the handgrips of her crutches.

Correct

8. Erica Anderson's crutch tips get wet, but she does not take the time to dry them before going into a shopping mall.

Incorrect

C. ACCESSIBILITY FOR PHYSICAL DISABILITIES
   Next to each of the following facilities, list the features you have observed that facilitate accessibility of individuals with a physical disability.

1. Schools
   Wheelchair acess, parking, bathrooms

2. Grocery stores
   Wheel chair acess, parking, bathrooms

3. Shopping malls
   Wheel chair acess, parking, bathrooms

4. Movie theaters
   Wheel chair acess, parking, designated seating, bathrooms

5. Restaurants
   Wheel chair acess, parking, designated seating, bathrooms

6. Medical offices
   Wheel chair acess, parking, bathrooms

7. Community parks
   Wheel chair acess, parking, bathrooms

D. CROSSWORD PUZZLE
Physical Agents to Promote Tissue Healing
Directions: Complete the crossword puzzle using the clues presented below.

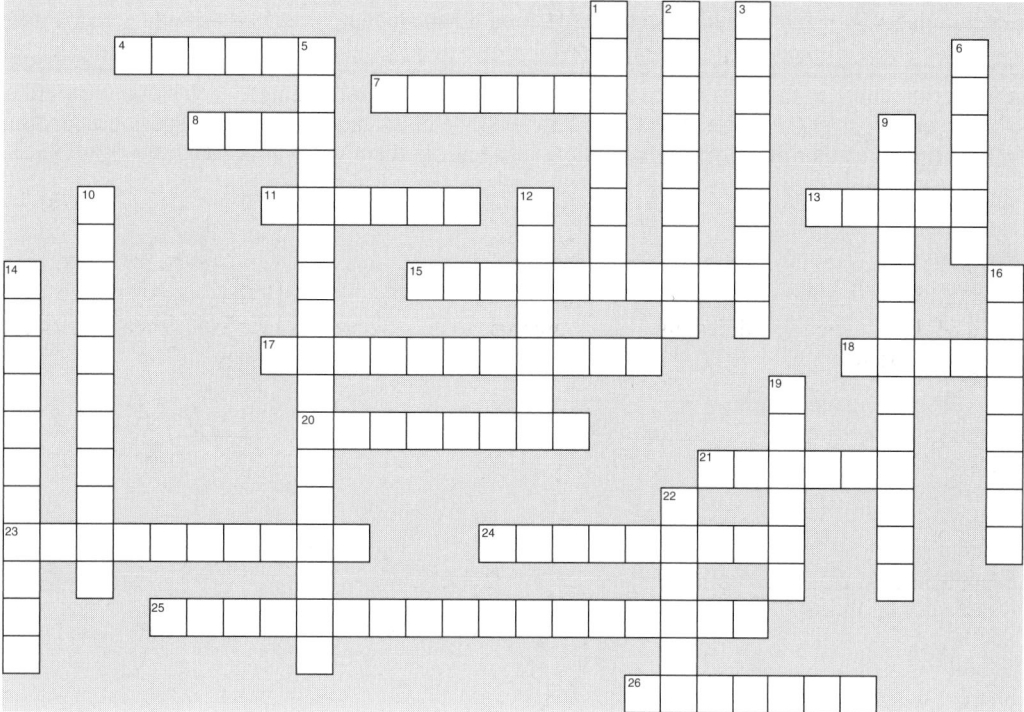

ACROSS
4 Example of dry cold
7 Are more sensitive to cold
8 Examples: standard, tripod, or quad
11 Overstretching of a muscle
13 Do not bend here to lift!
15 Walking
17 "Too long" crutches may cause this
18 Retention of fluid
20 Transfers weight from legs to arms
21 Needed after knee replacement
23 Broken leg crutch gait
24 Cold blood vessels do this
25 Do not use heat for this condition
26 Application of heat promotes this

DOWN
1 Red skin
2 Heat often prescribed for this condition
3 Slow crutch gait
5 Cane handle should be level with this
6 Maximum minutes for heat application
9 Elbow flexion for crutches
10 Prevents low back pain
12 Discharge
14 Pus formation
16 Condition that causes impaired circulation
19 Warm blood vessels do this
22 Cold prescribed for this condition

E. BONE AND JOINT CONDITIONS

1. It is National Bone and Joint Week. The mayor has asked you and your classmates to develop informative, creative, and colorful brochures for the community relating to bone and joint conditions. Choose a condition from the following list, and design a brochure using the blank FAQ (Frequently Asked Questions) brochure provided on pages 415-416 of the Student Study Guide. Each student in the class should select a different topic. On a separate sheet of paper, write three true-or-false questions relating to the information in your brochure.

2. Present your brochure to the class. After all the brochures have been presented, each student should ask his or her three questions to the entire class to see how well the class understands bone and joint conditions. (*Note:* You can take notes during the presentations and refer to them when answering the questions.)

    1. Bursitis
    2. Congenital hip dysplasia
    3. Epicondylitis
    4. Fibromyalgia
    5. Gout
    6. Hammer toe
    7. Herniated disc
    8. Juvenile rheumatoid arthritis
    9. Knee replacement surgery
    10. Kyphosis
    11. Osteoarthritis
    12. Osteomyelitis
    13. Osteoporosis
    14. Paget's disease
    15. Rheumatoid arthritis
    16. Scoliosis
    17. Sprain
    18. Strain
    19. Tendonitis

FAQ on:

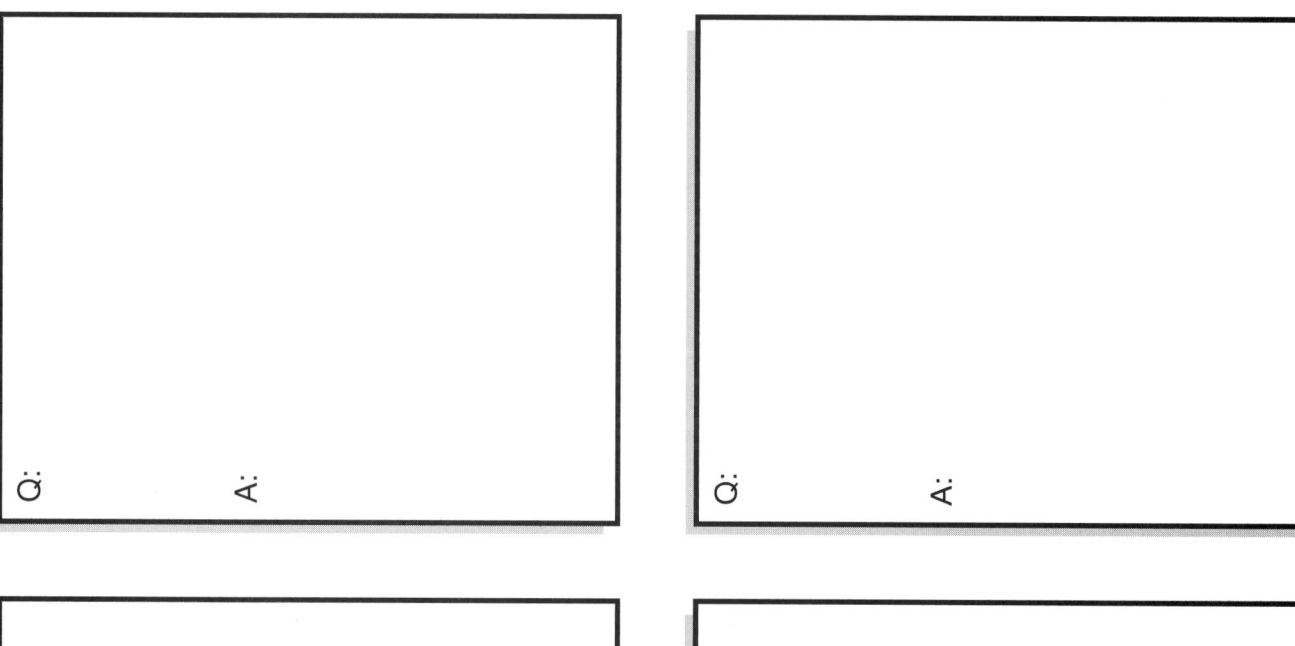

Q: A:

Q: A:

Q: A:

Q: A:

Q:

A:

Q:

A:

Illustration

Q:

A:

Q:

A:

PRACTICE FOR COMPETENCY

Local Application of Heat and Cold

Procedures 22-1, 22-2, and 22-3: Application of Heat. Apply the following heat treatments and record the procedure in the chart provided: Heating Pad, Hot Soak, Hot Compress, and Chemical Hot Pack.

Procedures 22-4, 22-5, and 22-6: Application of Cold. Apply the following cold treatments and record the results in the chart provided: Ice Bag, Cold Compress, and Chemical Cold Pack.

Ambulatory Aids

Procedure 22-7: Axillary Crutch Measurement. Measure an individual for axillary crutches and record the procedure in the chart provided.

Procedure 22-8: Crutch Gaits. Instruct an individual in mastering the following crutch gaits: four-point, two-point, three-point, swing-to, and swing-through. Record the procedure in the chart provided.

Procedure 22-9: Cane. Instruct an individual in the use of a cane and record the procedure in the chart provided.

Procedure 22-10: Walker. Instruct an individual in the use of a walker and record the procedure in the chart provided.

Date	CHART

CHART	
Date	

EVALUATION OF COMPETENCY

Procedure 22-1: Applying a Heating Pad

Name: _____   Date: _____

Evaluated By: _____   Score: _____

Performance Objective

Outcome:	Apply a heating pad.
Conditions:	Given a heating pad with a protective covering.
Standards:	Time: 5 minutes. Student completed procedure in _____ minutes.
	Accuracy: Satisfactory score on the Performance Evaluation Checklist.

Performance Evaluation Checklist

Trial 1	Trial 2	Point Value	Performance Standards
		●	Sanitized hands.
		●	Assembled equipment.
		●	Greeted the patient and introduced yourself.
		●	Identified the patient and explained the procedure.
		●	Placed the heating pad in protective covering.
		●	Connected the plug to electrical outlet and set selector switch to the proper setting.
		●	Placed heating pad on patient's affected body area and asked how the temperature felt.
		●	Instructed patient not to turn the temperature setting higher.
		▷	Stated why patient should be instructed not to lie on heating pad.
		▷	Explained why patient may want to increase the temperature.
		●	Checked patient's skin periodically.
		●	Administered treatment for the proper length of time as designated by physician.
		●	Sanitized hands.
		●	Charted the procedure correctly.
		●	Properly cared for and returned equipment to its storage place.
		★	Completed the procedure within 5 minutes.
			TOTALS

CHART	
Date	

Evaluation of Student Performance

EVALUATION CRITERIA			COMMENTS
Symbol	Category	Point Value	
＊	Critical Step	16 points	
●	Essential Step	6 points	
▷	Theory Question	2 points	

Score calculation: 100 points

– _____ points missed

_____ Score

Satisfactory score: 85 or above

CAAHEP Competencies Achieved:

Psychomotor (Skills)
☑ IV. 2. Report relevant information to others succinctly and accurately.
☑ IV. 6. Prepare a patient for procedures and/or treatments.

Affective (Behavior)
☑ I. 1. Apply critical thinking skills in performing patient assessment and care.

ABHES Competencies Achieved:

☑ 8. cc. Communicate on the recipient's level of comprehension.
☑ 9. d. Recognize and understand various treatment protocols.
☑ 9. l. Prepare patient for examinations and treatments.

EVALUATION OF COMPETENCY

Procedure 22-2: Applying a Hot Soak

Name: _____   Date: _____

Evaluated By: _____   Score: _____

Performance Objective

Outcome:	Apply a hot soak.
Conditions:	Given the following: soaking solution, bath thermometer, basin, and bath towels.
Standards:	Time: 10 minutes. Student completed procedure in ____ minutes.
	Accuracy: Satisfactory score on the Performance Evaluation Checklist.

Performance Evaluation Checklist

Trial 1	Trial 2	Point Value	Performance Standards
		●	Sanitized hands.
		●	Assembled equipment.
		●	Check the label on the solution container.
		●	Greeted the patient and introduced yourself.
		●	Identified the patient and explained the procedure.
		●	Filled basin half full with the warmed soaking solution.
		●	Checked temperature of the solution with a bath thermometer.
		▷	Stated the safe temperature range that should be used for an adult patient (105°F to 110°F).
		●	Assisted patient in finding a comfortable position and padded side of the basin with towel.
		●	Slowly and gradually immersed affected body part into the solution and asked patient how the temperature felt.
		●	Kept the solution at a constant temperature by removing cooler solution and adding hot solution.
		●	Placed a hand between patient and solution when adding more solution.
		●	Stirred the solution with your hand while pouring it.
		●	Checked patient's skin periodically.
		●	Applied hot soak for the proper length of time as designated by physician.
		●	Completely dried affected part.
		●	Sanitized hands.
		●	Charted the procedure correctly.

Trial 1	Trial 2	Point Value	Performance Standards
		●	Properly cared for and returned equipment to its storage place.
		✳	Completed the procedure within 10 minutes.
			TOTALS

CHART	
Date	

Evaluation of Student Performance

EVALUATION CRITERIA			COMMENTS
Symbol	**Category**	**Point Value**	
✳	Critical Step	16 points	
●	Essential Step	6 points	
▷	Theory Question	2 points	

Score calculation: 100 points

　　　　　−＿＿＿ points missed

　　　　　＿＿＿ Score

Satisfactory score: 85 or above

CAAHEP Competencies Achieved:

Psychomotor (Skills)
☑ IV. 2. Report relevant information to others succinctly and accurately.
☑ IV. 6. Prepare a patient for procedures and/or treatments.

Affective (Behavior)
☑ I. 1. Apply critical thinking skills in performing patient assessment and care.

ABHES Competencies Achieved:

☑ 8. cc. Communicate on the recipient's level of comprehension.
☑ 9. d. Recognize and understand various treatment protocols.
☑ 9. l. Prepare patient for examinations and treatments.

EVALUATION OF COMPETENCY

Procedure 22-3: Applying a Hot Compress

Name: _____   Date: _____

Evaluated By: _____   Score: _____

Performance Objective

Outcome:	Apply a hot compress.
Conditions:	Given the following: solution for the compresses, bath thermometer, basin, and washcloths.
Standards:	Time: 10 minutes. Student completed procedure in ____ minutes.
	Accuracy: Satisfactory score on the Performance Evaluation Checklist.

Performance Evaluation Checklist

Trial 1	Trial 2	Point Value	Performance Standards
		●	Sanitized hands.
		●	Assembled equipment.
		●	Checked the label on the solution container.
		●	Warmed the soaking solution.
		●	Greeted the patient and introduced yourself.
		●	Identified the patient and explained the procedure.
		●	Filled basin half full with the warmed solution.
		●	Checked temperature of the solution with a bath thermometer.
		▷	Stated the safe temperature range that should be used for an adult patient (105°F to 110°F).
		●	Completely immersed the compress in the solution.
		●	Squeezed excess solution from compress.
		●	Applied compress to affected body part and asked patient how the temperature felt.
		●	Placed additional compresses in the solution.
		●	Repeated the application every 2 to 3 minutes for the duration of time specified by physician.
		●	Checked patient's skin periodically.
		●	Checked temperature of the solution periodically, removed cooler fluid, and added hot fluid if needed.
			Administered treatment for proper length of time as designated by a physician.
		●	Thoroughly dried affected part.
		●	Sanitized hands.
		●	Charted the procedure correctly.

Trial 1	Trial 2	Point Value	Performance Standards
		●	Properly cared for and returned equipment to its storage place.
		✳	Completed the procedure within 10 minutes.
			TOTALS

CHART	
Date	

Evaluation of Student Performance

EVALUATION CRITERIA			COMMENTS
Symbol	Category	Point Value	
✳	Critical Step	16 points	
●	Essential Step	6 points	
▷	Theory Question	2 points	

Score calculation: 100 points

– _____ points missed

_____ Score

Satisfactory score: 85 or above

CAAHEP Competencies Achieved:

Psychomotor (Skills)
☑ IV. 2. Report relevant information to others succinctly and accurately.
☑ IV. 6. Prepare a patient for procedures and/or treatments.

Affective (Behavior)
☑ I. 1. Apply critical thinking skills in performing patient assessment and care.

ABHES Competencies Achieved:

☑ 8. cc. Communicate on the recipient's level of comprehension.
☑ 9. d. Recognize and understand various treatment protocols.
☑ 9. 1. Prepare patient for examinations and treatments.

EVALUATION OF COMPETENCY

Procedure 22-4: Applying an Ice Bag

Name: _____ Date: _____

Evaluated By: _____ Score: _____

Performance Objective

Outcome:	Apply an ice bag.
Conditions:	Given the following: ice bag and protective covering, and small pieces of ice.
Standards:	Time: 10 minutes. Student completed procedure in ____ minutes.
	Accuracy: Satisfactory score on the Performance Evaluation Checklist.

Performance Evaluation Checklist

Trial 1	Trial 2	Point Value	Performance Standards
		•	Sanitized hands.
		•	Assembled equipment.
		•	Greeted the patient and introduced yourself.
		•	Identified the patient and explained the procedure.
		•	Checked ice bag for leakage.
		•	Filled bag one-half to two-thirds full with small pieces of ice.
		▷	Explained why small pieces of ice are used.
		•	Expelled air from bag.
		▷	Explained the reason for expelling air from bag.
		•	Placed the bag in protective covering.
		▷	Stated the purpose of placing bag in protective covering.
		•	Placed bag on affected body area and asked patient how the temperature felt.
		•	Checked patient's skin periodically.
		▷	Listed skin changes that would warrant removal of bag.
		•	Refilled bag with ice and changed protective covering when needed.
		•	Administered treatment for the proper length of time as designated by physician.
		•	Sanitized hands.
		•	Charted the procedure correctly.
		•	Properly cared for and returned equipment to its storage place.
		*	Completed the procedure within 10 minutes.
			TOTALS

CHART	
Date	

Evaluation of Student Performance

EVALUATION CRITERIA			COMMENTS
Symbol	Category	Point Value	
✶	Critical Step	16 points	
●	Essential Step	6 points	
▷	Theory Question	2 points	
Score calculation: 100 points			
− _____ points missed			
_____ Score			
Satisfactory score: 85 or above			

CAAHEP Competencies Achieved:

Psychomotor (Skills)
☑ IV. 2. Report relevant information to others succinctly and accurately.
☑ IV. 6. Prepare a patient for procedures and/or treatments.

Affective (Behavior)
☑ I. 1. Apply critical thinking skills in performing patient assessment and care.

ABHES Competencies Achieved:

☑ 8. cc. Communicate on the recipient's level of comprehension.
☑ 9. d. Recognize and understand various treatment protocols.
☑ 9. l. Prepare patient for examinations and treatments.

EVALUATION OF COMPETENCY

Procedure 22-5: Applying a Cold Compress

Name: _____   Date: _____

Evaluated By: _____   Score: _____

Performance Objective

Outcome:	Apply a cold compress.
Conditions:	Given the following: ice cubes, a basin, and washcloths.
Standards:	Time: 10 minutes. Student completed procedure in ____ minutes.
	Accuracy: Satisfactory score on the Performance Evaluation Checklist.

Performance Evaluation Checklist

Trial 1	Trial 2	Point Value	Performance Standards
		●	Sanitized hands.
		●	Assembled equipment.
		●	Checked the label on the solution.
		●	Greeted the patient and introduced yourself.
		●	Identified the patient and explained the procedure.
		●	Placed large ice cubes in basin and added the solution until the basin is half full.
		▷	Explained why larger pieces of ice are used.
		●	Completely immersed the compress in the solution.
		●	Squeezed excess solution from compress.
		●	Applied compress to affected body part and asked patient how the temperature felt.
		●	Placed additional compresses in the solution.
		●	Repeated the application every 2 to 3 minutes for the duration of time specified by physician.
		●	Checked patient's skin periodically.
		●	Added ice if needed to keep the water cold.
		●	Administered treatment for proper length of time as designated by physician.
		●	Thoroughly dried affected part.
		●	Sanitized hands.
		●	Charted the procedure correctly.
		●	Properly cared for and returned equipment to its storage place.
		＊	Completed the procedure within 10 minutes.
			TOTALS

CHART	
Date	

Evaluation of Student Performance

EVALUATION CRITERIA			COMMENTS
Symbol	Category	Point Value	
$*$	Critical Step	16 points	
$\bullet$	Essential Step	6 points	
$\triangleright$	Theory Question	2 points	

Score calculation: 100 points

− _____ points missed

_____ Score

Satisfactory score: 85 or above

CAAHEP Competencies Achieved:

Psychomotor (Skills)
☑ IV. 2. Report relevant information to others succinctly and accurately.
☑ IV. 6. Prepare a patient for procedures and/or treatments.

Affective (Behavior)
☑ I. 1. Apply critical thinking skills in performing patient assessment and care.

ABHES Competencies Achieved:

☑ 8. cc. Communicate on the recipient's level of comprehension.
☑ 9. d. Recognize and understand various treatment protocols.
☑ 9. l. Prepare patient for examinations and treatments.

EVALUATION OF COMPETENCY

Procedure 22-6: Applying a Chemical Pack

Name: _____   Date: _____

Evaluated By: _____   Score: _____

Performance Objective

Outcome:	Apply a chemical cold and hot pack.
Conditions:	Given a chemical cold and hot pack.
Standards:	Time: 5 minutes. Student completed procedure in _____ minutes.
	Accuracy: Satisfactory score on the Performance Evaluation Checklist.

Performance Evaluation Checklist

Trial 1	Trial 2	Point Value	Performance Standards
		●	Sanitized hands.
		●	Assembled equipment.
		●	Greeted the patient and introduced yourself.
		●	Identified the patient and explained the procedure.
		●	Shook the crystals to the bottom of bag.
		●	Squeezed bag firmly to break inner water bag.
		●	Shook bag vigorously to mix the contents.
		●	Covered bag with a protective covering.
		●	Applied bag to affected area.
		●	Checked the patient's skin periodically.
		●	Administered treatment for the proper length of time.
		●	Discarded bag in an appropriate receptacle.
		●	Sanitized hands.
		●	Charted the procedure correctly.
		✳	Completed the procedure within 5 minutes.
			TOTALS
			CHART
Date			

Evaluation of Student Performance

EVALUATION CRITERIA			COMMENTS
Symbol	Category	Point Value	
∗	Critical Step	16 points	
●	Essential Step	6 points	
▷	Theory Question	2 points	

Score calculation: 100 points

– _____ points missed

_____ Score

Satisfactory score: 85 or above

CAAHEP Competencies Achieved:

Psychomotor (Skills)
☑ IV. 2. Report relevant information to others succinctly and accurately.
☑ IV. 6. Prepare a patient for procedures and/or treatments.

Affective (Behavior)
☑ I. 1. Apply critical thinking skills in performing patient assessment and care.

ABHES Competencies Achieved:

☑ 8. cc. Communicate on the recipient's level of comprehension.
☑ 9. d. Recognize and understand various treatment protocols.
☑ 9. l. Prepare patient for examinations and treatments.

EVALUATION OF COMPETENCY

(DVD) Procedure 22-7: Measuring for Axillary Crutches

Name: _____   Date: _____

Evaluated By: _____   Score: _____

Performance Objective

Outcome:	Measure a patient for axillary crutches.
Conditions:	Given the following: axillary crutches and a tape measure.
Standards:	Time: 10 minutes. Student completed procedure in _____ minutes.
	Accuracy: Satisfactory score on the Performance Evaluation Checklist.

Performance Evaluation Checklist

Trial 1	Trial 2	Point Value	Performance Standards
		●	Asked patient to stand erect.
		●	Positioned crutches with the tips at a distance of 2 inches in front of, and 4 to 6 inches to the side of each foot.
		●	Adjusted crutch length so that the shoulder rests were approximately 1½ to 2 inches below the axilla.
		●	Asked the patient to support his or her weight by the handgrips.
		●	Adjusted the handgrips so that patient's elbow was flexed approximately 30 degrees.
		●	Checked the fit of the crutches by placing two fingers between the top of crutch and patient's axilla.
		●	Charted the procedure correctly.
		✱	Completed the procedure within 10 minutes.
			TOTALS

CHART	
Date	

Evaluation of Student Performance

EVALUATION CRITERIA			COMMENTS
Symbol	Category	Point Value	
*	Critical Step	16 points	
•	Essential Step	6 points	
▷	Theory Question	2 points	

Score calculation: 100 points

− _____ points missed

_____ Score

Satisfactory score: 85 or above

CAAHEP Competencies Achieved:

Psychomotor (Skills)
☑ IV. 6. Prepare a patient for procedures and/or treatments.

Affective (Behavior)
☑ I. 1. Apply critical thinking skills in performing patient assessment and care.

ABHES Competencies Achieved:

☑ 5. b.Identify and respond appropriately when working/caring for patients with special needs.

EVALUATION OF COMPETENCY

Procedure 22-8: Instructing a Patient in Crutch Gaits

Name: _____   Date: _____

Evaluated By: _____   Score: _____

Performance Objective

Outcome:	Instruct an individual in the following crutch gaits: four-point, two-point, three-point, swing-to, and swing-through.
Conditions:	Given axillary crutches.
Standards:	Time: 15 minutes. Student completed procedure in ____ minutes.
	Accuracy: Satisfactory score on the Performance Evaluation Checklist.

Performance Evaluation Checklist

Trial 1	Trial 2	Point Value	Performance Standards
			TRIPOD POSITION
			Instructed the patient to:
		●	Stand erect and face straight ahead.
		●	Place the tips of crutches 4 to 6 inches in front of, and 4 to 6 inches to side of, each foot.
		▷	Stated one use of the tripod position.
			FOUR-POINT GAIT
			Instructed the patient to:
		●	Begin in the tripod position.
		●	Move the right crutch forward.
		●	Move the left foot forward to the level of the left crutch.
		●	Move the left crutch forward.
		●	Move the right foot forward to the level of the right crutch.
		●	Repeat the above sequence.
		▷	Stated one use of the four-point gait.
			TWO-POINT GAIT
			Instructed the patient to:
		●	Begin in the tripod position.
		●	Move the left crutch and the right foot forward at the same time.
		●	Move the right crutch and left foot forward at the same time.
		●	Repeat the above sequence.
		▷	Stated one use of the two-point gait.

Trial 1	Trial 2	Point Value	Performance Standards
			THREE-POINT GAIT
			Instructed the patient to:
		●	Begin in the tripod position.
		●	Move both crutches and the affected leg forward.
		●	Move the unaffected leg forward while balancing weight on both crutches.
		●	Repeat the above sequence.
		▷	Stated two uses of the three-point gait.
			SWING-TO GAIT
			Instructed the patient to:
		●	Begin in the tripod position.
		●	Move both crutches forward together.
		●	Lift and swing body to the crutches.
		●	Repeat the above sequence.
		▷	Stated one use of the swing-to gait.
			SWING-THROUGH GAIT
			Instructed the patient to:
		●	Begin in the tripod position.
		●	Move both crutches forward together.
		●	Lift and swing body past the crutches.
		●	Repeat the above sequence.
		▷	Stated one use of the swing-through gait.
		✶	Completed the procedure within 15 minutes.
			TOTALS

Evaluation of Student Performance

EVALUATION CRITERIA			COMMENTS
Symbol	Category	Point Value	
*	Critical Step	16 points	
•	Essential Step	6 points	
▷	Theory Question	2 points	

Score calculation: 100 points

−_____ points missed

_____ Score

Satisfactory score: 85 or above

CAAHEP Competencies Achieved:

Psychomotor (Skills)

☑ IV. 5. Instruct patients according to their needs to promote health maintenance and disease prevention.

☑ IV. 6. Prepare a patient for procedures and/or treatments.

Affective (Behavior)

☑ I. 2. Use language/verbal skills that enable patients' understanding.

☑ IV. 6. Demonstrate awareness of how an individual's personal appearance affects anticipated responses.

ABHES Competencies Achieved:

☑ **9.** q. Instruct patients with special needs.

Notes

EVALUATION OF COMPETENCY

Procedures 22-9 and 22-10: Instructing a Patient in the Use of a Cane and Walker

Name: ______________________________ Date: ______________

Evaluated By: ______________________________ Score: ______________

Performance Objective

Outcome: Instruct an individual in the use of a cane and walker.

Conditions: Given the following: a cane and a walker.

Standards: Time: 10 minutes. Student completed procedure in ____ minutes.

Accuracy: Satisfactory score on the Performance Evaluation Checklist.

Performance Evaluation Checklist

Trial 1	*Trial 2*	*Point Value*	*Performance Standards*
			CANE
			Instructed the patient to:
		•	Hold the cane on the strong side of body.
		•	Place tip of the cane 4 to 6 inches to the side of foot.
		•	Move the cane forward approximately 12 inches.
		•	Move the affected leg forward to the level of the cane.
		•	Move strong leg forward and ahead of the cane and weak leg.
		•	Repeat the above sequence.
		▷	Stated one condition for which a cane is used.
			WALKER
			Instructed the patient to:
		•	Pick up the walker and move it forward approximately 6 inches.
		•	Move the right foot and then the left foot up to the walker.
		•	Repeat the above sequence.
		▷	Stated one condition for which a walker is used.
		*	Completed the procedure within 10 minutes.
			TOTALS

Evaluation of Student Performance

EVALUATION CRITERIA			COMMENTS
Symbol	Category	Point Value	
∗	Critical Step	16 points	
●	Essential Step	6 points	
▷	Theory Question	2 points	

Score calculation: 100 points

− _____ points missed

_____ Score

Satisfactory score: 85 or above

CAAHEP Competencies Achieved:

Psychomotor (Skills)

☑ IV. 5. Instruct patients according to their needs to promote health maintenance and disease prevention.

☑ IV. 6. Prepare a patient for procedures and/or treatments.

Affective (Behavior)

☑ I. 2. Use language/verbal skills that enable patients' understanding.

☑ IV. 6. Demonstrate awareness of how an individual's personal appearance affects anticipated responses.

ABHES Competencies Achieved:

☑ **9.** q. Instruct patients with special needs.

23

The Gynecologic Examination and Prenatal Care

CHAPTER ASSIGNMENTS

√ After Completing	Date Due	Textbook Page(s)	TEXTBOOK ASSIGNMENTS	Possible Points	Points You Earned
		452-495	Read Chapter 23: The Gynecologic Examination and Prenatal Care		
		455 492	Read Case Study 1 Case Study 1 questions	5	
		473 493	Read Case Study 2 Case Study 2 questions	5	
		482 493	Read Case Study 3 Case Study 3 questions	5	
		488 493	Read Case Study 4 Case Study 4 questions	5	
			TOTAL POINTS		

√ After Completing	Date Due	Study Guide Page(s)	STUDY GUIDE ASSIGNMENTS (CTA: Critical Thinking Activity)	Possible Points	Points You Earned
		443	Pretest	10	
		444-445	Term Key Term Assessment	48	
		446-451	Evaluation of Learning questions	54	
		452	CTA A: Breast Cancer (5 pts/question)	30	
			CD Activity: Chapter 23 What's on Your Tray? (Record points earned)		
		453-455	CTA B: Methods of Contraception (3 pts/each method)	42	
		456	CTA C: Herpes and HPV (40 pts/brochure)	80	

√ After Completing	Date Due	Study Guide Page(s)	STUDY GUIDE ASSIGNMENTS (CTA: Critical Thinking Activity)	Possible Points	Points You Earned
		461	CTA D: Signs and Symptoms of Pregnancy	8	
		461	CTA E: Calculation of the EDD	5	
		462	CTA F: Nutrition during Pregnancy	8	
		463	CTA G: Minor Discomforts of Pregnancy	10	
		464	CTA H: Health Promotion during Pregnancy	7	
		464-465	CTA I: Breastfeeding	8	
		465	CTA J: Prenatal Ultrasound	5	
		466	CTA K: Crossword Puzzle	25	
			CD Activity: Chapter 23 Road to Recovery Game: OB/GYN Terminology (Record points earned)		
			CD Activity: Chapter 23 Animations	20	
			CD Activity: Chapter 23 Apply Your Knowledge questions (Record points earned)		
		443	Posttest	10	
			ADDITIONAL ASSIGNMENTS		
			TOTAL POINTS		

√ When Assigned by Your Instructor	Study Guide Page(s)	Practices Required	LABORATORY ASSIGNMENTS (Procedure Number and Name)	*Score
	467	5	**DVD** **Practice for Competency** 23-1: Breast Self-Examination Instructions Textbook reference: pp. 464-466	
	477-479		**Evaluation of Competency** 23-1: Breast Self-Examination Instructions	*
	469	5	**DVD** **Practice for Competency** 23-2: Assisting with a Gynecologic Examination Textbook reference: pp. 466-470	
	481-484		**Evaluation of Competency** 23-2: Assisting with a Gynecologic Examination	*
	471	5	**DVD** **Practice for Competency** 23-3: Assisting with a Return Prenatal Examination Textbook reference: pp. 489-491	
	485-487		**Evaluation of Competency** 23-3: Assisting with a Return Prenatal Examination	*
			ADDITIONAL ASSIGNMENTS	

Notes

Name _____   Date _____

?📄 PRETEST

True or False

_____ 1. A complete gynecologic examination consists of a breast examination and a pelvic examination.

_____ 2. The American Cancer Society recommends that a woman perform a breast self-examination weekly.

_____ 3. The purpose of the Pap test is for the early detection of cervical cancer.

_____ 4. The patient should be instructed to douche before having a Pap test.

_____ 5. Trichomoniasis produces a profuse frothy vaginal discharge.

_____ 6. Another name for candidiasis is a yeast infection.

_____ 7. _Prenatal care_ refers to the care of the pregnant woman before delivery of the infant.

_____ 8. During each return prenatal visit, the mother's urine is tested for glucose and protein.

_____ 9. The normal range for the fetal pulse rate is between 120 and 160 beats/min.

_____ 10. Amniocentesis can be used to diagnose certain genetically transmitted conditions.

?📄 POSTTEST

True or False

_____ 1. The patient position for a breast examination is the lithotomy position.

_____ 2. Most breast lumps are discovered by the physician.

_____ 3. Trichomoniasis is caused by a virus.

_____ 4. Chlamydia often occurs in association with syphilis.

_____ 5. In the absence of complications, the first prenatal visit should be scheduled after a woman has missed her first period.

_____ 6. True labor pains are referred to as Braxton Hicks contractions.

_____ 7. The purpose of measuring fundal height is to determine the degree of cervical dilation and effacement.

_____ 8. The fetal heart tones can first be detected between 4 and 6 weeks of gestation using a Doppler fetal pulse detector.

_____ 9. Obstetric ultrasound scanning is used to assess fetal lung maturity.

_____ 10. The perineum is the period of time in which the body systems are returning to their prepregnant state.

KEY TERM ASSESSMENT

The Gynecologic Examination

Directions: Match each medical term with its definition.

_____ 1. Adnexal

_____ 2. Amenorrhea

_____ 3. Atypical

_____ 4. Cervix

_____ 5. Colposcopy

_____ 6. Cytology

_____ 7. Dysmenorrhea

_____ 8. Dyspareunia

_____ 9. Dysplasia

_____ 10. Ectocervix

_____ 11. Endocervix

_____ 12. External os

_____ 13. Gynecology

_____ 14. Menopause

_____ 15. Menorrhagia

_____ 16. Metrorrhagia

_____ 17. Perimenopause

_____ 18. Perineum

_____ 19. Risk factor

_____ 20. Vulva

A. The opening of the cervical canal of the uterus into the vagina

B. The mucous membrane lining the cervical canal

C. Deviation from the normal

D. The external region between the vaginal orifice and the anus in a female and between the scrotum and the anus in a male

E. Adjacent

F. The absence or cessation of the menstrual period

G. The region of the external genital organs in the female

H. The science that deals with the study of cells, including their origin, structure, function, and pathology

I. The branch of medicine that deals with the diseases of the reproductive organs of women

J. The part of the cervix that projects into the vagina

K. Anything that increases an individual's chance of developing a disease

L. The growth of abnormal cells

M. Before the onset of menopause, the phase during which the woman with regular periods changes to irregular cycles and increased periods of amenorrhea

N. Pain in the vagina or pelvis experienced by a woman during sexual intercourse

O. Examination of the cervix using a lighted instrument with a magnifying lens

P. Bleeding between menstrual periods

Q. Excessive bleeding during a menstrual period

R. The lower narrow end of the uterus that opens into the vagina

S. Pain associated with the menstrual period

T. The permanent cessation of menstruation

Prenatal Care

Directions: Match each medical term with its definition.

_____ 1. Braxton Hicks contractions

_____ 2. Dilation (of the cervix)

_____ 3. EDD

_____ 4. Effacement

_____ 5. Embryo

_____ 6. Engagement

_____ 7. Fetal heart tones

_____ 8. Fetus

_____ 9. Fundus

_____ 10. Gestation

_____ 11. Gestational age

_____ 12. Infant

_____ 13. Lochia

_____ 14. Multigravida

_____ 15. Multipara

_____ 16. Nullipara

_____ 17. Obstetrics

_____ 18. Position

_____ 19. Postpartum

_____ 20. Preeclampsia

_____ 21. Prenatal

_____ 22. Presentation

_____ 23. Primigravida

_____ 24. Primipara

_____ 25. Puerperium

_____ 26. Quickening

_____ 27. Toxemia

_____ 28. Trimester

A. A woman who has completed two or more pregnancies to the age of viability regardless of whether they ended in live infants or stillbirths

B. The entrance of the fetal head or the presenting part into the pelvic inlet

C. Before birth

D. Three months, or one third, of the gestational period of pregnancy

E. The relation of the presenting part of the fetus to the maternal pelvis

F. The period of time, usually 4 to 6 weeks, in which the uterus and the body systems are returning to normal delivery

G. The dome-shaped upper portion of the uterus between the fallopian tubes

H. The first movements of the fetus in utero as felt by the mother

I. The child in utero, from the third month after conception to birth

J. A woman who has been pregnant more than once

K. Expected date of delivery, or due date

L. A woman who has carried a pregnancy to viability for the first time, regardless of whether the infant was stillborn or alive at birth

M. The stretching of the external os from an opening a few millimeters wide to an opening large enough to allow the passage of an infant (approximately 10 cm)

N. The period of intrauterine development from conception to birth

O. A discharge from the uterus after delivery consisting of blood, tissue, white blood cells, and some bacteria

P. The thinning and shortening of the cervical canal from its normal length of 1 to 2 cm to a structure with paper-thin edges in which there is no canal at all

Q. A woman who has not carried a pregnancy to the point of viability (20 weeks of gestation)

R. The branch of medicine concerned with the care of the woman during pregnancy, childbirth, and the postpartal period

S. A woman who is pregnant for the first time

T. Occurring after childbirth

U. Intermittent and irregular painless uterine contractions that occur throughout pregnancy

V. The heartbeat of the fetus as heard through the mother's abdominal wall

W. A child from birth to 12 months of age

X. The child in utero from the time of conception to the beginning of the first trimester

Y. The age of the fetus between conception and birth

Z. A major complication of pregnancy characterized by increasing hypertension, albuminuria, and edema

AA. Indication of the part of the fetus that is closest to the cervix and will be delivered first

BB. A condition occurring in pregnant women that includes preeclampsia and eclampsia

EVALUATION OF LEARNING

The Gynecologic Examination

Directions: Fill in each blank with the correct answer.

1. What is the purpose of the gynecologic examination?

   _____

   _____

   _____

2. What is the purpose of performing a breast examination?

   _____

   _____

   _____

3. How often should a woman perform a breast self-examination at home? When should it be performed in relation to the menstrual cycle and why?

   _____

   _____

   _____

4. What are the components of the pelvic examination?

   _____

   _____

5. What position is generally used for the pelvic examination?

   _____

6. How can the MA help the patient relax during the pelvic examination?

   _____

   _____

7. What is the function of a vaginal speculum?

   _____

   _____

8. Describe how you would lubricate the vaginal speculum when the physician performs the following:

   a. A Pap test using the direct-smear method: _____

   _____

   b. A Pap test using the liquid-based method: _____

   _____

9. What is the purpose of performing a visual examination of the vagina and the cervix?

   _____

   _____

10. What is the purpose of performing a Pap test?

   _____

   _____

11. Describe the schedule for having a Pap test as recommended by the American Cancer Society.

_____

_____

_____

12. Why should a specimen for a Pap test not be taken from a woman during her menstrual period?

_____

_____

13. Why should the MA instruct the patient not to douche or insert vaginal medications for 2 days before coming to the medical office to have a Pap test?

_____

_____

_____

_____

14. What are the three types of specimens that may be obtained for a Pap test? Where is each collected?

_____

_____

_____

15. Why must the slides be fixed immediately after collection of a specimen for the direct smear Pap test method?

_____

_____

_____

16. What are the advantages of using the liquid-based Pap test method?

_____

_____

_____

_____

17. List three conditions that the maturation index can help to evaluate.

_____

_____

_____

18. Why is the Bethesda system recommended for reporting the results of the Pap test?

_____

_____

_____

19. What is the purpose of performing the bimanual pelvic examination?

_____

_____

_____

20. What is the purpose of the rectal-vaginal examination?

_____

_____

21. Describe the laboratory procedure that can be used to identify *Trichomonas vaginalis* in the medical office.

_____

_____

_____

22. What medication is used to treat trichomoniasis? Why must the patient's sexual partner also be treated?

_____

_____

23. Describe the laboratory procedure that can be used to identify *Candida albicans* in the medical office.

_____

_____

_____

24. What medications are used to treat candidiasis?

_____

_____

25. What are the symptoms of PID? What complications can occur from PID?

_____

_____

26. How are chlamydia and gonorrhea usually diagnosed?

_____

_____

27. List the symptoms of each of the following sexually transmitted diseases (STDs):

   a. Trichomoniasis in the female

   _____

   _____

   _____

   _____

   b. Candidiasis in the female

   _____

   _____

   _____

   _____

   c. Chlamydia in the female and male

   _____

   _____

   _____

   _____

d. Gonorrhea in the female and male

_____

_____

_____

_____

Prenatal Care

Directions: Fill in each blank with the correct answer.

1. List the three categories of medical office visits for provision of prenatal and postnatal care of a pregnant woman.

_____

_____

_____

2. List the four components of the first prenatal visit.

_____

_____

_____

_____

3. What is the purpose of the prenatal record?

_____

_____

4. List two types of information included in the past medical history (of the prenatal record).

_____

_____

_____

5. List three types of information included in the present pregnancy history.

_____

_____

_____

6. What are the warning signs of a spontaneous abortion?

_____

_____

7. What is the purpose of the interval prenatal history?

_____

_____

8. Explain the importance of performing a physical examination on the prenatal patient.

_____

_____

_____

9. What examinations are included in the initial prenatal examination?

_____

_____

10. What is the importance of ensuring that a pregnant woman does not have gonorrhea before delivery of the infant?

_____

_____

11. Why is a pregnant woman tested for group B streptococcus (GBS)? When is the woman tested for GBS?

_____

_____

12. What is the purpose of performing a hemoglobin and hematocrit evaluation on a prenatal patient?

_____

_____

13. What is the importance of assessing the Rh factor and ABO blood type of a pregnant woman?

_____

_____

14. What is the purpose of performing a glucose challenge test on a pregnant woman?

_____

_____

15. What is the purpose of performing a rubella titer test on a pregnant woman?

_____

_____

16. Why does the CDC recommend that pregnant women have a blood test to screen for exposure to hepatitis B virus?

_____

_____

17. What is the purpose of the return prenatal visit? List the usual schedule for return prenatal visits.

_____

_____

_____

18. What tests are performed on the patient's urine specimen at each return visit, and why is each test performed?

_____

_____

_____

_____

19. List two purposes of measuring the fundal height.

_____

_____

20. What is the normal range for the fetal heart rate?

_____

21. What is the purpose of performing a vaginal examination as the patient nears term?

_____

_____

22. What is the purpose of performing each of the following special tests and procedures?

    a. Obstetric ultrasound scan: _____

    _____

    b. Amniocentesis: _____

    _____

    c. Fetal heart rate monitoring: _____

    _____

23. What conditions might warrant performing an amniocentesis?

_____

_____

_____

24. What conditions might warrant performing a fetal heart rate monitoring test?

_____

_____

_____

25. What occurs during the puerperium?

_____

_____

26. Explain the changes in the lochia that should normally occur during the puerperium.

_____

_____

_____

_____

27. List the procedures generally included in the 6 weeks–postpartum examination.

_____

_____

_____

_____

CRITICAL THINKING ACTIVITIES

A. BREAST CANCER

Select three of the following questions that interest you the most. Using the following Internet sites, answer these questions.

National Cancer Institute: www.cancer.gov

American Cancer Society: www.cancer.org

Cancer Facts: www.cancerfacts.com

1. Can a man develop breast cancer? Elaborate on your answer.

2. How does tamoxifen work in treating breast cancer?

3. What are the pros and cons of being tested for the breast cancer gene?

4. What methods are used to reconstruct the breast after a mastectomy?

5. What new diagnostic methods are currently being explored to detect breast cancer?

6. What complementary and alternative therapies are being used in the treatment of breast cancer?

Question # _____

_____

_____

_____

_____

_____

Question # _____

_____

_____

_____

_____

_____

Question # _____

_____

_____

_____

_____

_____

B. METHODS OF CONTRACEPTION

Patients coming to the medical office for gynecologic examinations frequently ask the medical assistant questions regarding methods of contraception. The medical assistant should have knowledge of the various types of contraceptives, how they work to prevent pregnancy, and the advantages and disadvantages of each. A list of common contraceptive methods is listed as follows. List the information requested for each in the spaces provided. The contraceptive Internet sites listed under **On the Web** at the end of Chapter 23 in your textbook can be used to complete this activity.

Contraceptive Method	Mode of Action	Advantages	Disadvantages
Oral contraceptive			
Contraceptive injections			
Contraceptive patch			
Male condom			

Contraceptive Method	Mode of Action	Advantages	Disadvantages
Female condom			
Spermicide			
Diaphragm			
Cervical cap			
Vaginal sponge			

Contraceptive Method	Mode of Action	Advantages	Disadvantages
Vaginal ring			
IUD			
Natural family planning			
Surgical sterilization			
Emergency contraception			

C. HERPES AND HPV

You are working at an OB/GYN office. Your physician is concerned about the increase in the numbers of patients contracting herpes and HPV. He asks you to design a colorful, creative, and informative brochure on herpes and HPV using the brochures provided on the following pages. These brochures will be published and placed in the waiting room to provide patients with education of these STDs. The STD Internet sites listed under **On the Web** at the end of Chapter 23 in your textbook can be used to complete this activity.

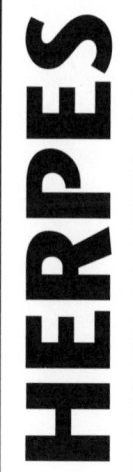

How common is herpes?

How can herpes be prevented?

What is herpes?

How do you get herpes?

How is herpes diagnosed?

What are the symptoms?

What causes herpes to recur?

How is herpes treated?

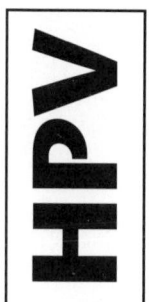

How common is HPV?

What are the complications of HPV?

What is HPV?

What are the symptoms?

How do you get HPV?

How is HPV diagnosed?

How is HPV tested?

How can HPV be prevented?

D. SIGNS AND SYMPTOMS OF PREGNANCY

Listed here are common signs and symptoms of pregnancy. Define each of them and, if possible, explain what causes the sign or symptom to occur. The pregnancy and childbirth Internet sites listed under **On the Web** at the end of Chapter 23 in your textbook can be used to obtain information to complete this activity.

1. Amenorrhea

_____

_____

2. Fatigue

_____

_____

3. Urinary frequency

_____

_____

4. Quickening

_____

_____

5. Goodell's sign

_____

_____

6. Hegar's sign

_____

_____

7. Braxton Hicks contractions

_____

_____

8. Skin changes: striae gravidarum, chloasma, linea nigra

_____

_____

_____

_____

E. CALCULATION OF THE EDD

Calculate the EDD of the following patients using Nägele's rule. The first day of each patient's last menstrual period (LMP) is listed here:

1. February 10, 2010. _____

2. April 28, 2010. _____

3. July 20, 2010. _____

4. October 2, 2010. _____

5. December 22, 2010. _____

F. NUTRITION DURING PREGNANCY

1. Brianna Flint is in your medical office for her first prenatal visit. This is her first pregnancy, and she is concerned about adequate nutrition during her pregnancy. Explain why the following nutrients are of particular importance during pregnancy, and provide good food sources of each. The pregnancy and childbirth Internet sites listed under **On the Web** at the end of Chapter 23 in your textbook can be used to obtain information to complete this activity.

2. In a classroom situation, select a partner. In a role-playing situation, one student takes the role of the MA and the other plays the role of the patient. Explain to the patient the importance of these nutrients and good food sources of each.

Nutrient	Importance during Pregnancy	Food Sources
Iron		
Calcium		
Protein		
Folic acid		

G. MINOR DISCOMFORTS OF PREGNANCY

1. Following is a list of the minor discomforts that a prenatal patient may experience during pregnancy. Indicate measures the patient can take to help prevent or relieve each discomfort. The pregnancy and childbirth Internet sites listed under **On the Web** at the end of Chapter 23 in your textbook can be used to obtain information to complete this activity.

2. In a classroom situation, select a partner. In a role-playing situation, one student takes the role of the MA and the other plays the role of the patient. The patient should indicate having a problem with each of these discomforts, and the MA should respond with the measures the patient could take to help prevent or relive each one.

   a. Nausea (morning sickness)

   _____

   _____

   b. Heartburn

   _____

   _____

   c. Fatigue

   _____

   _____

   d. Constipation

   _____

   _____

   e. Backache

   _____

   _____

   f. Breathing difficulties

   _____

   _____

   g. Varicose veins

   _____

   _____

   h. Hemorrhoids

   _____

   _____

   i. Leg cramps

   _____

   _____

   j. Swelling of the lower legs and feet

   _____

   _____

H. HEALTH PROMOTION DURING PREGNANCY

1. Obtain a prenatal guidebook, and list the information included in it regarding guidelines the patient should follow with respect to each of the areas listed. The pregnancy and childbirth Internet sites listed under **On the Web** at the end of Chapter 23 in your textbook can also be used to obtain information to complete this activity.

2. In a classroom situation, select a partner. In a role-playing situation, one student takes the role of the MA and the other plays the role of the patient. The patient should ask for guidance regarding each of these areas, and the MA should respond with appropriate information.

   a. Nutrition

   _____

   _____

   b. Employment

   _____

   _____

   c. Exercise

   _____

   _____

   d. Travel

   _____

   _____

   e. Smoking

   _____

   _____

   f. Alcohol

   _____

   _____

   g. Medication

   _____

   _____

I. BREASTFEEDING

1. Lucy Clark asks you for information regarding the advantages and disadvantages of breastfeeding and bottle-feeding. List these in the chart in the Student Study Guide. The pregnancy and childbirth Internet sites listed under **On the Web** at the end of Chapter 23 in your textbook can also be used to obtain information to complete this activity.

2. In a classroom situation, select a partner. In a role-playing situation, one student takes the role of the MA and the other plays the role of the patient. The patient should ask for information regarding the advantages and disadvantages of both methods, and the MA should respond with appropriate information.

Bottle-feeding	
Advantages	*Disadvantages*

Breastfeeding	
Advantages	*Disadvantages*

J. PRENATAL ULTRASOUND

View obstetric ultrasound scans at the following Internet site: www.ob-ultrasound.net/frames.htm. The following scans can be viewed at this site:

1. Gestational sac

2. Fetus at various gestational ages

3. Fetal measurements

4. Fetal organs

5. Three-dimensional images of the fetus

K. CROSSWORD PUZZLE
Gynecology and Obstetrics
Directions: Complete the crossword puzzle using the clues presented below.

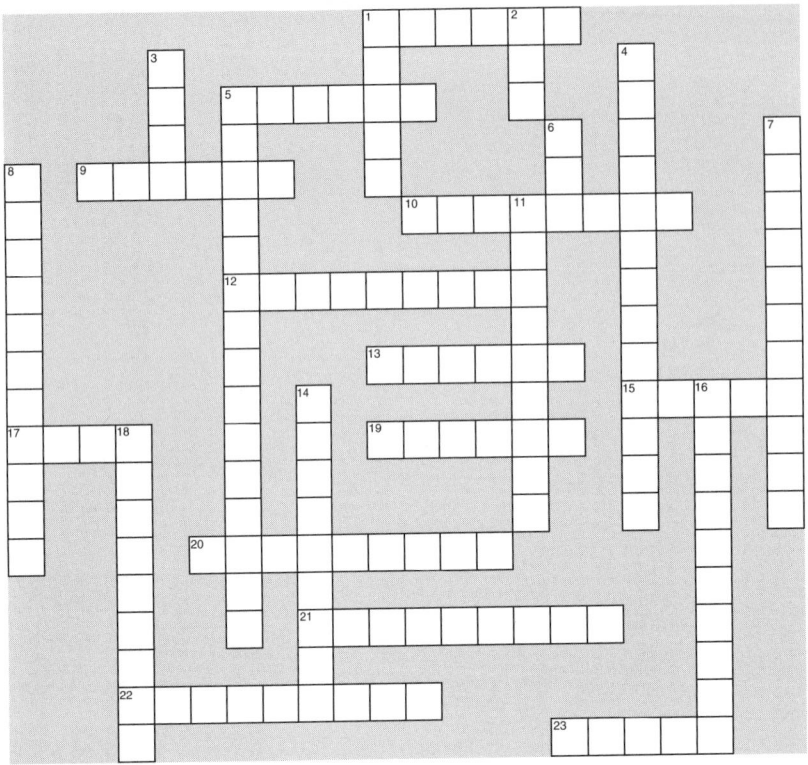

ACROSS

1 What most breast lumps are
5 STD preventer
9 Breast examination position
10 May not occur with STD, especially females
12 STD symptom
13 A viral STD
15 Slightly abnormal Pap cells
17 Definite minor Pap changes
19 Age to begin BSE
20 Breast radiograph
21 Growth of abnormal cells
22 Menstrual cycle ceases
23 Breast cancer increases (age)

DOWN

1 Collects both ectocervical and endocervical Pap specimen
2 Screening test for GDM
3 Warning sign of breast cancer
4 Phase before menopause
5 Causes vaginal yeast infection
6 Long-term use increases breast cancer risk
7 Spread of cancer
8 Serious STD complication
11 What all STDs can be
14 Antibiotics cure this STD
16 Examination of the cervix
18 Pelvic examination position

PRACTICE FOR COMPETENCY

Procedure 23-1: Breast Self-Examination. Instruct an individual about the procedure for performing a breast self-examination and record the procedure in the chart provided.

CHART	
Date	

CHART	
Date	

Procedure 23-2: Gynecological Examination.
1. Complete the cytology request form provided using a female classmate as the patient.
2. Practice the procedure for assisting with a gynecological examination. Record the vital signs and height and weight in the chart provided.

CHART	
Date	

GYN CYTOLOGY REQUISITION

THOMAS WOODSIDE, MD
501 MAIN ST
ST. LOUIS, MO 63146
(314) 883–0093

PATIENT INFO

Patient's Name (Last)	(First)	(MI)	Date of Birth MO	DAY	YR	Collection Time : AM PM	Collection Date MO	DAY	YR	Patient's ID #

Patient's Address   Phone

City   State   ZIP

RESP. PARTY

Name of Responsible Party (if different from patient)

Address of Responsible Party   APT #

City   State   ZIP

INSURANCE

Patient's Relationship to Responsible Party   ☐ 1. Self   ☐ 2. Spouse   ☐ 3. Child   ☐ 4. Other

Insurance Comany Name	Plan	Carrier Code

Subscriber/Member #   Location   Group #

Insurance Address   Physician's Provider #

City   State   ZIP

Employer's Name or Number   Insured SSN

Diagnosis/Signs/Symptoms in ICD-9 Format (Highest Specificity)

R E Q U I R E D

ICD-9 codes are the internationally accepted method of describing the clinical picture of the patient. All diagnoses should be provided by the ordering physician or his or her authorized designee. The following is a partial list of of common diagnoses in ICD-9 format. Most third party payers require an ICD-9 code to indicate the medical necessity of the test(s) and or profile(s) ordered. For a complete list of all ICD-9 codes, please refer to a current ICD-9 manual.

V76.2	Routine Cervical Pap Smear	616.0	Cervicitis	626.8	Abnormal Bleeding
V15.89	High Risk Cervical Screening	616.10	Vaginitis	627.1	Postmenopausal Bleeding
V22.2	Pregnancy	617.0	Endometriosis, Uterus	627.3	Atrophic Vaginitis
079.4	Human Papillomavirus	622.1	Dysplasia, Cervix	795.0	Abnormal Cervical Pap Smear
180.0	Malignant Neoplasm, Cervix	623.0	Dysplasia, Vagina		

COLLECTION METHOD	SOURCE OF SPECIMEN	COLLECTION TECHNIQUE
Liquid Based Prep **192055** ☐ Thin Prep Pap Test	☐ **Cervical**	☐ **Spatula**
192039 ☐ Thin Prep Pap Test w/reflex to HPV Hybrid Capture when ASC-US or SIL	☐ **Endocervical**	☐ **Brush**
192047 ☐ Thin Prep Pap Test w/reflex to high-risk only HPV Hybrid Capture when ASC-US	☐ **Vaginal**	☐ **Broom** ☐ **Other** _____
Pap Smear **009100** ☐ 1 Slide **009191** ☐ 2 Slides	**Date LMP** ___/___/___ Mo Day Year	
Pap Smear and Maturation Index **009209** ☐ 1 Slide **190074** ☐ 2 Slides		

PATIENT HISTORY	PREVIOUS TREATMENT	Date/Results
☐ **Pregnant** ☐ **PMP Bleeding**	☐ **None**	
☐ **Lactating** ☐ **Postpartum**	☐ **Colposcopy and Bx** _____	
☐ **Oral Contraceptives** ☐ **IUD**	☐ **Cryosurgery** _____	
☐ **Postmenopausal** ☐ **Postcoital Bleeding**	☐ **LEEP** _____	
☐ **Hormone Replacement Therapy** ☐ **DES Exposure** ☐ **Previous Abnormal Pap Test**	☐ **Laser Vaporization** _____	
☐ **Other** _____	☐ **Conization** _____	
	☐ **Hysterectomy** _____	
	☐ **Radiation** _____	
	☐ **Chemotherapy** _____	

(From Bonewit-West K: *Study guide for clinical procedures for medical assistants,* ed 7, St. Louis, 2008, Saunders.)

Procedure 23-3: Return Prenatal Examination.
1. Complete the prenatal health history form provided using a female classmate as the patient.
2. Prepare the patient and assist with a return prenatal examination. Record the results of procedures you performed on the chart provided.

CHART	
Date	

CHART

Date	

PRENATAL HEALTH HISTORY

PATIENT INFORMATION

Date: _____ EDD: _____   Referred By: _____

Name: _____   Phone (home): _____
       LAST   FIRST   MIDDLE   Phone (work): _____

Address: _____   Emergency Contact: _____

_____   Phone: _____
     CITY   STATE   ZIP

Date of Birth: ___/___/___ Age: ___ Marital Status: _____

Occupation: _____

Education: ☐ High School ☐ College ☐ Post-graduate

PAST MEDICAL HISTORY

	○ Neg + Pos	DETAIL POSITIVE REMARKS INCLUDE DATE AND TREATMENT		○ Neg + Pos	DETAIL POSITIVE REMARKS INCLUDE DATE AND TREATMENT
1. DIABETES			16. D (Rh) SENSITIZED		
2. HYPERTENSION			17. PULMONARY (TB, ASTHMA)		
3. HEART DISEASE			18. RHEUMATIC FEVER		
4. AUTOIMMUNE DISORDER			19. BLEEDING TENDENCY		
5. KIDNEY DISEASE/UTI			20. GYN SURGERY		
6. NEUROLOGIC/EPILEPSY					
7. PSYCHIATRIC			21. OPERATIONS/HOSPITALIZATIONS		
8. HEPATITIS/LIVER DISEASE			(YEAR AND REASON)		
9. VARICOSITIES/PHLEBITIS					
10. THYROID DYSFUNCTION			22. ANESTHETIC COMPLICATIONS		
11. TRAUMA/DOMESTIC VIOLENCE			23. HISTORY OF ABNORMAL PAP		
12. BLOOD TRANSFUSION			24. UTERINE ANOMALY/DES		

	AMT/DAY PREPREG.	AMT/DAY PREG.	# YEARS USE			
				25. INFERTILITY		
13. TOBACCO				26. SEXUALLY TRANSMITTED DISEASE		
14. ALCOHOL						
15. STREET DRUGS				27. OTHER		

IMMUNIZATIONS:

Mark an X next to those you have had.

☐ Influenza   ☐ Chickenpox

☐ Hepatitis B   ☐ Pneumococcal

☐ Hib   ☐ Tuberculin Test

☐ Polio   ☐ Tetanus Booster

☐ MMR

ALLERGIES:

List all allergies (foods, drugs, environment). ☐ None

_____

_____

_____

_____

_____

MENSTRUAL HISTORY

Menarche: Age of Onset _____   GYN Disorders (List): _____

Frequency: Q _____ Days

Duration: _____ Days   _____

Amount of Flow: ☐ Small ☐ Moderate ☐ Large   On contraceptive at conception? ☐ Yes ☐ No

(From Bonewit-West K: *Study guide for clinical procedures for medical assistants,* ed 7, St. Louis, 2008, Saunders.)

OBSTETRIC HISTORY

G _____ (Total Pregnancies)   T _____ (Term)   P _____ (Preterm)   A _____ (Abortions)?   L _____ (Living Children)

PREVIOUS PREGNANCIES:

DATE MONTH/ YEAR	WEEKS GEST.	LENGTH OF LABOR	BIRTH WEIGHT	SEX M/F	TYPE DELIVERY	ANES.	MATERNAL COMPLICATIONS	INFANT COMPLICATIONS

PRESENT PREGNANCY HISTORY

NAUSEA			ABDOMINAL PAIN	
VOMITING			URINARY COMPLAINTS	
FATIGUE			VAGINAL BLEEDING	
BREAST CHANGES			VAGINAL DISCHARGE	
INDIGESTION			PRURITIS	
CONSTIPATION			ACCIDENTS	
PERSISTENT HEADACHES			SURGERY	
DIZZINESS			X-RAYS	
VISUAL DISTURBANCE			RUBELLA EXPOSURE	
EDEMA (SPECIFY AREA)			OTHER VIRAL INFECTIONS	

LMP ____ / ____ / ____
    Mo   Day   Year

Amount of Flow: ☐ Small   ☐ Moderate   ☐ Large

CURRENT MEDICATIONS: (Include prescription, OTC, herbal, and vitamins). ☐ None

Medication _____   Frequency _____

INITIAL PHYSICAL EXAMINATION

DATE ____ / ____ / ____

1. HEENT ☐ NORMAL ☐ ABNORMAL	12. VULVA ☐ NORMAL	☐ CONDYLOMA	☐ LESIONS
2. FUNDI ☐ NORMAL ☐ ABNORMAL	13. VAGINA ☐ NORMAL	☐ INFLAMMATION	☐ DISCHARGE
3. TEETH ☐ NORMAL ☐ ABNORMAL	14. CERVIX ☐ NORMAL	☐ INFLAMMATION	☐ LESIONS
4. THYROID ☐ NORMAL ☐ ABNORMAL	15. UTERUS SIZE _____ WEEKS		☐ FIBROIDS
5. BREASTS ☐ NORMAL ☐ ABNORMAL	16. ADNEXA ☐ NORMAL	☐ MASS	
6. LUNGS ☐ NORMAL ☐ ABNORMAL	17. RECTUM ☐ NORMAL	☐ ABNORMAL	
7. HEART ☐ NORMAL ☐ ABNORMAL	18. DIAGONAL CONJUGATE ☐ REACHED	☐ NO	_____CM
8. ABDOMEN ☐ NORMAL ☐ ABNORMAL	19. SPINES ☐ AVERAGE	☐ PROMINENT	☐ BLUNT
9. EXTREMITIES ☐ NORMAL ☐ ABNORMAL	20. SACRUM ☐ CONCAVE	☐ STRAIGHT	☐ ANTERIOR
10. SKIN ☐ NORMAL ☐ ABNORMAL	21. SUBPUBIC ARCH ☐ NORMAL	☐ WIDE	☐ NARROW
11. LYMPH NODES ☐ NORMAL ☐ ABNORMAL	22. GYNECOID PELVIC TYPE ☐ YES	☐ NO	

COMMENTS (Number and explain abnormals): _____

_____

EXAM BY _____

(From Bonewit-West K: *Study guide for clinical procedures for medical assistants*, ed 7, St. Louis, 2008, Saunders.)

PATIENT'S NAME _____

INTERVAL PRENATAL HISTORY

Date 20___	Weeks Gestation	Height of Fundus (cm)	Weight	B/P	Urine Glucose	Urine Protein	FHT	Vaginal Examination	Presentation	Edema	Discharge	Bleeding	Contractions	Fetal Activity	NST	Next Appt.	Initials

PLANS/EDUCATION   (COUNSELED ✓)

☐ ANESTHESIA PLANS _____
☐ TOXOPLASMOSIS PRECAUTIONS (CATS/RAW MEAT) _____
☐ CHILDBIRTH CLASSES _____
☐ PHYSICAL/SEXUAL ACTIVITY _____
☐ LABOR SIGNS _____
☐ NUTRITION COUNSELING _____
☐ BREAST OR BOTTLE FEEDING _____
☐ NEWBORN CAR SEAT _____
☐ POSTPARTUM BIRTH CONTROL _____
☐ ENVIRONMENTAL/WORK HAZARDS _____

☐ TUBAL STERILIZATION _____
☐ VBAC COUNSELING _____
☐ CIRCUMCISION _____
☐ TRAVEL _____
☐ LIFESTYLE, TOBACCO, ALCOHOL _____

REQUESTS _____
_____
_____

TUBAL STERILIZATION	**DATE**	**INITIALS**
CONSENT SIGNED	___ / ___ / ___	_____

(From Bonewit-West K: *Study guide for clinical procedures for medical assistants*, ed 7, St. Louis, 2008, Saunders.)

LABORATORY		PATIENT'S NAME _____			
INITIAL LABS	**DATE**	**RESULTS**		**REVIEWED**	**COMMENTS**
BLOOD TYPE	/ /	A B AB O			
Rh FACTOR	/ /	☐ Pos ☐ Neg			
Rh ANTIBODY SCREEN	/ /	☐ Pos ☐ Neg			
HCT/HGB	/ /	_____ % _____ g/dL			
RUBELLA ANTIBODY TITER	/ /	Immune Nonimmune			
VDRL	/ /	☐ NR ☐ R			
HBsAg (HEPATITIS B)	/ /	☐ Pos ☐ Neg			
HIV	/ /	☐ Pos ☐ Neg ☐ Declined			
URINE CULTURE/SCREEN	/ /				
PAP TEST	/ /	☐ Normal ☐ Abnormal			
CHLAMYDIA (DNA PROBE)	/ /	☐ Pos ☐ Neg			
GONORRHEA (DNA PROBE)	/ /	☐ Pos ☐ Neg			
7–20 WEEK LABS (WHEN INDICATED/ELECTED)	**DATE**	**RESULTS**		**REVIEWED**	**COMMENTS**
ULTRASOUND #1 (7–13 WEEKS)	/ /	EDD:			
ULTRASOUND #2 (18–20 WEEKS)	/ /	EFW:			
TRIPLE SCREEN (15–20 WEEKS)	/ /				
CVS	/ /				
AMNIOCENTESIS	/ /				
24–28 WEEK LABS (WHEN INDICATED)	**DATE**	**RESULTS**		**REVIEWED**	**COMMENTS**
HCT/HGB	/ /	_____ % _____ g/dL			
GCT (24–28 WKS)	/ /	1 Hour _____			
GTT (IF SCREEN ABNORMAL)	/ /	_____ FBS _____ 1 Hour			
		_____ 2 Hour _____ 3 Hour			
D (Rh) ANTIBODY SCREEN	/ /				
D IMMUNE GLOBULIN (RhIG) GIVEN (28 WKS)	/ /	SIGNATURE			
32–36 WEEK LABS	**DATE**	**RESULTS**		**REVIEWED**	**COMMENTS**
HCT/HGB (32 WKS)	/ /	_____ % _____ g/dL			
ULTRASOUND #3 (34 WKS)	/ /	EFW:			
GROUP B STREP (35–37 WKS)	/ /	☐ Pos ☐ Neg			
ADDITIONAL LAB TESTS	**DATE**	**RESULTS**		**REVIEWED**	**COMMENTS**
	/ /				
	/ /				
	/ /				
	/ /				
	/ /				

(From Bonewit-West K: *Study guide for clinical procedures for medical assistants,* ed 7, St. Louis, 2008, Saunders.)

Trial 1	Trial 2	Point Value	Performance Standards
			3. In the Shower
		•	Gently lather each breast.
		▷	Explained why the breasts should be examined in the shower.
		•	Place right hand behind head.
		•	Use the finger pads of the middle three fingers of the left hand.
		•	Use small rotating motions and continuous firm pressure.
		•	Use your preferred pattern to thoroughly examine the right breast and underarm for lumps, hard knots, or thickening.
		•	Repeat the procedure on the left breast using the pads of your right fingers.
		•	Instructed the patient to report any lumps or changes to the physician immediately.
		▷	Explained why it is important to report changes immediately.
		•	Charted the procedure correctly.
		∗	Completed the procedure within 10 minutes.
			TOTALS

CHART	
Date	

Evaluation of Student Performance

EVALUATION CRITERIA			COMMENTS
Symbol	**Category**	**Point Value**	
∗	Critical Step	16 points	
•	Essential Step	6 points	
▷	Theory Question	2 points	

Score calculation: 100 points

−_____ points missed

_____ Score

Satisfactory score: 85 or above

CAAHEP Competencies Achieved:
Psychomotor (Skills)
☑ IV. 5. Instruct patients according to their needs to promote health maintenance and disease prevention.
☑ IV. 9. Document patient education.

Affective (Behavior)
☑ I. 2. Use language/verbal skills that enable patients' understanding.
☑ IV. 3. Use appropriate body language and other nonverbal skills in communicating with patients, family, and staff.

ABHES Competencies Achieved:
☑ 8. e. Locate resources and information for patients and employers.
☑ 8. cc. Communicate on the recipient's level of comprehension.
☑ 8. ii. Recognize and respond to verbal and non-verbal communication.
☑ 9. r. Teach patients methods of health promotion and disease prevention.

Notes

EVALUATION OF COMPETENCY

Procedure 23-2: Assisting with a Gynecological Examination

Name: _____   Date: _____

Evaluated By: _____   Score: _____

Performance Objective

Outcome:	Assist with a gynecologic examination.
Conditions:	Using an examining table.
	Given the following: disposable gloves, examining gown and drape, disposable vaginal speculum, lubricant, gauze pads, Hemoccult slide and developing solution, tissues, biohazard waste container, cytology request form, biohazard specimen transport bag.
	Direct Smear Method: Glass slides with frosted edge, cytology fixative, plastic spafula, endocervical brush, slide container.
	Liquid-Prep Method: ThinPrep Vial, plastic spatula and endocervical brush or cytology broom.
Standards:	Time: 15 minutes. Student completed procedure in ____ minutes.
	Accuracy: Satisfactory score on the Performance Evaluation Checklist.

Performance Evaluation Checklist

Trial 1	Trial 2	Point Value	*Performance Standards*
		●	Sanitized hands.
		●	Assembled equipment.
		●	Completed as much of the cytology request form as possible.
			Prepared the collection materials:
		●	***Pap Smear Method:*** Identified the slides on the frosted edge.
		●	***Liquid-Prep Method:*** Checked the expiration date and labeled the vial.
		●	Greeted the patient and introduced yourself.
		●	Identified the patient and explained the procedure.
		●	Escorted the patient to the examining room.
		●	Asked patient if she had any problems or concerns and chart the information.
		●	Completed the cytology request by asking necessary questions.
		●	Measured vital signs and height and weight and charted the results correctly.
			Prepared patient for the examination:
		●	Asked patient if she needed to empty bladder.
		▷	Explained why the bladder should be empty for the examination.

Trial 1	Trial 2	Point Value	Performance Standards
		●	Instructed the patient to undress and put on the examining gown with opening in front.
		●	Informed patient that physician would be in soon.
		●	Left the room to provide patient privacy.
		●	Made medical record available for review by the physician.
		●	Checked to make sure patient was ready.
		●	Informed physician that the patient was ready.
			Assisted the physician:
		●	Positioned and draped patient in a supine position for the breast examination.
		●	Positioned and draped patient in the lithotomy position for the pelvic examination.
		●	Prepared the vaginal speculum and handed it to the physician.
		▷	Explained how to prepare the speculum for the Pap smear method and the liquid-prep method.
		●	Prepared the light for physician.
		●	Handed vaginal speculum to physician.
		●	Reassured patient and helped her to relax during the examination.
		▷	Explained why patient should be relaxed during the examination.
			Assisted with collection of the Pap specimen:
		●	Applied gloves.
			1. Direct Smear Method
		●	Held each slide for the physician to smear the specimen on it.
		●	Immediately fixed the slides.
		●	Allowed slides to dry and placed them in a slide container.
			2 (a). Liquid-Prep Spatula and Brush Method
		●	Held the vial to receive the collection device from the physician.
		●	Correctly rinsed each collection device in the liquid preservative.
		▷	Explained why the collection device should be swirled vigorously.
		●	Discarded each collection device in a regular waste container.
		●	Tightened the cap on the vial.
			2 (b). Liquid-Prep Broom Method
		●	Held the vial to receive the broom from the physician.
		●	Correctly rinsed the broom in the liquid preservative.
		●	Discarded the broom in a biohazard waste container.
		●	Tightened the cap on the vial.
			3. SurePath Spatula and Brush Method
		●	Held the vial to receive each collection device from the physician.
		●	Broke off or disconnected tip of each collection device.
		●	Discarded each handle in a regular waste container.

Trial 1	Trial 2	Point Value	Performance Standards
		●	Tightened cap on the vial.
			Assisted with the remainder of the examination:
		●	Removed light source.
		●	Discarded vaginal speculum in a biohazard waste container.
		●	Provided the physician with lubricant for the bimanual and rectal-vaginal examinations.
		●	Assisted as required with the collection of the fecal occult blood specimen.
		●	Assisted the patient into a sitting position and allowed her to rest.
		▷	Explained why the patient should be allowed to rest.
		●	Offered the patient tissues to remove lubricant from the perineum.
		●	Assisted patient from the examining table.
		●	Instructed patient to get dressed.
		●	Informed patient of the method used by the medical office to relay test results.
		●	Tested the fecal occult blood specimen and charted the results.
		●	Prepared Pap specimen for transport to the laboratory.
		●	Placed specimen in a biohazard specimen bag and sealed the bag.
		●	Inserted the cytology requisition into the outside pocket of bag.
		●	Placed bag in appropriate location for pickup by the laboratory.
		●	Charted the transport of the Pap specimen to an outside laboratory.
		●	Cleaned the examining room.
		✱	Completed the procedure within 15 minutes.
			TOTALS

	CHART
Date	

Evaluation of Student Performance

EVALUATION CRITERIA			COMMENTS
Symbol	Category	Point Value	
✱	Critical Step	16 points	
●	Essential Step	6 points	
▷	Theory Question	2 points	
Score calculation: 100 points			
−_____ points missed			
_____ Score			
Satisfactory score: 85 or above			

CAAHEP Competencies Achieved:
Psychomotor (Skills)
☑ 1. 10. Assist physician with patient care.
☑ IV. 5. Instruct patients according to their needs to promote health maintenance and disease prevention.
☑ IV. 6. Prepare a patient for procedures and/or treatments.

Affective (Behavior)
☑ III. 3. Show awareness of patients' concerns.
☑ IV. 1. Demonstrate empathy in communicating with patients, family, and staff.

ABHES Competencies Achieved:
☑ 8. bb. Are impartial and show empathy when dealing with patients.
☑ 9. f. Screen and follow up patient test results.
☑ 9. k. Prepare and maintain examination and treatment area.
☑ 9. l. Prepare patient for examinations and treatments.
☑ 9. m. Assist physician with routine and specialty examinations and treatments.

GYN CYTOLOGY REQUISITION

THOMAS WOODSIDE, MD
501 MAIN ST
ST. LOUIS, MO 63146
(314) 883-0093

PATIENT INFO

Patient's Name (Last) | (First) | (MI) | Date of Birth MO DAY YR | Collection Time : AM PM | Collection Date MO DAY YR | Patient's ID #

Patient's Address | Phone

City | State | ZIP

RESP. PARTY

Name of Responsible Party (if different from patient)

Address of Responsible Party | APT #

City | State | ZIP

INSURANCE

Patient's Relationship to Responsible Party ☐ 1. Self ☐ 2. Spouse ☐ 3. Child ☐ 4. Other

Insurance Comany Name | Plan | Carrier Code

Subscriber/Member # | Location | Group #

Insurance Address | Physician's Provider #

City | State | ZIP

Employer's Name or Number | Insured SSN

Diagnosis/Signs/Symptoms in ICD-9 Format (Highest Specificity)

REQUIRED

ICD-9 codes are the internationally accepted method of describing the clinical picture of the patient. All diagnoses should be provided by the ordering physician or his or her authorized designee. The following is a partial list of of common diagnoses in ICD-9 format. Most third party payers require an ICD-9 code to indicate the medical necessity of the test(s) or profile(s) ordered. For a complete list of all ICD-9 codes, please refer to a current ICD-9 manual.

V76.2	Routine Cervical Pap Smear	616.0	Cervicitis	626.8	Abnormal Bleeding
V15.89	High Risk Cervical Screening	616.10	Vaginitis	627.1	Postmenopausal Bleeding
V22.2	Pregnancy	617.0	Endometriosis, Uterus	627.3	Atrophic Vaginitis
079.4	Human Papillomavirus	622.1	Dysplasia, Cervix	795.0	Abnormal Cervical Pap Smear
180.0	Malignant Neoplasm, Cervix	623.0	Dysplasia, Vagina		

COLLECTION METHOD

Liquid Based Prep
192055 ☐ Thin Prep Pap Test

192039 ☐ Thin Prep Pap Test w/reflex to HPV Hybrid Capture when ASC-US or SIL

192047 ☐ Thin Prep Pap Test w/reflex to high-risk only HPV Hybrid Capture when ASC-US

Pap Smear
009100 ☐ 1 Slide   009191 ☐ 2 Slides

Pap Smear and Maturation Index
009209 ☐ 1 Slide   190074 ☐ 2 Slides

SOURCE OF SPECIMEN

☐ Cervical
☐ Endocervical
☐ Vaginal

Date LMP
___ / ___ / ___
Mo   Day   Year

COLLECTION TECHNIQUE

☐ Spatula
☐ Brush
☐ Broom
☐ Other
_____

PATIENT HISTORY

☐ Pregnant
☐ Lactating
☐ Oral Contraceptives
☐ Postmenopausal
☐ Hormone Replacement Therapy

☐ PMP Bleeding
☐ Postpartum
☐ IUD
☐ Postcoital Bleeding
☐ DES Exposure
☐ Previous Abnormal Pap Test

☐ Other _____

PREVIOUS TREATMENT   Date/Results

☐ None
☐ Colposcopy and Bx _____
☐ Cryosurgery _____
☐ LEEP _____
☐ Laser Vaporization _____
☐ Conization _____
☐ Hysterectomy _____
☐ Radiation _____
☐ Chemotherapy _____

(From Bonewit-West K: *Study guide for clinical procedures for medical assistants*, ed 7, St. Louis, 2008, Saunders.)

EVALUATION OF COMPETENCY

Procedure 23-3: Assisting with a Return Prenatal Examination

Name: _____   Date: _____

Evaluated By: _____   Score: _____

Performance Objective

Outcome:	Prepare the patient and assist with a return prenatal examination.
Conditions:	Using an examining table.
	Given the following: centimeter tape measure, Doppler fetal pulse detector, ultrasound coupling agent, paper towel, disposable vaginal speculum, disposable gloves, lubricant, gauze pads, examining gown and drape, and a biohazard waste container.
Standards:	Time: 15 minutes. Student completed procedure in _____ minutes.
	Accuracy: Satisfactory score on the Performance Evaluation Checklist.

Performance Evaluation Checklist

Trial 1	Trial 2	Point Value	Performance Standards
		•	Sanitized hands.
		•	Set up the tray for the prenatal examination.
		•	Greeted the patient and introduced yourself.
		•	Identified the patient and explained the procedure.
		•	Asked the patient to obtain a urine specimen.
		•	Escorted the patient to the examining room and asked her to be seated.
		•	Asked the patient if she had experienced any problems since her last visit and recorded information in the prenatal record.
		•	Measured patient's blood pressure and charted the results correctly.
		•	Weighed the patient and charted the results correctly.
		▷	Stated the importance of weighing the patient.
		•	Instructed and prepared patient for the examination.
		•	Left room to provide patient with privacy.
		•	Made medical record available for review by the physician.
		•	Tested the urine specimen for glucose and protein and charted the results correctly.
		•	Checked to make sure the patient was ready to be seen by physician.
		•	Informed physician that patient was ready to be examined.
		•	Stated how the physician can be informed that the patient is ready.
		•	Assisted patient into a supine position and properly draped her.

Trial 1	Trial 2	Point Value	Performance Standards
			Assisted physician during the examination:
		•	Handed physician the tape measure for determination of fundal height.
		•	Applied coupling gel to the patient's abdomen and handed physician Doppler device.
		•	Removed gel from patient's abdomen.
		•	Cleaned the probe head of the Doppler device.
		•	Assisted patient into the lithotomy position if a vaginal specimen was to be obtained or if vaginal examination was to be performed.
			After completion of the examination:
		•	Assisted patient into a sitting position and allowed her to rest.
		•	Assisted patient from examining table.
		•	Provided patient teaching and explanation of physician's instructions as required.
		•	Escorted patient to the reception area.
		•	Cleaned the examining room in preparation for the next patient.
		•	Prepared any specimens collected for transport to an outside laboratory.
		∗	Completed the procedure within 15 minutes.
			TOTALS
			CHART
	Date		

Evaluation of Student Performance

EVALUATION CRITERIA			COMMENTS
Symbol	Category	Point Value	
∗	Critical Step	16 points	
•	Essential Step	6 points	
▷	Theory Question	2 points	
Score calculation: 100 points			
− ____ points missed			
____ Score			
Satisfactory score: 85 or above			

CAAHEP Competencies Achieved:

Psychomotor (Skills)

☑ 1. 10. Assist physician with patient care.
☑ II. 2. Maintain laboratory test results using flow sheets.
☑ IV. 1. Use reflection, restatement, and clarification techniques to obtain a patient history.
☑ IV. 5. Instruct patients according to their needs to promote health maintenance and disease prevention.
☑ IV. 6. Prepare a patient for procedures and/or treatments.
☑ IX. 7. Document accurately in the patient record.

Affective (Behavior)

☑ IV. 2. Apply active listening skills.
☑ IV. 8. Analyze communications in providing appropriate responses/feedback.

ABHES Competencies Achieved:

☑ 4. a. Document accurately.
☑ 8. e. Locate resources and information for patients and employers.
☑ 8. ff. Interview effectively.
☑ 9. f. Screen and follow up patient test results.
☑ 9. k. Prepare and maintain examination and treatment area.
☑ 9. l. Prepare patient for examinations and treatments.
☑ 9. m. Assist physician with routine and specialty examinations and treatments.
☑ 9. r. Teach patients methods of health promotion and disease prevention.

PATIENT'S NAME

INTERVAL PRENATAL HISTORY

Date 20__	Weeks Gestation	Height of Fundus (cm)	Weight	B/P	Urine Glucose	Urine Protein	FHT	Vaginal Examination	Presentation	Edema	Discharge	Bleeding	Contractions	Fetal Activity	NST	Next Appt.	Initials

(From Bonewit-West K: *Study guide for clinical procedures for medical assistants,* ed 7, St. Louis, 2008, Saunders.)

Notes

24

The Pediatric Examination

CHAPTER ASSIGNMENTS

√ After Completing	Date Due	Textbook Page(s)	TEXTBOOK ASSIGNMENTS	Possible Points	Points You Earned
		496-523	Read Chapter 24: The Pediatric Examination		
		498 521	Read Case Study 1 Case Study 1 questions	5	
		509 521-522	Read Case Study 2 Case Study 2 questions	5	
		513 522	Read Case Study 3 Case Study 3 questions	5	
			TOTAL POINTS		

√ After Completing	Date Due	Study Guide Page(s)	STUDY GUIDE ASSIGNMENTS (CTA: Critical Thinking Activity)	Possible Points	Points You Earned
		493	Pretest	10	
		494	Key Term Assessment	12	
		495-497	Evaluation of Learning questions	30	
		498	CTA A: Pediatric Weight	7	
			CD Activity: Chapter 24 Pounds and Ounces (Record points earned)		
		498	CTA B: Pediatric Length	8	
			CD Activity: Chapter 24 Inch by Inch (Record points earned)		
		498	CTA C: Growth Charts	18	
		499-501	CTA D: Motor and Social Development (5 pts/each category)	65	
		502	CTA E: Intramuscular Injection	15	

√ After Completing	Date Due	Study Guide Page(s)	STUDY GUIDE ASSIGNMENTS (CTA: Critical Thinking Activity)	Possible Points	Points You Earned
		502-503	CTA F: Vaccine Information Statement	10	
		503	CTA G: Locating and Interpreting a VIS	20	
		504	CTA H: Crossword Puzzle	30	
		505	CTA I: Choose-a-Clue Game (Record points earned)		
			🔵CD CD Activity: Chapter 24 Apply Your Knowledge questions (Record points earned)		
		493	📄 Posttest	10	
			ADDITIONAL ASSIGNMENTS		
			TOTAL POINTS		

√ When Assigned by Your Instructor	Study Guide Page(s)	Practices Required	LABORATORY ASSIGNMENTS (Procedure Number and Name)	*Score
	511	3	📀 **Practice for Competency** 24-A: Carrying an Infant Textbook reference: pp. 499-501	
	515-516		📖 **Evaluation of Competency** 24-A: Carrying an Infant	*
	512	5	📀 **Practice for Competency** 24-1: Measuring the Weight and Length of an Infant Textbook reference: pp. 503-504	
	517-518		📖 **Evaluation of Competency** 24-1: Measuring the Weight and Length of an Infant	*
	513	5	📀 **Practice for Competency** 24-2: Measuring Head and Chest Circumference of an Infant Textbook reference: pp. 504-505	
	519-520		📖 **Evaluation of Competency** 24-2: Measuring Head and Chest Circumference of an Infant	*
	512	5	📀 **Practice for Competency** 24-3: Calculating Growth Percentiles Textbook reference: pp. 505-507	
	521-522		📖 **Evaluation of Competency** 24-3: Calculating Growth Percentiles	*
	514	5	📀 **Practice for Competency** 24-4: Applying a Pediatric Urine Collector Textbook reference: pp. 510-511	
	523-525		📖 **Evaluation of Competency** 24-4: Applying a Pediatric Urine Collector	*
			ADDITIONAL ASSIGNMENTS	

Notes

Name _____   Date _____

? PRETEST

True or False

_____   1. A pediatrician is a physician who specializes in the diagnosis and treatment of disease in children.

_____   2. The first well-child visit is usually scheduled 1 week after birth.

_____   3. Length is measured with the child standing with his back to the measuring device.

_____   4. Blood pressure should be taken on a child starting at 8 years of age.

_____   5. It is best not to tell a child that an immunization will hurt.

_____   6. The vastus lateralis muscle site is recommended for administering an injection to an infant.

_____   7. An MMR injection includes the following immunizations: measles, meningitis, and rubella.

_____   8. A Vaccine Information Statement explains the benefits and risks of a vaccine in lay terminology.

_____   9. The hepatitis B vaccine can be given to a newborn.

_____   10. The blood specimen for a newborn screening test is obtained from the infant's earlobe.

? POSTTEST

True or False

_____   1. A well-child visit is also referred to as a health maintenance visit.

_____   2. A reason for weighing a child is to determine proper medication dosage of medication.

_____   3. Growth charts can be used to identify children with growth abnormalities.

_____   4. Measuring pediatric blood pressure helps to identify children at risk for developing type 1 diabetes.

_____   5. Using a blood pressure cuff that is too large for the child can result in a falsely low reading.

_____   6. The length of the needle used for a pediatric IM injection depends on the amount of medication being administered.

_____   7. The resistance of the body to pathogenic microorganisms or their toxins is known as _inflammation_.

_____   8. The recommended route of administration for an MMR is subcutaneous.

_____   9. Before administering a pediatric immunization, the NCVIA requires that the parent sign a consent form.

_____   10. If PKU is left untreated, it can lead to malnutrition.

Term KEY TERM ASSESSMENT

Directions: Match each medical term with its definition.

_____ 1. Immunity

_____ 2. Immunization

_____ 3. Infant

_____ 4. Length

_____ 5. Pediatrician

_____ 6. Pediatrics

_____ 7. Preschool child

_____ 8. School-age child

_____ 9. Toddler

_____ 10. Toxoid

_____ 11. Vaccine

_____ 12. Vertex

A. A medical doctor who specializes in the care and development of children and the diagnosis and treatment of children's diseases

B. A child from 1 to 3 years of age

C. The summit, or top, especially the top of the head

D. The resistance of the body to the effects of a harmful agent such as a pathogenic microorganism or its toxins

E. The branch of medicine that deals with the care and development of children and the diagnosis and treatment of children's diseases

F. A suspension of attenuated or killed microorganisms administered to an individual to prevent an infectious disease

G. The process of becoming immune or of rendering an individual immune through the use of a vaccine or toxoid

H. The measurement from the vertex of the head to the heel of the foot in a supine position

I. A toxin that has been treated by heat or chemicals to destroy its harmful properties

J. A child from birth to 12 months of age

K. A child from 3 to 6 years of age

L. A child from 6 to 12 years of age

D. MOTOR AND SOCIAL DEVELOPMENT

Using a reference source, describe the motor and social development of the age groups listed here. The first o
done for you.

AGE	MOTOR AND SOCIAL DEVELOPMENT
Birth to 3 months	Raises head but not stable, can turn head from side to side, activities are limited reflexes, cries when hungry, responsive social smile, coos, eyes can focus on an object and follow a moving object 180 degrees.
4 to 6 months	
7 to 9 months	
10 to 12 months	

AGE	MOTOR AND SOCIAL DEVELOPMENT
1 year	
2 years	
3 years	
4 years	
5 years	

I. CHOOSE-A-CLUE GAME

Object: To become familiar with childhood diseases

Directions

1. Cut out the game cards.
2. List three clues for each condition specified on the reverse of the card. Your clues should include information on symptoms, prevention, and treatment. The name of the disease *must not* be written on this side of the card.
3. Use the game cards as flash cards to study the diseases.
4. Get into a group of three students.
5. Place your game cards on the table in front of you with the clues facing up.
6. One of the players should name the first disease on the list presented below.
7. Each player places the appropriate game card on the table with the clues facing upward.
8. When all players have placed a card on the table, turn the cards over.
9. Award yourself 5 points if you have correctly determined the disease.
10. Review the information each player listed on his or her game card.
11. Keep track of your points on the score card provided.
12. Continue playing until all the diseases have been identified.

Good Internet reference sources to help you find clues include:

www.kidshealth.org

www.merck.com

Childhood Diseases

1. Conjunctivitis
2. Fifth disease
3. Head lice
4. Impetigo
5. Influenza
6. Meningococcal meningitis
7. Methicillin-resistant *Staphylococcus aureus* (MRSA)
8. Otitis media
9. Pertussis
10. Pinworms
11. Roseola
12. Respiratory syncytial virus (RSV)
13. Scarlet fever
14. Strep throat
15. Urinary tract infection
16. Varicella (chickenpox)

CHOOSE-A-CLUE
SCORE CARD

Name: _____

Recording Points:
Cross off a number each time you properly identify a disease (starting with 5 and continuing in sequence). Your total points will be equal to the last number you crossed off. Record this number in the space provided, and place a checkmark next to the level you achieved.

Points:	
5	75
10	80
15	85
20	90
25	95
30	100
35	105
40	110
45	115
50	120
55	125
60	130
65	135
70	140

TOTAL POINTS: _____

LEVEL:

☐ 75 points and above: **Free from Infection**
☐ 65 to 70 points: **Putting Up a Good Fight**
☐ 55 to 60 points: **Susceptible**
☐ 50 points and under: **Infected**

Conjunctivitis	Fifth disease
Head lice	Influenza
Meningitis	Mumps
Otitis media	Pertussis

Sym:

Prev:

Tx:

Sym:

Prev:

Tx:

Sym:

Prev:

Tx:

Sym:

Prev:

Tx:

Sym:

Prev:

Tx:

Sym:

Prev:

Tx:

Sym:

Prev:

Tx:

Sym:

Prev:

Tx:

Pinworms	Pneumonia
Roseola	Respiratory syncytial virus (RSV)
Scarlet fever	Strep throat
Urinary tract infection	Varicella (chicken pox)

Sym:

_____
_____

Prev:

_____
_____

Tx:

_____
_____

Sym:

_____
_____

Prev:

_____
_____

Tx:

_____
_____

Sym:

_____
_____

Prev:

_____
_____

Tx:

_____
_____

Sym:

_____
_____

Prev:

_____
_____

Tx:

_____
_____

Sym:

_____
_____

Prev:

_____
_____

Tx:

_____
_____

Sym:

_____
_____

Prev:

_____
_____

Tx:

_____
_____

Sym:

_____
_____

Prev:

_____
_____

Tx:

_____
_____

Sym:

_____
_____

Prev:

_____
_____

Tx:

_____
_____

PRACTICE FOR COMPETENCY

Procedure 24-A: Carrying an Infant. Practice the procedure for carrying an infant, using a pediatric training mannequin in the following positions: cradle and upright.

CARRYING POSITION	NUMBER OF PRACTICES

Procedures 24-1 and 24-3: Weight, Length, and Growth Charts.

1. **Weight and Length.** Measure the weight of an infant using a pediatric training mannequin. Record the results in the chart provided.
2. **Growth Charts.** Calculate growth percentiles on a growth chart using the values presented above. Assume these values were taken from the same (female) child over the course of her first year of life.

Age	Weight	Length
2 months	9 lb, 10 oz	21 ¾ inches
4 months	12 lb, 5 oz	24 ½ inches
6 months	16 lb, 2 oz	26 ¼ inches
9 months	20 lb, 8 oz	28 inches
12 months	22 lb, 6 oz	29 ½ inches

CHART	
Date	

Procedure 24-2: Head and Chest Circumference. Measure the head and chest circumference of an infant using a pediatric training mannequin. Record the results in the chart provided.

CHART	
Date	

Procedure 24-4: Pediatric Urine Collector. Practice the procedure for applying a pediatric urine collector, using a pediatric training mannequin. Record the procedure in the chart provided.

CHART	
Date	

EVALUATION OF COMPETENCY

Procedure 24-A: Carrying an Infant

Name: _____   Date: _____

Evaluated By: _____   Score: _____

Performance Objective

Outcome:	Carry an infant in the following positions: cradle and upright.
Conditions:	Given a pediatric training mannequin.
Standards:	Time: 5 minutes. Student completed procedure in _____ minutes.
	Accuracy: Satisfactory score on the Performance Evaluation Checklist.

Performance Evaluation Checklist

Trial 1	Trial 2	Point Value	Performance Standards
			Cradle Position
		●	Slid the left hand and arm under infant's back.
		●	Grasped infant's upper arm from behind.
		●	Encircled infant's upper arm with the thumb and fingers.
		●	Supported infant's head, shoulders, and back on your arm.
		●	Slipped the right arm up and under the infant's buttocks.
		●	Cradled infant in your arms with the infant's body resting against your chest.
			Upright Position
		●	Slipped the right hand under infant's head and shoulders.
		●	Spread the fingers apart to support infant's head and neck.
		●	Slipped the left forearm under infant's buttocks.
		●	Allowed infant to rest against your chest.
		∗	Completed the procedure within 5 minutes.
			TOTALS
CHART			
Date			

Evaluation of Student Performance

EVALUATION CRITERIA			COMMENTS
Symbol	**Category**	**Point Value**	
*	Critical Step	16 points	
●	Essential Step	6 points	
▷	Theory Question	2 points	

Score calculation: 100 points

−_____ points missed

_____ Score

Satisfactory score: 85 or above

CAAHEP Competencies Achieved:

Psychomotor (Skills)
☑ IV. 6. Prepare a patient for procedures and/or treatments.

Affective (Behavior)
☑ IV. 1. Demonstrate empathy in communicating with patients, family, and staff.

ABHES Competencies Achieved:

☑ 9. 1. Prepare patient for examinations and treatments.

EVALUATION OF COMPETENCY

Procedure 24-1: Measuring the Weight and Length of an Infant

Name: _____   Date: _____

Evaluated By: _____   Score: _____

Performance Objective

Outcome:	Measure the weight and length of an infant.
Conditions:	Using a pediatric training mannequin and a pediatric balance scale (table model).
	Given a paper protector.
Standards:	Time: 5 minutes. Student completed procedure in _____ minutes.
	Accuracy: Satisfactory score on the Performance Evaluation Checklist.

Performance Evaluation Checklist

Trial 1	Trial 2	Point Value	Performance Standards
			Weight
		•	Sanitized hands.
		•	Greeted the child's parent and introduced yourself.
		•	Identified the infant.
		•	Explained the procedure to the child's parent.
		•	Based on the medical office policy, asked parent to: a. Remove infant's clothing and put on a dry diaper, or b. Remove infant's clothing including the diaper.
		▷	Stated why the infant should not be weighed with a wet diaper.
		•	Unlocked pediatric scale and placed a clean paper protector on it.
		▷	Stated the purpose of the paper protector.
		•	Checked the balance scale for accuracy.
		▷	Stated the purpose for balancing the scale.
		•	Gently placed infant on his or her back on the scale.
		•	Placed one hand slightly above infant.
		•	Balanced scale.
		•	Read results while infant was lying still.
		•	Jotted down value or made a mental note of it.
		✲	The reading was identical to the evaluator's reading.
		•	Returned balance to its resting position and locked the scale.
			Length
		•	Placed the vertex of infant's head against the headboard at the zero mark.

Trial 1	Trial 2	Point Value	Performance Standards
		•	Asked parent to hold infant's head in position.
		•	Straightened infant's knees and placed soles of infant's feet firmly against the upright foot board.
		•	Read infant's length in inches from the measure.
		•	Jotted down value or made a mental note of it.
		✳	The reading was identical to the evaluator's reading.
		•	Removed infant from the scale and handed him or her to the parent.
		•	Returned foot board to its resting position.
		•	Sanitized hands.
		•	Charted the results correctly.
		✳	Completed the procedure within 5 minutes.
			TOTALS

CHART

Date	

Evaluation of Student Performance

EVALUATION CRITERIA			COMMENTS
Symbol	Category	Point Value	
✳	Critical Step	16 points	
•	Essential Step	6 points	
▷	Theory Question	2 points	

Score calculation: 100 points

− _____ points missed

_____ Score

Satisfactory score: 85 or above

CAAHEP Competencies Achieved:

Psychomotor (Skills)
☑ IV. 6. Prepare a patient for procedures and/or treatments.

Affective (Behavior)
☑ I. 2. Use language/verbal skills that enable patients' understanding.
☑ IV. 7. Demonstrate recognition of the patient's level of understanding in communications.

ABHES Competencies Achieved:

☑ 5. f. Identify and discuss developmental stages of life.
☑ 8. cc.Communicate on the recipient's level of comprehension.
☑ 9. l. Prepare patient for examinations and treatments.

✔ EVALUATION OF COMPETENCY

📀 Procedure 24-2: Measuring Head and Chest Circumference of an Infant

Name: _____ Date: _____

Evaluated By: _____ Score: _____

Performance Objective

Outcome:	Measure the head and chest circumference of an infant.
Conditions:	Given a flexible nonstretch tape measure (in centimeters).
Standards:	Time: 5 minutes. Student completed procedure in ____ minutes.
	Accuracy: Satisfactory score on the Performance Evaluation Checklist.

Performance Evaluation Checklist

Trial 1	Trial 2	Point Value	Performance Standards
			Measurement of Head Circumference
		•	Sanitized hands.
		•	Assembled equipment.
		•	Positioned the infant.
		▷	Stated what positions can be used to measure head circumference.
		•	Positioned the measuring device around the infant's head.
		•	The tape measure was placed slightly above the eyebrows and pinnae of the ears and around the occipital prominence at the back of the skull.
		•	Read the results in centimeters (or inches).
		•	Jotted down value or made a mental note of it.
		✳	The reading was identical to the evaluator's reading.
		•	Sanitized hands.
		•	Charted the results correctly.
			Measurement of Chest Circumference
		•	Positioned the infant on his or her back on the examining table.
		•	Encircled the tape around the infant's chest at the nipple line.
		•	Ensured that the tape was snug but not too tight.
		•	Read the results in centimeters (or inches).
		•	Jotted down this value or made a mental note of it.
		✳	The reading was identical to the evaluator's reading.
		•	Charted the results correctly.
		✳	Completed the procedure within 5 minutes.
			TOTALS

CHART	
Date	

Evaluation of Student Performance

EVALUATION CRITERIA			COMMENTS
Symbol	Category	Point Value	
＊	Critical Step	16 points	
●	Essential Step	6 points	
▷	Theory Question	2 points	

Score calculation: 100 points

−_____ points missed

_____ Score

Satisfactory score: 85 or above

CAAHEP Competencies Achieved:

Psychomotor (Skills)

☑ IV. 6. Prepare a patient for procedures and/or treatments.

Affective (Behavior)

☑ I. 1. Apply critical thinking skills in performing patient assessment and care.

ABHES Competencies Achieved:

☑ 9. 1. Prepare patient for examinations and treatments.

EVALUATION OF COMPETENCY

Procedure 24-3: Calculating Growth Percentiles

Name: _____   Date: _____

Evaluated By: _____   Score: _____

Performance Objective

Outcome:	Plot a pediatric growth value on a growth chart.
Conditions:	Given a pediatric growth chart.
Standards:	Time: 5 minutes. Student completed procedure in _____ minutes.
	Accuracy: Satisfactory score on the Performance Evaluation Checklist.

Performance Evaluation Checklist

Trial 1	Trial 2	Point Value	Performance Standards
		•	Selected the proper growth chart.
		•	Located the child's age in the horizontal column at the bottom of the chart.
		•	Located the growth value in the vertical column under the appropriate category.
		•	Drew an imaginary vertical line from the child's age mark and an imaginary horizontal line from the growth mark.
		•	Found the site at which the two lines intersected on the graph.
		•	Placed a dot on this site.
		•	Determined the percentile by following the curved percentile line upward.
		•	Read the value located on the right side of the chart.
		•	Estimated the results if the value did not fall exactly on a percentile line.
		•	Charted the results correctly.
		✳	The value was within ±2 percentage points of the evaluator's determination.
		✳	Completed the procedure within 5 minutes.
		TOTALS	

CHART	
Date	

Evaluation of Student Performance

EVALUATION CRITERIA			COMMEN
Symbol	**Category**	**Point Value**	
✶	Critical Step	16 points	
●	Essential Step	6 points	
▷	Theory Question	2 points	

Score calculation: 100 points

− _____ points missed

_____   Score

Satisfactory score: 85 or above

CAAHEP Competencies Achieved:

Psychomotor (Skills)
☑ II. 3. Maintain growth charts.

Affective (Behavior)
☑ II. 2. Distinguish between normal and abno‾   ‾ults.

ABHES Competencies Achieved:

☑ 8. hh. Receive, organize, prioriti‾   ‾ansmit information expediently.
☑ 5. f. Identify and discuss devel‾   ‾stages of life.

EVALUATION OF COMPETENCY

DVD **Procedure 24-4: Applying a Pediatric Urine Collector**

Name: _____   Date: _____

Evaluated By: _____   Score: _____

Performance Objective

Outcome:	Apply a pediatric urine collector.
Conditions:	Using a pediatric training mannequin.
	Given the following: disposable gloves, personal antiseptic wipes, pediatric urine collector bag, urine specimen container and label, and a waste container.
Standards:	Time: 10 minutes. Student completed procedure in _____ minutes.
	Accuracy: Satisfactory score on the Performance Evaluation Checklist.

Performance Evaluation Checklist

Trial 1	Trial 2	Point Value	Performance Standards
		●	Sanitized hands.
		●	Assembled equipment.
		●	Greeted the child's parent and introduced yourself.
		●	Identified the child and explained the procedure to the parent.
		●	Applied gloves.
		●	Positioned child on his or her back with legs spread apart.
			Cleansed the area and applied the bag:
			Females
		●	Cleansed each side of the meatus with a separate wipe using a front-to-back motion.
		●	Cleansed directly down the middle with a third wipe.
		●	Discarded each wipe after cleansing.
		▷	Stated the reason for cleansing the urinary meatus.
		●	Allowed the area to dry completely.
		▷	Explained why the area should be allowed to dry.
		●	Removed paper backing from urine collector bag.
		●	Placed the bottom of the adhesive ring on the perineum and worked upward.
		●	Firmly pressed the adhesive surface of the sponge ring firmly to the skin surrounding the external genitalia.
		●	Made sure there was no puckering.
		●	The opening of the bag was placed directly over the urinary meatus.
		●	The excess length of the bag was positioned toward the feet.

Trial 1	Trial 2	Point Value	Performance Standards
			Males
		•	Retracted the foreskin of the penis if the child is not circumcised.
		•	Cleansed each side of the urethral orifice with a separate wipe.
		•	Cleansed directly over the urethral orifice.
		•	Cleansed the scrotum.
		•	Discarded each wipe after cleansing.
		•	Allowed the area to dry completely.
		•	Removed the paper backing from urine collector bag.
		•	Positioned the bag so that child's penis and scrotum are projected through the opening of the bag.
		•	Firmly pressed the adhesive surface to the skin.
		•	The excess length of the bag was positioned toward the feet.
			Completed the procedure:
		•	Loosely diapered child.
		•	Checked bag every 15 minutes until urine specimen was obtained.
		•	Gently removed collector bag from top to bottom.
		•	Cleansed genital area with a personal antiseptic wipe and rediapered child.
		•	Transferred urine specimen into specimen container and tightly applied the lid.
		•	Applied label to container.
		•	Disposed of collector bag in a regular waste container.
		•	Tested the specimen or prepared it for transfer to an outside laboratory.
		▷	Explained why the urine specimen should not be allowed to stand at room temperature.
		•	Removed gloves and sanitized hands.
		•	Charted the procedure correctly.
		✳	Completed the procedure within 10 minutes.
			TOTALS
			CHART
Date			

Evaluation of Student Performance

EVALUATION CRITERIA			COMMENTS
Symbol	Category	Point Value	
∗	Critical Step	16 points	
●	Essential Step	6 points	
▷	Theory Question	2 points	
Score calculation: 100 points			
− _____ points missed			
_____ Score			
Satisfactory score: 85 or above			

CAAHEP Competencies Achieved:

Psychomotor (Skills)
☑ IV. 6. Prepare a patient for procedures and/or treatments.

Affective (Behavior)
☑ III. 2. Explain the rationale for performance of a procedure to the patient.

ABHES Competencies Achieved:

☑ 10. d. Collect, label, and process specimens.

Notes

25

Minor Office Surgery

CHAPTER ASSIGNMENTS

√ After Completing	Date Due	Textbook Page(s)	TEXTBOOK ASSIGNMENTS	Possible Points	Points You Earned
		524-570	Read Chapter 25: Minor Office Surgery		
		545 568	📖 Read Case Study 1 Case Study 1 questions	5	
		555 568-569	📖 Read Case Study 2 Case Study 2 questions	5	
		563 569	📖 Read Case Study 3 Case Study 3 questions	5	
			TOTAL POINTS		
√ After Completing	Date Due	Study Guide Page(s)	STUDY GUIDE ASSIGNMENTS (CTA: Critical Thinking Activity)	Possible Points	Points You Earned
		531	📝 Pretest	10	
		532	⚷Term Key Term Assessment	25	
		533-536	📋 Evaluation of Learning questions	40	
		536-537	CTA A: Medical and Surgical Asepsis	10	
		537-538	CTA B: Violation of Surgical Asepsis	10	
		539-540	CTA C: Surgical Instruments (2 points each)	22	
			💿 CD Activity: Chapter 25 It's Instrumental (Record points earned)		
			💿 CD Activity: Chapter 25 Keep It Sterile (Record points earned)		
		541	CTA D: Pioneers in Surgical Asepsis (5 points each)	15	

√ After Completing	Date Due	Study Guide Page(s)	STUDY GUIDE ASSIGNMENTS (CTA: Critical Thinking Activity)	Possible Points	Points You Earned
		542	CTA E: Crossword Puzzle	24	
		543	CTA F: Patient Instruction Sheet	20	
		547-548	CTA G: Road to Recovery Game: Surgical Asepsis (Record points earned)		
			CD Activity: Chapter 25 Apply Your Knowledge questions (Record points earned)		
		531	Posttest	10	
			ADDITIONAL ASSIGNMENTS		
			TOTAL POINTS		

√ When Assigned by Your Instructor	Study Guide Page(s)	Practices Required	LABORATORY ASSIGNMENTS (Procedure Number and Name)	*Score
	551	5	(DVD) **Practice for Competency** 25-1: Applying and Removing Sterile Gloves Textbook reference: pp. 532-534	
	553-554		**Evaluation of Competency** 25-1: Applying and Removing Sterile Gloves	*
	551	5	(DVD) **Practice for Competency** 25-2: Opening a Sterile Package Textbook reference: pp. 535-536	
	555-556		**Evaluation of Competency** 25-2: Opening a Sterile Package	*
	551	5	(DVD) **Practice for Competency** Using Commercially Prepared Sterile Packages Textbook reference: pp. 529-532	
	557-558		**Evaluation of Competency** Using Commercially Prepared Sterile Packages	*
	551	3	(DVD) **Practice for Competency** 25-3: Pouring a Sterile Solution Textbook reference: p. 536	
	559-560		**Evaluation of Competency** 25-3: Pouring a Sterile Solution	*
	551	5	(DVD) **Practice for Competency** 25-4: Changing a Sterile Dressing Textbook reference: pp. 539-541	
	561-563		**Evaluation of Competency** 25-4: Changing a Sterile Dressing	*
	551	Sutures: 3 Staples: 3	(DVD) **Practice for Competency** 25-5: Removing Sutures and Staples Textbook reference: pp. 545-547	
	565-567		**Evaluation of Competency** 25-5: Removing Sutures and Staples	*
	551	3	(DVD) **Practice for Competency** 25-6: Applying and Removing Adhesive Skin Closures Textbook reference: pp. 548-552	
	569-571		**Evaluation of Competency** 25-6: Applying and Removing Adhesive Skin Closures	*

√ When Assigned by Your Instructor	Study Guide Page(s)	Practices Required	LABORATORY ASSIGNMENTS (Procedure Number and Name)	*Score
	551	5	(DVD) **Practice for Competency** 25-7: Assisting with Minor Office Surgery Textbook reference: pp. 556-560	
	573-576		**Evaluation of Competency** 25-7: Assisting with Minor Office Surgery	*
	551	Each bandage turn: 3	(DVD) **Practice for Competency** 25-A: Applying Bandages Textbook reference: pp. 565-568	
	577-578		**Evaluation of Competency** 25-A: Applying Bandages	*
			ADDITIONAL ASSIGNMENTS	

Name _____   Date _____

? PRETEST

True or False

_____ 1. *Surgical asepsis* refers to practices that keep objects and areas free from all microorganisms.

_____ 2. Something that is sterile is contaminated if it comes in contact with a pathogen.

_____ 3. Reaching over a sterile field is a violation of sterile technique.

_____ 4. An incision is a jagged tearing of the tissues.

_____ 5. The skin is the first line of defense of the body.

_____ 6. One of the local signs of inflammation is fever.

_____ 7. Sutures approximate the edges of a wound until proper healing occurs.

_____ 8. A biopsy is usually performed to determine if an infection is present.

_____ 9. An ingrown toenail can be caused by shoes that are too tight.

_____ 10. One of the functions of a bandage is to hold a dressing in place.

? POSTTEST

True or False

_____ 1. Measuring a patient's temperature requires the use of surgical asepsis.

_____ 2. Hemostatic forceps are used to clamp off blood vessels.

_____ 3. An instrument with a ratchet should be kept in a closed position when not in use.

_____ 4. The physician would be most likely to order a tetanus booster for an abrasion.

_____ 5. Inflammation is the protective response of the body to trauma and the entrance of foreign substances.

_____ 6. A serous exudate is red in color.

_____ 7. Size 4-0 sutures have a smaller diameter than size 3 sutures.

_____ 8. Sebaceous cysts are commonly found on the palms of the hand.

_____ 9. Colposcopy is frequently used to evaluate lesions of the cervix.

_____ 10. Cryosurgery is used in the treatment of cervical cancer.

Term KEY TERM ASSESSMENT

Directions: Match each medical term with its definition.

M   1. Abrasion

E   2. Abscess

T   3. Absorbable suture

U   4. Approximation

V   5. Bandage

L   6. Biopsy

N   7. Capillary action

I   8. Colposcope

S   9. Colposcopy

B   10. Contaminate

K   11. Contusion

R   12. Cryosurgery

Y   13. Fibroblast

O   14. Forceps

J   15. Furuncle

F   16. Hemostasis

W   17. Incision

D   18. Infection

A   19. Inflammation

H   20. Laceration

X   21. Nonabsorbable suture

C   22. Puncture

G   23. Sterile

P   24. Surgical asepsis

Q   25. Wound

A. A protective response of the body to trauma and the entrance of foreign matter

B. To cause a sterile object or surface to become unsterile

C. A wound made by a sharp, pointed object piercing the skin

D. The condition in which the body is invaded by a pathogen

E. A collection of pus in a cavity surrounded by inflamed tissue

F. The arrest of bleeding by natural or artificial means

G. Free of all living microorganisms and bacterial spores

H. A wound in which the tissues are torn apart, leaving ragged and irregular edges

I. A lighted instrument with a binocular magnifying lens used to examine the vagina and cervix

J. A localized staphylococcal infection that originates deep within a hair follicle; also known as a boil

K. An injury to the tissues under the skin that causes blood vessels to rupture, allowing blood to seep into the tissues

L. The surgical removal and examination of tissue from the living body

M. A wound in which the outer layers of the skin are damaged

N. The action that causes liquid to rise along a wick, a tube, or a gauze dressing

O. A two-pronged instrument for grasping and squeezing

P. Practices that keep objects and areas sterile or free from microorganisms

Q. A break in the continuity of an external or internal surface caused by physical means

R. The therapeutic use of freezing temperatures to destroy abnormal tissue

S. The visual examination of the vagina and cervix using a lighted instrument with a magnifying lens

T. Suture material that is gradually digested by tissue enzymes and absorbed by the body

U. The process of bringing two parts, such as tissue, together, through the use of sutures or other means

V. A strip of woven material used to wrap or cover a part of the body

W. A clean cut caused by a cutting instrument

X. Suture material that is not absorbed by the body

Y. An immature cell from which connective tissue can develop

EVALUATION OF LEARNING

Directions: Fill in each blank with the correct answer.

1. List the responsibilities of the MA during a minor surgical operation.

   Set up the room for procedure, Assit patient, prepare patient, Assit physican

2. What is the function of a speculum?

   to assist in viewing in a canal

3. List five guidelines that should be followed in caring for instruments.

   Nandle carefully, Do not pile, Keep Sharp instruments seperate, Keep in open position, Rinse right away use proper technique when cleaning

4. What is the difference between a closed wound and an open wound?

   Closed wound is below Skin surface, Open wound - Skin is not intact

5. Why does a puncture wound encourage the growth of tetanus bacteria?

   Introduction of bacteria into wound directly

6. What is the purpose of inflammation?

   protective to inhibit foreign matter

7. List the four local signs that occur during inflammation.

   blood increase, redness, swelling, pain, warmth

8. What occurs during the inflammatory phase of wound healing?

   Increase blood supply bringing WBC & nutrients to site to assit in healing

9. What occurs during the granulation phase of wound healing?

   fibroblasts produce collagen

10. What occurs during the maturation phase of wound healing?

    Scar formation

11. What is an exudate?

    Drainage

12. Define the following types of exudates.
    a. Serous: _Clear_
    b. Sanguineous: _red with RBC_
    c. Purulent: _Pus_

13. List two functions of a sterile dressing.
    Protect wound and speed healing

14. Following are listed the names and sizes of sutures. For each, circle the suture that has the smaller diameter.
    a. (4-0 surgical silk)
       00 surgical silk
    b. 0 chromic gut
       (3-0 chromic gut)
    c. (2-0 polypropylene)
       2 polypropylene

15. List five examples of materials used for nonabsorbable sutures.
    Silk, cotton, nylon, polyester, prolene,
    Stainless Steel, Surgical Steel Staples

16. What is a swaged needle? List advantages of using a swaged needle.
    Suture and needle are one unit -
    does not slip

17. Why are sutures inserted in the head and neck generally removed sooner than other sutures?
    more blood Supply to area -
    faster healing

18. List two advantages of using surgical skin staples to approximate a wound.
    faster closure - less trama to tissue
    Easier for closing large wounds

19. List three advantages of adhesive skin closures.
    Eliminate need for sutures and
    local anesthetic. Easy to apply
    and remove

20. What is the purpose of preparing the patient's skin before minor office surgery?
    Cleanse bacteria -

21. What is the purpose of a fenestrated drape?
    Keep area isolated and as
    Sterile as possible

22. List the names of two local anesthetics commonly used in the medical office during minor office surgery.

Xylocaine and Novocaine

23. Explain how an instrument should be handed to the physician during minor office surgery.

Handle first

24. What is a sebaceous cyst, and what causes it to form?

Closed sac that contains secretions from oil gland. forms due to obstruction.

25. What is the purpose of using a rubber Penrose drain after incising a localized infection?

Keep the edges of tissue apart - facilitates drainage of exudate

26. What is the purpose of a needle biopsy?

removal and examination of tissue from body for examination

27. What is an ingrown toenail?

the edge of the toenail grows deeply into nail groove

28. List three causes of an ingrown toenail.

tight shoes, trama, improper clipping

29. List three indications for performing a colposcopy.

abnormal pap, look for cervical lesion, or after treatment for cervical cancer

30. What is the purpose of performing a cervical punch biopsy?

remove cervical tissue for examination

31. List the postoperative instructions that must be relayed to a patient after a cervical punch biopsy.

minimal amount of bleeding, discarge is expected, come back in 1 week for check up

32. List two uses of cryosurgery.

Chronic cervicitis and cervical erosion

33. List the postoperative instructions that must be relayed to a patient after cervical cryosurgery.

Discharge, nothing in vaginal for 4 weeks, return 6 weeks after for check up

34. List three functions of a bandage.

Control bleeding, protect wound, hold dressing in place, immobolize injured part of body.

35. List four guidelines to follow when applying a bandage.

medical asepsis

not too tight

Bandage body part in normal body position

36. List four signs that may indicate a bandage is too tight.

Coldness, pallor, numbness, cyanosis of nailbed

37. Why should the MA be careful when applying an elastic bandage?

it is easy to apply too tightly

38. What is the purpose of reversing the spiral during a spiral-reverse turn?

Smoother fit and prevents gaping

39. List two uses of the figure-eight bandage turn.

hold dressing in place

Support and immobilize

40. What type of bandage turn is used to anchor a bandage?

recurrent turn

CRITICAL THINKING ACTIVITIES

A. MEDICAL AND SURGICAL ASEPSIS

Refer to Chapter 17 and describe the difference between medical asepsis and surgical asepsis.

practices that are employed to reduce pathogens / reduce pathogens during a surgical procedure

Which technique (medical asepsis or surgical asepsis) would be employed during the following procedures? In the procedures requiring surgical asepsis, indicate which of the following reasons necessitate the use of surgical asepsis: caring for broken skin, the penetration of a skin surface, or entering a body cavity that is normally sterile.

1. Administering oral medication

   Medical asepsis

2. Inserting sutures

   Surgical asepsis

3. Measuring oral temperature

   medical asepsis

4. Applying a bandage to the forearm

   medical asepsis

5. Performing a needle biopsy

   Surgical asepsis

6. Removing a sebaceous cyst

   Surgical asepsis

7. Obtaining a Pap smear

   medical asepsis

8. Inserting a urinary catheter

   Surgical asepsis

9. Incision and drainage of an abscess

   Surgical asepsis

10. Applying a dressing to an open wound

    Surgical asepsis

B. VIOLATION OF SURGICAL ASEPSIS

In the following situations, the principles of surgical asepsis have been violated. Explain why the techniques should not be performed in this manner.

1. Not checking the sterilization indicator on a sterile package before opening it

   Could contaminate patient

2. Wearing rings during the application of sterile gloves

Could tear or put holes in gloves

3. Talking over a sterile field

Could contaminate field

4. Reaching over a sterile field

Contaminate field

5. Holding sterile gauze below waist level

Contaminate gauze

6. Not palming the label when pouring an antiseptic solution

Not clairifying solution

7. Spilling an antiseptic solution on the sterile field

Contaminat field

8. Passing a soiled dressing over the sterile field

Contaminate field

9. Placing a vial of Xylocaine on the sterile field

Contaminate field

10. Using bare hands to arrange articles on the sterile field

Contaminate field

C. SURGICAL INSTRUMENTS

State the name and use of each of the following types of surgical instruments. Identify any of the following parts present on each instrument by labeling the instrument: box lock, spring handle, ratchets, serrations, cutting edge, and teeth.

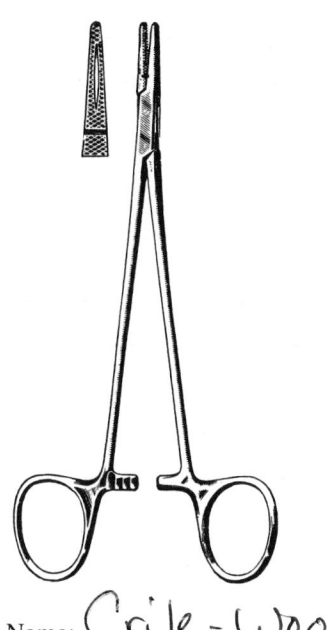

1. Name: Crile-Wood needle holde
   Use: insert sutures

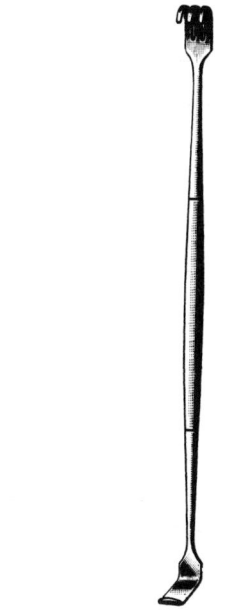

2. Name: retractor
   Use: Hold tissues back

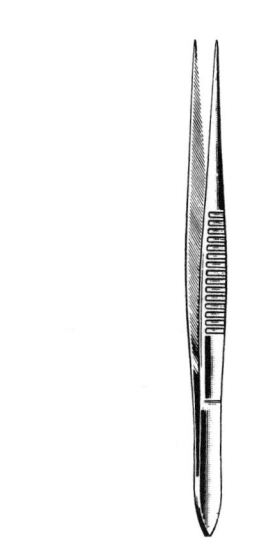

3. Name: Splinter forceps
   Use: Suture remover

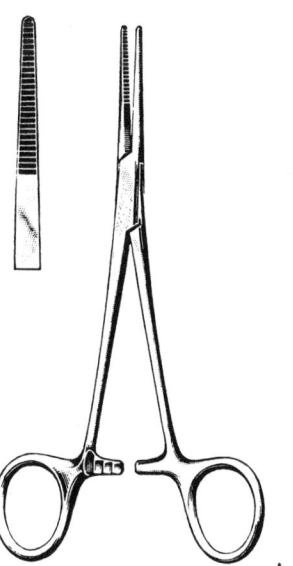

4. Name: Hemostatic forceps
   Use: retrieving tissues

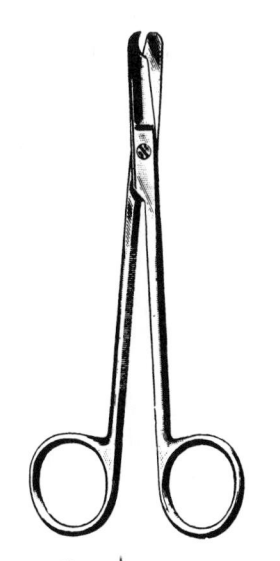

5. Name: Suture siccors
   Use: Clip sutures

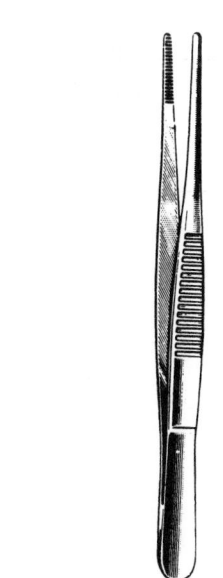

6. Name: thumb foreceps
   Use:

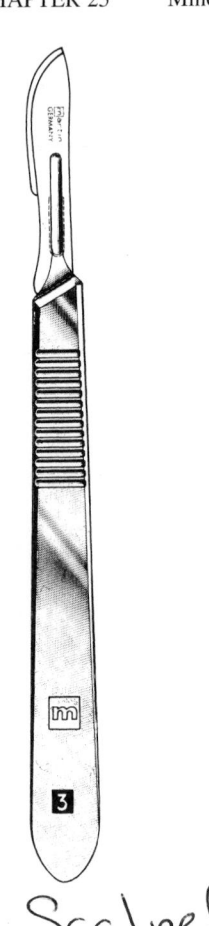

7. Name: <u>Scalpel</u>
   Use: <u>incision</u>

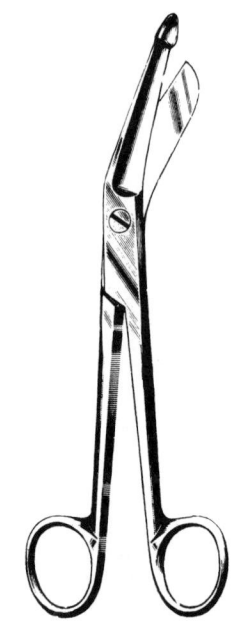

8. Name: <u>Bandage Siccors</u>
   Use: <u>remove bandage</u>

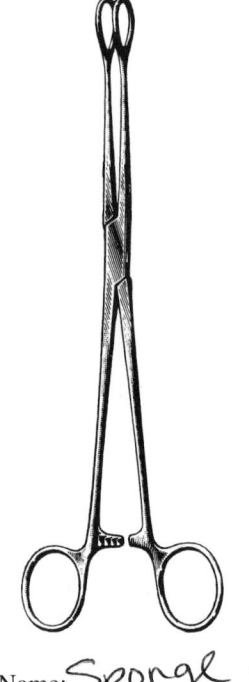

9. Name: <u>Sponge forceps</u>
   Use: <u>Uterine</u>

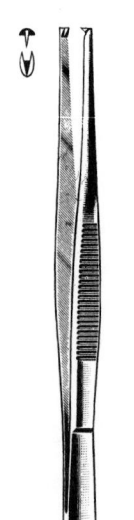

10. Name: <u>Tissue</u>
    Use: <u>grasping</u>

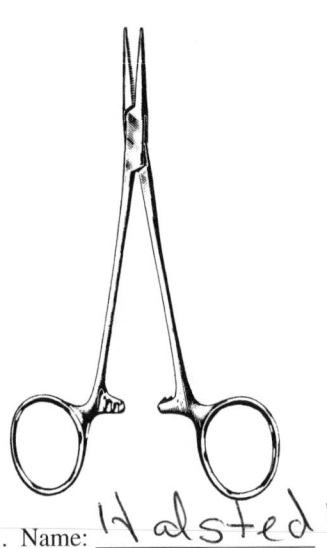

11. Name: <u>Halsted Mosquito forceps</u>
    Use: <u>Clamp</u>

D. PIONEERS IN SURGICAL ASEPSIS
Using a reference source, describe the contributions the following men made to medicine, especially regarding surgical asepsis.

1. Ignaz Semmelweis

    _____

    _____

    _____

2. Louis Pasteur

    _____

    _____

    _____

3. Joseph Lister

    _____

    _____

    _____

E. CROSSWORD PUZZLE
Minor Office Surgery
Directions: Complete the crossword puzzle using the clues presented below.

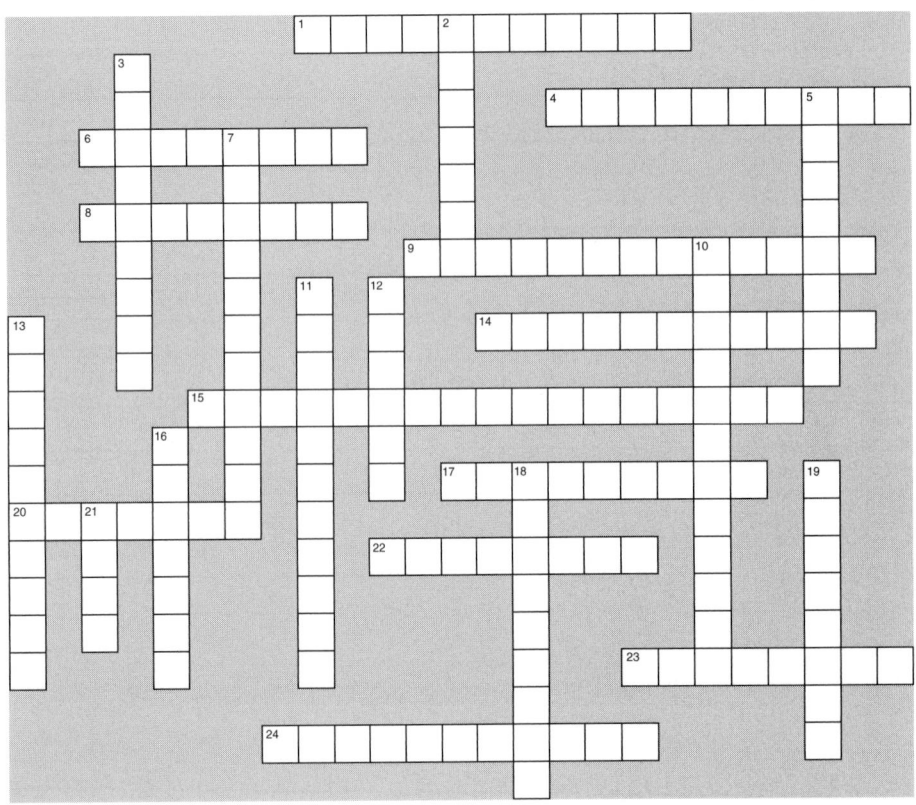

(From Bonewit-West K: *Study guide for clinical procedures for medical assistants,* ed 7, St. Louis, 2008, Saunders.)

ACROSS

1 Drape with a hole
4 Produces collagen
6 Clean, smooth cut
8 Boil
9 Sac containing oil secretions
14 Pus formation
15 Clamps off blood vessels
17 Local anesthetic brand name
20 Pus in a cavity
22 Tetanus may grow here
23 Local sign of inflammation
24 Bring together

DOWN

2 Free of all microorganisms and spores
3 Bruise
5 Scrape
7 Exudate containing blood
10 Suture/needle combination
11 Treatment for chronic cervicitis
12 Father of modern surgery
13 Ragged and irregular wound
16 Discovered penicillin
18 Position for colposcopy
19 Antiseptic brand name
21 Nonabsorbable suture material

F. PATIENT INSTRUCTION SHEET

1. You are working for a surgeon, and she would like you to develop a patient instruction sheet for a minor surgery. Select one of the minor surgeries listed. Using the instruction sheet, develop a sheet that would be informative and visually appealing to a patient. Be as creative as possible in designing your sheet.

2. Select a partner. Have your partner play the role of a patient who is going to have the minor surgery performed, and explain the information in the sheet. Ask the patient to sign the sheet, and witness the patient's signature.

   Minor Office Surgeries:

   a. Sebaceous cyst removal

   b. Needle biopsy

   c. Ingrown toenail removal

   d. Colposcopy and biopsy

   e. Cervical cryosurgery

Notes

PATIENT INSTRUCTION SHEET

NAME OF THE PROCEDURE:

DESCRIPTION OF PROCEDURE:

PURPOSE OF THE PROCEDURE:

HOW TO PREPARE FOR THE PROCEDURE:

WHAT TO DO FOLLOWING THE PROCEDURE:

I have received and understand the above instructions:

Patient's Signature _____

Witness: _____ Date: _____

(From Bonewit-West K: *Study guide for clinical procedures for medical assistants,* ed 7, St. Louis, 2008, Saunders.)

G. ROAD TO RECOVERY GAME: SURGICAL ASEPSIS

Object   To lead your "patient" to recovery by correctly determining if an action violates sterile technique or does
                    not violate sterile technique

Needed   **Road to Recovery** game board (located at the end of this manual)
                    Game cards
                    A token for each player (such as a button or coin)
                    Dice (1)
                    Playing cards
                    Score card

Directions

1. Get into a group of four students. Make a list of 16 actions that violate *(V)* surgical asepsis and 16 actions that do
   not violate *(NV)* surgical asepsis. You can use the information in Critical Thinking Activity B for some of your
   actions that violate surgical asepsis. Each student should take four *V* actions and four *NV* actions and write them on
   his or her game cards, making sure to use the appropriate *V* or *NV* card.
2. Cut out the game cards, and trade your group's set of game cards with another group.
3. Place one complete set of cards on the game board with the action facing up (and the *V* or *NV* designation
   facing down).
4. Play **Road to Recovery** following the directions on the reverse side of the game board. A player should pick up a
   card and read the action and respond by indicating whether the action *violates* sterile technique or does *not violate*
   sterile technique. Turn your card over to determine if you answered correctly. If you did, award yourself 5 points. If
   you answered incorrectly, you receive 0 points. If time permits, trade your set of cards with another group and
   continue playing. If a question arises as to the correct answer, consult your instructor for assistance.
5. Keep track of your points using the score card provided.

ROAD TO RECOVERY
SCORE CARD

Name: _____

Recording Points:

Using the Game Card Points box, cross off a number each time you answer a game card correctly (starting with 5 and continuing in sequence). Your total game card points will be equal to the last number you crossed off. Record this number in the space provided (1). Record any extra points you were awarded during the game (2), and any points that were deducted (3). To determine your total points, add (1) and (2) together and deduct (3). Record this number in the Total Points Earned space provided. Compare your score with the other players and determine where you placed. Place a check mark next to the level of recovery your patient attained.

Game Card Points:			
5	75	145	215
10	80	150	220
15	85	155	225
20	90	160	230
25	95	165	235
30	100	170	240
35	105	175	245
40	110	180	250
45	115	185	255
50	120	190	260
55	125	195	265
60	130	200	270
65	135	205	275
70	140	210	280

Calculation of Points:

(1) Total Game Card Points: _____

(2) Additional Points Awarded: _____

(3) Deducted Points: _____

TOTAL POINTS EARNED: _____

LEVEL OF RECOVERY:

Patient's Name: _____

☐ First Place: **Fully Recovered**
☐ Second Place: **Almost Recovered**
☐ Third Place: **Still Recovering**
☐ Fourth Place: **Gasping for Air**

Action:

Action:

Action:

Action:

Action:

Action:

Action:

Action:

V

V

V

V

NV

NV

NV

NV

PRACTICE FOR COMPETENCY

Sterile Technique

Procedure 25-1: Applying and Removing Sterile Gloves. Apply and remove sterile gloves.

Procedure 25-2: Sterile Package. Open a sterile package.

Commercially Prepared Sterile Packages. Add a sterile article to a sterile field using a peel-apart package. Practice each of the methods used to transfer articles to a sterile field as shown in Figure 25-3 of your textbook.

Procedure 25-3: Sterile Solution. Pour a sterile solution into a container on a sterile field.

Minor Surgical Procedures

Procedure 25-4: Sterile Dressing. Change a sterile dressing and record the procedure in the chart provided.

Procedure 25-5: Suture and Staple Removal. Practice the procedure for removing sutures and staples and record the procedure in the chart provided.

Procedure 25-6: Adhesive Skin Closures. Practice the procedure for applying and removing adhesive skin closures and record the procedure in the chart provided.

Procedure 25-7: Assisting with Minor Office Surgery. Obtain eight index cards. For each of the following minor office surgeries, indicate (on one side of the card) the equipment and supplies required for the side table. On the other side of the card, indicate the equipment and supplies required for the sterile tray setup. Set up a surgical tray for the procedures listed below using your index cards. In the chart provided, record the instructions relayed to the patient following the surgery.

a. Suture insertion

b. Sebaceous cyst removal

c. Incision and drainage of a localized infection

d. Needle biopsy

e. Ingrown toenail removal

f. Colposcopy

g. Cervical punch biopsy

h. Cervical cryosurgery

Procedure 25-A: Applying Bandages. Practice the following bandage turns:

a. Circular turn

b. Spiral turn

c. Spiral-reverse turn

d. Figure-eight turn

e. Recurrent turn

CHART	
Date	

CHART	
Date	

☑ EVALUATION OF COMPETENCY

📀 Procedure 25-1: Applying and Removing Sterile Gloves

Name: _____   Date: _____

Evaluated By: _____   Score: _____

Performance Objective

Outcome:	Apply and remove sterile gloves.
Conditions:	Given the appropriate sized sterile gloves.
	Using a clean, flat surface.
Standards:	Time: 5 minutes. Student completed procedure in _____ minutes.
	Accuracy: Satisfactory score on the Performance Evaluation Checklist.

Performance Evaluation Checklist

Trial 1	Trial 2	Point Value	Performance Standards
			Application of Gloves
		•	Removed rings and washed hands with an antimicrobial soap.
		▷	Explained why the hands should be washed.
		•	Selected appropriately sized gloves.
		▷	Explained what might occur if the gloves are to small or too large.
		•	Placed the glove package on a clean, flat surface.
		•	Opened the sterile glove package without touching the inside of the wrapper.
		•	Picked up the first glove on the inside of the cuff without contaminating.
		▷	Explained why the inside of the cuff can be touched with the bare hand.
		•	Did not touch the outside of the glove with the bare hand.
		•	Stepped back and pulled on glove and allowed the cuff to remain turned back on itself.
		•	Picked up the second glove by slipping sterile gloved fingers under its cuff and grasping the opposite side with the thumb.
		▷	Stated how the above step prevents contamination.
		•	Pulled the glove on and turned back the cuff.
		•	Turned back the cuff of the first glove without contaminating.
		•	Adjusted the gloves to a comfortable position.
		•	Inspected the gloves for tears.
		▷	Explained what should be done if a glove is torn.

Trial 1	Trial 2	Point Value	*Performance Standards*
			Removal of Gloves
		•	Grasped the outside of the right glove 1 to 2 inches from the top with the gloved left hand.
		•	Slowly pulled right glove off the hand.
		•	Pulled the right glove free and scrunched it into a ball with the gloved left hand.
		•	Placed index and middle fingers of the right hand on the inside of left glove.
		•	Did not allow the clean hand to touch the outside of the glove.
		•	Pulled the glove off the left hand, enclosing the balled-up right glove.
		•	Discarded both gloves in an appropriate waste container.
		▷	Stated how to discard gloves if they are visibly contaminated with blood.
		•	Sanitized hands.
		✳	Completed the procedure within 5 minutes.
			TOTALS

Evaluation of Student Performance

EVALUATION CRITERIA			COMMENTS
Symbol	**Category**	**Point Value**	
✳	Critical Step	16 points	
•	Essential Step	6 points	
▷	Theory Question	2 points	

Score calculation: 100 points

−____ points missed

____ Score

Satisfactory score: 85 or above

CAAHEP Competencies Achieved:

Psychomotor (Skills)
☑ III. 3. Select appropriate barrier/personal protective equipment (PPE) for potentially infectious situations.

ABHES Competencies Achieved:

☑ 9. b. Apply principles of aseptic techniques and infection control.
☑ 9. i. Use standard precautions.

EVALUATION OF COMPETENCY

DVD **Procedure 25-2: Opening a Sterile Package**

Name: _____   Date: _____

Evaluated By: _____   Score: _____

Performance Objective

Outcome:	Open a sterile package.
Conditions:	Given a sterile package.
	Using a clean, flat surface.
Standards:	Time: 5 minutes. Student completed procedure in ____ minutes.
	Accuracy: Satisfactory score on the Performance Evaluation Checklist.

Performance Evaluation Checklist

Trial 1	Trial 2	Point Value	Performance Standards
		•	Sanitized hands.
		•	Assembled equipment.
		•	Checked pack to make sure it is not wet, torn, or opened.
		•	Checked the autoclave tape on the pack.
		▷	Stated the purpose of autoclave tape.
		•	Positioned the pack on the table so that the top flap of wrapper will open away from the body.
		•	Removed the fastener on wrapped package and discarded it.
		•	Opened the first flap away from the body.
		•	Opened the left and right flaps without contaminating contents.
		•	Opened the flap closest to the body.
		•	In all cases, only touched the outside of the wrapper.
		•	In all cases, did not reach over the sterile contents of the package.
		▷	Stated why the medical assistant should not reach over the contents of the package.
		•	Adjusted the sterile wrapper by the corners as needed.
		•	Checked the sterilization indicator on the inside of the pack.
		✶	Completed the procedure within 5 minutes.
			TOTALS

Evaluation of Student Performance

EVALUATION CRITERIA			COMMENTS
Symbol	Category	Point Value	
✱	Critical Step	16 points	
●	Essential Step	6 points	
▷	Theory Question	2 points	

Score calculation: 100 points

– _____ points missed

_____ Score

Satisfactory score: 85 or above

CAAHEP Competencies Achieved:

Psychomotor (Skills)

☑ I. 10. Assist physician with patient care.

ABHES Competencies Achieved:

☑ 9. n. Assist physician with minor office surgical procedures.

EVALUATION OF COMPETENCY

Using Commercially Prepared Sterile Packages

Name: _____   Date: _____

Evaluated By: _____   Score: _____

Performance Objective

Outcome:	Add a sterile article to a sterile field from a peel-apart package by ejecting its contents onto the field.
Conditions:	Given the following: peel-apart package and a sterile field.
Standards:	Time: 3 minutes. Student completed procedure in _____ minutes.
	Accuracy: Satisfactory score on the Performance Evaluation Checklist.

Performance Evaluation Checklist

Trial 1	Trial 2	Point Value	Performance Standards
		•	Sanitized hands.
		•	Grasped the two unsterile flaps of the peel-pack between thumbs.
		•	Pulled the package apart using a rolling-outward motion.
		▷	Stated what parts of the peel-pack must remain sterile.
		•	Stepped back slightly from the sterile field.
		▷	Explained the reason for stepping back.
		•	Gently ejected contents of the peel-pack onto the sterile field.
		✳	Completed the procedure within 3 minutes.
		TOTALS	

Evaluation of Student Performance

EVALUATION CRITERIA			COMMENTS
Symbol	Category	Point Value	
✳	Critical Step	16 points	
•	Essential Step	6 points	
▷	Theory Question	2 points	
Score calculation: 100 points			
− _____ points missed			
_____ Score			
Satisfactory score: 85 or above			

CAAHEP Competencies Achieved:

Psychomotor (Skills)
☑ I. 10. Assist physician with patient care.

ABHES Competencies Achieved:

☑ 9. n. Assist physician with minor office surgical procedures.

EVALUATION OF COMPETENCY

Procedure 25-3: Pouring a Sterile Solution

Name: _____   Date: _____

Evaluated By: _____   Score: _____

Performance Objective

Outcome:	Pour a sterile solution.
Conditions:	Given the following: sterile solution, sterile container, and a sterile towel.
Standards:	Time: 5 minutes Student completed procedure in _____ minutes.
	Accuracy: Satisfactory score on the Performance Evaluation Checklist.

Performance Evaluation Checklist

Trial 1	Trial 2	Point Value	Performance Standards
		•	Checked the label of the solution.
		•	Checked the expiration date on the solution.
		•	Checked the solution label a second time.
		•	Palmed the label of the bottle.
		▷	Explained why the label should be palmed.
		•	Removed cap and placed it on a flat surface with the open end up.
		▷	Stated why cap should be placed with the open end up.
		•	Rinsed the lip of the bottle.
		▷	Explained why the lip of the bottle should be rinsed.
		•	Poured the proper amount of solution into a sterile container.
		•	Did not allow the neck of the bottle to come in contact with container.
		•	Did not allow any of the solution to splash onto the sterile field.
		▷	Explained why the sterile solution should not be allowed to splash onto the sterile field.
		•	Replaced cap on container without contaminating.
		•	Checked the label a third time.
		*	Completed the procedure within 5 minutes.
			TOTALS

Evaluation of Student Performance

EVALUATION CRITERIA			COMMENTS
Symbol	Category	Point Value	
∗	Critical Step	16 points	
●	Essential Step	6 points	
▷	Theory Question	2 points	
Score calculation: 100 points			
− _____ points missed			
_____ Score			
Satisfactory score: 85 or above			

CAAHEP Competencies Achieved:

Psychomotor (Skills)
☑ I. 10. Assist physician with patient care.

ABHES Competencies Achieved:

☑ 9. n. Assist physician with minor office surgical procedures.

EVALUATION OF COMPETENCY

Procedure 25-4: Changing a Sterile Dressing

Name: _____   Date: _____

Evaluated By: _____   Score: _____

Performance Objective

Outcome:	Change a sterile dressing.
Conditions:	Given the following: clean disposable gloves, antiseptic swabs, sterile gloves, plastic waste bag, adhesive tape and scissors, biohazard waste container, sterile dressing, and thumb forceps.
Standards:	Time: 10 minutes. Student completed procedure in _____ minutes.
	Accuracy: Satisfactory score on the Performance Evaluation Checklist.

Performance Evaluation Checklist

Trial 1	Trial 2	Point Value	Performance Standards
		•	Washed hands with an antimicrobial soap.
		•	Assembled equipment.
		•	Set up unsterile items.
		•	Positioned the plastic waste bag in a convenient location.
		•	Greeted the patient and introduced yourself.
		•	Identified the patient and explained the procedure.
		•	Instructed patient not to move during procedure.
		•	Adjusted the light.
		•	Applied clean gloves.
		•	Loosened the tape and carefully removed soiled dressing.
		•	Did not touch inside of dressing next to the wound.
		▷	Explained why the inside of the dressing should not be touched.
		▷	Described what should be done if the dressing is stuck to the wound.
		•	Placed soiled dressing in the waste bag without touching outside of bag.
		•	Inspected the wound.
		▷	Stated what type of inspection should be performed.
		•	Opened the antiseptic swabs and placed the pouch in a convenient location or held them.
		•	Applied the antiseptic to the wound.
		•	Used a new swab for each motion.
		•	Discarded each contaminated swab in the waste bag after use.

Trial 1	Trial 2	Point Value	Performance Standards
		●	Removed gloves and discarded them without contaminating.
		●	Sanitized hands and prepared the sterile field.
		●	Opened sterile glove package and applied sterile gloves.
		●	Picked up sterile dressing from the tray using sterile gloves or sterile forceps.
		●	Placed sterile dressing over the wound by lightly dropping it in place.
		▷	Explained why the dressing should be dropped onto the wound.
		●	Did not move dressing after dropping it in place.
		▷	Stated why the dressing should not be moved.
		●	Discarded gloves (and forceps) in the waste bag.
		●	Applied hypoallergenic tape to hold sterile dressing in place.
		●	Instructed patient in wound care.
		▷	Described the wound care that should be relayed to the patient.
		●	Provided the patient with written instructions.
		●	Asked patient to sign instruction sheet.
		●	Witnessed the patient's signature.
		●	Gave a signed copy to the patient.
		●	Filed original in the patient's medical record.
		●	Returned equipment.
		●	Disposed of plastic bag in a biohazard waste container.
		●	Sanitized hands.
		●	Charted the procedure correctly.
		✳	Completed the procedure within 10 minutes.
			TOTALS

	CHART
Date	

Evaluation of Student Performance

EVALUATION CRITERIA			COMMENTS
Symbol	**Category**	**Point Value**	
＊	Critical Step	16 points	
●	Essential Step	6 points	
▷	Theory Question	2 points	

Score calculation: 100 points

−＿＿＿＿＿ points missed

＿＿＿＿ Score

Satisfactory score: 85 or above

CAAHEP Competencies Achieved:

Psychomotor (Skills)

☑ IV. 5. Instruct patients according to their needs to promote health maintenance and disease prevention.
☑ IV. 6. Prepare a patient for procedures and/or treatments.
☑ IV. 8. Document patient care.
☑ IV. 9. Document patient education.

Affective (Behavior)

☑ III. 2. Explain the rationale for performance of a procedure to the patient.
☑ III. 3. Show awareness of patients' concerns regarding their perceptions related to the procedure being performed.

ABHES Competencies Achieved:

☑ 4. a. Document accurately.
☑ 8. cc. Communicate on the recipient's level of comprehension.
☑ 9. l. Prepare patient for examinations and treatments.
☑ 9. r. Teach patients methods of health promotion and disease prevention.

Notes

EVALUATION OF COMPETENCY

Procedure 25-5: Removing Sutures and Staples

Name: _____ Date: _____

Evaluated By: _____ Score: _____

Performance Objective

Outcome:	Remove sutures and staples.
Conditions:	Given the following: antiseptic swabs, clean disposable gloves, sterile 4 × 4 gauze, surgical tape, biohazard waste container, suture removal kid, and staple removal kit.
Standards:	Time: 10 minutes. Student completed procedure in ____ minutes.
	Accuracy: Satisfactory score on the Performance Evaluation Checklist.

Performance Evaluation Checklist

Trial 1	Trial 2	Point Value	Performance Standards
		●	Washed hands with an antimicrobial soap.
		●	Assembled equipment.
		●	Greeted the patient and introduced yourself.
		●	Identified the patient and explained the procedure.
		●	Positioned the patient as required.
		●	Adjusted the light.
		●	Checked to make sure the sutures (or staples) were intact.
		●	Checked to make sure the incision line was approximated and free from infection.
		▷	Explained what to do if the incision line is not approximated.
		●	Opened the suture or staple removal kit.
		●	Applied clean gloves.
		●	Cleaned the incision line with antiseptic swabs using a new swab for each motion.
		●	Allowed the skin to dry.
			Removed sutures as follows:
		●	Informed the patient that he or she would feel a pulling sensation.
		●	Picked up the knot of suture with thumb forceps.
		●	Placed curved tip of suture scissors under the suture.
		●	Cut suture below the knot on the side of suture closest to the skin.
		●	Gently pulled suture out through the outer skin orifice, using a smooth continuous motion.

Trial 1	Trial 2	Point Value	Performance Standards
		•	Did not allow any portion of suture previously on the outside to be pulled through the skin lying beneath the incision line.
		•	Placed the suture on the gauze.
		•	Repeated above sequence until all sutures were removed.
			Removed staples as follows:
		•	Gently placed the jaws of the staple remover under the staple.
		•	Squeezed the staple handles until they were closed.
		•	Lifted the staple remover upward to remove the staple.
		•	Placed staple on gauze.
		•	Continued until all the staples were removed.
		•	Counted number of sutures or staples and checked number with chart.
		•	Cleansed the site with an antiseptic swab.
		•	Applied adhesive skin closures if directed by physician.
		•	Applied DSD, if directed to do so by physician.
		•	Disposed of all sutures or staples and gauze in biohazard waste container.
		•	Removed gloves and sanitized hands.
		•	Charted the procedure correctly.
		✳	Completed the procedure within 10 minutes.
			TOTALS
			CHART
	Date		

Evaluation of Student Performance

EVALUATION CRITERIA			COMMENTS
Symbol	Category	Point Value	
✳	Critical Step	16 points	
●	Essential Step	6 points	
▷	Theory Question	2 points	

Score calculation: 100 points

−_____ points missed

_____ Score

Satisfactory score: 85 or above

CAAHEP Competencies Achieved:

Psychomotor (Skills)
☑ IV. 5. Instruct patients according to their needs to promote health maintenance and disease prevention.
☑ IV. 6. Prepare a patient for procedures and/or treatments.
☑ IV. 8. Document patient care.

Affective (Behavior)
☑ III. 3. Show awareness of patients' concerns regarding their perceptions related to the procedure being performed.
☑ IV. 1. Demonstrate empathy in communicating with patients, family, and staff.

ABHES Competencies Achieved:

☑ 4. a. Document accurately.
☑ 8. bb. Are impartial and show empathy when dealing with patients.
☑ 8. cc. Communicate on the recipient's level of comprehension.
☑ 9. l. Prepare patient for examinations and treatments.
☑ 9. r. Teach patients methods of health promotion and disease prevention.

Notes

☑ EVALUATION OF COMPETENCY

📀 Procedure 25-6: Applying and Removing Adhesive Skin Closures

Name: _____   Date: _____

Evaluated By: _____   Score: _____

Performance Objective

Outcome:	Apply and remove adhesive skin closures.
Conditions:	Given the following: clean disposable gloves, sterile gloves, antiseptic solution, surgical scrub brush, antiseptic swabs, tincture of benzoin, sterile cotton-tipped applicator, adhesive skin closure strips, sterile 4 × 4 gauze pads, surgical tape, and a biohazard waste container.
Standards:	Time: 10 minutes. Student completed procedure in _____ minutes.
	Accuracy: Satisfactory score on the Performance Evaluation Checklist.

Performance Evaluation Checklist

Trial 1	Trial 2	Point Value	Performance Standards
			Application of Adhesive Skin Closures
		•	Washed hands with an antimicrobial soap.
		•	Assembled equipment.
		•	Greeted the patient and introduced yourself.
		•	Identified patient and explained the procedure.
		•	Positioned the patient as required.
		•	Adjusted the light.
		•	Applied clean gloves.
		•	Inspected the wound.
		•	Scrubbed the wound with an antiseptic solution.
		•	Allowed the skin to dry or patted dry.
		•	Applied antiseptic using a new swab for each motion.
		•	Allowed the skin to dry.
		•	Applied tincture of benzoin without letting it touch the wound.
		▷	Stated the purpose of tincture of benzoin.
		•	Allowed the skin to dry.
		•	Removed gloves and washed hands.
		•	Opened the package of adhesive strips and laid them on a flat surface.
		•	Applied sterile gloves and tore tab off card of strips.
		•	Peeled a strip of tape off the card.
		•	Checked to make sure the skin surface was dry.

Trial 1	Trial 2	Point Value	Performance Standards
		•	Secured one end of the strip to the skin by pressing down firmly.
		•	Stretched the strip across the incision until the edges of the wound were approximated.
		•	Secured the strip to the skin on the other side of the wound.
		•	Applied the next strip on one side of center strip at an ⅛-inch interval.
		•	Applied a third strip at an ⅛-inch interval on the other side of the center strip.
		•	Continued applying the strips at ⅛-inch intervals until the edges of the wound were approximated.
		▷	Explained why the strips should be spaced at ⅛-inch intervals.
		•	Applied two closures approximately ½-inch from the ends of the strips.
		▷	Stated the purpose of applying a strip along each edge.
		•	Applied a sterile dressing over the strips if indicated by the physician.
		•	Removed gloves and sanitized hands.
		•	Instructed the patient in wound care and provided written instructions.
		•	Charted the procedure correctly.
			Removal of Adhesive Skin Closures
		•	Sanitized hands.
		•	Greeted the patient and introduced yourself.
		•	Identified the patient and explained the procedure.
		•	Positioned the patient as required.
		•	Checked to make sure the incision line was approximated and free from infection.
		•	Positioned a 4 × 4 gauze pad in a convenient location.
		•	Applied clean gloves.
		•	Peeled off each half of the strip from the outside toward the wound margin.
		•	Lifted the strip away from the wound and placed on the gauze.
		•	Continued until all closures were removed.
		•	Cleansed the site with an antiseptic swab.
		•	Applied a sterile dressing if indicated by the physician.
		•	Disposed of strips and gauze in a biohazard waste container.
		•	Removed gloves and sanitized hands.
		•	Charted the procedure correctly.
		∗	Completed the procedure within 10 minutes.
			TOTALS

CHART	
Date	

Evaluation of Student Performance

EVALUATION CRITERIA			COMMENTS
Symbol	Category	Point Value	
✳	Critical Step	16 points	
●	Essential Step	6 points	
▷	Theory Question	2 points	

Score calculation: 100 points

−_____ points missed

_____ Score

Satisfactory score: 85 or above

CAAHEP Competencies Achieved:

Psychomotor (Skills)
☑ IV. 5. Instruct patients according to their needs to promote health maintenance and disease prevention.
☑ IV. 6. Prepare a patient for procedures and/or treatments.
☑ IV. 8. Document patient care.

Affective (Behavior)
☑ III. 2. Explain the rationale for performance of a procedure to the patient.
☑ III. 3. Show awareness of patients' concerns regarding their perceptions related to the procedure being performed.

ABHES Competencies Achieved:

☑ 4. a. Document accurately.
☑ 8. bb. Are impartial and show empathy when dealing with patients.
☑ 8. cc. Communicate on the recipient's level of comprehension.
☑ 9. l. Prepare patient for examinations and treatments.
☑ 9. r. Teach patients methods of health promotion and disease prevention.

Notes

EVALUATION OF COMPETENCY

Procedure 25-7: Assisting with Minor Office Surgery

Name: _____   Date: _____

Evaluated By: _____   Score: _____

Performance Objective

Outcome:	Set up the surgical tray and assist with minor office surgery.
Conditions:	Given the instruments and supplies required for a specific minor office surgery as designed by the instructor.
Standards:	Time: 15 minutes. Student completed procedure in _____ minutes.
	Accuracy: Satisfactory score on the Performance Evaluation Checklist.

Performance Evaluation Checklist

Trial 1	Trial 2	Point Value	Performance Standards
		•	Determined the type of minor office surgery to be performed.
		•	Prepared examining room.
		•	Sanitized hands.
		•	Set up articles required that are not sterile on a side table or counter.
		•	Labeled the specimen container (if included).
		•	Washed hands with an antimicrobial soap.
		•	Set up the minor office surgery tray on a clean, dry, flat surface, using the principles of surgical asepsis.
			Prepackaged sterile setup:
		•	Selected the appropriate package from supply shelf and placed it on a flat surface.
		•	Opened the setup using the inside of wrapper as the sterile field.
		•	Checked the sterilization indicator on inside of pack.
		•	Added any additional articles required for the surgery and covered tray setup with a standard towel.
			Transferred articles to a sterile field:
		•	Placed sterile towel on a flat surface by two corner ends, making sure not to contaminate it.
		•	Transferred sterile articles to the field, using peel-apart packages.
		•	Applied sterile glove.
		•	Arranged articles neatly on the sterile field with sterile glove.
		•	Checked to make sure all articles were available on the sterile field.

Trial 1	Trial 2	Point Value	Performance Standards
		●	Covered the tray setup with a sterile towel without allowing arms to pass over the sterile field.
			Prepared the patient:
		●	Greeted the patient and introduced yourself.
		●	Identified the patient, explained the procedure, and reassured the patient.
		●	Asked patient if he or she needs to void before the surgery.
		●	Instructed patient on clothing removal.
		●	Instructed patient not to move during procedure or to talk, laugh, sneeze, or cough over the sterile field.
		●	Positioned patient as required for the type of surgery to be performed.
		●	Adjusted the light so that it was focused on the operative site.
			Prepared the patient's skin:
		●	Applied clean disposable gloves.
		●	Shaved skin (if required).
		●	Cleansed skin with an antiseptic solution.
		●	Rinsed and dried the area.
		●	Applied antiseptic using antiseptic swabs.
		●	Allowed the skin to dry.
		●	Removed gloves and sanitized hands.
		●	Checked to make sure that everything was ready and informed physician.
			Assisted the physician:
		●	Uncovered the tray setup.
		●	Opened the outer glove wrapper for physician.
		●	Held the vial while physician withdrew the local anesthetic.
		●	Adjusted the light as required.
		●	Restrained patient.
		●	Relaxed and reassured patient.
		●	Handed instruments and supplies to physician. (Sterile gloves required.)
		●	Kept the sterile field neat and orderly. (Sterile gloves required.)
		●	Held basin for physician to deposit soiled instruments and supplies. (Clean gloves required.)
		●	Retracted tissue. (Sterile gloves required.)
		●	Sponged blood from operative site. (Sterile gloves required.)
		●	Added instruments and supplies as necessary to the sterile field.
		●	Held specimen container to accept specimen. (Clean gloves required.)
		●	Cut ends of suture material after insertion by physician. (Sterile gloves required.)
			Following the surgery:
		●	Applied sterile dressing to the surgical wound if ordered by physician.

Trial 1	Trial 2	Point Value		Performance Standards
		●		Stayed with patient as a safety precaution.
		●		Assisted and instructed patient as required.
		●		Verified that patient understood postoperative instructions.
		●		Provided patient with verbal and written wound care instructions.
		▷		Stated the patient instructions that should be relayed for wound and suture care.
		●		Relayed information regarding the return visit.
		●		Assisted patient off table.
		●		Instructed patient to get dressed.
		●		Transferred any specimens collected to the laboratory with a completed biopsy request.
		●		Charted correctly.
		●		Cleaned examining room.
		●		Discarded disposable contaminated articles in a biohazard waste container.
		●		Sanitized and sterilized instruments.
		∗		Completed the procedure within 15 minutes.
				TOTALS
			CHART	
Date				

Evaluation of Student Performance

EVALUATION CRITERIA			COMMENTS
Symbol	**Category**	**Point Value**	
∗	Critical Step	16 points	
●	Essential Step	6 points	
▷	Theory Question	2 points	
Score calculation: 100 points			
−_____ points missed			
_____ Score			
Satisfactory score: 85 or above			

CAAHEP Competencies Achieved:

Psychomotor (Skills)
☑ I. 10. Assist physician with patient care.
☑ IV. 5. Instruct patients according to their needs to promote health maintenance and disease prevention.
☑ IV. 6. Prepare a patient for procedures and/or treatments.
☑ IV. 8. Document patient care.
☑ IX. 1. Respond to issues of confidentiality.

Affective (Behavior)
☑ III. 2. Explain the rationale for performance of a procedure to the patient.
☑ III. 3. Show awareness of patients' concerns regarding their perceptions related to the procedure being performed.
☑ IV. 6. Demonstrate awareness of how an individual's personal appearance affects anticipated responses.
☑ IX. 3. Recognize the importance of local, state, and federal legislation and regulations in the practice setting.

ABHES Competencies Achieved:

☑ 4. a. Document accurately.
☑ 4. f. Comply with federal, state, and local health laws and regulations.
☑ 8. bb. Are impartial and show empathy when dealing with patients.
☑ 8. cc. Communicate on the recipient's level of comprehension.
☑ 9. e. Recognize emergencies and treatments and minor office surgical procedures.
☑ 9. l. Prepare patient for examinations and treatments.
☑ 9. n. Assist physician with minor office surgical procedures
☑ 9. r. Teach patients methods of health promotion and disease prevention.

EVALUATION OF COMPETENCY

Procedure 25-A: Applying Bandages

Name: _____   Date: _____

Evaluated By: _____   Score: _____

Performance Objective

Outcome:	Apply the following bandage turns: circular, spiral, spiral-reverse, figure-eight, and recurrent.
Conditions:	Given the following: a roller bandage and an elastic bandage.
Standards:	Time: 15 minutes. Student completed procedure in ____ minutes.
	Accuracy: Satisfactory score on the Performance Evaluation Checklist.

Performance Evaluation Checklist

Trial 1	Trial 2	Point Value	Performance Standards
			Circular Turn
		●	Placed the end of a bandage on a slant.
		●	Encircled the body part while allowing the corner of the bandage to extend.
		●	Turned down corner of bandage.
		●	Made another circular turn around the body part.
		▷	Stated a use of the circular turn.
			Spiral Turn
		●	Anchored bandage using a circular turn.
		●	Encircled the body part while keeping bandage at a slant.
		●	Carried each spiral turn upward at a slight angle.
		●	Overlapped each previous turn by one half to two thirds the width of bandage.
		▷	Stated a use of the spiral turn.
			Spiral-Reverse Turn
		●	Anchored bandage using a circular turn.
		●	Encircled the body part while keeping bandage at a slant.
		●	Reversed the spiral turn using the thumb or index finger.
		●	Directed bandage downward and folded it on itself.
		●	Kept bandage parallel to the lower edge of the previous turn.
		●	Overlapped each previous turn by two thirds the width of the bandage.
		▷	Stated a use of the spiral-reverse turn.

Trial 1	Trial 2	Point Value	Performance Standards
			Figure-Eight Turn
		●	Anchored bandage using a circular turn.
		●	Slanted bandage turns to alternately ascend and descend around the body part.
		●	Crossed the turns over one another in the middle to resemble a figure eight.
		●	Overlapped each previous turn by two thirds the width of bandage.
		▷	Stated a use of the figure-eight turn.
			Recurrent Turn
		●	Anchored bandage using two circular turns.
		●	Passed bandage back and forth over the tip of the body part being bandaged.
		●	Overlapped each previous turn by two thirds of the width of the bandage.
		▷	Stated a use of the recurrent turn.
		✳	Completed the procedure within 15 minutes.
			TOTALS

	CHART
Date	

Evaluation of Student Performance

EVALUATION CRITERIA			COMMENTS
Symbol	Category	Point Value	
✳	Critical Step	16 points	
●	Essential Step	6 points	
▷	Theory Question	2 points	

Score calculation: 100 points

− _____ points missed

_____ Score

Satisfactory score: 85 or above

CAAHEP Competencies Achieved:

Psychomotor (Skills)
☑ IV. 5. Instruct patients according to their needs to promote health maintenance and disease prevention.
☑ IV. 6. Prepare a patient for procedures and/or treatments.

Affective (Behavior)
☑ I. 1. Apply critical thinking skills in performing patient assessment and care.

ABHES Competencies Achieved:

☑ 9. l. Prepare patient for examinations and treatments.
☑ 9. r. Teach patients methods of health promotion and disease prevention.

26

Administration of Medication and Intravenous Therapy

CHAPTER ASSIGNMENTS

√ After Completing	Date Due	Textbook Page(s)	TEXTBOOK ASSIGNMENTS	Possible Points	Points You Earned
		571-635	Read Chapter 26: Administration of Medication and Intravenous Therapy		
		578 633	Read Case Study 1 Case Study 1 questions	5	
		596 633	Read Case Study 2 Case Study 2 questions	5	
		617 633	Read Case Study 3 Case Study 3 questions	5	
			TOTAL POINTS		
√ After Completing	Date Due	Study Guide Page(s)	STUDY GUIDE ASSIGNMENTS (CTA: Critical Thinking Activity)	Possible Points	Points You Earned
		585	Pretest	10	
		586-587	Key Term Assessment	30	
		587-593	Evaluation of Learning questions	80	
		593-596	CTA A: Using the PDR	34	
		596-597	CTA B: Locating Information in a Drug Insert	12	
		597	CTA C: Drug Classifications (3 points each)	30	
		598	CTA D: Seven Rights of Medication Administration	35	
			CD Activity: Chapter 26 Script It! (Record points earned)		

√ After Completing	Date Due	Study Guide Page(s)	STUDY GUIDE ASSIGNMENTS (CTA: Critical Thinking Activity)	Possible Points	Points You Earned
		599	CTA E: Liquid Measurement	11	
		599	CTA F: Parts of a Needle and Syringe	11	
			CD Activity: Chapter 26 Take the Plunge (Record points earned)		
		599-600	CTA G: Hypodermic Syringe Calibrations	10	
			CD Activity: Chapter 26 Which Needle? (Record points earned)		
		600	CTA H: Insulin Syringe Calibrations	20	
		600-601	CTA I: Tuberculin Syringe Calibrations	14	
			CD Activity: Chapter 26 Draw It Up! (Record points earned)		
		601	CTA J: Syringe and Needle Labels (3 points each)	12	
		601	CTA K: Angle of Insertion for Injections	3	
		601-602	CTA L: Preparing and Administering Parenteral Medication	18	
		602-603	CTA M: Anaphylactic Reaction	20	
		604-605	CTA N: Mantoux Test Results	30	
		605-615	CTA O: Researching Drugs (5 points/drug)	200	
		616	CTA P: Crossword Puzzle	40	
			CD Activity: Chapter 26 Road to Recovery Game: Drug Categories (Record points earned)		
			CD Activity: Chapter 26 Animations	20	
			CD Activity: Chapter 26 Apply Your Knowledge questions (Record points earned)		
		585	Posttest	10	
			ADDITIONAL ASSIGNMENTS		
			TOTAL POINTS		

√ After Completing	Date Due	Study Guide Page(s)	STUDY GUIDE ASSIGNMENTS: DRUG DOSAGE CALCULATION: SUPPLEMENTAL EDUCATION FOR CHAPTER 26	Possible Points	Points You Earned
		637	**Unit 1: The Metric System** A. Units of Measurement	10	
		638	**Unit 1: The Metric System** B. Metric Abbreviations	7	
		638	**Unit 1: The Metric System** C. Metric Notation	20	
		639	**Unit 2: The Apothecary System** A. Units of Measurement	14	
		639	**Unit 2: The Apothecary System** B. Apothecary Abbreviations	10	
		640	**Unit 2: The Apothecary System** C. Apothecary Notation	20	
		640	**Unit 3: The Household System** A. Units of Measurement	4	
		641	**Unit 4: Medication Orders** A. Medical Abbreviations	30	
		641-643	**Unit 4: Medication Orders** B. Interpreting Medication Orders (3 points each)	30	
		643-644	**Unit 5: Converting Units of Measurement** A. Using Conversion Tables (2 points each)	50	
		644-646	**Unit 5: Converting Units of Measurement** B. Converting Units within the Metric System (2 points each)	40	
		646-648	**Unit 5: Converting Units of Measurement** C. Converting Units within the Apothecary System (2 points each)	50	
		648-650	**Unit 5: Converting Units of Measurement** D. Converting Units within the Household System (2 points each)	20	
		650-652	**Unit 6: Ratio and Proportion** A. Ratio and Proportion Guidelines (6 points each)	48	
		652-654	**Unit 6: Ratio and Proportion** B. Converting Units Using Ratio and Proportion (2 points each)	40	

√ After Completing	Date Due	Study Guide Page(s)	STUDY GUIDE ASSIGNMENTS: DRUG DOSAGE CALCULATION: SUPPLEMENTAL EDUCATION FOR CHAPTER 26	Possible Points	Points You Earned
		654-660	**Unit 7: Determining Drug Dosage** A. Oral Administration: Oral Solid Medications (2 points each)	20	
		654-660	**Unit 7: Determining Drug Dosage** A. Oral Administration: Oral Liquid Medications (2 points each)	10	
		660-663	**Unit 7: Determining Drug Dosage** B. Parenteral Administration (2 points each)	20	

√ When Assigned by Your Instructor	Study Guide Page(s)	Practices Required	LABORATORY ASSIGNMENTS (Procedure Number and Name)	*Score
	617	5	**Practice for Competency** 26-1: Administering Oral Medication Textbook reference: pp. 599-600	
	619-620		**Evaluation of Competency** 26-1: Administering Oral Medication	*
	617	Vial: 5 Ampule: 5	**Practice for Competency** 26-2: Preparing an Injection Textbook reference: pp. 608-611	
	621-623		**Evaluation of Competency** 26-2: Preparing an Injection	*
	617	3	**Practice for Competency** 26-3: Reconstituting Powdered Drugs Textbook reference: pp. 611-612	
	625-626		**Evaluation of Competency** 26-3: Reconstituting Powdered Drugs	*
	617	5	**Practice for Competency** 26-4: Administering a Subcutaneous Injection Textbook reference: pp. 612-614	
	627-628		**Evaluation of Competency** 26-4: Administering a Subcutaneous Injection	*
	617	5	**Practice for Competency** 26-5: Administering an Intramuscular Injection Textbook reference: pp. 614-616	
	629-630		**Evaluation of Competency** 26-5: Administering an Intramuscular Injection	*
	617	5	**Practice for Competency** 26-6: Z-Track Intramuscular Injection Technique Textbook reference: p. 617	
	631-632		**Evaluation of Competency** 26-6: Z-Track Intramuscular Injection Technique	*
	617	5	**Practice for Competency** 26-7: Administering an Intradermal Injection Textbook reference: pp. 625-627	
	633-635		**Evaluation of Competency** 26-7: Administering an Intradermal Injection	*

√ When Assigned by Your Instructor	Study Guide Page(s)	Practices Required	LABORATORY ASSIGNMENTS (Procedure Number and Name)	*Score
			ADDITIONAL ASSIGNMENTS	

Name _____ Date _____

PRETEST

True or False

_____ 1. A drug is a chemical that is used for treatment, prevention, or diagnosis of disease.

_____ 2. The generic name of a drug is assigned by the pharmaceutical manufacturer that develops the drug.

_____ 3. The Rx symbol comes from the Latin word *recipe* and means "take."

_____ 4. An anaphylactic reaction can be life threatening.

_____ 5. The dorsogluteal site is the most common site for administering injections in infants.

_____ 6. A subcutaneous injection is given into muscle tissue.

_____ 7. The purpose of aspirating when administering an injection is to make sure the needle is not in a blood vessel.

_____ 8. The Mantoux tuberculin test is administered through a subcutaneous injection.

_____ 9. The peripheral veins of the arm and hand are used most often for administering IV therapy.

_____ 10. Chemotherapy is the use of chemicals to treat disease.

POSTTEST

True or False

_____ 1. OSHA is responsible for determining if drugs are safe before release for human use.

_____ 2. An enteric-coated tablet does not dissolve until it reaches the intestines.

_____ 3. The apothecary system is most often used to administer medication in the medical office.

_____ 4. The parenteral route of administering medications is used when the patient is allergic to the oral form of the drug.

_____ 5. Hypodermic syringes are calibrated in cubic centimeters.

_____ 6. The maximum amount of medication that can be administered through the subcutaneous route is 2 cc.

_____ 7. A patient with latent tuberculosis infection has a negative reaction to a TB test.

_____ 8. A tuberculin skin test result should be read 15 to 20 minutes after administering.

_____ 9. Intermittent IV administration involves the administration of IV medication over a specific amount of time at specified intervals.

_____ 10. Immune globulin consists of pooled human plasma that contains clotting factors.

KEY TERM ASSESSMENT

Directions: Match each medical term with its definition.

_____ 1. Adverse reaction

_____ 2. Allergen

_____ 3. Allergy

_____ 4. Ampule

_____ 5. Anaphylactic reaction

_____ 6. Autoimmune disease

_____ 7. Chemotherapy

_____ 8. Controlled drug

_____ 9. Dose

_____ 10. Drug

_____ 11. Enteral nutrition

_____ 12. Gauge

_____ 13. Hemophilia

_____ 14. Immune globulins

_____ 15. Induration

_____ 16. Infusion

_____ 17. Inhalation administration

_____ 18. Intradermal injection

_____ 19. Intramuscular injection

_____ 20. Intravenous therapy

_____ 21. Oral administration

_____ 22. Parenteral

_____ 23. Pharmacology

_____ 24. Prescription

_____ 25. Subcutaneous injection

_____ 26. Sublingual administration

_____ 27. Topical administration

_____ 28. Transfusion

A. Application of a drug to a particular spot, usually for a local action

B. Introduction of medication into the dermal layer of the skin

C. A small, sealed glass container that holds a single dose of medication

D. A physician's order authorizing the dispensing of drugs by a pharmacist

E. An unintended and undesirable effect produced by a drug

F. An abnormal hypersensitivity of the body to substances that are ordinarily harmless

G. The administration of a liquid agent directly into a patient's vein where it is distributed throughout the body by way of the circulatory system

H. A small raised area of the skin

I. Introduction of medication beneath the skin, into the subcutaneous or fatty layer of the body

J. An area of hardened tissue

K. A closed glass container with a rubber stopper that holds medication

L. The administration of medication by way of air or other vapor being drawn into the lungs

M. A serious allergic reaction that requires immediate treatment

N. Administration of medication by mouth

O. A drug that has restrictions placed on it by the federal government because of its potential for abuse

P. Introduction of medication into the muscular layer of the body

Q. Administration of medication by placing it under the tongue

R. The quantity of a drug to be administered at one time

S. A substance that is capable of causing an allergic reaction

T. A chemical used for the treatment, prevention, or diagnosis of disease

U. The diameter of the lumen of a needle used to administer medication

V. Administration of medication by injection

W. The study of drugs

X. A condition in which the body's immune system produces antibodies that attack the body's own cells

Y. The use of chemicals to treat disease; most often used to refer to the treatment of cancer using antineoplastic medications

Z. The delivery of nutrients through a tube inserted into the GI tract

AA. An inherited bleeding disorder caused by a deficiency of a clotting factor needed for proper coagulation of the blood

_____ 29. Vial

_____ 30. Wheal

BB. A blood product consisting of pooled human plasma containing antibodies

CC. The administration of fluids, medications, or nutrients into a vein

DD. The administration of whole blood or blood products through the intravenous route

EVALUATION OF LEARNING

Directions: Fill in each blank with the correct answer.

Administration of Medication

1. What is the difference between administering, prescribing, and dispensing medication at the medical office?

_____

_____

_____

_____

2. What is the difference between the generic name and the brand name of a drug?

_____

_____

_____

_____

3. What is a liniment?

_____

_____

4. What is a spray?

_____

_____

5. What is a syrup?

_____

_____

6. What is a tablet?

_____

7. What is the purpose of scoring a tablet?

_____

8. List two drugs that come in the form of chewable tablets.

_____

9. List two reasons for enterically coating a tablet.

_____

_____

10. What is a capsule?

_____

11. Why must a suppository have a cylindric or conical shape?

_____

_____

12. What is a transdermal patch?

_____

_____

13. Why is the metric system used most often to administer medication?

_____

_____

14. Define the term *volume*.

_____

15. Describe the use of the household system of measurement.

_____

_____

16. When is conversion required?

_____

_____

17. What is a controlled drug?

_____

18. In what forms can a prescription be authorized?

_____

_____

_____

19. What requirements must be followed when writing a prescription for a schedule II drug?

_____

_____

_____

20. List five brand names of schedule II analgesics.

_____

_____

21. What requirements must be followed when writing a prescription for a schedule III drug?

_____

_____

_____

22. What is a schedule IV drug?

_____

_____

23. List three brand names of schedule IV analgesics.

_____

_____

24. List four brand names of schedule IV antianxiety agents.

_____

_____

25. What is included in each of the following parts of a prescription?

   a. Superscription: _____

   b. Inscription: _____

   c. Subscription: _____

   d. Signatura: _____

26. Why is it important for the patient's age to be indicated on a prescription?

_____

_____

27. What types of medications should be recorded on a medication record form?

_____

28. List three factors that affect the action of drugs in the body.

_____

_____

_____

29. What are the symptoms and treatment of an anaphylactic reaction?

_____

_____

30. What are the advantages and disadvantages of using the parenteral route of administration?

_____

_____

_____

_____

31. How do safety-engineered syringes reduce the risk of a needlestick injury?

_____

32. What is the purpose of using a filter needle when withdrawing medication from an ampule?

_____

33. What sites are used most frequently to administer an SC injection?

_____

_____

34. List three medications commonly administered through an SC injection.

_____

35. Why is medication absorbed faster through the IM route than through the SC route?

_____

_____

36. List the four IM injection sites, and explain why these sites must be used to administer an IM injection.

_____

_____

_____

37. What types of medication are given using the Z-track technique?

_____

_____

38. What sites are used most frequently to administer an intradermal injection?

_____

39. What is the most frequent use of an intradermal injection?

_____

40. What are the symptoms of active pulmonary tuberculosis?

_____

41. What is latent tuberculosis infection?

_____

42. Who should have a tuberculin test?

_____

43. What is induration, and what causes it?

_____

_____

44. What procedures are performed if a patient has a positive reaction to a tuberculin skin test?

_____

_____

45. List 10 examples of common allergens.

_____

_____

_____

_____

2. How can this section assist the user?

_____

_____

Product Information

Under which heading would you look in this section to find information on:

1. Conditions the drug is approved to treat by the FDA

_____

_____

2. Information to relay to the patient to ensure safe and effective use of the drug

_____

_____

3. Route of administration

_____

4. Symptoms associated with an overdose of the drug

_____

_____

_____

5. Situations that require special consideration when the drug is used

_____

_____

6. Generic name of the drug

_____

7. How the drug functions in the body to produce its therapeutic effect

_____

_____

8. Situations in which the drug should not be used

_____

_____

9. Recommended adult dosage and duration of treatment

_____

10. How to pronounce the brand name of the drug

_____

11. Handling and storage conditions

_____

_____

_____

12. Serious adverse reactions that may occur with the drug

_____

_____

_____

13. Symptoms associated with an overdose of ...ug

_____   _____

_____   _____

_____   _____

14. Unintended and undesirable effec... ... may occur with the use of the drug

_____   _____

_____   _____

_____   _____

15. Modification of dosage n... ...for children

_____   _____

B. LOCATING INF... ...ON IN A DRUG INSERT

Obtain a dru... ...prescription drug, and answer the following questions.

1. What is ... ...e of the drug?

_____

2. ... ...eneric name of the drug?

_____

...is the drug category of this medication?

_____

What are the dosage forms for this drug?

_____

5. What is the route of administration of this medication?

_____

6. What are the indications and usage for this medication?

_____

_____

_____

7. What are the contraindications for this medication?

_____

_____

_____

8. List the warnings for this drug.

_____

_____

_____

9. What are the general precautions for this medication?

_____

_____

_____

10. What information should be relayed to patients for this medication?

_____

_____

_____

11. What are the adverse reactions for this medication?

_____

_____

_____

12. What is the dosage and administration for this medication?

_____

_____

C. DRUG CLASSIFICATIONS

Inspect the package labels of 10 drugs (or use other means) to assess the classification of each drug based on preparation and action. List the name of each drug along with its appropriate category in the spaces provided. Compare results. *Example:* Drug: Tylenol Elixir. Classification based on preparation: elixir. Classification based on action: analgesic, antipyretic.

Classification Based On:

Drug	Preparation	Action
1. _____	_____	_____
2. _____	_____	_____
3. _____	_____	_____
4. _____	_____	_____
5. _____	_____	_____
6. _____	_____	_____
7. _____	_____	_____
8. _____	_____	_____
9. _____	_____	_____
10. _____	_____	_____

D. SEVEN RIGHTS OF MEDICATION ADMINISTRATION

You are the office manager at a large clinic. Six new MAs were just hired. Your physician asks you to design an illustrated poster portraying the seven rights of medication administration to remind the new employees of the importance of following these guidelines. Use the diagram below to design your poster.

Follow the Seven "Rights"	
Right Drug	Right Dose
Right Time	Right Patient
Right Route	Right Technique
Right Documentation	

ANAPHYLACTIC REACTION

N. MANTOUX TEST RESULTS

1. In the space provided, indicate whether the following Mantoux test results are positive, doubtful, or negative:

   a. 12 mm of induration: _____

   b. 7 mm of induration: _____

   c. 5 mm of induration (the patient is infected with HIV): _____

   d. 2 mm of induration: _____

   e. Erythema: 6 mm wide (no induration): _____

2. Complete a tuberculosis test record card for each of the above results. (Use patient names of your choice. The brand name of the Mantoux test is Tubersol 5 TU.)

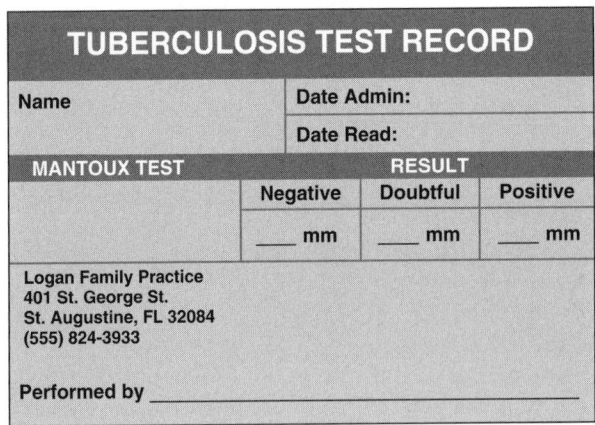

(From Bonewit-West K: *Study guide for clinical procedures for medical assistants,* ed 7, St. Louis, 2008, Saunders.)

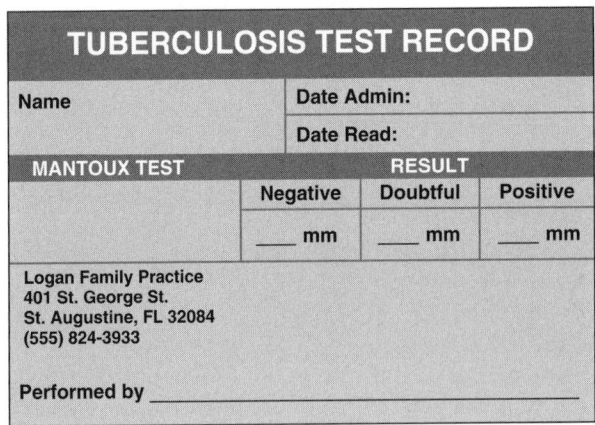

(From Bonewit-West K: *Study guide for clinical procedures for medical assistants,* ed 7, St. Louis, 2008, Saunders.)

TUBERCULOSIS TEST RECORD

| Name | Date Admin: |
| | Date Read: |

MANTOUX TEST	RESULT		
	Negative	Doubtful	Positive
	____ mm	____ mm	____ mm

Logan Family Practice
401 St. George St.
St. Augustine, FL 32084
(555) 824-3933

Performed by _____

(From Bonewit-West K: *Study guide for clinical procedures for medical assistants,* ed 7, St. Louis, 2008, Saunders.)

TUBERCULOSIS TEST RECORD

| Name | Date Admin: |
| | Date Read: |

MANTOUX TEST	RESULT		
	Negative	Doubtful	Positive
	____ mm	____ mm	____ mm

Logan Family Practice
401 St. George St.
St. Augustine, FL 32084
(555) 824-3933

Performed by _____

(From Bonewit-West K: *Study guide for clinical procedures for medical assistants,* ed 7, St. Louis, 2008, Saunders.)

TUBERCULOSIS TEST RECORD

| Name | Date Admin: |
| | Date Read: |

MANTOUX TEST	RESULT		
	Negative	Doubtful	Positive
	____ mm	____ mm	____ mm

Logan Family Practice
401 St. George St.
St. Augustine, FL 32084
(555) 824-3933

Performed by _____

(From Bonewit-West K: *Study guide for clinical procedures for medical assistants,* ed 7, St. Louis, 2008, Saunders.)

O. RESEARCHING DRUGS
   Obtain a drug reference book, and look up the following information for each of the drugs listed on the Pharmacology Drug Sheets: generic name and drug classification, indications, patient teaching. Record this information in the appropriate space on the Pharmacology Drug Sheets.

Pharmacology Drug Sheet

Name: _____

Generic Name and Drug Classification	Indications	Patient Teaching
Accupril		
Adderall		
Adrenalin		
Ambien		

Pharmacology Drug Sheet

Name: _____

Generic Name and Drug Classification	Indications	Patient Teaching
Amoxil		
Bentyl		
Cardizem		
Catapres		

Pharmacology Drug Sheet

Name: _____

Generic Name and Drug Classification	Indications	Patient Teaching
Celebrex		
Cipro		
Coumadin		
Cozaar		

Pharmacology Drug Sheet

Name: _____

Generic Name and Drug Classification	Indications	Patient Teaching
Depo-Medrol		
Diflucan		
Dilantin		
Flagyl		

Pharmacology Drug Sheet

Name: _____

Generic Name and Drug Classification	Indications	Patient Teaching
Flexeril		
Fosamax		
Glucotrol XL		
Inderal		

Pharmacology Drug Sheet

Name: _____

Generic Name and Drug Classification	Indications	Patient Teaching
INFeD		
Lanoxin		
Lasix		
Levoxyl		

Pharmacology Drug Sheet

Name: _____

Generic Name and Drug Classification	Indications	Patient Teaching
Lipitor		
Lomotil		
Mexate		
Nitro-Bid		

Pharmacology Drug Sheet

Name: _____

Generic Name and Drug Classification	Indications	Patient Teaching
Phenergan		
Plavix		
Prevacid		
Prozac		

Pharmacology Drug Sheet

Name: _____

Generic Name and Drug Classification	Indications	Patient Teaching
Singulair		
Tessalon		
Viagra		
Vicodin		

Pharmacology Drug Sheet

Name: _____

Generic Name and Drug Classification	Indications	Patient Teaching
Xanax		
Zithromax		
Zyloprim		
Zyrtec		

P. CROSSWORD PUZZLE
Administration of Medication
Directions: Complete the crossword puzzle using the clues presented below.

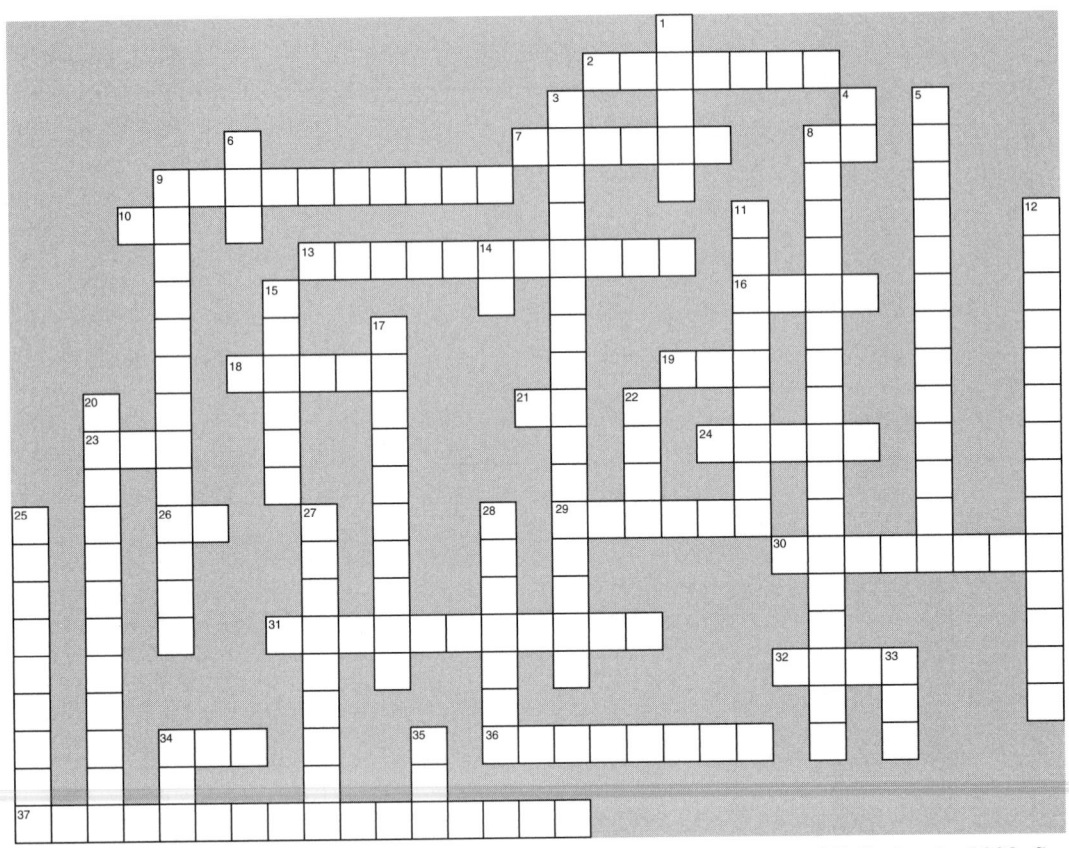

(From Bonewit-West K: *Study guide for clinical procedures for medical assistants,* ed 7, St. Louis, 2008, Saunders.)

ACROSS

2 Discovered penicillin
7 Most aggressive Hymenoptera
8 1 ml = 1 _____
9 Present with a Mantoux
10 Right ear
13 Used to treat anaphylactic reaction
16 Metric weight unit
18 Ranges between 18 and 27
19 Aspirin
21 Every day
23 Available without a prescription
24 Needle opening
26 Before meals
29 Symptoms: wheezing and dyspnea
30 Allergy to molds and pollen
31 Conditions a drug is approved to treat
32 Immediately!
34 Tuberculin is made of this
36 Causes house dust allergy
37 Runny and inflamed allergic nose

DOWN

1 Slant of the needle
3 Do not use this drug!
4 Route of administration for allergy injection
5 Drug to discontinue before allergy testing
6 Approves drugs
8 Poison ivy causes this
9 Abnormal or peculiar reaction
11 Means "label" in Latin
12 Calibrated in units
14 By mouth
15 Prevents syringe from rolling
17 This drug may cause an allergic reaction
20 Site for deep IM injection
22 Blood test for allergies
25 Hives
27 Prescription requirement for controlled drug
28 Maximum of 1 cc at this site
33 Three times a day
34 Drug reference (ex)
35 As needed

DRUG DOSAGE CALCULATION: SUPPLEMENTAL EDUCATION FOR CHAPTER 26

This section is designed as supplemental education for Chapter 26 (Administration of Medication) in your textbook. Completion of the exercises in this section will enable you to calculate drug dosage effectively and accurately, which is essential for administering the proper amount of medication to patients and preventing medication errors. This section is organized so that each unit builds on the next one; therefore, it is important that you are completely familiar with each step before proceeding to the next.

Learning Objectives

After completing this chapter, you should be able to:

1. Identify metric abbreviations.

2. Indicate dose quantity using metric notation guidelines.

3. Identify apothecary abbreviations.

4. Indicate dose quantity using apothecary notations.

5. Identify common medical abbreviations used in writing medication orders.

6. Interpret medication orders.

7. Convert units of measurement within the following systems: metric, apothecary, and household.

8. Convert units of measurement using ratio and proportion.

9. Convert units of measurement between the metric, apothecary, and household systems.

10. Determine oral drug dosage.

11. Determine parenteral drug dosage.

UNIT 1: THE METRIC SYSTEM

A. Units of Measurement

The basic units of measurement in the metric system are the gram, liter, and meter. The gram is a unit of weight used to measure solids; the liter is a unit of measure used to measure liquids; and the meter is a unit of linear measure used to measure length or distance.

Practice Problems: Units of Measurement

Directions: In the space provided below, indicate whether each of the following metric units of measurement is a unit of weight (W), volume (V), or length (L).

_____ 1. milligram

_____ 2. cubic centimeter

_____ 3. meter

_____ 4. kilogram

_____ 5. liter

_____ 6. milliliter

_____ 7. kiloliter

_____ 8. millimeter

_____ 9. microgram

_____ 10. gram

B. Metric Abbreviations

Practice Problems: Metric Abbreviations

Review the metric abbreviations in your textbook before completing these problems.

Directions: In the space provided, indicate the correct abbreviation for each of the metric units of measurement listed below.

_____ 1. milligram

_____ 2. gram

_____ 3. kilogram

_____ 4. liter

_____ 5. cubic centimeter

_____ 6. microgram

_____ 7. milliliter

C. Metric Notation

Practice Problems: Metric Notations

In order to read prescriptions and medication orders, to record medication administration, and to avoid medication errors, the MA must be familiar with and be able to use metric notation guidelines. Review the Metric Notation Guidelines on page 586 of your textbook before completing the following practice problems.

Directions: In the space provided, use metric notation guidelines to indicate the following dose quantities.

_____ 1. 25 milligrams

_____ 2. 5 grams

_____ 3. 1 ½ liters

_____ 4. 1 cubic centimeter

_____ 5. 10 milliliters

_____ 6. ½ gram

_____ 7. 50 milligrams

_____ 8. ½ cubic centimeter

_____ 9. 4 milliliters

_____ 10. 2 kilograms

_____ 11. 120 milliliters

_____ 12. 3 cubic centimeters

_____ 13. ¼ gram

_____ 14. 250 milligrams

_____ 15. ½ liter

_____ 16. 500 milliliters

_____ 17. 1 cubic centimeter

_____ 18. 5 kilograms

_____ 19. 2 ½ grams

_____ 20. 10 milligrams

UNIT 2: THE APOTHECARY SYSTEM

A. Units of Measurement

The basic units of measurement in the apothecary system are the grain, minim, and inch. The grain is a unit of weight used to measure solids; the minim is a unit of measure used to measure liquids; and the inch is a unit of linear measure used to measure length or distance.

Practice Problems: Units of Measurement

Directions: In the space provided, indicate whether each of the following units of measurement is a unit of weight (W), volume (V), or length (L).

_____   1. grain

_____   2. inch

_____   3. minim

_____   4. fluid dram

_____   5. foot

_____   6. quart

_____   7. ounce

_____   8. gallon

_____   9. yard

_____   10. fluid ounce

_____   11. pound

_____   12. pint

_____   13. dram

_____   14. mile

B. Apothecary Abbreviations

Practice Problems: Apothecary Abbreviations

Review the apothecary abbreviations in your textbook before completing these problems.
Directions: In the space provided, indicate the correct abbreviation or symbol for each of the apothecary units of measurement listed below.

_____   1. grain

_____   2. dram

_____   3. ounce

_____   4. minim

_____   5. fluid dram

_____   6. fluid ounce

_____   7. pint

_____   8. quart

_____   9. gallon

_____   10. inch

C. Apothecary Notation

Practice Problems: Apothecary Notation

Although the apothecary system is used less frequently than the metric system, the MA must still be familiar with and be able to use apothecary notation guidelines. Review the Apothecary Notation Guidelines on page 587 of your textbook before completing the following practice problems.

Directions: In the space provided, use apothecary notations to indicate the following dose quantities.

_____   1. 4 ounces

_____   2. 10 grains

_____   3. 5 drams

_____   4. ½ ounce

_____   5. 6 fluid drams

_____   6. 7 ½ grains

_____   7. 3 ½ ounces

_____   8. 10 minims

_____   9. 3 fluid ounces

_____   10. 2 drams

_____   11. ¼ grain

_____   12. 16 ounces

_____   13. 12 minims

_____   14. 1 dram

_____   15. 9 fluid drams

_____   16. 4 grains

_____   17. 8 drams

_____   18. 32 fluid ounces

_____   19. 30 minims

_____   20. 8 ounces

UNIT 3: THE HOUSEHOLD SYSTEM

The household system is more complicated and less accurate for administering medication than the metric and apothecary systems. However, most individuals are familiar with this system because of its frequent use in the United States. Thus, this unit of measurement may be the only one the patient can fully relate to and therefore may safely use to administer liquid medication at home.

A. Units of Measurement

Volume is the only household unit of measurement used to administer medication. The basic unit of liquid volume is the drop. The remaining units, in order of increasing volume, are the teaspoon, tablespoon, ounce, cup, and glass.

Practice Problems: Units of Measurement

Directions: In the space provided, indicate the correct abbreviation for each of the household units of measurement listed below.

_____   1. drop

_____   2. teaspoon

_____   3. tablespoon

_____   4. ounce

UNIT 4: MEDICATION ORDERS

To safely administer medication, the MA should be completely familiar with common medical abbreviations. Review Table 26-5 in your textbook before completing the following practice problems.

A. Medical Abbreviations

Practice Problems: Medical Abbreviations

Directions: In the space provided, write the meaning of the following medical abbreviations.

_____   1. NPO

_____   2. prn

_____   3. AS

_____   4. hs

_____   5. tab

_____   6. OD

_____   7. ac

_____   8. pc

_____   9. qid

_____   10. c̄

_____   11. OU

_____   12. s̄

_____   13. bid

_____   14. tid

_____   15. qh

_____   16. gtts

_____   17. qd

_____   18. q4h

_____   19. AU

_____   20. qs

_____   21. IM

_____   22. caps

_____   23. qod

_____   24. po

_____   25. OS

_____   26. ad lib

_____   27. āā

_____   28. DAW

_____   29. INH

_____   30. OTC

B. Interpreting Medication Orders

Practice Problems: Interpreting Medication Orders

To safely administer medication and instruct patients on administering medication at home, the MA should be able to interpret medication orders.

Directions: Interpret the following medication orders. Using a drug reference, indicate the drug category based on action and a brand name for each medication.

1. tetracycline 250 mg po qid × 10 days

_____

Drug category: _____

Brand name: _____

2. lansoprazole 30 mg po qd ac

_____

Drug category: _____

Brand name: _____

3. alprazolam 0.25 mg po tid

_____

Drug category: _____

Brand name: _____

4. diltiazem 50 mg po q4h

_____

Drug category: _____

Brand name: _____

5. ciprofloxacin 500 mg q12h

_____

Drug category: _____

Brand name: _____

6. hydrocodone/acetaminophen 5 mg q4h prn

_____

Drug category: _____

Brand name: _____

7. furosemide 40 mg po qAM

_____

Drug category: _____

Brand name: _____

8. paroxetine 20 mg po qd in AM

_____

Drug category: _____

Brand name: _____

9. cetirizine 5 mg po qd

_____

Drug category: _____

Brand name: _____

10. cyclobenzaprine 10 mg po tid × 1 wk

_____

Drug category: _____

Brand name: _____

UNIT 5: CONVERTING UNITS OF MEASUREMENT

A. Using Conversion Tables

Changing from one unit of measurement to another is known as conversion. Conversion is required when medication is ordered in one unit of measurement and the medication label expresses the drug strength in a different unit. The dose quantity must be mathematically translated or converted to the unit of measurement of the medication on hand. For example, if the physician orders 5 grams of an oral solid medication and the medication label expresses the drug strength in milligrams, the MA will need to convert the grams into milligrams to know how much medication to administer.

Converting units of measurement can be classified into the following categories:

1. Conversion of units within a measurement system.

2. Conversion of units from one measurement system to another.

Converting units within a measurement system allows a quantity to be expressed in a different but equal unit of measurement within the same system. An example of converting between units of weight within the metric system is as follows: 1 gram is equal to 1000 milligrams.

Converting from one measurement system to another allows a quantity to be expressed in a unit of measurement of another system. An example of a conversion between the apothecary and metric systems is as follows: 1 grain (apothecary system) is equivalent to 60 milligrams (metric system). Methods used to convert units of measurement are presented in this unit and in Unit 6.

Conversion requires the use of a conversion table to indicate the equivalent values between units of measurement. The practice problems that follow will assist you in attaining competency in conversion table utilization.

Practice Problems: Conversion Tables

Refer to the conversion tables at the end of this chapter. Locate and record the equivalent value for each of the units of measurement listed on the following page. In the space provided, indicate the conversion table you used to locate the equivalent value (e.g., metric, apothecary, metric to apothecary).

		ANSWER	CONVERSION TABLE
1. 1 g	=	_____ mg	_____
2. 1 ounce	=	_____ drams	_____
3. 1 tablespoon	=	_____ teaspoons	_____
4. 1 grain	=	_____ mg	_____
5. 1 liter	=	_____ ml	_____
6. 1 dram	=	_____ grains	_____
7. 1 pint	=	_____ fluid ounces	_____
8. 1 teaspoon	=	_____ drops	_____
9. 1 ml	=	_____ cc	_____
10. 1 ml	=	_____ minims	_____
11. 1 fluid ounce	=	_____ ml	_____
12. 1 kg	=	_____ g	_____
13. 1 fluid dram	=	_____ minims	_____

14. 1 gallon   =   _____ quarts   _____

15. 1 ounce   =   _____ tablespoons   _____

16. 1 quart   =   _____ pints   _____

17. 1 fluid dram   =   _____ ml   _____

18. 1 g   =   _____ grains   _____

19. 1 quart   =   _____ ml   _____

20. 1 drop   =   _____ minims   _____

21. 1 fluid ounce   =   _____ tablespoons   _____

22. 1 fluid dram   =   _____ teaspoons   _____

23. 1 tablespoon   =   _____ fluid drams   _____

24. 1 kg   =   _____ pounds   _____

25. 1 glass   =   _____ ml   _____

B. Converting Units within the Metric System

Drug administration often requires conversion within the metric system to prepare the correct dosage. Metric conversion involves either converting a larger unit to a smaller unit (e.g., grams to milligrams) or converting a smaller unit to a larger unit (e.g., milliliters to liters).

Methods used to convert one metric unit to another are described as follows.

Converting a Larger Unit to a Smaller Unit

Converting a larger unit to a smaller unit within the metric system can be accomplished using one of three methods of conversion, outlined below. The method you use is based on your personal preference as well as the level of difficulty of the conversion problem; for example, more difficult problems will require the use of ratio and proportion as the method of conversion.

Examples of converting a larger unit to a smaller unit are as follows:

1. grams to milligrams
2. liters to milliliters
3. kilograms to grams

METHOD OF CONVERSION: To convert a larger unit to a smaller unit within the metric system:

Method 1: Multiply the unit to be changed by 1000.
Method 2: Move the decimal point of the unit to be changed three places to the right.
Method 3: Ratio and proportion (see Unit 6).

GUIDELINE: If you are converting a larger unit to a smaller unit, you should expect the quantity to become larger. Use this guideline as a reference to assist in making accurate conversions. Refer to the example problems below as an illustration of this guideline.

Examples

PROBLEM   2 L = _____ ml
Method 1:   Multiply the unit to be changed by 1000.
     $2 \times 1000 = 2000$ ml
Method 2:   Move the decimal point of the unit to be changed three places to the right.
     2.0 0 0. = 2000 ml

Answer	2 L = 2000 ml

PROBLEM   4 g = _____ mg
Method 1:   Multiply the unit to be changed by 1000.

$4 \times 1000 = 4000$ mg

Method 2:   Move the decimal point of the unit to be changed three places to the right.
4.0 0 0. = 4000 mg

Answer	4 g = 4000 mg

Converting a Smaller Unit to a Larger Unit

Converting a smaller unit to a larger unit within the metric system can be accomplished using one of three methods of conversion as outlined below.

Examples of converting a smaller unit to a larger unit are as follows:
1. milligrams to grams
2. milliliters to liters
3. grams to kilograms

> METHOD OF CONVERSION: To convert a smaller unit to a larger unit within the metric system:
>
> *Method 1:* Divide the unit to be changed by 1000.
> *Method 2:* Move the decimal point of the unit to be changed three places to the left.
> *Method 3:* Ratio and proportion (see Unit 6).
>
> GUIDELINE: If you are converting a smaller unit to a larger unit, you should expect the quantity to become smaller. Refer to the problems below as an illustration of this guideline.

Examples

PROBLEM   250 mg = _____ g
Method 1:   Divide the unit to be changed by 1000.
$250 \div 1000 = 0.25$ g
Method 2:   Move the decimal point of the unit to be changed three places to the left.
.2 5 0. = 0.25 g

Answer	250 mg = 0.25 g

PROBLEM   1500 ml = _____ L
Method 1:   Divide the unit to be changed by 1000.
$1500 \div 1000 = 1.5$ L
Method 2:   Move the decimal point of the unit to be changed three places to the left.
1.5 0 0. = 1.5 L

Answer	1500 ml = 1.5 L

Practice Problems: Converting Units within the Metric System

Directions: Convert the following metric units of measurement using either Method 1 or Method 2. In the space provided, indicate if the conversion is going from a larger to smaller unit (L→S) or smaller to larger unit (S→L).

		ANSWER	DIRECTION OF CONVERSION
1. 1 g	=	_____ mg	_____
2. 750 mg	=	_____ g	_____
3. 2 kg	=	_____ g	_____
4. 1000 g	=	_____ kg	_____
5. 1.5 L	=	_____ ml	_____

6. 250 ml   =   _____ L   _____

7. 5 g   =   _____ mg   _____

8. 0.25 kg   =   _____ g   _____

9. 1000 mg   =   _____ g   _____

10. 2.5 g   =   _____ mg   _____

11. 475 ml   =   _____ L   _____

12. 0.05 g   =   _____ mg   _____

13. 0.5 L   =   _____ ml   _____

14. 1000 ml   =   _____ L   _____

15. 500 g   =   _____ kg   _____

16. 50 mg   =   _____ g   _____

17. 1 L   =   _____ ml   _____

18. 40 g   =   _____ mg   _____

19. 50 ml   =   _____ L   _____

20. 1 kg   =   _____ g   _____

C. Converting Units within the Apothecary System

Drug administration may sometimes require conversion within the apothecary system to prepare the correct dosage. Apothecary conversion involves converting a larger unit to a smaller unit (e.g., drams to grains) or converting a smaller unit to a larger unit (e.g., ounces to pounds). Methods used to convert one apothecary unit to another are described below.

Converting a Larger Unit to a Smaller Unit

Converting a larger unit to a smaller unit within the apothecary system is accomplished through either the equivalent value method or the ratio and proportion method. Examples of converting a larger unit to a smaller unit are as follows:

Weight:
drams to grains
ounces to drams
pounds to ounces

Volume:
fluid drams to minims
fluid ounces to fluid drams
pints to fluid ounces
quarts to pints
gallons to quarts

METHOD OF CONVERSION: To convert a larger unit to a smaller unit within the apothecary system:

Method 1:
a. Look at the Apothecary Conversion Table at the end of this chapter to determine the equivalent value between the two units of measurement.
b. Multiply the equivalent value by the number next to the larger unit of measurement.
Method 2: Ratio and proportion (see Unit 6).

Examples
PROBLEM   4 drams = _____ grains
Method 1:
a. Look at the conversion table to determine the equivalent value:
   1 dram = 60 grains
   60 = the equivalent value

b. Multiply the equivalent value by the number next to the larger unit of measurement:
    $4 \times 60 = 240$ grains

> ***Answer***   4 drams = 240 grams

PROBLEM   1 ½ pints = _____ fluid ounces
Method 1:
a. Look at the conversion table to determine the equivalent value:
    1 pint = 16 fluid ounces
    16 = the equivalent value
b. Multiply the equivalent value by the number next to the larger unit of measurement:
    $1.5 \times 16 = 24$ fluid ounces

> ***Answer***   1 ½ pints = 24 fluid ounces

Converting a Smaller Unit to a Larger Unit

Converting a smaller unit to a larger unit within the apothecary system can also be accomplished using either the equivalent value method or the ratio and proportion method. Examples of converting from a smaller unit to a larger unit are as follows:

Weight:	*Volume:*
grains to drams	minims to fluid drams
drams to ounces	fluid drams to fluid ounces
ounces to pounds	fluid ounces to pints
	pints to quarts
	quarts to gallons

> METHOD OF CONVERSION: To convert a smaller unit to a larger unit within the
>   apothecary system:
>
> *Method 1:*
> a. Look at the Apothecary Conversion Table at the end of this chapter to determine the
>   equivalent value between the two units of measurement.
> b. Divide the equivalent value into the number next to the smaller unit of measurement.
> *Method 2:* Ratio and proportion (see Unit 6).

Examples
PROBLEM   30 grains = _____ drams
Method 1:
a. Look at the conversion table to determine the equivalent value:
    60 grains = 1 dram
    60 = the equivalent value
b. Divide the equivalent value into the number next to the smaller unit of measurement:
    $30 \div 60 = ½$ dram

> ***Answer***   30 grains = ½ dram

PROBLEM   16 fluid drams = _____ fluid ounces
Method 1:
a. Look at the conversion table to determine the equivalent value:
    8 fluid drams = 1 fluid ounce
    8 = the equivalent value
b. Divide the equivalent value into the number next to the smaller unit of measurement:
    $16 \div 8 = 2$ fluid ounces

> ***Answer***   16 fluid drams = 2 fluid ounces

Practice Problems: Converting Units within the Apothecary System

Convert the following apothecary units of measurement using the equivalent value method of conversion. In the space provided, indicate the equivalent value for each problem.

		ANSWER	EQUIVALENT VALUE
1. 2 quarts	=	_____ pints	_____
2. 4 drams	=	_____ grains	_____
3. ½ ounce	=	_____ drams	_____
4. 300 grains	=	_____ drams	_____
5. 2 fluid drams	=	_____ minims	_____
6. 8 pints	=	_____ quarts	_____
7. 16 drams	=	_____ ounces	_____
8. 24 fluid drams	=	_____ fluid ounces	_____
9. 18 ounces	=	_____ pounds	_____
10. 32 fluid ounces	=	_____ pints	_____
11. ½ quart	=	_____ pints	_____
12. ½ dram	=	_____ grains	_____
13. 3 ounces	=	_____ drams	_____
14. 210 grains	=	_____ drams	_____
15. 4 ½ fluid drams	=	_____ minims	_____
16. 3 pints	=	_____ quarts	_____
17. 4 drams	=	_____ ounces	_____
18. 24 ounces	=	_____ pounds	_____
19. 8 fluid ounces	=	_____ pints	_____
20. 2 quarts	=	_____ gallons	_____
21. 120 minims	=	_____ fluid drams	_____
22. 2 fluid ounces	=	_____ fluid drams	_____
23. ½ pound	=	_____ ounces	_____
24. 4 pints	=	_____ fluid ounces	_____
25. 2 gallons	=	_____ quarts	_____

D. Converting Units within the Household System

Household system conversion involves converting a larger unit to a smaller unit (e.g., tablespoons to teaspoons) or converting a smaller unit to a larger unit (e.g., tablespoons to ounces). Methods used to convert one unit to another are described below.

Converting a Larger Unit to a Smaller Unit

Converting a larger unit to a smaller unit within the household system is accomplished using either the equivalent value method or the ratio and proportion method. The method you use is based upon your personal preference as well as the level of difficulty of the conversion problem. Examples of converting a larger unit to a smaller unit are as follows:

Volume:
teaspoons to drops
tablespoons to teaspoons
ounces to teaspoons
ounces to tablespoons
teacup to ounces
glass to ounces

METHOD OF CONVERSION: To convert a larger unit to a smaller unit with the
household system:

Method 1:
a. Look at the Household Conversion Table at the end of this chapter to determine the
   equivalent value between the two units of measurement.
b. Multiply the equivalent value by the number next to the larger unit of measurement.
Method 2: Ratio and proportion (see Unit 6).

Examples
PROBLEM   2 tablespoons = _____ teaspoons
Method 1:
   a. Look at the conversion table to determine the equivalent value:
      1 tablespoon = 3 teaspoons
      3 = the equivalent value
   b. Multiply the equivalent value by the number next to the larger unit of measurement:
      $2 \times 3 = 6$ teaspoons

> *Answer*   2 tablespoons = 6 teaspoons

PROBLEM   ½ teaspoon = _____ drops
Method 1:
   a. Look at the conversion table to determine the equivalent value:
      1 teaspoon = 60 drops
      60 = the equivalent value
   b. Multiply the equivalent value by the number next to the larger unit of measurement:
      $\frac{1}{2} \times 60 = 30$ drops

> *Answer*   ½ teaspoon = 30 drops

Converting a Smaller Unit to a Larger Unit

Converting a smaller unit to a larger unit within the household system is accomplished using either the equivalent value
method or the ratio and proportion method. Examples of converting from a smaller unit to a larger unit are as follows:
   Volume:
   drops to teaspoons
   teaspoons to tablespoons
   teaspoons to ounces
   tablespoons to ounces
   ounces to teacups
   ounces to glasses

METHOD OF CONVERSION: To convert a smaller unit to a larger unit within the household system:

Method 1:
a. Look at the Household Conversion Table at the end of this chapter to determine the equivalent
   value between the two units of measurement.
b. Divide the equivalent value into the number next to the smaller unit of measurement.
Method 2: Ratio and proportion (see Unit 6).

Examples

PROBLEM   4 tablespoons = _____ ounces

Method 1:

   a. Look at the conversion table to determine the equivalent value:

      1 ounce = 2 tablespoons

      2 = the equivalent value

   b. Divide the equivalent value into the number next to the smaller unit of measurement:

      4 ÷ 2 = 2 ounces

> ***Answer***   4 tablespoons = 2 ounces

PROBLEM   24 ounces = _____ glasses

Method 1:

   a. Look at the conversion table to determine the equivalent value:

      1 glass = 8 ounces

      8 = the equivalent value

   b. Divide the equivalent value into the number next to the smaller unit of measurement:

      24 ÷ 8 = 3 glasses

> ***Answer***   24 ounces = 3 glasses

Practice Problems: Converting Units within the Household System

Directions: Convert the following household units of measurement using the equivalent value method of conversion. In the space provided, indicate the equivalent value for each problem.

			ANSWER	EQUIVALENT VALUE
1.	12 teaspoons	=	_____ ounces	_____
2.	4 ounces	=	_____ glasses	_____
3.	90 drops	=	_____ teaspoons	_____
4.	½ ounce	=	_____ tablespoons	_____
5.	6 teaspoons	=	_____ tablespoons	_____
6.	3 tablespoons	=	_____ ounces	_____
7.	18 ounces	=	_____ teacups	_____
8.	½ ounce	=	_____ teaspoons	_____
9.	3 tablespoons	=	_____ teaspoons	_____
10.	½ teaspoon	=	_____ drops	_____

UNIT 6: RATIO AND PROPORTION

Ratio and proportion are also used to convert units of measurement. This method of conversion has the advantage of clarifying the mathematical rationale for the methods of conversion previously presented. It is also useful in converting units of measurement that are more difficult to calculate, such as converting between systems, for example, when converting an apothecary unit of measurement to a metric unit of measurement.

A. Ratio and Proportion Guidelines

   Some basic guidelines must be followed when using ratio and proportion. These guidelines are described below.

   1. A **ratio** is composed of two related numbers separated by a colon. It indicates the relationship between two quantities or numbers. The ratio example below shows a relationship between milligrams and grams, i.e., 1000 mg = 1 g.

      EXAMPLE   1000 mg : 1 g

2. A **proportion** shows the relationship between two equal ratios. The proportion consists of two ratios separated by an equal sign (=) which indicates that the two ratios are equal. This proportion example shows the relationship between two equal ratios of milligrams and grams.

EXAMPLE   1000 mg : 1 g = 2000 mg : 2 g

3. The units of measurement in the two ratios of a proportion must be expressed in the same sequence. The correct sequencing in the proportion example below is mg: g = mg: g, *not* mg: g = g: mg.

EXAMPLE   *Correct:*   1000 mg : 1 g = 2000 mg : 2 g
              Incorrect: 1000 mg : 1 g = 2 g : 2000 mg

4. The numbers on the ends of a proportion are called the **extremes** while the numbers in the middle of the proportion are known as the **means**. In this example, the means consist of 1 g and 2000 mg and the extremes are 1000 mg and 2 g.

EXAMPLE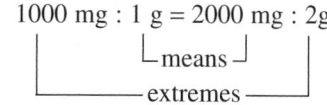
              1000 mg : 1 g = 2000 mg : 2g

5. The product of the means equals the product of the extremes. The calculation of the product of the means in the example is as follows: $1 \times 2000 = 2000$. The calculation of the product of the extremes is as follows: $1000 \times 2 = 2000$. Hence, the product of the means equals the product of the extremes or $2000 = 2000$.

EXAMPLE   1000 mg : 1 g = 2000 mg : 2 g
              $1 \times 2000 = 1000 \times 2$
              $2000 = 2000$

6. In setting up a proportion, one side of the equation consists of the known quantities and the other side of the equation consists of the unknown quantity. The letter **x** is commonly used to express the unknown quantity. To be consistent, the known quantities are indicated on the left side of the equation and the unknown quantity is indicated on the right side of the equation. Using the above proportion, but inserting an unknown quantity, or **x**, the equation is set up as follows:

EXAMPLE   1000 mg : 1 g   =   x mg : 2 g
              (known quantities)   (unknown quantity)

Practice Problems: Ratio and Proportion Guidelines

Answer the following questions:

1. What is a ratio?   _____

   _____

2. In the space provided, place a check mark next to each correct example of a ratio.

   _____ a. 15 drops : 15 minims : 1 ml

   _____ b. 1000 ml = 1 L

   _____ c. 1 ounce : 8 drams

   _____ d. 60 minims/1 fluid dram

   _____ e. 1 dram : 60 grains

   _____ f. 1 ml : 1 cc

3. What is a proportion?

   _____

   _____

   _____

4. In the space provided, place a check mark next to each correct example of a proportion.

   _____ a. 1 ml : 1 cc

   _____ b. 1 grain : 60 mg = 4 grains : 240 mg

_____ c. 2x = 60 mg

_____ d. 1000 ml : 1 L = 500 ml : 0.5 L

_____ e. 1000 mg : 1 grain = 1000 ml : 1 L

5. In the space provided, place a check mark next to each proportion that has correct sequencing for the units of measurement.

_____ a. 1000 g : 1 kg = 1500 g : 1.5 kg

_____ b. 60 grains : 1 dram = 2 drams : 120 grains

_____ c. 1000 mg : 1 g = 2000 mg : x g

6. Circle the means and underline the extremes in each of the following proportions:

   a. 1000 mg : 1 g = 500 mg : 0.5 g

   b. 2 pints : 1 quart = 4 pints : 2 quarts

   c. 1 ml : 1 cc = 2 ml : 2 cc

7. In each of the following proportions, what is the product of the means and the product of the extremes?

   a. 1000 g : 1 kg = 1500 g : 1.5 kg

   _____ product of the means

   _____ product of the extremes

   b. 60 minims : 1 fluid dram = 120 minims : 2 fluid drams

   _____ product of the means

   _____ product of the extremes

   c. 60 mg : 1 grain = 300 mg : 5 grains

   _____ product of the means

   _____ product of the extremes

8. In each of the following proportions, circle the known quantities and underline the unknown quantity.

   a. 1000 mg : 1 g = 500 mg : x g

   b. 1 g : 15 grains = 2 g : x grains

   c. 8 drams : 1 ounce = x drams : 4 ounces

B. Converting Units Using Ratio and Proportion

The method to follow to convert units using ratio and proportion is outlined below.

METHOD OF CONVERSION: To convert a unit of measurement using ratio and proportion:

   a. Look at the appropriate conversion table at the end of this chapter to determine what is known about the two units of measurement (equivalent value).
   b. State the known quantities as a ratio.
   c. Determine the unknown quantity.
   d. State the unknown quantity as a ratio.
   e. Set up the proportion with the known quantities on the left side and the unknown quantity on the right side of the equation.
   f. Solve the equation as follows: Multiply the product of the means and the product of the extremes. Divide the equation by the number(s) before the x.
   g. Include the unit of measure corresponding to x in the original equation with the answer.

Examples

PROBLEM   2 g = _____ mg

a. Look at the metric conversion table to determine what is known about the two units of measurement:

1000 mg = 1 g

b. State the known quantities as a ratio:

1000 mg : 1 g

c. Determine the unknown quantity:

2 g = x mg

d. State the unknown quantity as a ratio using the correct unit of measurement sequencing:

x mg : 2 g

e. Set up the proportion with the known quantities on the left side and the unknown quantity on the right side of the equation:

1000 mg : 1 g = x mg : 2 g

f. Solve the equation by multiplying the product of the means and the product of the extremes and dividing the equation by the number before the x:

1000 mg : 1 g = x mg : 2 g
$1 \times x = 1000 \times 2$
1x = 2000
x = 2000

g. Include the unit of measure corresponding to x in the original equation with the answer:

x = 2000 mg

> **Answer**   2 g = 2000 mg

PROBLEM

300 mg = _____ grains

The steps outlined above are followed here also. However, they are combined as they would be in working an actual conversion problem.

60 mg : 1 grain = 300 mg : x grains
$1 \times 300 = 60 \times x$
300 = 60x
$300 \div 60 = 60x \div 60$
x = 5 grains

> **Answer**   300 mg = 5 grains

Practice Problems: Converting Units Using Ratio and Proportion

Directions: Use ratio and proportion to convert between the apothecary, metric, and household systems by completing the problems below. In the space at the right, indicate what is known regarding the two units of measurement.

		ANSWER	KNOWN QUANTITIES
1. 30 minims	=	_____ ml	_____
2. 4 kg	=	_____ pounds	_____
3. 90 ml	=	_____ fluid ounces	_____
4. 30 mg	=	_____ grains	_____
5. 60 mg	=	_____ ounces	_____

6.	250 ml	=	_____ pints	_____
7.	6 g	=	_____ drams	_____
8.	1 ½ quarts	=	_____ ml	_____
9.	3 g	=	_____ grains	_____
10.	5 fluid drams	=	_____ ml	_____
11.	80 pounds	=	_____ kg	_____
12.	500 ml	=	_____ quarts	_____
13.	8 ml	=	_____ teaspoons	_____
14.	4 grains	=	_____ mg	_____
15.	32 ml	=	_____ fluid drams	_____
16.	120 mg	=	_____ grains	_____
17.	30 ml	=	_____ tablespoons	_____
18.	60 drops	=	_____ ml	_____
19.	1 ½ fluid ounces	=	_____ tablespoons	_____
20.	½ fluid ounce	=	_____ ml	_____

UNIT 7: DETERMINING DRUG DOSAGE

A. Oral Administration

Dosage refers to the amount of medication to be administered to the patient. Each medication has a certain dosage range or range of quantities that produce therapeutic effects. It is important to administer the exact drug dosage. If the dose is too small, it will not produce a therapeutic effect, whereas too large a dose could be harmful or even fatal to the patient.

The steps to follow in determining drug dosage depend on the unit of measurement in which the drug is ordered and the unit of measurement of the drug you have available, or the dose on hand. A general discussion of the method for determining drug dosage is as follows:

1. If the dose on hand is the same as that which has been ordered, no calculation is required. In this example, both the dose ordered and the dose on hand are in the same unit of measurement, and one tablet is administered to the patient.

EXAMPLE   The physician orders 50 mg of a medication po.
The drug label reads 50 mg/tablet.

2. If the dosage ordered is in the same unit of measurement as that indicated on the medication label, only one calculation step is required. In this example, both the dose ordered and the dose on hand are in the same unit of measurement, or grains. The calculation step performed will be to determine the number of tablets to administer to the patient.

EXAMPLE   The physician orders gr v̄ of a medication po.
The drug label reads gr x̄ tablet.

3. If the dosage ordered is in a different unit of measurement than indicated on the drug label, two calculation steps are required to determine the amount of medication to administer to the patient. In this example, the dose ordered and the dose on hand are stated in different units of measurement, or in grams and milligrams. The first step requires conversion of the dose ordered to the unit of measurement of the dose on hand; in this example, grams must be converted to milligrams. The second step is to determine the number of tablets to administer to the patient.

EXAMPLE   The physician orders 1 g of a medication po.
The drug label reads 500 mg/tablet.

A detailed discussion of determining drug dosage for administration of oral medication follows. The method used to calculate drug dosage when the units of measurement are the same is presented first, followed by the method used when the units of measurement are different.

Determining Drug Dosage with the Same Units of Measurement

Determining the correct drug dosage to be administered when the units of measurement are the same requires the use of a formula that is explained below.

DRUG DOSAGE FORMULA

$$\frac{D\ (\textit{dose ordered})}{H\ (\textit{on hand})} \times V\ (\textit{vehicle}) = x\ (\text{Amount of medication to be administered})$$

D (*dose ordered*): This is the amount of medication ordered by the physician.

H (*drug strength on hand*): This is the dosage strength available as indicated on the medication label or the dose on hand.

V (*vehicle*): The vehicle refers to the type of preparation containing the dose on hand (e.g., tablet, capsule, liquid).

x: The letter x is used to express the unknown quantity or the amount of medication to be administered.

GUIDELINES
1. The units of measurement must be included when setting up the problem.
2. The values for D and H must be in the same unit of measurement.
3. The value of x is expressed in the same unit as V.
4. When determining the drug dosage for oral liquid medication, the vehicle must also include the amount of liquid in which the available drug is contained. For example, if the medication label reads 250 mg/5 ml, the value of V is 5 ml.

The method to follow to determine drug dosage using this formula is outlined below. The first example illustrates determining dosage for oral solid medication.

Examples

PROBLEM   *Oral Solid Medication:*
The physician orders 50 mg of a medication po.
The medication label reads 25 mg/tablet.
How much medication should be administered to the patient?

Drug Dosage Formula:

$$\frac{D}{H} \times V = x$$

a. Identify the dose ordered.
   D = 50 mg

b. Identify the strength of the drug on hand.
   H = 25 mg

c. Determine the vehicle containing the dose on hand.
   V = 1 tablet

d. Calculate the amount of medication to administer to the patient. The units of measurement must be included when setting up the problem, and the values for D and H must be in the same unit of measurement. The value of x is expressed in the same unit as V; in this problem V = 1 tablet.

   $$\frac{50\ mg}{25\ mg} \times 1\ tablet = x$$

   $(50 \div 25 = 2) \times 1\ tablet = x$

   $2 \times 1\ tablet = x$

   $x = 2\ tablets$

Answer   2 tablets are administered to the patient.

The next problem illustrates the determination of drug dosage for oral liquid medication. The steps outlined above are followed; however, they are combined as should be done when working out drug dosage problems. Remember, with oral liquid medication, the vehicle must also include the amount of liquid in which the available drug is contained; in the problem below, V = 5 ml.

PROBLEM   *Oral Liquid Medication:*
               The physician orders 500 mg of a medication.
               The medication label reads 250 mg/5 ml.
               How much medication should be administered to the patient?

$$\frac{D}{H} \times V = x$$

$$\frac{500 \text{ mg}}{250 \text{ mg}} \times 5 \text{ ml} = x$$

$(500 \div 250 = 2) \times 5 \text{ ml} = x$

$2 \times 5 \text{ ml} = x$

$x = 10 \text{ ml}$

> **Answer**   10 ml of medication is administered to the patient.

Determining Drug Dosage with Different Units of Measurement

At times the medication ordered is in a different unit of measurement than indicated on the drug label. In this case, the desired dose quantity must be converted to the unit of measurement of the dose on hand before the drug dosage is determined. The method you use to convert a unit of measurement is based on your personal preference. Refer to Units 5 and 6 to review methods of conversion before completing this section.

> The following steps are required to determine drug dosage when the units of measurement are different:
> *Step 1:*   Convert the dose quantities to the same unit of measurement. For consistency, it is best to convert to the unit of measurement of the drug on hand.
> *Step 2:*   Determine the amount of medication to administer to the patient, using the drug dosage formula.

Examples
PROBLEM   *Oral Solid Medication:*
               The physician orders gr $\bar{x}$ of medication po.
               The medication label reads 300 mg/tablet.
               How much medication should be administered to the patient?

Step 1: The dosage ordered must be converted to the unit of measurement of the medication on hand. In this problem, 10 grains must be converted to milligrams. The ratio and proportion method of conversion is used to make the conversion.

gr $\bar{x}$ = _____ mg
1 grain : 60 mg = 10 grains : x mg
600 = 1x
x = 600 mg

> **Answer**   gr $\bar{x}$ = 600 mg

The medication ordered is now in the same unit of measurement as the medication on-hand.
Step 2: Determine the amount of medication to administer to the patient using the drug dosage formula.

$$\frac{D}{H} \times V = x$$

$$\frac{600 \text{ mg}}{300 \text{ mg}} \times 1 \text{ tablet} = x$$

$(600 \div 300 = 2) \times 1$ tablet = x
2×1 tablet = x
x = 2 tablets

> *Answer*   2 tablets are administered to the patient.

PROBLEM   *Oral Liquid Medication:*
The physician order gr $\overline{xv}$ of a medication po.
The medication label reads 300 mg/fluid dram.
How much medication should be administered to the patient?

Step 1: Convert 15 grains to milligrams using ratio and proportion:
gr $\overline{xv}$ = _____ mg
60 mg : 1 grain = x mg : 15 grains
1x = 900 mg
x = 900 mg

> *Answer*   gr $\overline{xv}$ = 900 mg

Step 2: Determine the amount of medication to administer to the patient using the drug dosage formula.
$$\frac{D}{H} \times V = x$$
$$\frac{900 \text{ mg}}{300 \text{ mg}} \times 1 \text{ fluid dram} = x$$
$(900 \div 300 = 3) \times 1$ fluid dram = x
3×1 fluid dram = x
x = 3 fluid drams

> *Answer*   3 fluid drams of medication are administered to the patient.

Practice Problems: Oral Administration

Directions: Determine the drug dosage to be administered for each of the following oral medication orders and record your answer below. In the space provided, indicate the drug category based on action for each medication using a drug reference.

Oral Solid Medications:

1. The physician orders Inderal 160 mg po.
   Medication label:

Inderal
propranolol
80 mg/capsule

How much medication should be administered? _____

Drug category: _____

2. The physician orders Tagamet gr $\overline{v}$ po.
   Medication label:

Tagament
cimetidine
300 mg/tablet

How much medication should be administered? _____

Drug category: _____

3. The physician orders Amoxil 0.5 g po.
   Medication label:

   Amoxil
   amoxicillin

   250 mg/capsule

How much medication should be administered? _____

Drug category: _____

4. The physician orders Lasix 80 mg po.
   Medication label:

   Lasix
   furosemide

   40 mg/tablet

How much medication should be administered? _____

Drug category: _____

5. The physician orders Lomotil 5 mg po.
   Medication label:

   Lomotil
   diphenoxylate/atropine

   2.5 mg/tablet

How much medication should be administered? _____

Drug category: _____

6. The physician orders Zithromax 0.5 g po.
   Medication label:

   Zithromax
   azithromycin

   250 mg/tablet

How much medication should be administered? _____

Drug category: _____

7. The physician orders Calan grtt po.
   Medication label:

   Calan
   verapamil

   40 mg/tablet

How much medication should be administered? _____

Drug category: _____

    8. The physician orders Xanax 0.5 mg po.
      Medication label:

> Xanax
> alprazolam
>
> 0.25 mg/tablet

How much medication should be administered? _____

Drug category: _____

    9. The physician orders Phenergan 25 mg po.
      Medication label:

> Phenergan
> promethazine
>
> 12.5 mg/tablet

How much medication should be administered? _____

Drug category: _____

    10. The physician orders Procardia XL gr $\overline{ss}$ po.
      Medication label:

> Procardia
> nifedipine
>
> 10 mg/tablet

How much medication should be administered? _____

Drug category: _____

Oral Liquid Medications:

    1. The physician orders Sumycin Suspension 250 mg po.
      Medication label:

> Sumycin Suspension
> tetracycline
>
> 125 mg/5 ml

How much medication should be administered? _____

Drug category: _____

    2. The physician orders Tagamet liquid 300 mg po.
      Medication label:

> Tagamet
> cimetidine liquid
>
> 300 mg/5 ml

How much medication should be administered? _____

Drug category: _____

3. The physician orders Tylenol Elixir grt po.
   Medication label:

> Tylenol Elixir
> acetaminophen
>
> 120 mg/5 ml

How much medication should be administered? _____

Drug category: _____

4. The physician orders Amoxil Suspension 0.5 g po.
   Medication label:

> Amoxil Suspension
> amoxicillin
>
> 125 mg/5 ml

How much medication should be administered? _____

Drug category: _____

5. The physician orders Gantanol Suspension 1 g po.
   Medication label:

> Gantanol Suspension
> sulfamethoxazole
>
> 500 mg/5 ml

How much medication should be administered? _____

Drug category: _____

B. Parenteral Administration

Medications for parenteral administration must be suspended in solution. The medication label indicates the amount of the drug contained in each milliliter of solution. For example, if a medication label reads 10 mg/ml, this means that there are 10 mg of medication for each ml of liquid volume. Some medications, such as penicillin, insulin, and heparin, are ordered and measured in terms of units (e.g., 300,000 units/ml). This refers to their biological activity in animal tests or the amount of the drug which is required to produce a particular response.

Parenteral medication is available in a number of dispensing forms, which include ampules, single-dose vials, and multiple-dose vials. Once the proper drug dosage has been determined, the medication is drawn into a syringe from the dispensing unit. Since most syringes are calibrated in cubic centimeters (cc), it is important to remember the equivalent value between ml and cc, or 1 ml is equal to 1 cc.

Determining drug dosage for parenteral administration is calculated in a similar manner as that for oral liquid medication as explained below. The first problem illustrates the determination of drug dosage when the medication is ordered in a different unit of measurement from the dose on-hand, requiring two calculation steps.

Examples

PROBLEM   The physician orders 0.5 g of a medication IM.
                 The medication label reads 250 mg/2 ml.
                 How much medication should be administered?

Step 1: Convert 0.5 gram to milligrams.
0.5 g = _____ mg
1000 mg : 1 g = x mg : 0.5 g
1x = 500
x = 500 mg

> **Answer**   0.5 g = 500 mg

Step 2: Determine the amount of medication to administer to the patient:

$\dfrac{D}{H} \times V = x$

$\dfrac{500 \text{ mg}}{250 \text{ mg}} \times 2 \text{ ml} = x$

$(500 \div 250 = 2) \times 2 \text{ ml} = x$

$2 \times 2 \text{ ml} = x$

$x = 4 \text{ ml (cc)}$

> **Answer**   4 cc of medication are administrated to the patient.

The next problem illustrates the determination of drug dosage with a medication ordered in units. Note that both the dose ordered and the dose on hand are in the same unit of measurement; therefore, conversion of units of measurement is not necessary.

PROBLEM   The physician orders 600,000 units of a medication IM.
                 The medication label reads 300,000 units/ml.
                 How much medication should be administered?

$\dfrac{D}{H} \times V = x$

$\dfrac{600,000 \text{ units}}{300,000 \text{ units}} \times 1 \text{ ml} = x$

$(600,000 \div 300,000 = 2) \times 1 \text{ ml} = x$

$x = 2 \text{ ml (cc)}$

> **Answer**   2 cc of medication are administrated to the patient.

Practice Problems: Parenteral Administration

Determine the drug dosage to be administered for each of the following parenteral medication orders and record your answer below. In the space provided, indicate the drug category based on action using a drug reference.

1. The physician orders Vistaril 75 mg IM.
   Medication label:

> Vistaril
> hydroxyzine injection
>
> 50 mg/ml

How much medication should be administered? _____

Drug category: _____

2. The physician orders Cobex (vitamin B$_{12}$) 200 mcg IM.
Medication label:

> Cobex
> cyanocobalamin injection
>
> 100 mcg/ml

How much medication should be administered? _____

Drug category: _____

3. The physician orders Depo-Medrol 40 mg IM.
Medication label:

> Depo-Medrol
> methylprednisolone injection
>
> 80 mg/ml

How much medication should be administered? _____

Drug category: _____

4. The physician orders Wycillin 600,000 units IM.
Medication label:

> Wycillin
> procaine penicillin G injection
>
> 300,000 units/ml

How much medication should be administered? _____

Drug category: _____

5. The physician orders Rocephin 100 mg IM.
Medication label:

> Rocephin
> ceftriaxone injection
>
> 1 g/ml

How much medication should be administered? _____

Drug category: _____

6. The physician orders INFeD 100 mg IM.
   Medication label:

> INFeD
> iron dextran injection
>
> 50 mg/ml

How much medication should be administered? _____

Drug category: _____

7. The physician orders Bicillin 1.2 million units IM.
   Medication label:

> Bicillin
> benzathine penicillin G injection
> 600,000 units/ml

How much medication should be administered? _____

Drug category: _____

8. The physician orders Depo-Provera 150 mg IM.
   Medication label:

> Depo-Provera
> medroxyprogesterone
>
> 150 mg/ml

How much medication should be administered? _____

Drug category: _____

9. The physician orders Pronestyl 0.25 g IM.
   Medication label:

> Pronestyl
> procainamide injection
>
> 500 mg/ml

How much medication should be administered? _____

Drug category: _____

10. The physician orders Compazine 7 mg IM.
    Medication label:

> Compazine
> prochlorperazine injection
>
> 5 mg/ml

How much medication should be administered? _____

Drug category: _____

Table 26-1. Metric System Conversion of Equivalent Values

WEIGHT

1000 micrograms = 1 milligram
1000 milligrams = 1 gram
1000 grams = 1 kilogram

VOLUME

1000 milliliters = 1 liter
1000 liters = 1 kiloliter
1 milliliter = 1 cubic centimeter

Table 26-2. Apothecary System: Conversion of Equivalent Values

WEIGHT

60 grains = 1 dram
8 drams = 1 ounce
12 ounces = 1 pound

VOLUME

60 minims = 1 fluid dram
8 fluid drams = 1 fluid ounce
16 fluid ounces = 1 pint
2 pints = 1 quart
4 quarts = 1 gallon

Table 26-3. Household System: Conversion of Equivalent Values

ABBREVIATIONS

drop: gtt
teaspoon: tsp
tablespoon: T
ounce: oz
cup: c

VOLUME

60 drops = 1 teaspoon
3 teaspoons = 1 tablespoon
6 teaspoons = 1 ounce
2 tablespoons = 1 ounce
6 ounces = 1 teacup
8 ounces = 1 glass
8 ounces = 1 cup

27

Cardiopulmonary Procedures

CHAPTER ASSIGNMENTS

√ After Completing	Date Due	Textbook Page(s)	TEXTBOOK ASSIGNMENTS	Possible Points	Points You Earned
		636-656	Read Chapter 27: Cardiopulmonary Procedures		
		642 655	Read Case Study 1 Case Study 1 questions	5	
		651 655	Read Case Study 2 Case Study 2 questions	5	
		653 655	Read Case Study 3 Case Study 3 questions	5	
			TOTAL POINTS		
√ After Completing	Date Due	Study Guide Page(s)	STUDY GUIDE ASSIGNMENTS (CTA: Critical Thinking Activity)	Possible Points	Points You Earned
		671	Pretest	10	
		672	Key Term Assessment	15	
		674-678	Evaluation of Learning questions	25	
		678	CTA A: Chest Leads	5	
			CD Activity: Chapter 27 Find That Lead (Record points earned)		
		679	CTA B: ECG Cycle	10	
		680	CTA C: GO TO! Game (Record points earned)		
			CD Activity: Chapter 27 It's a Cycle (Individual Player) (Record points earned)		

√ After Completing	Date Due	Study Guide Page(s)	STUDY GUIDE ASSIGNMENTS (CTA: Critical Thinking Activity)	Possible Points	Points You Earned
			CD Activity: Chapter 27 It's an Artifact (Record points earned)		
		687	CTA D: Artifacts	30	
		687	CTA E: Myocardial Infarction	20	
		691	CTA F: Crossword Puzzle	27	
		692	CTA G: Road to Recovery Game: Cardiopulmonary Procedures (Record points earned)		
			CD Activity: Chapter 27 Animations	20	
			CD Activity: Chapter 27 Apply Your Knowledge questions (Record points earned)		
		671	Posttest	10	
			ADDITIONAL ASSIGNMENTS		
			TOTAL POINTS		

√ When Assigned by Your Instructor	Study Guide Page(s)	Practices Required	LABORATORY ASSIGNMENTS (Procedure Number and Name)	*Score
	695	3	🔵 **Practice for Competency** 27-1: Running a 12-Lead, Three-Channel Electrocardiogram Textbook reference: pp. 646-648	
	697-699		📋 **Evaluation of Competency** 27-1: Running a 12-Lead, Three-Channel Electrocardiogram	*
	695	3	🔵 **Practice for Competency** 27-2: Spirometry Testing Textbook reference: pp. 653-654	
	701-703		📋 **Evaluation of Competency** 27-2: Spirometry Testing	*
			ADDITIONAL ASSIGNMENTS	

Notes

Name_____ Date _____

PRETEST

True or False

_____ 1. The cardiac cycle represents one complete heartbeat.

_____ 2. The portion of the ECG between two waves is known as a *segment*.

_____ 3. A standard ECG consists of 10 leads.

_____ 4. An electrolyte facilitates the transmission of electrical impulses.

_____ 5. Leads V_1 through V_6 are known as the *augmented leads*.

_____ 6. Electrodes that are too loose can cause an alternating current artifact.

_____ 7. When running an ECG, the medical assistant should work on the left side of the patient.

_____ 8. An ECG that is within normal limits is said to have a normal sinus rhythm.

_____ 9. The purpose of a pulmonary function test is to assess cardiac functioning.

_____ 10. In spirometry, the predicted value means what the results should be for a patient with COPD.

POSTTEST

True or False

_____ 1. An electrocardiogram is a recording of the electrical activity of the heart.

_____ 2. An amplifier is a device placed on the skin that picks up electrical impulses released by the heart.

_____ 3. The P wave represents the contraction of the ventricles.

_____ 4. If the electrocardiograph is standardized, the standardization mark will be 20 mm high.

_____ 5. Electrocardiograms are normally recorded with the paper moving at a speed of 25 mm/second.

_____ 6. A muscle artifact can be identified by its fuzzy, irregular baseline.

_____ 7. The left leg electrode is used as a ground reference when running an ECG.

_____ 8. Holter monitor electrocardiography is used to detect intermittent cardiac dysrhythmias.

_____ 9. A spirometer measures how much air is exhaled by the lungs and how fast it is exhaled.

_____ 10. Spirometry can be used to assess a patient with emphysema.

KEY TERM ASSESSMENT

Directions: Match each medical term with its definition.

_____   1. Artifact

_____   2. Atherosclerosis

_____   3. Baseline

_____   4. Cardiac cycle

_____   5. Dysrhythmia

_____   6. ECG cycle

_____   7. Electrocardiogram

_____   8. Electrocardiograph

_____   9. Electrode

_____ 10. Electrolyte

_____ 11. Interval

_____ 12. Ischemia

_____ 13. Normal sinus rhythm

_____ 14. Segment

_____ 15. Spirometer

A. A chemical substance that promotes conduction of an electrical current

B. The flat horizontal line that separates the various waves of the electrocardiogram cycle

C. The instrument used to record the electrical activity of the heart

D. Additional electrical activity picked up by the electrocardiograph that interferes with the normal appearance of the electrocardiogram cycles

E. Refers to an electrocardiogram that is within normal limits

F. One complete heartbeat

G. The graphic representation of the electrical activity of the heart

H. The length of a wave or the length of a wave with a segment

I. The graphic representation of a heartbeat

J. A conductor of electricity, which is used to promote contact between the body and the electrocardiograph

K. The portion of the electrocardiogram between two waves

L. Deficiency of blood in a body part

M. An instrument for measuring air taken into and expelled from the lungs

N. Buildup of fibrous plaques of fatty deposits and cholesterol on the inner walls of the coronary arteries

O. An irregular heart rhythm

Notes

EVALUATION OF LEARNING

Directions: Fill in each blank with the correct answer.

1. What is the purpose of electrocardiography?

   _____

   _____

   _____

2. What is the cardiac cycle?

   _____

3. Label the following on the ECG cycle:

   P wave   P-R segment

   QRS complex   S-T segment

   T wave   P-R interval

   Q-T interval

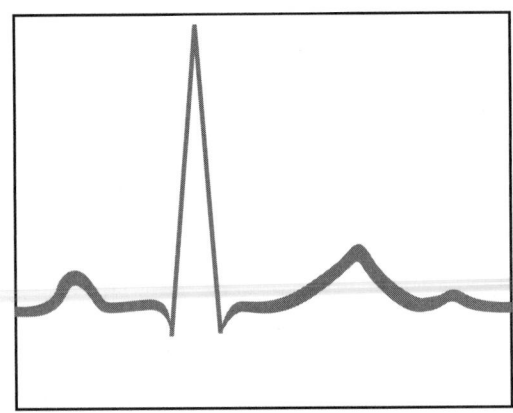

(From Bonewit-West K: *Study guide for clinical procedures for medical assistants,* ed 7, St. Louis, 2008, Saunders.)

4. Explain what each component of the ECG cycle represents.

   P wave: _____

   QRS complex: _____

   T wave: _____

   P-R segment: _____

   S-T segment: _____

   P-R interval: _____

   Q-T interval: _____

5. What is the purpose of standardizing the electrocardiograph?

_____

_____

_____

6. How high should the standardization mark be when the ECG is standardized?

_____

7. What is the function of an electrode?

_____

_____

8. Why must an electrolyte be used when recording an ECG?

_____

_____

_____

9. Diagram the bipolar leads on the following illustration:

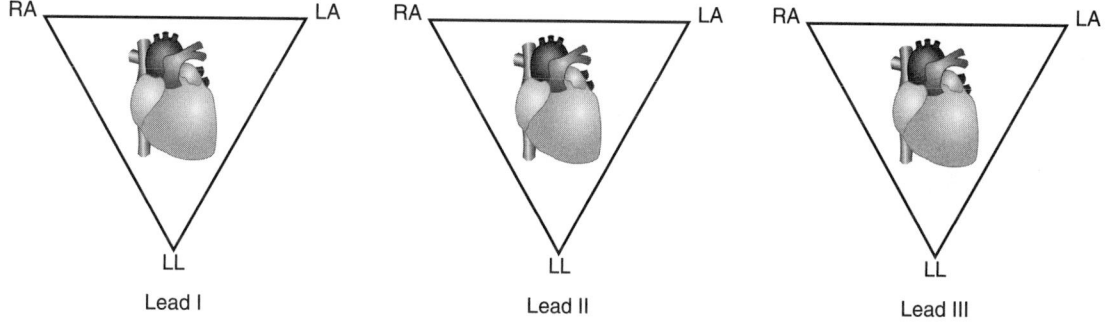

| Lead I | Lead II | Lead III |

(From Bonewit-West K: *Study guide for clinical procedures for medical assistants,* ed 7, St. Louis, 2008, Saunders.)

10. Locate and label the location of the chest leads on the following illustration:

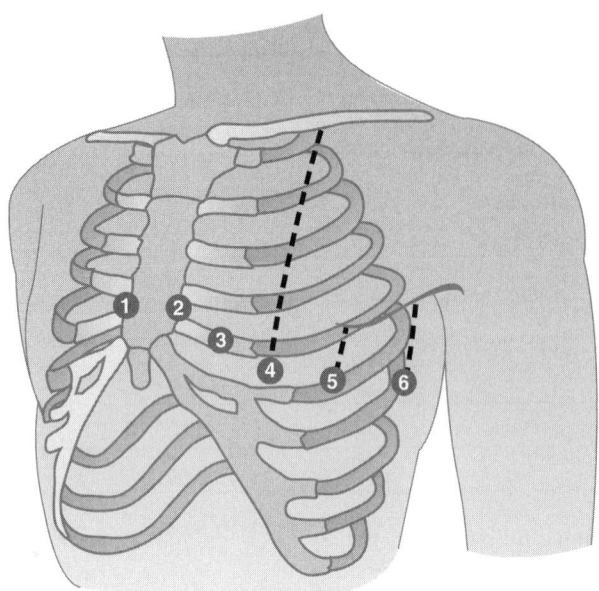

(From Bonewit-West K: *Study guide for clinical procedures for medical assistants,* ed 7, St. Louis, 2008, Saunders.)

11. A normal ECG is recorded with the paper moving at a speed of:

_____

12. What is the difference between a three-channel and a single-channel electrocardiograph?

_____

_____

_____

13. What is the purpose of each of the following electrocardiograph capabilities?

a. Teletransmission

_____

_____

b. Interpretive capability

_____

_____

14. Why should artifacts be eliminated if they occur in an ECG recording?

_____

_____

_____

15. What is the function of an artifact filter?

_____

16. List three possible causes of muscle artifacts.

_____
_____
_____

17. List two possible causes of wandering baseline.

_____
_____

18. List three possible causes of AC artifacts.

_____
_____
_____

19. List three uses of Holter monitor electrocardiography.

_____
_____
_____
_____
_____

20. List examples of cardiac dysrhythmias.

_____
_____
_____
_____

21. What is the purpose of a pulmonary function test?

_____

22. What are the indications for performing spirometry?

_____
_____
_____

23. What is forced vital capacity?

_____
_____

24. What patient preparation is required for spirometry?

_____
_____
_____

25. What is the purpose of postbronchodilator spirometry?

_____

_____

CRITICAL THINKING ACTIVITIES

A. CHEST LEADS

Practice locating the six chest leads on five different individuals. Try to select individuals of both sexes of various ages and body contours. Record each individual's name here after you have successfully located the chest leads. Also record any problems you encountered locating the leads.

1. _____

2. _____

3. _____

4. _____

5. _____

B. ECG CYCLE

Attach part of an ECG graph from a recording. Identify and label the various waves, intervals, and segments making up an ECG cycle on two different leads.

C. GO TO! GAME

Object To show your knowledge of locating the waves, intervals, and segments on an ECG cycle and answering questions relating to the ECG cycle

Needed GO TO! game board
Game cards
A small token for each player (such as a button or coin)
Score card

Directions

1. Cut out the **GO TO!** game cards.
2. Review the components of the ECG cycle.
3. Get into a group of three players.
4. Place one complete set of the game cards on the game board with the **GO TO!** question facing up and the answer facing down.
5. In turn, a player selects a game card and goes to the site indicated on the card.
6. If the player goes to the correct site, he or she is awarded 5 points. If there is a question regarding the correct site, consult your instructor.
7. The player answers the question on the game card. If the answer is correct, the player is awarded another 5 points.
8. Keep track of your points on the score card provided.
9. Continue playing until all the game cards have been used.
10. Calculate your points, and determine the knowledge level you attained.
11. If time permits, shuffle the game cards and play the game again.

GO TO!
SCORE CARD

Name: _____

Recording Points:
Cross off a number each time you go to a site correctly. Cross off another number each time you answer a question correctly. Your total points will be equal to the last number you crossed off. Record this number in the space provided and determine the knowledge level you attained.

Points:	
5	75
10	80
15	85
20	90
25	95
30	100
35	105
40	110
45	115
50	120
55	125
60	130
65	135
70	140

TOTAL POINTS: _____

LEVEL:

☐ 95 points and above: **Sheer genius!**
☐ 75 to 90 points: **Shows great promise**
☐ 55 to 70 points: **Time to study**
☐ 50 points and below: **Brain freeze**

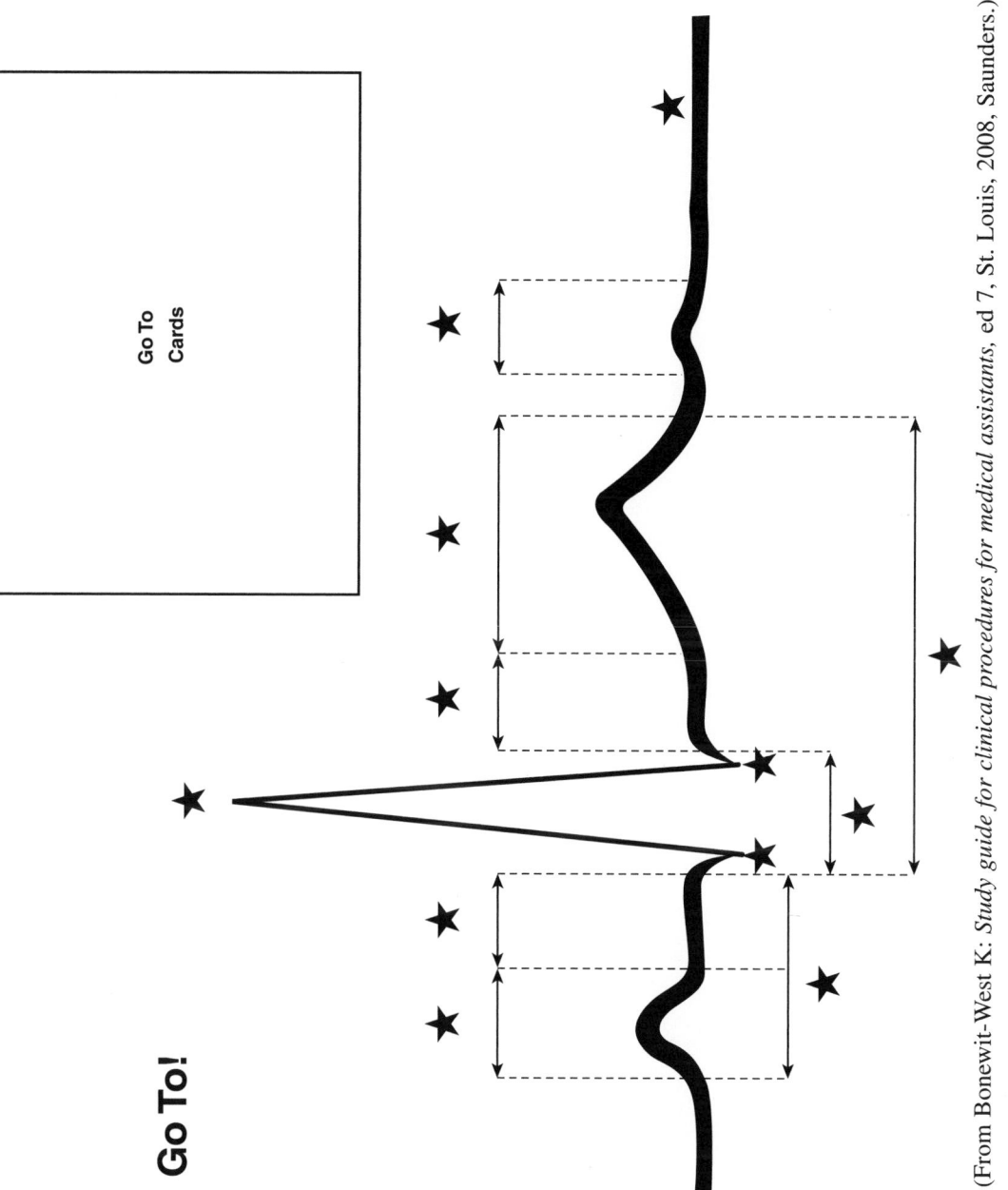

Go To!

Go To
Cards

(From Bonewit-West K: *Study guide for clinical procedures for medical assistants,* ed 7, St. Louis, 2008, Saunders.)

Notes

GO TO:

P WAVE

Q: What are the cuspid valves
doing right now?

GO TO:

Q WAVE

Q: Which heart chamber pumps blood
from the heart and out into the body?

GO TO:

R WAVE

**You're on top of the world.
Answer your question and
take another turn.**

Q: State the location of V_5.

GO TO:

S WAVE

Q: State the location of V_2.

GO TO:

T WAVE

Q: What is happening in the heart
during this time?

GO TO:

U WAVE

Q: State the location of V_1.

GO TO:

P-R SEGMENT

Q: What does this time lapse represent?

GO TO:

P-R INTERVAL

Q: What does this time lapse represent?

A: Left ventricle

A: The cuspid valves are open.

A: Fourth intercostal space at left margin of sternum

A: At horizontal level of V_4 at left anterior axillary line

A: Fourth intercostal space at right margin of sternum

A: The muscle cells of the heart are recovering in preparation for another impulse.

A: The time interval from the beginning of the atrial depolarization to the beginning of ventricular depolarization

A: The time interval from the end of the atrial depolarization to the beginning of ventricular depolarization

GO TO:

QRS COMPLEX

Q: What are the atria doing right now?

GO TO:

S-T SEGMENT

Q: What does this time interval represent?

GO TO:

Q-T INTERVAL

Q: What does this time interval represent?

GO TO:

WHERE THE ATRIA ARE CONTRACTING

Q: What are the semilunar valves doing right now?

GO TO:

WHERE THE IMPULSE IS BEING DELAYED AT THE AV NODE

Q: Why is the impulse being delayed at the AV node?

GO TO:

WHERE THE VENTRICLES ARE CONTRACTING

Q: What are the cuspid valves doing right now?

GO TO:

WHERE THE VENTRICLES ARE RECOVERING

Q: State the location of V_3.

GO TO:

WHERE THE HEART RESTS
Take a rest. Answer this question, but you lose your next turn.

Q: State the location of V_4.

A: The time interval from the end of
the ventricular depolarization to
the beginning of repolarization
of the ventricles

A: The atria are resting.

A: The semilunar valves are closed.

A: The time interval from the beginning
of the ventricular depolarization
to the end of repolarization
of the ventricles

A: The cuspid valves are closed.

A: To give the ventricles a chance
to fill with blood from the atria

A: Fifth intercostal space at
junction of the left midclavicular line

A: Midway between
V_2 and V_4 clavicular line

D. ARTIFACTS

If possible, attach examples of the following types of artifacts here:

1. Muscle artifact

2. Wandering baseline

3. Alternating current artifact

E. MYOCARDIAL INFARCTION

You are working for a cardiologist. Your physician is concerned about the increase in the numbers of patients having heart attacks. He asks you to design a colorful, creative, and informative brochure on heart attacks using the brochure provided on the following page. This brochure will be published and placed in the waiting room to provide patients with education on heart attacks. The heart disease Internet sites listed under **On the Web** in your textbook can be used to complete this activity.

Notes

FAQ
on:

Q: A:

Q: A:

Q: A:

Q: A:

Q:

A:

Q:

A:

Illustration

Q:

A:

Q:

A:

F. CROSSWORD PUZZLE
Cardiopulmonary Procedures
Directions: Complete the crossword puzzle using the clues presented below.

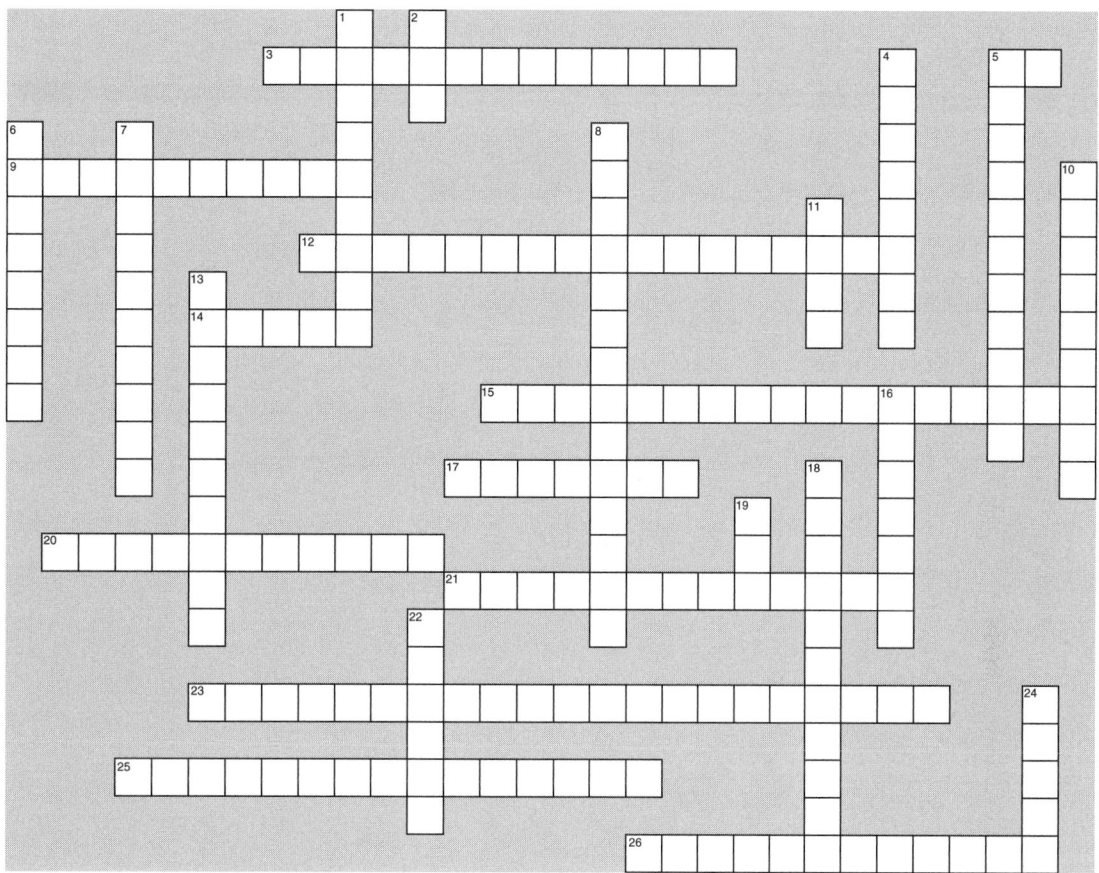

ACROSS
3 Ambulatory 24-hour ECG
5 Ground electrode
9 Small, straight, spiked lines
12 ECG within normal limits
14 Atria contract
15 "Too loose" electrodes can cause this
17 Leads I, II, III
20 Helps transmit heart's impulse
21 Drug for angina
23 ECG on a treadmill
25 Coronary artery plaque condition
26 One complete heartbeat

DOWN
1 Picks up heart's impulse
2 ECG std mark in mm
4 Not enough blood
5 Long recording of lead II
6 ECG horizontal line
7 Contraction of the ventricles
8 Drug that opens air passages
10 Damaged alveoli disease
11 Fourth intercostal to the left
13 "How well can you breathe?" test
16 Primary cause of COPD
18 Rhythm not normal
19 Take a deep breath and blow it all out!
22 Artifact from a moving patient
24 The ventricles are recovering

G. ROAD TO RECOVERY GAME: CARDIOPULMONARY PROCEDURES

Object   To lead your "patient" to recovery by correctly answering questions relating to cardiopulmonary procedures

Needed   **Road to Recovery** game board (located at the end of this manual)
                   Game cards
                   A token for each player (such as a button or coin)
                   Dice (1)
                   Score card

Directions
1. Select three other classmates to be in your group (total of four in each group).
2. Cut out the **Road to Recovery** game cards.
3. Each person in the group selects a different category from the textbook as listed below:
   a. Electrocardiography
   b. Cardiac Dysrhythmias and Highlight on Stress Testing
   c. Holter Monitor and Patient Teaching for Angina
   d. Pulmonary Function Tests and Highlight on Smoking Cessation
4. Make up 16 true/false questions for your category. Write the question on one side of the card and the answer on the opposite side (T or F).
5. Put all of the game cards together and shuffle them.
6. Place the game cards on the board with the question facing up (and the answer facing down).
7. Play **Road to Recovery** following the directions on the reverse side of the game board. (*Note:* It is all right to answer a question from your own card.) If there are questions regarding the correct answer, consult your instructor.
8. Keep track of your points using the score card provided.

**ROAD TO RECOVERY
SCORE CARD**

Name: _____

Recording Points:
Using the Game Card Points box, cross off a number each time you answer a game card correctly (starting with 5 and continuing in sequence). Your total game card points will be equal to the last number you crossed off. Record this number in the space provided (1). Record any extra points you were awarded during the game (2), and any points that were deducted (3). To determine your total points, add (1) and (2) together and deduct (3). Record this number in the Total Points Earned space provided. Compare your score with the other players and determine where you placed. Place a check mark next to the level of recovery your patient attained.

Game Card Points:			
5	75	145	215
10	80	150	220
15	85	155	225
20	90	160	230
25	95	165	235
30	100	170	240
35	105	175	245
40	110	180	250
45	115	185	255
50	120	190	260
55	125	195	265
60	130	200	270
65	135	205	275
70	140	210	280

Calculation of Points:

(1) Total Game Card Points: _____

(2) Additional Points Awarded: _____

(3) Deducted Points: _____

TOTAL POINTS EARNED: _____

LEVEL OF RECOVERY:

Patient's Name: _____

☐ First Place: **Fully Recovered**
☐ Second Place: **Almost Recovered**
☐ Third Place: **Still Recovering**
☐ Fourth Place: **Gasping for Air**

Question:	Question:	Question:	Question:
Question:	Question:	Question:	Question:
Question:	Question:	Question:	Question:
Question:	Question:	Question:	Question:

Answer:	Answer:	Answer:	Answer:
Answer:	Answer:	Answer:	Answer:
Answer:	Answer:	Answer:	Answer:
Answer:	Answer:	Answer:	Answer:

PRACTICE FOR COMPETENCY

Procedure 27-1: 12-Lead Electrocardiogram. Practice the procedure for running a 12-lead electrocardiogram, and record the procedure in the chart provided.

Procedure 27-2: Spirometry. Practice the procedure for performing a spirometry test, and record the procedure in the chart provided.

CHART	
Date	

CHART	
Date	

EVALUATION OF COMPETENCY

Procedure 27-1: Running a 12-Lead, Three-Channel Electrocardiogram

Name: _____ Date: _____

Evaluated By: _____ Score: _____

Performance Objective

Outcome:	Record a 12-lead electrocardiogram.
Conditions:	Using a three-channel electrocardiograph.
	Given ECG paper and disposable electrodes.
Standards:	Time: 15 minutes. Student completed procedure in _____ minutes.
	Accuracy: Satisfactory score on the Performance Evaluation Checklist.

Performance Evaluation Checklist

Trial 1	Trial 2	Point Value	Performance Standards
		●	Worked in a quiet atmosphere away from sources of electrical interference.
		●	Sanitized hands.
		●	Greeted the patient and introduced yourself.
		●	Identified the patient and explained the procedure.
		●	Instructed the patient that he/she will need to lie still and not talk during the procedure.
		▷	Explained why the patient should lie still and not talk.
		●	Asked patient to remove appropriate clothing.
		●	Assisted patient into a supine position on the table.
		●	Made sure that patient's arms and legs were adequately supported on the table.
		●	Draped patient properly.
		●	Positioned the electrocardiograph with the power cord pointing away from patient and not passing under the table.
		●	Worked on the left side of the patient.
		●	Prepared the patient's skin for application of the disposable electrodes.
		▷	Explained why the patient's skin must be prepared properly.
		●	Applied the limb electrodes.
		●	Properly located each chest position and applied the chest electrodes.
		▷	Explained why the tabs of the electrodes should be positioned correctly.
		●	Connected the lead wires to the electrodes.

Trial 1	Trial 2	Point Value	Performance Standards
		•	Arranged lead wires to follow body contour.
		▷	Explained why the lead wires should follow body contour.
		•	Plugged the patient cable into machine and properly supported the cable.
		•	Turned on the electrocardiograph.
		•	Entered patient data using the soft-touch keypad.
		▷	Stated the purpose of entering patient data.
		•	Reminded patient to lie still and pressed the AUTO button to run the recording.
		•	Checked to make sure the standardization mark is 10 mm high.
		•	Checked to make sure the R wave has a positive deflection.
		▷	Stated what would cause the R wave to have a negative deflection.
		•	Checked the recording for artifacts and corrected them if they occurred.
		•	Informed the patient that he/she can move and talk.
		•	Turned off the electrocardiograph.
		•	Disconnected the lead wires.
		•	Removed and discarded the disposable electrodes.
		•	Assisted patient from the table.
		•	Sanitized hands.
		•	Charted the procedure correctly.
		•	Placed the recording in the appropriate place to be reviewed by physician.
		•	Returned equipment to proper place.
		∗	Completed the procedure within 15 minutes.
			TOTALS

	CHART
Date	

Evaluation of Student Performance

EVALUATION CRITERIA			COMMENTS
Symbol	Category	Point Value	
✳	Critical Step	16 points	
●	Essential Step	6 points	
▷	Theory Question	2 points	

Score calculation: 100 points

– _____ points missed

_____ Score

Satisfactory score: 85 or above

CAAHEP Competencies Achieved:

Psychomotor (Skills)
☑ I. 5. Perform electrocardiography.

Affective (Behavior)
☑ I.2. Use language/verbal skills that enable patients' understanding.
☑ XI. 1. Recognize the effects of stress on all persons involved in emergency situations.

ABHES Competencies Achieved:

☑ 8. cc. Communicate on the recipient's level of comprehension.
☑ 9. o. Perform: (1) Electrocardiograms.

Notes

EVALUATION OF COMPETENCY

(DVD) **Procedure 27-2: Spirometry Testing**

Name: _____ Date: _____

Evaluated By: _____ Score: _____

Performance Objective

Outcome:	Perform a spirometry test.
Conditions:	Using a monitor.
	Given the following: disposable tubing, disposable mouthpiece, disposable nose clips, waste container.
Standards:	Time: 20 minutes. Student completed procedure in _____ minutes.
	Accuracy: Satisfactory score on the Performance Evaluation Checklist.

Performance Evaluation Checklist

Trial 1	Trial 2	Point Value	Performance Standards
		●	Sanitized hands.
		●	Assembled and prepared equipment.
		●	Calibrated the spirometer.
		▷	Stated the reason for calibrating the spirometer.
		●	Applied a disposable mouthpiece to the mouthpiece holder.
		●	Greeted the patient and introduced yourself.
		●	Identified the patient and explained the procedure.
		●	Asked the patient if he/she prepared properly.
		●	Asked the patient to remove heavy or restrictive clothing and to loosen tight clothing.
		▷	Explained why tight clothing should be loosened.
		●	Measured the patient's weight and height.
		▷	Explained the reason for measuring weight and height.
		●	Asked the patient to sit near the machine.
		●	Entered patient data into the computer database of the spirometer.
			Described and demonstrated the breathing maneuver:
		●	Relax and take the deepest breath possible.
		●	Place the mouthpiece in your mouth and seal your lips tightly around it.
		●	Blow out as hard as you can for as long as possible.

Trial 1	Trial 2	Point Value	Performance Standards
		●	Do not block the opening of the mouthpiece with your tongue.
		●	Remove the mouthpiece from your mouth.
		▷	Explained why the lips should be tightly sealed around the mouthpiece.
		●	Told the patient the instructions would be repeated during the test.
		●	Encouraged the patient to remain calm.
		●	Gently applied the nose clips.
		▷	Stated the purpose of the nose clips.
		●	Handed mouthpiece to patient.
		●	Began the test and actively coached the patient.
		●	Informed patient of modifications needed if breathing maneuver was not performed correctly.
		●	Continued the test until three acceptable efforts were obtained.
		●	Gently removed the nose clips from patient's nose.
		●	Removed the mouthpiece from its holder.
		●	Disposed of nose clips and mouthpiece in a waste container.
		●	Allowed the patient to remain seated for a few minutes.
		●	Sanitized your hands.
		●	Printed the report and labeled it.
		●	Charted the procedure correctly.
		●	Placed the spirometry report in appropriate location for review by the physician.
		●	Cleaned the spirometer.
		∗	Completed the procedure within 20 minutes.
			TOTALS

	CHART
Date	

Evaluation of Student Performance

EVALUATION CRITERIA			COMMENTS
Symbol	Category	Point Value	
*	Critical Step	16 points	
•	Essential Step	6 points	
▷	Theory Question	2 points	

Score calculation: 100 points

−_____ points missed

_____ Score

Satisfactory score: 85 or above

CAAHEP Competencies Achieved:

Psychomotor (Skills)
☑ I. 4. Perform pulmonary function testing.

Affective (Behavior)
☑ I.2. Use language/verbal skills that enable patients' understanding.

ABHES Competencies Achieved:

☑ 8. cc. Communicate on the recipient's level of comprehension.
☑ 9. o. Perform: (2) Respiratory testing.

Notes

28

Specialty Examinations and Procedures:
Colon Procedures
Male Reproductive Health
Radiology and Diagnostic Imaging

CHAPTER ASSIGNMENTS

√ After Completing	Date Due	Textbook Page(s)	TEXTBOOK ASSIGNMENTS	Possible Points	Points You Earned
		657-680	Read Chapter 28: Specialty Examinations and Procedures: Colon Procedures, Male Reproductive Health, and Radiology and Diagnostic Imaging		
		662 678	📝 Read Case Study 1 Case Study 1 questions	5	
		668 678-679	📝 Read Case Study 2 Case Study 2 questions	5	
		677 679	📝 Read Case Study 3 Case Study 3 questions	5	
			TOTAL POINTS		

√ After Completing	Date Due	Study Guide Page(s)	STUDY GUIDE ASSIGNMENTS (CTA: Critical Thinking Activity)	Possible Points	Points You Earned
		709	❓ Pretest	10	
		710	🔑 Key Term Assessment	22	
		711-715	📋 Evaluation of Learning questions	47	
		716	CTA A: FOBT Diet and Medication Modifications Game (Record points earned)		

√ After Completing	Date Due	Study Guide Page(s)	STUDY GUIDE ASSIGNMENTS (CTA: Critical Thinking Activity)	Possible Points	Points You Earned
		721	CTA B: FOBT Patient Preparation	10	
		721	CTA C: Sigmoidoscopy	10	
		721	CTA D: Dear Gabby	10	
		722	CTA E: Crossword Puzzle	24	
		723	CTA F: Lower GI	5	
		723	CTA G: Intravenous Pyelogram (IVP)	5	
		723-724	CTA H: Magnetic Resonance Imaging	7	
		725	CTA I: Crossword Puzzle	21	
			💿 CD Activity: Chapter 28 Animations	20	
			💿 CD Activity: Chapter 28 Apply Your Knowledge questions (Record points earned)		
		709	📰 Posttest	10	
			ADDITIONAL ASSIGNMENTS		
			TOTAL POINTS		

√ When Assigned by Your Instructor	Study Guide Page(s)	Practices Required	LABORATORY ASSIGNMENTS (Procedure Number and Name)	*Score
	727	5	**(DVD) Practice for Competency** 28-1 and 28-2: Fecal Occult Blood Testing: Guaiac Slide Test Method Textbook reference: pp. 662-665	
	729-731		**Evaluation of Competency** 28-1 and 28-2: Fecal Occult Blood Testing: Guaiac Slide Test Method	*
	727	3	**Practice for Competency** 28-A: Preparation for Radiology Examinations Textbook reference: pp. 671-674	
	733-734		**Evaluation of Competency** 28-A: Preparation for Radiology Examinations	*
	727	3	**Practice for Competency** 28-B: Preparation for Diagnostic Imaging Procedures Textbook reference: pp. 674-678	
	735-736		**Evaluation of Competency** 28-B: Preparation for Diagnostic Imaging Procedures	*
			ADDITIONAL ASSIGNMENTS	

Notes

Name _____   Date _____

? PRETEST

True or False

_____ 1. Invisible blood in the stool is termed *melena*.

_____ 2. Colorectal cancer is a common form of cancer in individuals older than 40 years.

_____ 3. If a Hemoccult test is positive, the physician may order a coronary angiogram.

_____ 4. Prostate screening is recommended once a year for men older than 50.

_____ 5. The most common sign of testicular cancer is a small, hard, painless lump on the testicle.

_____ 6. The permanent record of the picture produced on x-ray film is a sonogram.

_____ 7. Mammography can be used to detect breast calcifications.

_____ 8. An IVP is a radiograph of the kidneys and urinary tract.

_____ 9. Ultrasonography allows for continuous viewing of a structure.

_____ 10. A patient does not need to remove metal before having an MRI.

? POSTTEST

True or False

_____ 1. Consuming red meat may cause a false-positive result on a Hemoccult test.

_____ 2. The Hemoccult test should be stored in the refrigerator after applying a stool specimen to it.

_____ 3. A flexible sigmoidoscopy can be used to diagnose colorectal cancer.

_____ 4. There are often no symptoms in the early stages of prostate cancer.

_____ 5. A PSA level of 20 is within normal range.

_____ 6. Bone is an example of a radiolucent structure.

_____ 7. Patient movement during a radiographic examination causes confusing shadows on the film.

_____ 8. The breasts are compressed during mammography to prevent radiation burns.

_____ 9. CT produces a series of cross-sectional images.

_____ 10. A radioactive material is introduced into the body before a nuclear medicine imaging procedure is performed.

Term KEY TERM ASSESSMENT

Directions: Match each medical term with its definition.

_____ 1. Biopsy

_____ 2. Colonoscopy

_____ 3. Contrast medium

_____ 4. Echocardiogram

_____ 5. Endoscope

_____ 6. Enema

_____ 7. Fluoroscope

_____ 8. Fluoroscopy

_____ 9. Insufflate

_____ 10. Melena

_____ 11. Occult blood

_____ 12. Peroxidase

_____ 13. Radiograph

_____ 14. Radiography

_____ 15. Radiologist

_____ 16. Radiology

_____ 17. Radiolucent

_____ 18. Radiopaque

_____ 19. Sigmoidoscope

_____ 20. Sigmoidoscopy

_____ 21. Sonogram

_____ 22. Ultrasonography

A. The visualization of the entire colon using a colonoscope

B. Blood occurring in such a small amount that it is not visually detectable by the unaided eye

C. The surgical removal and examination of tissue from the living body

D. The visual examination of the rectum and sigmoid colon using a sigmoidoscope

E. The darkening of the stool caused by the presence of blood in an amount of 50 ml or greater

F. An instrument that consists of a tube and an optical system that is used for direct visual inspection of organs or cavities

G. A substance that is able to transfer oxygen from hydrogen peroxide to oxidize guaiac, causing the guaiac to turn blue

H. An endoscope that is specially designed for passage through the anus to permit visualization of the rectum and sigmoid colon

I. To blow a powder, vapor, or gas (such as air) into a body cavity.

J. A permanent record of a picture of an internal body organ or structure produced on radiographic film

K. A medical doctor who specializes in the diagnosis and treatment of disease using radiant energy such as x-rays, radium, and radioactive material

L. A substance used to make a particular structure visible on a radiograph

M. The record obtained with ultrasonography

N. An injection of fluid into the rectum to aid in the elimination of feces from the colon

O. The branch of medicine that deals with the use of radiant energy in the diagnosis and treatment of disease

P. An instrument used to view internal organs and structures directly

Q. Describing a structure that obstructs the passage of x-rays

R. The taking of permanent records of internal body organs and structures by passing x-rays through the body to act on a specially sensitized film

S. Describing a structure that permits the passage of x-rays

T. Examination of a patient with a fluoroscope

U. An ultrasound examination of the heart

V. The use of high-frequency sound waves to produce an image of an organ or tissue

EVALUATION OF LEARNING

Colon Procedures and Male Reproductive Health

Fill in each blank with the correct answer.

1. List five causes of blood in the stool.

   _____

   _____

   _____

2. Define the term *melena*, and explain what causes it.

   _____

   _____

   _____

   _____

3. What is the primary reason for screening patients for the presence of fecal occult blood?

   _____

   _____

4. Why must three stool specimens be obtained for the guaiac slide test?

   _____

   _____

   _____

5. List two reasons for placing a patient on a high-fiber diet when testing for fecal occult blood.

   _____

   _____

   _____

6. List examples of medications that must be discontinued before guaiac slide testing.

   _____

   _____

7. List two factors that could cause false-positive test results on a guaiac slide test.

   _____

   _____

8. List three examples of diagnostic tests that may be performed if the guaiac slide test is positive.

   _____

   _____

   _____

9. Why is it important to perform quality control methods when developing the guaiac slide test?

   _____

   _____

10. What is the purpose of performing a sigmoidoscopy?

_____

_____

_____

11. Describe the advance patient preparation that may be required for a sigmoidoscopy.

_____

_____

_____

_____

12. What is the purpose of the digital rectal examination?

_____

_____

_____

13. What is the purpose of insufflating air into the colon during a sigmoidoscopy?

_____

_____

14. What is the purpose of suctioning during sigmoidoscopy?

_____

_____

15. What is the recommended patient position for flexible fiberoptic sigmoidoscopy?

_____

16. Where is the prostate gland located?

_____

_____

17. What are the symptoms of prostate cancer?

_____

_____

_____

18. How is the digital rectal examination used for the early detection of prostate cancer?

_____

_____

19. What is the purpose of the PSA test?

_____

_____

20. What is the PSA level for each of the following?

   a. Normal range: _____

b. Slightly elevated range: _____

c. Moderately elevated range: _____

d. Highly elevated: _____

21. What patient preparation is required for a PSA test?

_____

_____

22. What tests may be ordered by the physician if the patient has positive prostate screening results?

_____

_____

23. What are the risk factors for testicular cancer?

_____

_____

24. What is the most common sign of testicular cancer?

_____

_____

Radiology and Diagnostic Imaging
Directions: Fill in each blank with the correct answer.

1. Who discovered x-rays?

_____

2. What is the function of x-rays?

_____

_____

3. Why is it so important for a patient to prepare properly for a radiographic examination?

_____

_____

4. What is the function of a radiopaque contrast medium?

_____

_____

5. What is the purpose of mammography?

_____

_____

_____

6. Why must the breasts be compressed during mammography?

_____

_____

7. What is the purpose of the upper GI radiographic examination?

_____

_____

_____

8. Why must the GI tract be free of food and fluid before an upper GI is performed?

_____

_____

9. A lower GI radiographic examination assists in the diagnosis of what conditions?

_____

_____

10. Why is it important to remove gas and fecal material from the colon before a lower GI radiographic examination is performed?

_____

_____

11. What is an intravenous pyelogram?

_____

_____

12. What type of patient preparation is required for an IVP?

_____

_____

_____

_____

13. Define the following:

a. Angiocardiogram

_____

_____

b. Bronchogram

_____

_____

c. Coronary angiogram

_____

_____

d. Cerebral angiogram

_____

_____

e. Cystogram

_____

_____

14. What are the primary uses of ultrasonography?

_____

_____

15. What are the advantages of ultrasonography?

_____

_____

_____

16. What is the purpose of performing an obstetric US?

_____

_____

_____

17. What are the primary uses of computed tomography?

_____

_____

_____

18. What type of images are produced by computed tomography?

_____

_____

19. What type of patient preparation is required for computed tomography?

_____

_____

_____

_____

20. What are the primary uses of MRI?

_____

_____

_____

21. What material is used with a nuclear medicine diagnostic imaging procedure?

_____

22. What are the most common nuclear medicine diagnostic imaging procedures?

_____

_____

23. What are the advantages of digital imaging technology?

_____

_____

_____

CRITICAL THINKING ACTIVITIES

A. FOBT DIET AND MEDICATION MODIFICATIONS GAME

Object To show your knowledge of foods and medications that are permitted and not permitted before and during an FOBT using a guaiac slide test

Needed Game cards

Directions

1. Cut out the game cards.
2. Determine if each food and medication is permitted or not permitted before and during FOBT using the guaiac slide test.
3. On one side of the card, indicate if it is permitted by placing a *P* on the card. If it is not permitted, place an *NP* on the reverse side of the card.
4. Choose a partner, and place one complete set of game cards on a flat surface between both players with the food or medication facing up.
5. Taking turns, select a game card, and indicate if the food or medication is permitted or not permitted before and during an FOBT.
6. If the player gives the correct answer, he or she is awarded 5 points. If there is a question regarding an answer, consult your instructor.
7. Keep track of your points on the score card provided. Continue playing until all the game cards have been used.
8. Calculate your points, and determine the knowledge level you attained.
9. If time permits, shuffle the game cards, and play the game again.

**FOBT
SCORE CARD**

Name: _____

Recording Points:
Cross off a number each time you go to a site correctly. Cross off another number each time you answer a question correctly. Your points will be equal to the last number you crossed off. Record this number in the space provided and determine the knowledge level you attained.

Points:	
5	75
10	80
15	85
20	90
25	95
30	100
35	105
40	110
45	115
50	120
55	125
60	130
65	135
70	140

TOTAL POINTS: _____

LEVEL OF KNOWLEDGE:

☐ 75 points and above: **Sheer genius!**
☐ 55 to 70 points: **Shows great promise**
☐ 35 to 50 points: **Time to study**
☐ Below 35 points: **Brain freeze**

Vitamin C	Corticosteroid	Turnip	Bacon
Iron Supplement	Bran Cereal	Green Beans	Oatmeal
Aspirin	Pear	Vitamin A	Carrots
Popcorn	Horseradish	Calcium Supplement	Lamb

Chicken	Celery	Apple	Whole Wheat Bread
Fish	Corn	Radish	Melon
Liver	Spinach	Cauliflower	Peach
Red Meat	Lettuce	Broccoli	Banana

B. FOBT PATIENT PREPARATION

Frank Morrison has been given a Hemoccult slide kit for an FOBT. In the space provided, plan a breakfast, lunch, and dinner meal for him following the FOBT patient preparation guidelines on page 661 of your textbook.

_____

_____

_____

_____

_____

_____

C. SIGMOIDOSCOPY

Ken Hofmann has been scheduled to have a sigmoidoscopy. He asks for your help in planning a light evening meal containing low-residue foods. In the space provided, plan a balanced evening meal for Mr. Hofmann.

_____

_____

_____

_____

_____

D. DEAR GABBY

Gabby broke her wrist while skating and wants you to fill in for her. Respond to the following letter using the knowledge you have acquired in this chapter.

Dear Gabby:

I am 15 years old and my mom just took me to a new doctor for a sports physical examination. I am going to play football this fall at my high school. Before this, I had always gone to the doctor I had since I was little, but I had to switch since I am getting older. After the doctor did my physical, he told me that I needed to examine my testicles every month, and that the medical assistant would be in to explain how it is done.

Gabby, I was totally shocked, and you can bet I got out of that office before she had a chance to do that. I am too embarrassed to ask my parents about this. Gabby, what is going on? I am only 15 years old. Are my parents taking me to a quack, and should I report this to someone?

Signed,

Don't Know What to Do

_____

_____

_____

_____

_____

_____

_____

_____

_____

_____

E. CROSSWORD PUZZLE
Colon Procedures and Male Reproductive Health
Directions: Complete the crossword puzzle using the clues presented below.

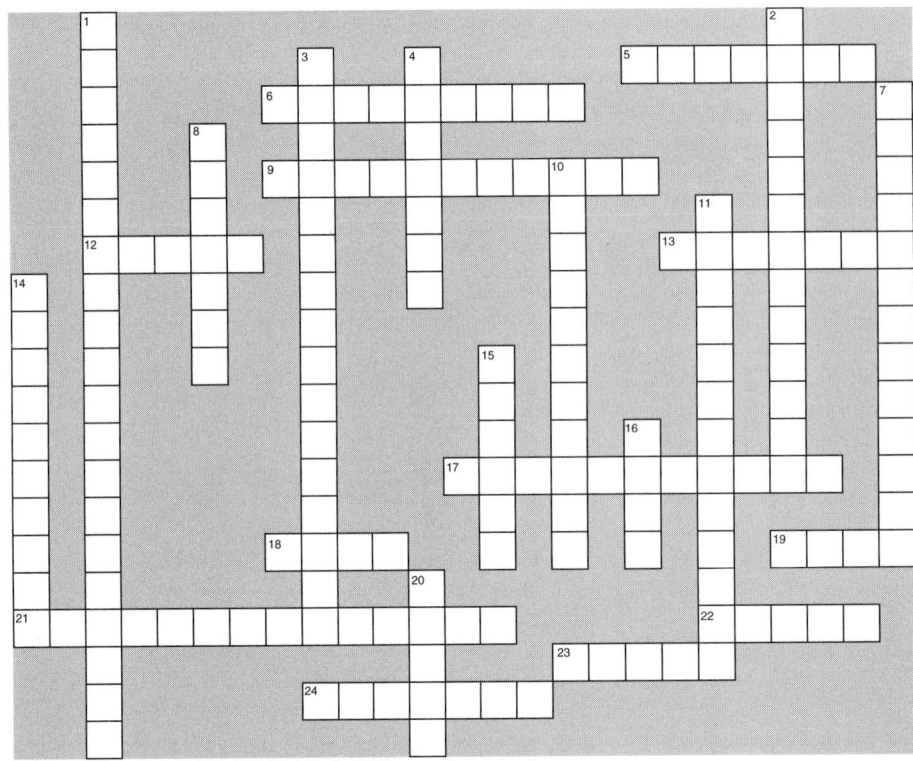

(From Bonewit-West K: *Study guide for today's medical assistant,* ed 7, St. Louis, 2008, Saunders.)

ACROSS	DOWN
5 Med to avoid during FOBT	**1** Testicular CA risk factor
6 How to clean sigmoidoscope	**2** Secretes fluid that transports sperm
9 Visualization of colon	**3** Increases PSA level
12 Pt prep for flex sigmoid	**4** Cause of CRC
13 Age to start TSE	**7** Increases risk of CRC
17 Can cause blood in the stool	**8** Can cause false-positive result on FOBT
18 Pt position for flex sig	**10** Nonvisible blood
19 Color of positive Hemoccult	**11** May be done after a positive FOBT
21 Symptom of CRC	**14** Leading cause of CA deaths
22 CRC often starts from this	**15** Black and tarlike stool
23 CRC increases after this age	**16** May be done after elevated PSA
24 Prostate CA screening test	**20** Prostate CA increases after this age

F. LOWER GI

Trent Douglas has been having pain in his lower abdomen and occult blood in his stool. Dr. Hartman tells you to schedule him for a lower GI radiographic examination at Grant Hospital. Explain how you would instruct Mr. Douglas to prepare for this examination. Include the patient preparation and the reason for each of the measures.

_____

_____

_____

_____

_____

_____

G. INTRAVENOUS PYELOGRAM (IVP)

Dr. Tristen instructs you to schedule Ellie Ray for an intravenous pyelogram (IVP) at Grant Hospital. After you have explained to Ms. Ray the instructions for preparing for the examination, she asks you the following questions. Respond to them in the space provided.

1. What body structures will be x-rayed during the examination?

_____

_____

_____

2. Why must gas and fecal material be removed from the intestines?

_____

_____

_____

3. Why will iodine be injected into my veins?

_____

_____

_____

4. Will I feel anything when the iodine is injected?

_____

_____

_____

5. What is done if an individual is allergic to iodine?

_____

_____

H. MAGNETIC RESONANCE IMAGING

Jason Zindra, a college baseball player, has been experiencing pain in his left shoulder joint. Dr. Baker schedules him for MRI of the left shoulder. Jason asks you the following questions regarding this procedure. Respond to them in the space provided.

1. Is this a safe procedure?

_____

_____

2. Will there be any pain involved with this procedure?

_____

_____

3. Will I be exposed to x-rays?

_____

_____

4. What should I wear to the test?

_____

_____

5. May I wear my watch during the procedure to keep track of the time?

_____

_____

6. Does the MRI machine make any noise?

_____

_____

7. Will the technician be in the room with me?

_____

_____

I. CROSSWORD PUZZLE
Radiology and Diagnostic Imaging
Directions: Complete the crossword puzzle using the clues provided below.

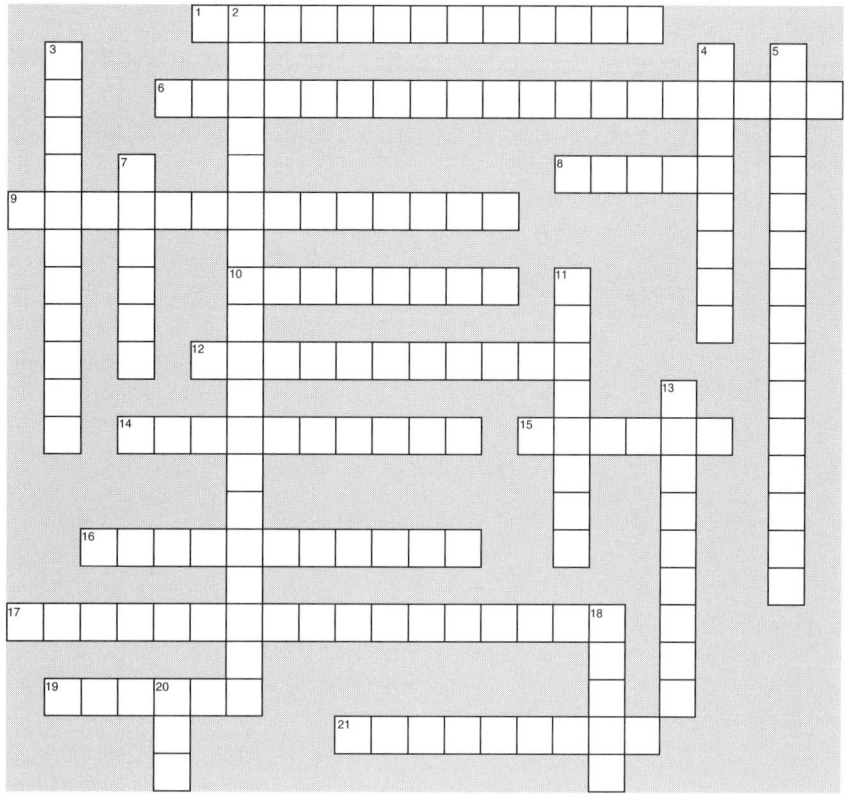

ACROSS
1 Radiograph of bile ducts
6 Can tell if it is twins
8 Color of radiolucent structure
9 US of heart
10 US recording
12 For direct viewing of internal organs
14 Obstructs x-rays
15 Produces cross-sectional images
16 X-ray doctor
17 Radiograph of coronary arteries
19 Lower GI contrast medium
21 Radiograph of urinary bladder

DOWN
2 Radiograph of uterus and fallopian tubes
3 Radiograph of the lungs
4 Detects a stress fracture
5 Radiograph of the heart
7 IVP contrast medium
11 Discovered x-rays
13 Breast radiograph
18 Remove during an MRI
20 Used to diagnose kidney stones

Notes

PRACTICE FOR COMPETENCY

Procedure 28-1 and 28-2: Hemoccult Slide Test
1. **Patient Instructions.** Instruct an individual in the specimen collection procedure for a Hemoccult slide test. Record patient instructions in the chart provided.
2. **Developing the Test.** Develop a Hemoccult test, and record the results in the chart provided.

Procedure 28-A: Radiology Examinations. Instruct a patient in the proper preparation required for each of the following types of radiographic examinations: Mammogram, Upper GI, Lower GI, and Intravenous Pyelogram. Record the procedure in the chart provided.

Procedure 28-B: Diagnostic Imaging Procedures. Instruct a patient in the proper preparation required for each of the following types of diagnostic imaging procedures: Ultrasonography, Computed Tomography, Magnetic Resonance Imaging, and Nuclear Medicine. Record the procedure in the chart provided.

CHART	
Date	

CHART	
Date	

EVALUATION OF COMPETENCY

Procedures 28-1 and 28-2: Fecal Occult Blood Testing: Guaiac Slide Test Method

Name: _____   Date: _____

Evaluated By: _____   Score: _____

Performance Objective

Outcome:	Instruct an individual in the specimen collection procedure for a Hemoccult slide test and develop the test.
Conditions:	Given the following: Hemoccult slide testing kit, developing solution, reference card, and a waste container.
Standards:	Time: 15 minutes. Student completed procedure in ____ minutes.
	Accuracy: Satisfactory score in the Performance Evaluation Checklist.

Performance Evaluation Checklist

Trial 1	Trial 2	Point Value	Performance Standards
			Instructions for the Hemoccult Slide Test
		●	Obtained the Hemoccult slide testing kit.
		●	Checked expiration date on the slides.
		▷	Described what might occur if the slides are outdated.
		●	Greeted the patient and introduced yourself.
		●	Identified the patient and explained purpose of the test.
		●	Informed patient when the test should not be performed.
		●	Instructed patient in the proper preparation required for the test.
		●	Encouraged patient to adhere to the diet modifications.
		▷	Explained why the patient should follow the diet modifications.
		●	Provided patient with the Hemoccult slide test kit.
		●	Instructed patient in completion of the information on the front flap of each card.
		●	Provided instructions on the proper care and storage of the slides.
		▷	Explained why the slides must be stored properly.
			Instructed the patient in the initiation of the test by:
		●	Beginning the diet modifications.
		●	Collecting a stool specimen from the first bowel movement after the 3-day preparatory period.
			Instructed the patient in the proper collection of the stool specimen:
		●	Fill in the collection date on the front flap.

Trial 1	Trial 2	Point Value	*Performance Standards*
		●	Use a clean, dry container to collect the stool specimen.
		●	Collect the stool sample before it comes in contact with toilet bowl water.
		●	Use the wooden applicator to obtain specimen from one part of the stool.
		●	Open the front flap of the first cardboard slide.
		●	Spread a thin smear of the specimen over the filter paper in the square labeled "A."
		●	Obtain another specimen from a different area of the stool, using the other end of the applicator.
		●	Spread a thin smear of the specimen over the filter paper in the square labeled "B."
		●	Close the front flap of the cardboard slide and fill in the date.
		●	Discard the applicator in a waste container.
		▷	Explained why a sample is collected from two different parts of the stool.
		●	Instructed patient to place slides in a regular envelope to air-dry overnight.
		●	Instructed patient to continue the testing period on 3 different days until all three specimens have been obtained.
		●	Instructed patient to place the cardboard slides in the foil envelope and return them to the medical office.
		●	Provided patient with an opportunity to ask questions.
		●	Made sure the patient understood the instructions.
		●	Charted in the patient's record.
			Developing the Hemoccult Slide Test
		●	Assembled equipment.
		●	Checked expiration date on the developing solution bottle.
		▷	Explained how the solution should be stored.
		●	Sanitized hands and applied gloves.
		●	Opened the back flap of the cardboard slides.
		●	Applied two drops of the developing solution to the guaiac test paper underlying the back of each smear.
		●	Did not allow the developing solution to come in contact with skin or eyes.
		●	Read results within 60 seconds.
		●	The results were identical to the evaluator's results.
		▷	Explained why the slides should be read within 60 seconds.
		●	Performed the quality-control procedure on each slide.
		●	Read the quality-control results after 10 seconds.
		▷	Described what is observed during a normal positive and negative control reaction.

Trial 1	Trial 2	Point Value	Performance Standards
		▷	Stated the purpose of the quality-control procedure.
		●	Properly disposed of the slides in a regular waste container.
		●	Removed gloves and sanitized hands.
		●	Charted the results correctly.
		✳	Completed the procedure within 15 minutes.
			TOTALS

CHART	
Date	

Evaluation of Student Performance

EVALUATION CRITERIA			COMMENTS
Symbol	Category	Point Value	
✳	Critical Step	16 points	
●	Essential Step	6 points	
▷	Theory Question	2 points	

Score calculation: 100 points

−_____ points missed

_____ Score

Satisfactory score: 85 or above

CAAHEP Competencies Achieved:

Psychomotor (Skills)
☑ I. 11. Perform quality control measures.
☑ IV. 5. Instruct patients according to their needs to promote health maintenance and disease prevention.

Affective (Behavior)
☑ III. 1. Display sensitivity to patient rights and feelings in collecting specimens.

ABHES Competencies Achieved:

☑ 8. cc. Communicate on the recipient's level of comprehension.
☑ 10. b. Perform selected CLIA-waived tests that assist with diagnosis and treatment: (6) Kit testing.
☑ 10. f. Instruct patients in the collection of a fecal specimen.

Notes

EVALUATION OF COMPETENCY

Procedure 28-A: Preparation for Radiology Examinations

Name: _____   Date: _____

Evaluated By: _____   Score: _____

Performance Objective

Outcome:	Instruct a patient in the proper preparation required for each of the following radiographic examinations: mammogram, upper GI, lower GI, and intravenous pyelogram.
Conditions:	Given a patient instruction sheet for each radiographic examination.
Standards:	Time: 15 minutes. Student completed procedure in _____ minutes.
	Accuracy: Satisfactory score in the Performance Evaluation Checklist.

Performance Evaluation Checklist

Trial 1	Trial 2	Point Value	Performance Standards
		●	Greeted and identified patient.
		●	Introduced yourself.
			Instructed patient in the proper preparation for each of the following radiographic examinations:
		●	Mammogram
		●	Upper GI
		●	Lower GI
		●	Intravenous pyelogram
		●	Charted the procedure correctly.
		✳	Completed the procedure within 15 minutes.
			TOTALS

CHART	
Date	

Evaluation of Student Performance

EVALUATION CRITERIA			COMMENTS
Symbol	Category	Point Value	
∗	Critical Step	16 points	
●	Essential Step	6 points	
▷	Theory Question	2 points	

Score calculation: 100 points

　　　　　　　 −_____ points missed

　　　　　　　 _____ Score

Satisfactory score: 85 or above

CAAHEP Competencies Achieved:

Psychomotor (Skills)
☑ IV. 6. Prepare a patient for procedures and/or treatments.

Affective (Behavior)
☑ I. 2. Use language/verbal skills that enable patient's understanding.

ABHES Competencies Achieved:

☑ 8. cc. Communicate on the recipient's level of comprehension.
☑ 9.1. Prepare patient for examinations and treatments.

EVALUATION OF COMPETENCY

Procedure 28-B: Preparation for Diagnostic Imaging Procedures

Name: _____   Date: _____

Evaluated By: _____   Score: _____

Performance Objective

Outcome:	Instruct a patient in the proper preparation required for each of the following diagnostic imaging procedures: ultrasonography, computed tomography, and magnetic resonance imaging.
Conditions:	Given a patient instruction sheet for each diagnostic imaging procedure.
Standards:	Time: 15 minutes. Student completed procedure(s) in _____ minutes.
	Accuracy: Satisfactory score in the Performance Evaluation Checklist.

Performance Evaluation Checklist

Trial 1	Trial 2	Point Value	Performance Standards
		●	Greeted and identified the patient.
		●	Introduced yourself.
			Instructed patient in the proper preparation for each of the following diagnostic imaging procedures:
		●	Ultrasonography
		●	Computed tomography
		●	Magnetic resonance imaging
		●	Nuclear medicine
		●	Charted the procedure correctly.
		＊	Completed the procedure within 15 minutes.
			TOTALS
CHART			
Date			

Evaluation of Student Performance

EVALUATION CRITERIA			COMMENTS
Symbol	Category	Point Value	
✳	Critical Step	16 points	
●	Essential Step	6 points	
▷	Theory Question	2 points	

Score calculation: 100 points

− _____ points missed

____ Score

Satisfactory score: 85 or above

CAAHEP Competencies Achieved:

Psychomotor (Skills)
☑ IV. 6. Prepare a patient for procedures and/or treatments.

Affective (Behavior)
☑ I. 2. Use language/verbal skills that enable patient's understanding.

ABHES Competencies Achieved:

☑ 8. cc. Communicate on the recipient's level of comprehension.
☑ 9.1. Prepare patient for examinations and treatments.

29

Introduction to the Clinical Laboratory

CHAPTER ASSIGNMENTS

√ After Completing	Date Due	Textbook Page(s)	TEXTBOOK ASSIGNMENTS	Possible Points	Points You Earned
		681-699	Read Chapter 29: Introduction to the Clinical Laboratory		
		691 698	📖 Read Case Study 1 Case Study 1 questions	5	
		692 698	📖 Read Case Study 2 Case Study 2 questions	5	
		692 698-699	📖 Read Case Study 3 Case Study 3 questions	5	
			TOTAL POINTS		

√ After Completing	Date Due	Study Guide Page(s)	STUDY GUIDE ASSIGNMENTS (CTA: Critical Thinking Activity)	Possible Points	Points You Earned
		741	📝 Pretest	10	
		742	🔑 Key Term Assessment	10	
		743-745	📋 Evaluation of Learning questions	18	
		745	CTA A: Laboratory Directory Information	10	
		746	CTA B: Specimen Requirements	15	
		746	CTA C: Identifying Abnormal Values	10	
		746-747	CTA D: Laboratory Report	25	
		748	CTA E: Crossword Puzzle	22	
			💿 CD Activity: Chapter 29 Apply Your Knowledge questions (Record points earned)		
		741	📝 Posttest	10	

√ After Completing	Date Due	Study Guide Page(s)	STUDY GUIDE ASSIGNMENTS (CTA: Critical Thinking Activity)	Possible Points	Points You Earned
			ADDITIONAL ASSIGNMENTS		
			TOTAL POINTS		

√ When Assigned by Your Instructor	Study Guide Page(s)	Practices Required	LABORATORY ASSIGNMENTS (Procedure Number and Name)	*Score
	749	3	**Practice for Competency** 29-1: Collecting a Specimen for Transport to an Outside Laboratory Textbook reference: pp. 693-695	
	751-752		📖 **Evaluation of Competency** 29-1: Collecting a Specimen for Transport to an Outside Laboratory	*
			ADDITIONAL ASSIGNMENTS	

Notes

Name _____   Date _____

PRETEST

True or False

_____ 1. When the body is in homeostasis, an imbalance exists in the body.

_____ 2. A routine test is performed to assist in the early detection of disease.

_____ 3. The laboratory request form provides the outside laboratory with information needed to test the specimen.

_____ 4. The clinical diagnosis is indicated on a laboratory request to correlate laboratory data with the needs of the physician.

_____ 5. The purpose of a laboratory report is to indicate the patient's diagnosis.

_____ 6. A patient who is fasting in preparation for a laboratory test is permitted to drink diet soda.

_____ 7. A small sample taken from the body to represent the nature of the whole is known as a *specimen*.

_____ 8. A laboratory report marked QNS means that the patient did not prepare properly.

_____ 9. Fecal occult blood testing is an example of a CLIA-waived test.

_____ 10. The purpose of quality control is to prevent accidents in the laboratory.

POSTTEST

True or False

_____ 1. Laboratory tests are most frequently ordered by the physician to assist in the diagnosis of pathologic conditions.

_____ 2. A laboratory directory indicates the patient preparation required for laboratory tests.

_____ 3. Laboratory tests termed *profiles* contain a number of different tests.

_____ 4. A lipid profile includes a test for glucose.

_____ 5. The purpose of patient preparation for a laboratory test is to ensure the test results fall within normal range.

_____ 6. A comprehensive metabolic profile requires that the patient fast.

_____ 7. Antibiotics taken by the patient prior to the collection of a throat specimen for culture may result in a false-positive result.

_____ 8. The purpose of CLIA is to prevent exposure of employees to bloodborne pathogens.

_____ 9. If a POL is performing moderate-complexity tests, CLIA requires that two levels of controls be run daily.

_____ 10. *In vitro* means occurring in the living body.

Directions: Match each medical term with its definition.

_____ 1. Fasting

_____ 2. Homeostasis

_____ 3. Laboratory test

_____ 4. Normal range

_____ 5. Plasma

_____ 6. Profile

_____ 7. Quality control

_____ 8. Routine test

_____ 9. Serum

_____ 10. Specimen

A. A certain established and acceptable parameter or reference range within which the laboratory test results of a healthy individual are expected to fall

B. The clear, straw-colored part of the blood (plasma) that remains after the solid elements and the clotting factor fibrinogen have been separated out of it

C. The state in which body systems are functioning normally and the internal environment of the body is in equilibrium

D. A number of laboratory tests providing related or complementary information used to determine the health of a patient

E. Abstaining from food or fluids (except water) for a specified amount of time before the collection of a specimen

F. The clinical analysis and study of materials, fluids, or tissues obtained from patients to assist in diagnosing and treating disease

G. Laboratory test performed routinely on apparently healthy patients to assist in the early detection of disease

H. The liquid part of the blood, consisting of a clear, yellowish fluid that makes up approximately 55% of the blood volume

I. A small sample of something taken to show the nature of the whole

J. The application of methods to ensure that test results are reliable and valid and errors are detected and eliminated

☑ EVALUATION OF LEARNING

Directions: Fill in each blank with the correct answer.

1. What is the general purpose of a laboratory test?

   _____

   _____

2. List five specific uses of laboratory test results.

   _____

   _____

   _____

   _____

3. What is the purpose of performing a routine test?

   _____

   _____

4. What information is included in a laboratory directory?

   _____

   _____

   _____

   _____

5. What is the purpose of a laboratory request?

   _____

   _____

6. What is the reason for indicating the following information on the laboratory request form?
   a. Patient's age and gender

   _____

   _____

   b. Date and time of collection of the specimen

   _____

   _____

   c. Source of the specimen

   _____

   _____

   d. Physician's clinical diagnosis

   _____

   _____

   e. Any medications the patient is taking

   _____

   _____

7. What tests are included in the following profiles?

   a. Comprehensive metabolic profile

     _____

     _____

   b. Hepatic profile

     _____

     _____

   c. Prenatal profile

     _____

     _____

   d. Lipid profile

     _____

     _____

8. What information is included on laboratory reports?

     _____

     _____

     _____

     _____

9. Why must the test results of specimens tested by an outside laboratory be compared with the normal ranges supplied by the laboratory?

     _____

     _____

10. Why do some laboratory tests require advance patient preparation?

     _____

     _____

11. Why is it important to explain the reason for the advance preparation to the patient?

     _____

     _____

12. What is a specimen?

     _____

     _____

13. List 10 examples of specimens.

     _____

     _____

     _____

     _____

     _____

14. Why must a specimen be properly handled and stored?

_____

_____

15. What are the six basic steps involved in testing a specimen?

_____

_____

_____

_____

_____

_____

16. What is the purpose of quality control?

_____

_____

_____

17. List four quality control methods that should be employed in testing a specimen.

_____

_____

_____

_____

18. List 10 laboratory safety guidelines that should be followed in the medical office to prevent accidents from occurring.

_____

_____

_____

_____

_____

CRITICAL THINKING ACTIVITIES

A. LABORATORY DIRECTORY INFORMATION

Look at a laboratory directory (from an outside medical laboratory), and list the categories of information included in it (e.g., normal range of laboratory tests).

_____

_____

_____

_____

_____

_____

B. SPECIMEN REQUIREMENTS

Refer to Table 29-1 in your textbook, and list the specimen requirements for each of the following tests:

1. Albumin, serum: _____

2. ALT: _____

3. Bilirubin, total: _____

4. Blood group (ABO): _____

5. BUN, serum: _____

6. Calcium: _____

7. CBC (with differential): _____

8. CPK: _____

9. Glucose, plasma: _____

10. LD: _____

11. Sedimentation rate (ESR): _____

12. Thyroxine (T_4): _____

13. Triglycerides: _____

14. Uric acid, serum: _____

15. Urinalysis: _____

C. IDENTIFYING ABNORMAL VALUES

Refer to the laboratory report in your textbook (Figure 29-2), and circle any abnormal values using a red pen.

D. LABORATORY REPORT

Refer to the laboratory report in your textbook (Figure 29-2). Using the normal values listed on this report, determine if the following tests fall within normal range or if they are high or low. Mark each test according to the following: N = normal, H = high, L = low. Your patient is a woman.

1. Glucose: 140 mg/dL: _____

2. BUN: 15 mg/dL: _____

3. Creatinine: 1.7 mg/dL: _____

4. Calcium: 10.2 mg/dL: _____

5. Magnesium: 0.4 mmol/L: _____

6. Sodium: 156 mmol/L: _____

7. Potassium: 5.5 mmol/L: _____

8. Chloride: 84 mmol/L: _____

9. Carbon dioxide: 18 mmol/L: _____

10. Uric acid: 5.2 mg/dL: _____

11. Total protein: 4.0 g/dL: _____

12. Albumin: 3.5 g/dL: _____

13. Total bilirubin: 0.8 mg/dL: _____

14. Alkaline phosphatase: 80 U/L: _____

15. LD: 132 U/L: _____

16. AST: 24 U/L: _____

17. ALT: 44 U/L: _____

18. Total cholesterol: 260 mg/dL: _____

19. HDL cholesterol: 57 mg/dL: _____

20. LDL cholesterol: 165 mg/dL: _____

21. WBC: 15.5 ($\times 10^3$/mm^3): _____

22. Hemoglobin: 10.4 g/dL: _____

23. Hematocrit: 34%: _____

24. Prothrombin time: 10 seconds: _____

25. Neutrophils: 84%: _____

E. CROSSWORD PUZZLE
Introduction to the Clinical Laboratory
Directions: Complete the crossword puzzle using the clues presented below.

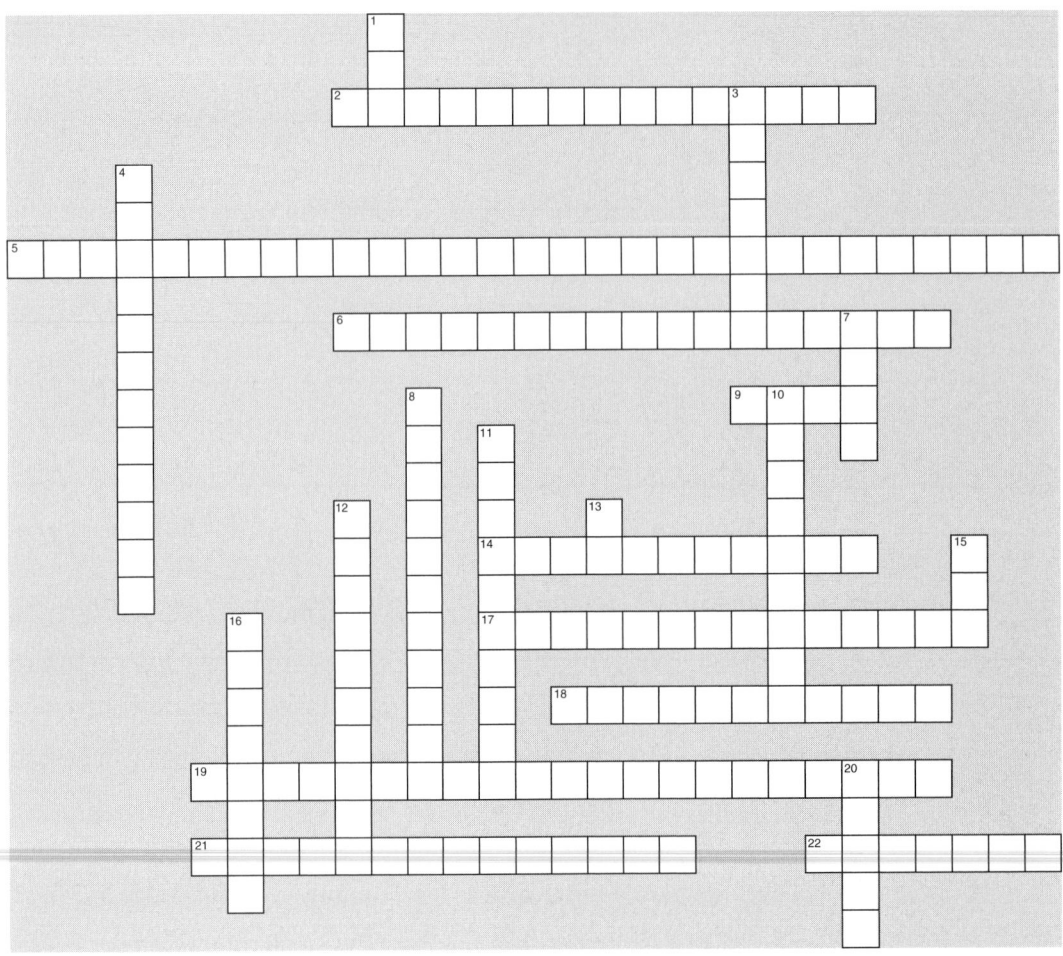

ACROSS
2 Pregnant lady tests
5 General health screen tests
6 Tentative diagnosis
9 To improve quality of laboratory testing
14 Detects disease early
17 Accurate and reliable test results
18 Healthy body
19 Which disease is it?
21 Lots of liver tests
22 More than one laboratory test

DOWN
1 Syphilis test
3 No food or fluid
4 CHD tests
7 As soon as possible
8 Where test results fall for a healthy person
10 What are the results?
11 Order a laboratory test
12 Exempt from CLIA
13 CLIA requires three times/year for MC tests
15 In-house laboratory
16 Sample of the body
20 Plasma minus fibrinogen

PRACTICE FOR COMPETENCY

Procedure 29-1: Collecting Specimen for Transport to an Outside Laboratory.
1. **Laboratory Requisition**. Complete the Laboratory Request Form on the following page using a classmate as a patient. The tests that have been ordered by the physician include the following: CBC (with differential), total cholesterol, HDL cholesterol, and plasma glucose.
2. **Specimen Collection**. Practice the procedure for collecting a specimen for transport to an outside laboratory and record the procedure in the chart provided.

CHART	
Date	

LABORATORY REQUISITION
Biomedical Laboratories, Inc.
100 Main Street
Athens, Georgia 45760

☐ Fax	Send additional copy of report to:	( )
☐ Call	Client Number/Physician's Name	Phone/Fax number
☐ Mail	Physician's Address	City, State, Zip

Patient's Name (Last)	(First)	(MI)	Sex	Date of Birth MO | DAY | YEAR	Collection Time : AM PM	Fasting YES NO	Collection Date MO | DAY | YEAR

NPI/UPIN	Physician's ID #	Patient's SS #	Patient's ID #	Urine hrs/vol hrs___ vol___

PATIENT / RESP. PARTY

Physician's Name (Last, First)	Physician's Signature	Patient's Address	Phone
Medicare # (Include prefix/suffix)	☐ Primary ☐ Secondary	City	State ZIP
Medicaid # State	Physician's Provider #	Name of Responsible Party (if different from patient)	
Diagnosis/Signs/Symptoms in ICD-9 Format (Highest Specificity) **REQUIRED**		Address of Responsible Party (if different from patient) APT #	
		City State ZIP	

INSURANCE

Patient's Relationship to Responsible Party ■ 1–Self ■ 2–Spouse ■ 3–Child ■ 4–Other			Performance Lab ☐	Carrier	Group #	Employee #	Mem
Insurance Company Name	Plan	Carrier Code					
Subscriber/Member #	Location	Group #	I hereby authorize the release of medical information related to the service subscribed herein and authorize payment directed to LabCorp. X _____ Patient's Signature ____ Date				
Insurance Address	Physician's Provider #		**MEDICARE ADVANCE BENEFICIARY NOTICE**				
City	State	ZIP	I have read the ABN on the reverse. If Medicare denies payment, I agree to pay for the identified test(s). X _____ Patient's Signature ____ Date				
Employer's Name or Number	Insured SS # (If not patient)	Worker's Comp ☐ Yes ☐ No					

NOTE: WHEN ORDERING TESTS FOR WHICH MEDICARE OR MEDICAID REIMBURSEMENT WILL BE SOUGHT, PHYSICIANS SHOULD ONLY ORDER TESTS THAT ARE MEDICALLY NECESSARY FOR THE DIAGNOSIS OR TREATMENT OF THE PATIENT. COMPONENTS OF THE ORGAN OR DISEASE PANELS/COMBINATIONS PRINTED BELOW ARE SHOWN ON THE REVERSE SIDE AND MAY ALSO BE ORDERED INDIVIDUALLY BELOW. COMPONENTS MAY BE BILLED SEPARATELY PER CARRIER POLICY.

PROFILES (See reverse for components)			**ALPHABETICAL TESTS CON'T**			**ALPHABETICAL TESTS CON'T**			**MICROBIOLOGY** See Reverse Side
80049	Basic Metabolic Profile	SST	84520	BUN	SST	83002	LH	SST	■ENDOCERVICAL ■THROAT ■URINE
80054	Comp Metabolic Profile	SST	82310	Calcium	SST	83690	Lipase	SER	■STOOL ■URETHRAL INDICATE SOURCE
80051	Electrolyte Profile	SST	80156	Carbamazepine (Tegretol®)	SER	80178	Lithium (Eskalith®)	SER	87070 Aerobic Bacterial Culture Bact Trnspt
80058	Hepatic Profile	SST	82378	CEA	SST	83735	Magnesium, Serum	SST	87490 87590 Chlamydia/GC DNA Probe w/ Confirmation on Positives Probe Trnspt
80059	Hepatitis Profile	SST	82465	Cholesterol, Total	SST	80184	Phenobarbital (Luminal®)	SER	87490 87590 Chlamydia/GC DNA Probe Without Confirmation Probe Trnspt
80061	Lipid Profile	SST	82565	Creatinine	SST	80185	Phenytoin (Dilantin®)	SER	87490 Chlamydia DNA Probe Probe Trnspt
80091	Thyroid Profile	SST	80162	Digoxin	SER	84132	Potassium	SST	87081 Genital, Beta-Hemolytic Strep Cult, Group B Bact Trnspt
80055	Prenatal Profile	RED LAV	82670	Estradiol	SST	84146	Prolactin, Serum	SST	87070 Genital Culture, Routine Bact Trnspt
80072	Rheumatoid Profile	SST	82728	Ferritin, Serum	SST	84153	Prostate-Specific Antigen	SST	87070 Lower Respiratory Culture Steril Trnspt
HEMATOLOGY			82985	Fructosamine	SST	84066	Prostatic Acid Phos	SST	87590 N. gonorrhoeae DNA Probe Probe Trnspt
85025	CBC w Diff	LAV	83001	FSH	SST	84155	Protein, Total	SST	87015 87211 Ova and Parasites O & P Kit
85027	CBC w/o Diff	LAV	83001 83002	FSH and LH	SST	85610	Prothrombin Time (PT)	BLU	87081 X2 87045 Stool Culture Fecal Trnspt
85014	Hematocrit	LAV	82977	GGT	SST	85610 85730	PT and PTT Activated	BLU	87081 Throat, Beta-Hemolytic Strep Cult, Group A Bact Trnspt
85018	Hemoglobin	LAV	82947	Glucose, Plasma	GRY	85730	PTT Activated	BLU	87060 Upper Respiratory Culture, Routine Bact Trnspt
85595	Platelet Count	LAV	82947	Glucose, Serum	SST	86431	Rheumatoid Arthritis Factor	SST	87086 Urine Culture, Routine Urn Cul Trnspt
85041	RBC Count	LAV	82950	Glucose, 2-hr. PP	SST	86592	RPR	SST	
85048	WBC Count	LAV	83036	Glycohemoglobin, Total	LAV	86762	Rubella Antibodies, IgG	SST	Clinical Information/Comments
85007	WBC Differential	LAV	84703	hCG, Beta Subunit, Qual	SST	85651	Sed Rate	LAV	
89190	Nasal Smear, Eosin	Nasal Smear	84702	hCG, Beta Subunit, Quant	SST	84295	Sodium	SST	
85060	Pathologist Consult– Peripheral Smear	LAV	83718	HDL Cholesterol	SST	84403	Testosterone	SST	
ALPHABETICAL/COMBINATION TESTS			86677	Helicobacter pylori, IgG	SST	80198	Theophylline	SER	
86900 86901	ABO and Rh	LAV	86706	Hep B Surface Antibody	SST	84436	Thyroxine (T4)	SST	**OTHER TESTS/INDIVIDUAL COMPONENTS**
82040	Albumin	SST	87340	Hep B Surface Antigen	SST	84478	Triglycerides	SST	TEST # TEST NAMES
84075	Alkaline Phosphatase	SST	86803	Hep C Antibody	SST	84480	Triiodothyronine (T3)	SST	
84460	ALT (SGPT)	SST	83036	Hemoglobin A1C	LAV	84443	TSH, High Sensitivity	SST	
82150	Amylase, Serum	SST	86701	HIV Antibodies	SST	84550	Uric Acid	SST	
86038	Antinuclear Antibodies	SST	83540	Iron, Total	SST	81003	Urinalysis Microscopic on Positives	URN	
84450	AST (SGOT)	SST	83540 83550	Iron and IBC	SST	81001	Urinalysis with Microscopic	URN	
82607 82746	B12 and Folate	SST	83615	LDH	SST	80164	Valproic Acid (Depakene®)	SER	
82250	Bilirubin, Total	SST							

LAB USE ONLY	STAT ☐998074	VENIPUNCTURE ☐998085	TRAVEL ☐998096	NON LABCORP ☐998239	VERBAL ORDER ☐998250	CHART ORDER ☐998261	HANDWRITTEN ☐998272	24 HR TUV ☐998283	PST/PSC #

CONTAINERS RECEIVED	SST SPUN	USST UNSPUN	SER SERUM TRNSPT	FRZ FRZ TRNS	RED RED	LAV LAVENDER	SLD SLIDE	BLU LT. BLUE	GRY GREY	GRN GREEN	RYB RYL BLU	YEL ACD	PLS PLASMA	URN URINE	24U 24 HR URINE	TA-U TART. ACID	FL FLUID	OT OTHER	BACT TRNSP	O & P KIT	PROBE TRNSP	URN CULT TRNSP	STERIL TRNSP	FECAL TRNSP	VIRAL TRNSP

300-0384

(From Bonewit-West K: *Study guide for clinical procedures for medical assistants*, ed 7, St. Louis, 2008, Saunders.)

EVALUATION OF COMPETENCY

Procedure 29-1: Collecting a Specimen for Transport to an Outside Laboratory

Name: _____   Date: _____

Evaluated By: _____   Score: _____

Performance Objective

Outcome:	Collect a specimen for transport to an outside laboratory.
Conditions:	Given the appropriate supplies for the specimen collection and transport (will be based upon the type of specimen collected).
Standards:	Time: 10 minutes. Student completed procedure in ____ minutes.
	Accuracy: Satisfactory score in the Performance Evaluation Checklist.

Performance Evaluation Checklist

Trial 1	Trial 2	Point Value	Performance Standards
		●	Informed patient of any advance preparation or special instructions.
		▷	Explained why patient should prepare properly.
		●	Reviewed requirements in the laboratory directory for the collection and handling of the specimen.
		●	Completed laboratory request form.
		●	Sanitized hands.
		●	Assembled equipment and supplies.
		●	Labeled the tubes and containers with patient's name, date, and initials.
		●	Greeted patient and introduced yourself.
		●	Identified patient and explained procedure.
		▷	Stated why it is important to correctly identify patient.
		●	Determined if patient prepared properly for test.
			Collected specimen incorporating the following guidelines:
		●	Followed the OSHA standard.
		●	Collected specimen using proper technique.
		●	Collected the proper type and amount of specimen required for the test.
		●	Processed specimen further if required by the outside laboratory.
		●	Placed the lid tightly on specimen container.
			Prepared specimen for transport:
		●	Placed specimen in biohazard specimen bag.
		●	Placed laboratory request in outside pocket of bag.
		●	Properly handled and stored specimen.
		●	Charted the procedure correctly.

Trial 1	Trial 2	Point Value	Performance Standards
			Processed laboratory report:
		●	Reviewed laboratory report when it was returned.
		●	Notified physician of any abnormal results.
		●	Filed laboratory report in patient's chart after review by physician.
		✳	Completed the procedure within 10 minutes.
			TOTALS

CHART	
Date	

Evaluation of Student Performance

EVALUATION CRITERIA			COMMENTS
Symbol	Category	Point Value	
✳	Critical Step	16 points	
●	Essential Step	6 points	
▷	Theory Question	2 points	

Score calculation: 100 points

    − _____ points missed

    _____ Score

Satisfactory score: 85 or above

CAAHEP Competencies Achieved:

Psychomotor (Skills)
☑ I. 11. Perforom quality control measures.
☑ I. 16. Screen test results.
☑ II. 2. Maintain laboratory test results using flow sheets.

Affective (Behavior)
☑ III. 1. Display sensitivity to patient rights and feelings in collecting specimens.

ABHES Competencies Achieved:

☑ 9. f. Screen and follow up patient test results.
☑ 10. a. Practice quality control.
☑ 10. d. Collect, label, and process specimens.

30

Urinalysis

CHAPTER ASSIGNMENTS

√ After Completing	Date Due	Textbook Page(s)	TEXTBOOK ASSIGNMENTS	Possible Points	Points You Earned
		700-728	Read Chapter 30: Urinalysis		
		702 726	📖 Read Case Study 1 Case Study 1 questions	5	
		707 726-727	📖 Read Case Study 2 Case Study 2 questions	5	
		724 727	📖 Read Case Study 3 Case Study 3 questions	5	
			TOTAL POINTS		

√ After Completing	Date Due	Study Guide Page(s)	STUDY GUIDE ASSIGNMENTS (CTA: Critical Thinking Activity)	Possible Points	Points You Earned
		757	📝 Pretest	10	
		758	🖊 Key Term Assessment	17	
		759-761	📋 Evaluation of Learning questions	32	
		761	CTA A: First-Voided Specimen	2	
		762	CTA B: Clean-Catch Specimen	4	
		762	CTA C: Urine Testing Kit Instructions	6	
			💿 CD Activity: Chapter 30 Chemical Testing of Urine (Record points earned)		
		763	CTA D: Crossword Puzzle	20	
			💿 CD Activity: Chapter 30 Road to Recovery Game: Urinalysis Terminology (Record points earned)		
			💿 CD Activity: Chapter 30 Animations		

√ After Completing	Date Due	Study Guide Page(s)	STUDY GUIDE ASSIGNMENTS (CTA: Critical Thinking Activity)	Possible Points	Points You Earned
			ⓒᴰ CD Activity: Chapter 30 Apply Your Knowledge questions (Record points earned)		
		757	🖼 Posttest	10	
			ADDITIONAL ASSIGNMENTS		
			TOTAL POINTS		

√ When Assigned by Your Instructor	Study Guide Page(s)	Practices Required	LABORATORY ASSIGNMENTS (Procedure Number and Name)	*Score
	765	3	**⊙ Practice for Competency** 30-1: Clean-Catch Midstream Specimen Collection Instructions Textbook reference: pp. 704-705	
	769-771		**Evaluation of Competency** 30-1: Clean-Catch Midstream Specimen Collection Instructions	*
	765	5	**Practice for Competency** 30-A: Assess the Color and Appearance of a Urine Specimen Textbook reference: pp. 705-706	
	773-774		**Evaluation of Competency** 30-A: Assess the Color and Appearance of a Urine Specimen	*
	765	5	**⊙ Practice for Competency** 30-2: Chemical Testing of Urine with the Multistix 10 SG Reagent Strip Textbook reference: pp. 714-716	
	775-777		**Evaluation of Competency** 30-2: Chemical Testing of Urine with the Multistix 10 SG Reagent Strip	*
	765	2	**Practice for Competency** 30-3: Prepare a Urine Specimen for Microscopic Examination: Kova Method Textbook reference: pp. 721-723	
	779-781		**Evaluation of Competency** 30-3: Prepare a Urine Specimen for Microscopic Examination: Kova Method	*
	765	2	**⊙ Practice for Competency** 30-4: Performing a Urine Pregnancy Test Textbook reference: pp. 725-726	
	783-784		**Evaluation of Competency** 30-4: Performing a Urine Pregnancy Test	*
			ADDITIONAL ASSIGNMENTS	

Notes

Name _____   Date _____

PRETEST

True or False

_____ 1. Approximately 95% of urine consists of water.

_____ 2. Frequency is the condition of having to urinate often.

_____ 3. An excessive increase in urine output is termed *polyuria*.

_____ 4. A clean-catch midstream urine specimen is required for a urine culture.

_____ 5. Urinalysis consists of a physical, chemical, and microscopic examination of urine.

_____ 6. A urine specimen that is light yellow in color indicates that bacteria are present in the specimen.

_____ 7. The pH of most urine specimens is neutral.

_____ 8. Blood may normally be present in the urine due to menstruation.

_____ 9. *Hematuria* refers to the presence of blood in the urine.

_____ 10. HCG is a hormone that is present in the urine and blood of a pregnant woman.

POSTTEST

True or False

_____ 1. Urea is a waste product derived from the breakdown of glucose.

_____ 2. A normal adult excretes approximately 250 ml of urine each day.

_____ 3. Vomiting can result in oliguria.

_____ 4. The distal urethra normally contains microorganisms.

_____ 5. A 24-hour urine specimen may be collected to assist in the diagnosis of a UTI.

_____ 6. If a urine specimen is allowed to stand for more than 1 hour at room temperature, the pH becomes more acidic.

_____ 7. If a freshly voided specimen is cloudy, this may mean that a UTI is present.

_____ 8. The normal specific gravity of urine ranges from 1.003-1.030.

_____ 9. Dysuria is the inability to control urination at night.

_____ 10. Casts are formed in the urinary bladder.

KEY TERM ASSESSMENT

Directions: Match each medical term with its definition.

_____ 1. Bilirubinuria

_____ 2. Glycosuria

_____ 3. Ketonuria

_____ 4. Ketosis

_____ 5. Micturition

_____ 6. Nephron

_____ 7. Oliguria

_____ 8. pH

_____ 9. Polyuria

_____ 10. Proteinuria

_____ 11. Refractive index

_____ 12. Refractometer

_____ 13. Renal threshold

_____ 14. Specific gravity

_____ 15. Supernatant

_____ 16. Urinalysis

_____ 17. Void

A. Decreased or scanty output of urine
B. The presence of protein in the urine
C. The clear liquid that remains at the top after a precipitate settles
D. The presence of bilirubin in the urine
E. Increased output of urine
F. The concentration at which a substance in the blood that is not normally excreted by the kidneys begins to appear in the urine
G. The presence of sugar in the urine
H. The physical, chemical, and microscopic analysis of urine
I. The presence of ketone bodies in the urine
J. The act of voiding urine
K. An accumulation of large amounts of ketone bodies in the tissues and body fluids
L. The weight of a substance compared with the weight of an equal volume of a substance known as the standard
M. The unit that describes the acidity or alkalinity of a solution
N. The functional unit of the kidney
O. An instrument used to measure the refractive index of urine, which is an indirect measurement of the specific gravity of urine
P. The ratio of the velocity of light in air to the velocity of light in a solution
Q. To empty the bladder

EVALUATION OF LEARNING

Directions: Fill in each blank with the correct answer.

1. Most of the urine (95%) is composed of what substance?

_____

_____

2. List two conditions that may cause polyuria.

_____

_____

3. List two conditions that may cause oliguria.

_____

_____

4. What is the term used to describe painful urination?

_____

5. What is the term used to describe a condition of frequent urination?

_____

6. What is the term used to describe excessive (voluntary) urination during the night?

_____

7. The inability to retain urine is known as:

_____

8. What type of urine specimen is required for the detection of a UTI?

_____

9. List three changes that may occur in a urine specimen if it is allowed to stand for more than 1 hour.

_____

_____

10. Why is a first-voided morning specimen often preferred for urine testing?

_____

_____

11. A 24-hour urine specimen is often used to diagnose what condition?

_____

_____

12. Why does concentrated urine tend to be dark in color?

_____

_____

13. List two factors that may cause a urine specimen to become cloudy.

_____

_____

14. What type of odor would a urine specimen that has been allowed to stand out for a long time have?

_____

15. What is the purpose of testing the specific gravity of urine?

_____

16. What is the normal range for the specific gravity of urine?

_____

17. What is the difference between a qualitative test and a quantitative test?

_____

_____

_____

18. What may cause an increase in the pH of the urine?

_____

_____

19. Why does urine become more alkaline if it is not preserved?

_____

_____

_____

20. What may cause glycosuria?

_____

_____

21. What may cause ketosis?

_____

_____

22. What may cause blood to appear in the urine?

_____

_____

23. Why should a nitrite test not be performed on a urine specimen that has been left standing out?

_____

_____

24. How should urine reagent strips be stored?

_____

_____

25. What is the purpose of performing a microscopic examination of the urine?

_____

_____

_____

26. Why is a first-voided urine specimen recommended for a microscopic examination of the urine?

_____

_____

27. What effect does concentrated urine have on red blood cells present in it?

_____

_____

28. What is a urinary cast?

_____

_____

29. What conditions may cause yeast cells to appear in the urine?

_____

30. List three reasons for performing a pregnancy test.

_____

31. What is the name of the hormone that is present only in the urine and blood of a pregnant woman?

_____

32. List five guidelines that should be followed when performing a pregnancy test.

_____

_____

_____

_____

CRITICAL THINKING ACTIVITIES

A. FIRST-VOIDED SPECIMEN

You have instructed Jim Pratt to collect a first-voided morning urine specimen, to be brought to the medical office for testing. Respond to the following questions posed by Mr. Pratt.

1. Why is a first-voided specimen desired?

_____

_____

2. Why must the specimen be preserved until it is brought to the medical office?

_____

_____

B. CLEAN-CATCH SPECIMEN

You have just instructed Ann Berger to obtain a clean-catch midstream specimen at the medical office. Respond to the following questions posed by Mrs. Berger.

1. What is the purpose of cleansing the urinary meatus?

   _____

   _____

2. Why must a front-to-back motion be used to clean the urinary meatus?

   _____

   _____

3. Why must a small amount of urine first be voided into the toilet?

   _____

   _____

4. Why should the inside of the specimen cup not be touched?

   _____

   _____

C. URINE TESTING KIT INSTRUCTIONS

Obtain the instructions that come with any type of commercially prepared diagnostic kit for the chemical testing of urine (e.g., Multistix 10 SG). Using the instructions, answer the following questions. (*Note:* A package insert for Multistix 10 SG can be obtained on the Internet by entering the following address: http://diagnostics.siemens.com/siemens/en_GLOBAL/gg_diag_FBAs/files/urinalysis_pdf/clinitek_status/clinitek_status_multistix_10.pdf

1. What is the brand name of the test?

   _____

2. This test assists in the diagnosis of what conditions?

   _____

   _____

   _____

3. What type of urine specimen is recommended for this test?

   _____

   _____

   _____

4. This test is used to detect the presence of what substances?

   _____

   _____

   _____

5. Explain the proper storage and handling of this test.

   _____

   _____

   _____

6. List any substances or techniques that may interfere with obtaining an accurate reading (e.g., not reading the test at the prescribed time).

   _____

   _____

   _____

D. CROSSWORD PUZZLE
Urinalysis
Directions: Complete the crossword puzzle using the clues presented below.

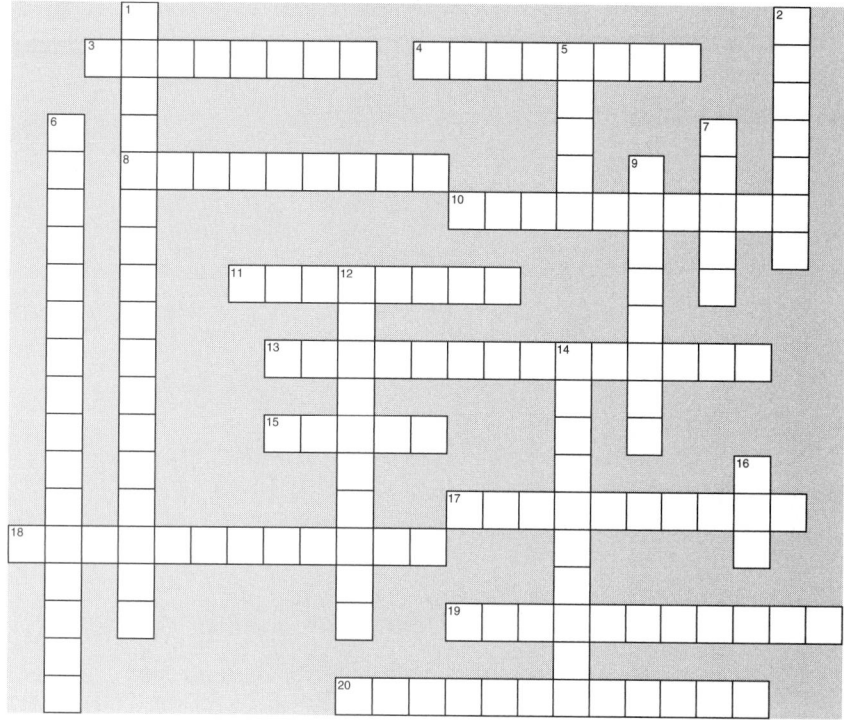

ACROSS

3 Cause of oliguria
4 Cause of glycosuria
8 Yellow urine pigment
10 Treatment for UTI
11 Deteriorates urine strips
13 Security for urine drug testing
15 Neutral pH
17 Specimen for C & S
18 Normal cause of hematuria
19 Specimen for pregnancy test
20 24-hour specimen can diagnose cause of this

DOWN

1 Bedwetting
2 Symptom of UTI
5 URI bacteria
6 Exactly!
7 Most of urine
9 This drug causes polyuria
12 Cause of ketonuria
14 Physical, chemical, and microscopic
16 Makes pregnancy test positive

Notes

PRACTICE FOR COMPETENCY

Procedure 30-1: Clean-Catch Midstream Urine Specimen. Collection Instructions. Instruct an individual in the procedure for collecting a clean-catch midstream specimen and record the procedure in the chart provided.

Procedure 30-A: Color and Appearance of a Urine Specimen. Assess the color and appearance of a urine specimen and record the results in the chart provided.

Procedure 30-2: Chemical Testing of Urine with the Multistix 10 SG Reagent Strip. Perform a chemical assessment of a urine specimen using a Multistix 10 SG reagent strip. Record the results on the laboratory report form provided. Circle any abnormal results.

Procedure 30-3: Prepare a Urine Specimen for Microscopic Examination: Kova Method. Practice the procedure for preparing a urine specimen for a microscopic analysis of the urine sediment. Examine the specimen and record the results in the chart provided.

Procedure 30-4: Urine Pregnancy Test. Perform a urine pregnancy test and record results in the chart provided.

Cʜᴀʀᴛ	
Date	

CHART	
Date	

CHARTING EXAMPLE

Multistix® 10 SG Reagent Strips for Urinalysis

PATIENT

DATE   TIME

LEUKOCYTES	NEGATIVE ☐		TRACE ☐	SMALL + ☐	MODERATE ☐ ++	LARGE +++ ☐
NITRITE	NEGATIVE ☐		POSITIVE ☐	POSITIVE ☐	(Any degree of uniform pink color is found)	
UROBILINOGEN	NORMAL 0.2 ☐	NORMAL 1 ☐	mg/dL 2 ☐	4 ☐	8 ☐ (1mg = approx. 1 BU)	
PROTEIN	NEGATIVE ☐	TRACE ☐	mg/dL 30 * ☐	100 ++ ☐	300 +++ ☐	2000 OR MORE ☐
pH	5.0 ☐	6.0 ☐	6.5 ☐	7.0 ☐	7.5 ☐	8.0 ☐	8.5 ☐
BLOOD	NEGATIVE ☐	NON-HEMOLYZED ☐ TRACE	NON-HEMOLYZED ☐ MODERATE	HEMOLYZED TRACE ☐	SMALL + ☐	MODERATE ++ ☐	LARGE +++ ☐
SPECIFIC GRAVITY	1.000 ☐	1.006 ☐	1.010 ☐	1.015 ☐	1.020 ☐	1.025 ☐	1.030 ☐
KETONE	NEGATIVE ☐	mg/dL	TRACE 5 ☐	SMALL 15 ☐	MODERATE 40 ☐	LARGE 80 ☐	LARGE 160 ☐
BILIRUBIN	NEGATIVE ☐		SMALL + ☐	MODERATE ++ ☐	LARGE +++ ☐	
GLUCOSE	NEGATIVE ☐	g/L (%) mg/dL	1/10 tr.) 100 ☐	1/6 250 ☐	1/2 500 ☐	1 1000 ☐	2 or more 2000 or more ☐

(Modified and printed by permission of Siemens Healthcare Diagnostics, Deerfield, Ill, 60015.)

CHARTING EXAMPLE

Multistix® 10 SG Reagent Strips for Urinalysis

PATIENT

DATE   TIME

LEUKOCYTES	NEGATIVE ☐		TRACE ☐	SMALL + ☐	MODERATE ☐ ++	LARGE +++ ☐
NITRITE	NEGATIVE ☐		POSITIVE ☐	POSITIVE ☐	(Any degree of uniform pink color is found)	
UROBILINOGEN	NORMAL 0.2 ☐	NORMAL 1 ☐	mg/dL 2 ☐	4 ☐	8 ☐ (1mg = approx. 1 BU)	
PROTEIN	NEGATIVE ☐	TRACE ☐	mg/dL 30 * ☐	100 ++ ☐	300 +++ ☐	2000 OR MORE ☐
pH	5.0 ☐	6.0 ☐	6.5 ☐	7.0 ☐	7.5 ☐	8.0 ☐	8.5 ☐
BLOOD	NEGATIVE ☐	NON-HEMOLYZED ☐ TRACE	NON-HEMOLYZED ☐ MODERATE	HEMOLYZED TRACE ☐	SMALL + ☐	MODERATE ++ ☐	LARGE +++ ☐
SPECIFIC GRAVITY	1.000 ☐	1.006 ☐	1.010 ☐	1.015 ☐	1.020 ☐	1.025 ☐	1.030 ☐
KETONE	NEGATIVE ☐	mg/dL	TRACE 5 ☐	SMALL 15 ☐	MODERATE 40 ☐	LARGE 80 ☐	LARGE 160 ☐
BILIRUBIN	NEGATIVE ☐		SMALL + ☐	MODERATE ++ ☐	LARGE +++ ☐	
GLUCOSE	NEGATIVE ☐	g/L (%) mg/dL	1/10 tr.) 100 ☐	1/6 250 ☐	1/2 500 ☐	1 1000 ☐	2 or more 2000 or more ☐

(Modified and printed by permission of Siemens Healthcare Diagnostics, Deerfield, Ill, 60015.)

CHARTING EXAMPLE

Multistix® 10 SG Reageant Strips for Urinalysis

PATIENT

DATE   TIME

LEUKOCYTES	NEGATIVE ☐		TRACE ☐	SMALL ☐ +	MODERATE ☐ ++	LARGE ☐ +++	
NITRITE	NEGATIVE ☐		POSITIVE ☐	POSITIVE ☐	(Any degree of uniform pink color is found)		
UROBILINOGEN	NORMAL ☐ 0.2	NORMAL ☐ 1	mg/dL ☐ 2	4 ☐	8 ☐ (1mg = approx. 1 BU)		
PROTEIN	NEGATIVE ☐	TRACE ☐	mg/dL ☐ 30 *	100 ☐ ++	300 ☐ +++	2000 OR MORE ☐	
pH	5.0 ☐	6.0 ☐	6.5 ☐	7.0 ☐	7.5 ☐	8.0 ☐	8.5 ☐
BLOOD	NEGATIVE ☐	NON-HEMOLYZED ☐ TRACE	NON-HEMOLYZED ☐ MODERATE	HEMOLYZED ☐ TRACE	SMALL ☐ +	MODERATE ☐ ++	LARGE ☐ +++
SPECIFIC GRAVITY	1.000 ☐	1.006 ☐	1.010 ☐	1.015 ☐	1.020 ☐	1.025 ☐	1.030 ☐
KETONE	NEGATIVE ☐	mg/dL	TRACE ☐ 5	SMALL ☐ 15	MODERATE ☐ 40	LARGE ☐ 80	LARGE ☐ 160
BILIRUBIN	NEGATIVE ☐		SMALL ☐ +	MODERATE ☐ ++	LARGE ☐ +++		
GLUCOSE	NEGATIVE ☐	g/L (%) mg/dL	1/10 tr.) ☐ 100	1/6 ☐ 250	1/2 ☐ 500	1 ☐ 1000	2 or more ☐ 2000 or more

(Modified and printed by permission of Siemens Healthcare Diagnostics, Deerfield, Ill, 60015.)

CHARTING EXAMPLE

Multistix® 10 SG Reageant Strips for Urinalysis

PATIENT

DATE   TIME

LEUKOCYTES	NEGATIVE ☐		TRACE ☐	SMALL ☐ +	MODERATE ☐ ++	LARGE ☐ +++	
NITRITE	NEGATIVE ☐		POSITIVE ☐	POSITIVE ☐	(Any degree of uniform pink color is found)		
UROBILINOGEN	NORMAL ☐ 0.2	NORMAL ☐ 1	mg/dL ☐ 2	4 ☐	8 ☐ (1mg = approx. 1 BU)		
PROTEIN	NEGATIVE ☐	TRACE ☐	mg/dL ☐ 30 *	100 ☐ ++	300 ☐ +++	2000 OR MORE ☐	
pH	5.0 ☐	6.0 ☐	6.5 ☐	7.0 ☐	7.5 ☐	8.0 ☐	8.5 ☐
BLOOD	NEGATIVE ☐	NON-HEMOLYZED ☐ TRACE	NON-HEMOLYZED ☐ MODERATE	HEMOLYZED ☐ TRACE	SMALL ☐ +	MODERATE ☐ ++	LARGE ☐ +++
SPECIFIC GRAVITY	1.000 ☐	1.006 ☐	1.010 ☐	1.015 ☐	1.020 ☐	1.025 ☐	1.030 ☐
KETONE	NEGATIVE ☐	mg/dL	TRACE ☐ 5	SMALL ☐ 15	MODERATE ☐ 40	LARGE ☐ 80	LARGE ☐ 160
BILIRUBIN	NEGATIVE ☐		SMALL ☐ +	MODERATE ☐ ++	LARGE ☐ +++		
GLUCOSE	NEGATIVE ☐	g/L (%) mg/dL	1/10 tr.) ☐ 100	1/6 ☐ 250	1/2 ☐ 500	1 ☐ 1000	2 or more ☐ 2000 or more

(Modified and printed by permission of Siemens Healthcare Diagnostics, Deerfield, Ill, 60015.)

EVALUATION OF COMPETENCY

Procedure 30-1: Clean-Catch Midstream Specimen Collection Instructions

Name: _____   Date: _____

Evaluated By: _____   Score: _____

Performance Objective

Outcome:	Instruct a patient in the procedure for collecting a clean-catch midstream urine specimen.
Conditions:	Given the following: sterile specimen container and personal antiseptic towelettes, and tissues.
Standards:	Time: 10 minutes. Student completed procedure in _____ minutes.
	Accuracy: Satisfactory score on the Performance Evaluation Checklist.

Performance Evaluation Checklist

Trial 1	Trial 2	Point Value	Performance Standards
		•	Sanitized hands.
		•	Greeted the patient and introduced yourself.
		•	Identified the patient and explained the procedure.
		•	Assembled equipment.
		•	Labeled specimen container.
			Instructed the female patient by telling her to:
		•	Wash hands and open antiseptic towelettes.
		•	Remove lid from specimen container without touching inside of container or lid.
		•	Pull down undergarments and sit on the toilet.
		•	Expose the urinary meatus by spreading the labia apart with one hand.
		•	Cleanse each side of the urinary meatus with a front-to-back motion using a separate towelette on each side of the meatus.
		▷	Explained why a front-to-back motion should be used.
		•	After use, discard each towelette in toilet.
		•	Cleanse directly across the meatus using a third towelette and discard it.
		•	Void a small amount of urine into the toilet, while continuing to hold the labia apart.
		▷	Explained the purpose of voiding into the toilet.
		•	Collect the next amount of urine by voiding into the sterile container without touching the inside of the container.
		•	Fill container approximately half full with urine.
		•	Void the last amount of urine into the toilet.
		•	Replace specimen container lid.

Trial 1	Trial 2	Point Value	Performance Standards
		●	Wipe area dry with a tissue, flush the toilet, and wash hands.
			Instructed the male patient by telling him to:
		●	Wash hands and open antiseptic towelettes, and remove lid from specimen container.
		●	Pull down undergarments and stand in front of toilet.
		●	Retract the foreskin of the penis if uncircumcised.
		●	Cleanse area around the meatus and the urethral opening by wiping each side of the meatus with a separate antiseptic towelette.
		●	Cleanse directly across the meatus using a third antiseptic towelette.
		●	Discard each towelette in the toilet after use.
		●	Void a small amount of urine into the toilet.
		●	Collect the next amount of urine by voiding into the sterile container without touching the inside of the container.
		●	Fill container approximately half full with urine.
		●	Void the last amount of urine into the toilet.
		●	Replace lid on specimen container.
		●	Wipe area dry with a tissue and wash hands.
			Performed the following:
		●	Provided patient with instructions on what to do with specimen.
		●	Completed a laboratory requisition, if required.
		●	Charted the procedure correctly.
		●	Tested specimen or prepared it for transport to an outside laboratory.
		✶	Completed the procedure within 10 minutes.
			TOTALS

CHART	
Date	

Evaluation of Student Performance

EVALUATION CRITERIA			COMMENTS
Symbol	Category	Point Value	
*	Critical Step	16 points	
•	Essential Step	6 points	
▷	Theory Question	2 points	

Score calculation: 100 points

– _____ points missed

_____ Score

Satisfactory score: 85 or above

CAAHEP Competencies Achieved:

Psychomotor (Skills)

☑ IV. 2. Report relevant information to others succinctly and accurately.

Affective (Behavior)

☑ III. 1. Display sensitivity to patient rights and feelings in collecting specimens.
☑ III. 2. Explain the rationale for performance of a procedure to the patient.

ABHES Competencies Achieved:

☑ 8. cc. Communicate on the recipient's level of comprehension.
☑ 10. e. Instruct patients in the collection of a clean-catch midstream urine specimen.

Notes

EVALUATION OF COMPETENCY

Procedure 30-A: Assessing Color and Appearance of a Urine Specimen

Name: _____ Date: _____

Evaluated By: _____ Score: _____

Performance Objective

Outcome:	Assess the color and appearance of a urine specimen.
Conditions:	Given a transparent container and a urine specimen.
Standards:	Time: 5 minutes. Student completed procedure in ____ minutes.
	Accuracy: Satisfactory score on the Performance Evaluation Checklist.

Performance Evaluation Checklist

Trial 1	Trial 2	Point Value	Performance Standards
			Color
		•	Sanitized hands and applied gloves.
		•	Transferred urine specimen to a transparent container.
		•	Assessed the color of the urine specimen.
		*	The assessment was identical to the evaluator's assessment.
		•	Charted the results correctly.
			Appearance
		•	Assessed the appearance of the urine specimen in the transparent container.
		*	Confirmed that the assessment was identical to the evaluator's assessment.
		•	Charted the results correctly.
		•	Properly disposed of urine specimen.
		•	Sanitized hands and removed gloves.
		*	Completed the procedure within 5 minutes.
			TOTALS
			CHART
Date			

Evaluation of Student Performance

EVALUATION CRITERIA			COMMENTS
Symbol	Category	Point Value	
*	Critical Step	16 points	
●	Essential Step	6 points	
▷	Theory Question	2 points	

Score calculation: 100 points

      – _____ points missed

      _____ Score

Satisfactory score: 85 or above

CAAHEP Competencies Achieved:

Psychomotor (Skills)
☑ I. 14. Perform urinalysis.

Affective (Behavior)
☑ II. 2. Distinguish between normal and abnormal test results.

ABHES Competencies Achieved:

☑ 10. b. Perform selected CLIA-waived tests that assist with diagnosis and treatment: (1) Urinalysis.

EVALUATION OF COMPETENCY

Procedure 30-2: Chemical Testing of Urine with the Multistix 10 SG Reagent Strip

Name: _____   Date: _____

Evaluated By: _____   Score: _____

Performance Objective

Outcome:	Perform a chemical assessment of a urine specimen.
Conditions:	Given the following: disposable gloves, Multistix 10 SG reagent strips, urine container, laboratory report form, and a waste container.
Standards:	Time: 5 minutes. Student completed procedure in _____ minutes.
	Accuracy: Satisfactory score on the Performance Evaluation Checklist.

Performance Evaluation Checklist

Trial 1	Trial 2	Point Value	Performance Standards
		•	If necessary, performed a quality control procedure.
		▷	Stated when a quality control procedure should be performed.
		•	Obtained a freshly voided urine specimen from patient.
		▷	Explained why the container used to collect specimen should be clean.
		•	Sanitized hands.
		•	Assembled equipment.
		•	Checked expiration date of the reagent strips.
		▷	Stated why expiration date should be checked.
		•	Applied gloves.
		•	Removed a reagent strip from container and recapped immediately.
		▷	Explained why container should be recapped immediately.
		•	Did not touch the test areas with fingers.
		•	Explained why the test areas should not be touched with fingers.
		•	Mixed the urine specimen thoroughly.
		•	Removed the lid and completely immersed the reagent strip in urine specimen.
		•	Removed the strip immediately and ran the edge against the rim of urine container. Started the timer.
		▷	Explained why excess urine should be removed from the strip.
		•	Held the reagent strip in a horizontal position and placed it as close as possible to the corresponding color blocks on color chart.
		▷	Explained why the strip should be held in a horizontal position.

Trial 1	Trial 2	Point Value	*Performance Standards*
		●	Read the results at the exact reading times specified on color chart.
		▷	Explained why the results must be read at specified times.
		∗	The results were identical to the evaluator's results.
		●	Disposed of the strip in a regular waste container.
		●	Removed gloves and sanitized hands.
		●	Charted the results correctly.
		∗	Completed the procedure within 5 minutes.
			TOTALS

CHART

Date	

Evaluation of Student Performance

EVALUATION CRITERIA			COMMENTS
Symbol	Category	Point Value	
∗	Critical Step	16 points	
●	Essential Step	6 points	
▷	Theory Question	2 points	

Score calculation: 100 points

− _____ points missed

_____ Score

Satisfactory score: 85 or above

CAAHEP Competencies Achieved:

Psychomotor (Skills)
☑ I. 11. Perform quality control measures.
☑ I. 14. Perform urinalysis.

Affective (Behavior)
☑ II. 2. Distinguish between normal and abnormal test results.

ABHES Competencies Achieved:

☑ 10. a. Practice quality control.
☑ 10. b. Perform selected CLIA-waived tests that assist with diagnosis and treatment : (1) Urinalysis, (6) Kit testing, (c) Dip sticks.

CHARTING EXAMPLE

Multistix® *10 SG Reageant Strips for Urinalysis*

PATIENT

DATE   TIME

LEUKOCYTES	NEGATIVE ☐		TRACE ☐	SMALL + ☐	MODERATE ☐ ++	LARGE +++ ☐
NITRITE	NEGATIVE ☐		POSITIVE ☐	POSITIVE ☐	(Any degree of uniform pink color is found)	
UROBILINOGEN	NORMAL 0.2 ☐	NORMAL 1 ☐	mg/dL 2 ☐	4 ☐	8 ☐ (1mg = approx. 1 BU)	
PROTEIN	NEGATIVE ☐	TRACE ☐	mg/dL 30 * ☐	100 ++ ☐	300 +++ ☐ 2000 OR MORE ☐	
pH	5.0 ☐	6.0 ☐	6.5 ☐	7.0 ☐	7.5 ☐	8.0 ☐ 8.5 ☐
BLOOD	NEGATIVE ☐	NON-HEMOLYZED TRACE ☐	NON-HEMOLYZED MODERATE ☐	HEMOLYZED TRACE ☐	SMALL + ☐ MODERATE ++ ☐	LARGE +++ ☐
SPECIFIC GRAVITY	1.000 ☐	1.006 ☐	1.010 ☐	1.015 ☐	1.020 ☐ 1.025 ☐	1.030 ☐
KETONE	NEGATIVE ☐	mg/dL	TRACE 5 ☐	SMALL 15 ☐	MODERATE 40 ☐ LARGE 80 ☐	LARGE 160 ☐
BILIRUBIN	NEGATIVE ☐		SMALL ☐	MODERATE ++ ☐	LARGE +++ ☐	
GLUCOSE	NEGATIVE ☐	g/L (%) mg/dL	1/10 tr.) 100 ☐	1/6 250 ☐	1/2 500 ☐ 1 1000 ☐	2 or more 2000 or more ☐

(Modified and printed by permission of Siemens Healthcare Diagnostics, Deerfield, Ill, 60015.)

CHARTING EXAMPLE

Multistix® *10 SG Reageant Strips for Urinalysis*

PATIENT

DATE   TIME

LEUKOCYTES	NEGATIVE ☐		TRACE ☐	SMALL + ☐	MODERATE ☐ ++	LARGE +++ ☐
NITRITE	NEGATIVE ☐		POSITIVE ☐	POSITIVE ☐	(Any degree of uniform pink color is found)	
UROBILINOGEN	NORMAL 0.2 ☐	NORMAL 1 ☐	mg/dL 2 ☐	4 ☐	8 ☐ (1mg = approx. 1 BU)	
PROTEIN	NEGATIVE ☐	TRACE ☐	mg/dL 30 * ☐	100 ++ ☐	300 +++ ☐ 2000 OR MORE ☐	
pH	5.0 ☐	6.0 ☐	6.5 ☐	7.0 ☐	7.5 ☐	8.0 ☐ 8.5 ☐
BLOOD	NEGATIVE ☐	NON-HEMOLYZED TRACE ☐	NON-HEMOLYZED MODERATE ☐	HEMOLYZED TRACE ☐	SMALL + ☐ MODERATE ++ ☐	LARGE +++ ☐
SPECIFIC GRAVITY	1.000 ☐	1.006 ☐	1.010 ☐	1.015 ☐	1.020 ☐ 1.025 ☐	1.030 ☐
KETONE	NEGATIVE ☐	mg/dL	TRACE 5 ☐	SMALL 15 ☐	MODERATE 40 ☐ LARGE 80 ☐	LARGE 160 ☐
BILIRUBIN	NEGATIVE ☐		SMALL ☐	MODERATE ++ ☐	LARGE +++ ☐	
GLUCOSE	NEGATIVE ☐	g/L (%) mg/dL	1/10 tr.) 100 ☐	1/6 250 ☐	1/2 500 ☐ 1 1000 ☐	2 or more 2000 or more ☐

(Modified and printed by permission of Siemens Healthcare Diagnostics, Deerfield, Ill, 60015.)

Notes

EVALUATION OF COMPETENCY

Procedure 30-3: Prepare a Urine Specimen for Microscopic Examination: Kova Method

Name: _____   Date: _____

Evaluated By: _____   Score: _____

Performance Objective

Outcome:	Prepare a urine specimen for microscopic analysis by the physician under the microscope.
Conditions:	Given the following: disposable gloves; first-voided morning urine specimen; Kova urine centrifuge tube, cap, pipet, slide, and stain; test tube rack; urine centrifuge; mechanical stage microscope; and waste container.
Standards:	Time: 15 minutes. Student completed procedure in _____ minutes.
	Accuracy: Satisfactory score on the Performance Evaluation Checklist.

Performance Evaluation Checklist

Trial 1	Trial 2	Point Value	Performance Standards
		•	Sanitized hands.
		•	Assembled equipment.
		•	Applied gloves.
		•	Mixed urine specimen with pipet.
		▷	Stated the purpose of mixing the specimen.
		•	Poured urine specimen into urine centrifuge tube to the 12-ml mark.
		•	Capped the tube.
		•	Centrifuged specimen for 5 minutes.
		▷	Stated the purpose of centrifuging the specimen.
		•	Removed the tube from the centrifuge without disturbing the sediment.
		•	Removed the cap.
		•	Inserted Kova pipet into the urine tube and seated it firmly.
		•	Poured off the supernatant fluid.
		•	Removed pipet from the tube.
		•	Added one drop of Kova stain to the tube.
		▷	Stated the purpose of the stain.
		•	Placed pipet back in tube and mixed specimen thoroughly.
		•	Placed urine tube in test tube rack.
		•	Transferred a sample of the specimen to the Kova slide.

Trial 1	Trial 2	Point Value	Performance Standards
		•	Did not overfill or underfill the well of the Kova slide.
		•	Placed pipet in the urine tube.
		•	Allowed specimen to sit for 1 minute.
		▷	Explained the purpose of allowing the specimen to sit 1 minute.
		•	Properly focused the specimen under the microscope for the physician.
		•	When the physician is finished examining the specimen, removed the slide from the stage.
		•	Disposed of the slide and pipet in a regular waste container.
		•	Flushed the remaining urine down the sink.
		•	Capped the empty urine tube and disposed of it in a regular waste container.
		•	Removed gloves and sanitized hands.
		✳	Completed the procedure within 15 minutes.
			TOTALS

CHART

Date	

Evaluation of Student Performance

EVALUATION CRITERIA			COMMENTS
Symbol	Category	Point Value	
✳	Critical Step	16 points	
•	Essential Step	6 points	
▷	Theory Question	2 points	

Score calculation: 100 points

− _____ points missed

_____ Score

Satisfactory score: 85 or above

CAAHEP Competencies Achieved:

Psychomotor (Skills)

☑ I. 11. Perform quality control measures.

☑ I. 14. Perform urinalysis.

Affective (Behavior)

☑ III. 2. Explain the rationale for performance of a procedure to the patient.

ABHES Competencies Achieved:

☑ 10. a. Practice quality control.

☑ 10. b. Perform selected CLIA-waived tests that assist with diagnosis and treatment: (1) Urinalysis.

Notes

EVALUATION OF COMPETENCY

Procedure 30-4: Performing a Urine Pregnancy Test

Name: _____   Date: _____

Evaluated By: _____   Score: _____

Performance Objective

Outcome:	Perform a urine pregnancy test.
Conditions:	Given the following: disposable gloves, urine pregnancy testing kit, first-voided morning urine specimen, waste container.
Standards:	Time: 5 minutes. Student completed procedure in _____ minutes.
	Accuracy: Satisfactory score on the Performance Evaluation Checklist.

Performance Evaluation Checklist

Trial 1	Trial 2	Point Value	Performance Standards
			Preparing the Specimen
		•	Sanitized hands.
		•	Assembled equipment.
		•	Checked the expiration date on the pregnancy test.
		▷	Explained why the expiration date should be checked.
		•	If necessary, ran controls on the pregnancy test.
		▷	Stated when controls should be run.
		•	Applied gloves.
		•	Mixed the urine specimen.
		•	Removed the test cassette from its pouch.
		•	Placed the test cassette on a clean, dry, level surface.
		•	Added 3 drops of urine to the well on the test cassette.
		•	Disposed of the pipet in a regular waste container.
		•	Waited 3 minutes and read the results.
		•	Interpreted the test results.
		✳	The results were identical to the evaluator's results.
		▷	Described the appearance of a positive and a negative test result.
		▷	Explained what should be done if a blue control line does not appear.
		•	Disposed of the test cassette in a regular waste container.

Trial 1	Trial 2	Point Value	Performance Standards
		●	Removed gloves and sanitized hands.
		●	Charted the results correctly.
		✱	Completed the procedure within 5 minutes.
			TOTALS

CHART

Date	

Evaluation of Student Performance

EVALUATION CRITERIA			COMMENTS
Symbol	Category	Point Value	
✱	Critical Step	16 points	
●	Essential Step	6 points	
▷	Theory Question	2 points	

Score calculation: 100 points

− _____ points missed

_____ Score

Satisfactory score: 85 or above

CAAHEP Competencies Achieved:

Psychomotor (Skills)
☑ I. 11. Perform quality control measures.
☑ I. 16. Screen test results.

Affective (Behavior)
☑ II. 2. Distinguish between normal and abnormal test results.

ABHES Competencies Achieved:

☑ 10. a. Practice quality control.
☑ 10. b. Perform selected CLIA-waived tests that assist with diagnosis and treatment: (6) Kit Testing, (a) Pregnancy.

31

Phlebotomy

CHAPTER ASSIGNMENTS

√ After Completing	Date Due	Textbook Page(s)	TEXTBOOK ASSIGNMENTS	Possible Points	Points You Earned
		729-766	Read Chapter 31: Phlebotomy		
		736 765	Read Case Study 1 Case Study 1 questions	5	
		747 765	Read Case Study 2 Case Study 2 questions	5	
		753 765-766	Read Case Study 3 Case Study 3 questions	5	
			TOTAL POINTS		

√ After Completing	Date Due	Study Guide Page(s)	STUDY GUIDE ASSIGNMENTS (CTA: Critical Thinking Activity)	Possible Points	Points You Earned
		789	Pretest	10	
		790	Key Term Assessment	16	
		791-794	Evaluation of Learning questions	32	
		794	CTA A: Antecubital Veins	5	
			CD Activity: Chapter 31 Got Blood? (Record points earned)		
		794-795	CTA B: Venipuncture: Vacuum Tube Method	15	
		795-796	CTA C: Venipuncture Situations	7	
		796-797	CTA D: Skin Puncture	8	
		797	CTA E: Crossword Puzzle	23	
			CD Activity: Chapter 31 Apply Your Knowledge questions (Record points earned)		
		789	Posttest	10	

√ After Completing	Date Due	Study Guide Page(s)	STUDY GUIDE ASSIGNMENTS (CTA: Critical Thinking Activity)	Possible Points	Points You Earned
			ADDITIONAL ASSIGNMENTS		
			TOTAL POINTS		

√ When Assigned by Your Instructor	Study Guide Page(s)	Practices Required	LABORATORY ASSIGNMENTS (Procedure Number and Name)	*Score
	799	5	**Practice for Competency** 31-1: Venipuncture: Vacuum Tube Method Textbook reference: pp. 742-746	
	801-803		**Evaluation of Competency** 31-1: Venipuncture: Vacuum Tube Method	*
	799	5	**Practice for Competency** 31-2: Venipuncture: Butterfly Method Textbook reference: pp. 748-753	
	805-808		**Evaluation of Competency** 31-2: Venipuncture: Butterfly Method	*
	799	3	**Practice for Competency** 31-3: Skin Puncture: Disposable Semiautomatic Lancet Device Textbook reference: pp. 760-762	
	809-810		**Evaluation of Competency** 31-3: Skin Puncture: Disposable Semiautomatic Lancet Device	*
	799	3	**Practice for Competency** 31-4: Skin Puncture: Reusable Semiautomatic Lancet Device Textbook reference: pp. 762-764	
	811-812		**Evaluation of Competency** 31-4: Skin Puncture: Reusable Semiautomatic Lancet Device	*
			ADDITIONAL ASSIGNMENTS	

Notes

Name _____   Date _____

PRETEST

True or False

_____ 1. An individual who collects blood specimens is known as a *vampire*.

_____ 2. The purpose of applying a tourniquet when performing venipuncture is to make the patient's veins stand out.

_____ 3. The tourniquet should be left on the patient's arm for at least 2 minutes before performing a venipuncture.

_____ 4. Serum is obtained from whole blood that has been centrifuged.

_____ 5. A 25-gauge needle is recommended for performing venipuncture.

_____ 6. The size of the evacuated tube used to obtain a venous blood specimen depends on the size of the patient's veins.

_____ 7. A correct order of draw for the vacuum tube method of venipuncture is red, lavender, gray, and green.

_____ 8. Veins are most likely to collapse in patients with large veins and thick walls.

_____ 9. Hemolysis of a blood specimen results in inaccurate test results.

_____ 10. When obtaining a capillary specimen, the first drop of blood should be used for the test.

POSTTEST

True or False

_____ 1. Venous reflux can be prevented by filling the evacuated tube to the exhaustion of the vacuum.

_____ 2. If the tourniquet is applied too tightly, inaccurate test results may occur.

_____ 3. The median cubital vein is the best vein to use for venipuncture.

_____ 4. Upon standing, a blood specimen to which an anticoagulant has been added separates into plasma, buffy coat, and blood cells.

_____ 5. Whole blood is obtained by using a tube containing an anticoagulant.

_____ 6. An evacuated glass tube with a lavender stopper contains EDTA.

_____ 7. A red-stoppered tube is used to collect a blood specimen for most blood chemistries.

_____ 8. Not filling a tube to the exhaustion of the vacuum can result in hemolysis of the blood specimen.

_____ 9. If the needle is removed from the arm before removing the tourniquet, the evacuated tube will not fill completely.

_____ 10. If a fibrin clot forms in the serum layer of a blood specimen, it will lead to inaccurate test results.

Term KEY TERM ASSESSMENT

Directions: Match each medical term with its definition.

_____ 1. Antecubital space

_____ 2. Anticoagulant

_____ 3. Buffy coat

_____ 4. Evacuated tube

_____ 5. Hematoma

_____ 6. Hemoconcentration

_____ 7. Hemolysis

_____ 8. Osteochondritis

_____ 9. Osteomyelitis

_____ 10. Phlebotomist

_____ 11. Phlebotomy

_____ 12. Plasma

_____ 13. Serum

_____ 14. Venipuncture

_____ 15. Venous reflux

_____ 16. Venous stasis

A. The liquid part of blood, consisting of a clear, yellowish fluid that makes up approximately 55% of the total blood volume
B. A substance that inhibits blood clotting
C. A health professional trained in the collection of blood specimens
D. The breakdown of blood cells
E. A closed glass or plastic tube that contains a premeasured vacuum
F. The temporary cessation or slowing of the venous blood flow
G. A thin, light-colored layer of white blood cells and platelets that lays between a top layer of plasma and a bottom layer of red blood cells when an anticoagulant has been added to a blood specimen
H. The surface of the arm in front of the elbow
I. Inflammation of bone and cartilage
J. An increase in the concentration of the nonfilterable blood components
K. Plasma from which the clotting factor fibrinogen has been removed
L. Incision of a vein for the removal or withdrawal of blood
M. Inflammation of the bone due to bacterial infection
N. A swelling or mass of coagulated blood caused by a break in a blood vessel
O. Puncturing of a vein
P. The backflow of blood (from an evacuated tube) into the patient's vein

EVALUATION OF LEARNING

Directions: Fill in each blank with the correct answer.

1. List the three major areas of blood collection included in phlebotomy.

   _____

   _____

2. What is the purpose of performing a venipuncture?

   _____

   _____

3. List the methods that can be used to perform a venipuncture.

   _____

   _____

   _____

4. What are the advantages of using the vacuum tube method of venipuncture?

   _____

   _____

5. When would the butterfly method of venipuncture be preferred over the vacuum tube method?

   _____

   _____

   _____

6. Explain how to prevent venous reflux.

   _____

   _____

7. What is the purpose of the tourniquet?

   _____

   _____

8. After locating a suitable vein for venipuncture, what three qualities should be determined with respect to the vein?

   _____

   _____

9. Why are the antecubital veins preferred for performing a venipuncture?

   _____

   _____

   _____

10. List four techniques that can be used to make veins more prominent.

    _____

    _____

    _____

    _____

11. Why should the veins of the hand be used only as a last resort when performing a venipuncture?

_____

_____

_____

12. How is a serum specimen obtained?

_____

_____

13. How is a whole blood specimen obtained?

_____

_____

14. List the three layers into which the blood separates when it is mixed with an anticoagulant.

_____

_____

15. List the layers into which the blood separates when an anticoagulant is not added to it.

_____

_____

16. List four OSHA safety precautions that must be followed when performing a venipuncture and separating serum or plasma from whole blood.

_____

_____

17. What is the range for the gauge and size of the needle used for the vacuum tube method of venipuncture?

_____

_____

18. What is the purpose of the flange on the plastic holder of the vacuum tube system?

_____

_____

19. What type of additive is present in each of the following evacuated tubes?

Red: _____

Lavender: _____

Gray: _____

Light blue: _____

Green: _____

20. What color stopper must be used to collect the blood specimen for each of the tests listed?

Complete blood count: _____

Prothrombin time (PT): _____

Glucose tolerance test: _____

Most blood chemistry tests: _____

Blood gas determinations: _____

21. Why is it important to use the correct order of draw when performing a venipuncture?

_____

_____

22. Why is it important to mix a tube containing an anticoagulant immediately after drawing it?

_____

_____

23. What is the range for the gauge and size of needle used for the butterfly method of venipuncture?

_____

_____

24. List four ways to prevent a blood specimen from becoming hemolyzed.

_____

_____

_____

_____

25. List examples of dissolved substances contained in the serum of blood.

_____

_____

_____

26. What is the purpose of performing laboratory tests on serum?

_____

_____

_____

27. List the proper size tube that must be used to obtain the following serum specimens.

2 ml of serum: _____

6 ml of serum: _____

4 ml of serum: _____

28. What is a fibrin clot, and why should it be avoided in a serum specimen?

_____

_____

_____

29. How does a serum separator tube function in the collection of a serum specimen?

_____

_____

_____

30. What is the preferred site for a skin puncture for the following individuals?

a. Adult: _____

b. Infant: _____

31. Give two examples of microcollection devices.

_____

_____

32. Why should a finger puncture not be performed on the index finger?

_____

_____

CRITICAL THINKING ACTIVITIES

A. ANTECUBITAL VEINS

Practice palpating the antecubital veins on at least five individuals. Use a tourniquet applied to each individual's arm, and ask the individual to clench his or her fist. Record the individual's name and which vein would be considered the best to use on each individual when performing venipuncture.

NAME   SUITABLE VEIN

1. _____

2. _____

3. _____

4. _____

5. _____

B. VENIPUNCTURE: VACUUM TUBE METHOD

Using the principles outlined in the vacuum tube venipuncture procedure, state what might happen under the following circumstances:

1. An evacuated tube is used that is past its expiration date.

_____

_____

2. The vacuum tube is not labeled.

_____

_____

3. The tourniquet is not applied tightly enough.

_____

_____

4. The tourniquet is left on for more than 1 minute.

_____

_____

5. The area that has just been cleansed with an antiseptic is not allowed to dry before the venipuncture is made.

_____

_____

6. The evacuated tube is inserted past the indentation in the plastic holder before the vein is entered.

_____

_____

7. An angle of less than 15 degrees is used when performing venipuncture.

_____

_____

8. An angle of more than 15 degrees is used when performing venipuncture.

_____

_____

9. The needle is moved after insertion.

_____

_____

10. Venous reflux occurs when using an EDTA evacuated tube.

_____

_____

11. The vacuum tube is removed before it has filled to the exhaustion of the vacuum.

_____

_____

12. The needle is removed from the arm before the tourniquet has been removed.

_____

_____

13. A gauze pad is not placed slightly above the puncture site before removing the needle.

_____

_____

14. The patient bends the arm at the elbow after the needle is removed.

_____

_____

15. The patient lifts a heavy object after the procedure.

_____

_____

C. VENIPUNCTURE SITUATIONS

You are responsible for performing the venipunctures in your medical office. Explain what you would do in each of the following situations:

1. The patient asks you if the venipuncture will hurt.

_____

_____

2. On palpating the patient's vein, you find that it feels stiff and hard.

_____

_____

3. You have attempted one venipuncture in a patient with small veins using the vacuum tube method of venipuncture; however, the vein collapsed and you were unable to obtain blood.

_____

_____

4. The patient moves during the procedure, causing the needle to come out of the arm.

_____

_____

5. You have inserted the needle into the vein but notice a sudden swelling around the puncture site.

_____

_____

6. You inadvertently puncture the brachial artery after inserting the needle.

_____

_____

7. The patient begins to sweat and tells you that she feels warm and light-headed.

_____

_____

D. SKIN PUNCTURE

The MA is performing a skin puncture on an adult patient to obtain a capillary blood specimen for a hemoglobin test. For each of the following situations, write *C* if the technique is correct and *I* if the technique is incorrect. If the technique is correct, explain the rationale for performing it that way; if incorrect, explain what might happen if the technique were performed in the incorrect manner.

_____ 1. Before making the puncture, the MA asks the patient to rinse his or her hand in warm water.

_____

_____

_____ 2. The puncture is made with the patient in a standing position.

_____

_____

_____ 3. The site is allowed to dry thoroughly after it is cleansed with an antiseptic wipe.

_____

_____

_____ 4. The specimen is collected from the lateral part of the tip of the ring finger.

_____

_____

_____ 5. The puncture is made perpendicular to the lines of the fingerprint.

_____

_____

_____ 6. The depth of the puncture is 4 mm.

_____

_____

_____ 7. The first drop of blood is wiped away.

_____

_____

_____ 8. The puncture site is squeezed to obtain the blood specimen.

_____

_____

E. CROSSWORD PUZZLE
Phlebotomy
Directions: Complete the crossword puzzle using the clues presented below.

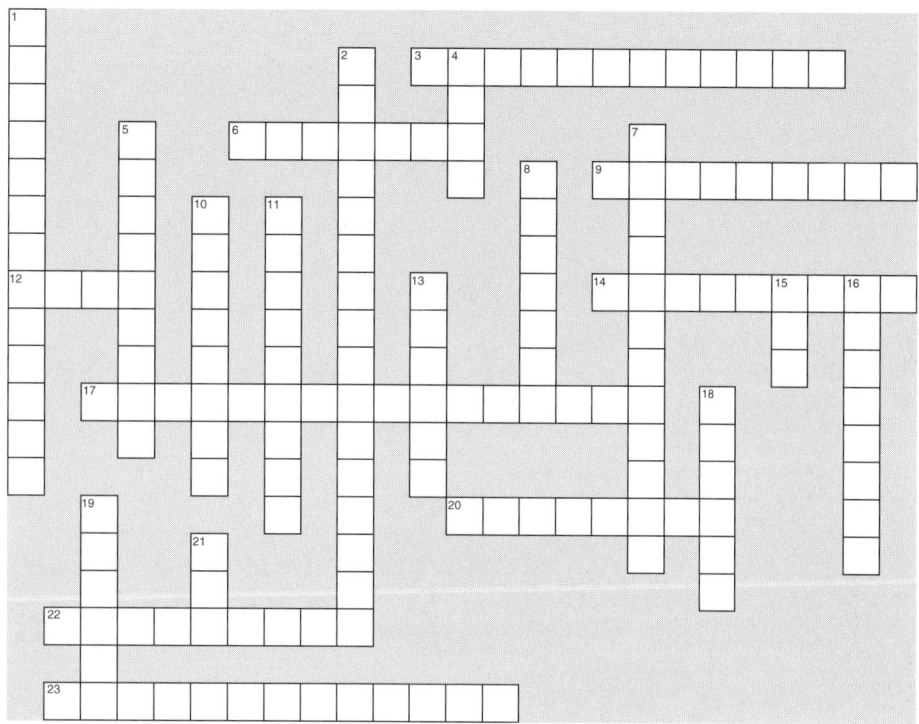

ACROSS
- **3** Collects blood
- **6** VP angle of insertion (degrees)
- **9** Broken RBCs
- **12** Fluoride/oxalate tube
- **14** For small veins
- **17** Fainting
- **20** Outdated tube problem
- **22** PT tube
- **23** Best VP vein

DOWN
- **1** Inhibits blood clotting
- **2** In front of the elbow
- **4** Last-choice veins
- **5** WBCs and platelets
- **7** Backflow of blood
- **8** Rolling vein
- **10** Bad bruise
- **11** What blood pressure does during fainting
- **13** Liquid part of the blood
- **15** No additive tube
- **16** EDTA tube
- **18** Fainting warning signal
- **19** Faint position
- **21** Contains a "separating" gel

Notes

PRACTICE FOR COMPETENCY

Procedure 31-1: Venipuncture—Vacuum Tube Method. Practice the procedure for collecting a venous blood specimen using the vacuum tube method. Record the procedure in the chart provided.

Procedure 31-2: Venipuncture—Butterfly Method. Practice the procedure for collecting a venous blood specimen using the butterfly method. Record the procedure in the chart provided.

Procedure 31-3: Disposable Lancet. Obtain a capillary blood specimen using a disposable semiautomatic lancet device.

Procedure 31-4: Reusable Lancet. Obtain a capillary blood specimen using a reusable semiautomatic lancet.

CHART	
Date	

CHART	
Date	

EVALUATION OF COMPETENCY

Procedure 31-1: Venipuncture—Vacuum Tube Method

Name: _____ Date: _____

Evaluated By: _____ Score: _____

Performance Objective

Outcome:	Perform a venipuncture using the vacuum tube method.
Conditions:	Given the following: disposable gloves, tourniquet, antiseptic wipe, double-pointed needle, plastic holder, evacuated tubes with labels, gauze pad, adhesive bandage, biohazard sharps container.
Standards:	Time: 10 minutes. Student completed procedure in ____ minutes.
	Accuracy: Satisfactory score on the Performance Evaluation Checklist.

Performance Evaluation Checklist

Trial 1	Trial 2	Point Value	Performance Standards
		●	Sanitized hands.
		●	Greeted the patient and introduced yourself.
		●	Identified the patient.
		●	Asked patient if he/she prepared properly.
			Prepared the equipment:
		●	Assembled equipment.
		●	Selected the proper evacuated tubes.
		●	Checked the expiration date of the tubes.
		▷	Stated the purpose of checking the expiration date.
		●	Labeled the evacuated tubes.
		●	Completed a laboratory request form, if necessary.
		●	Screwed the plastic holder onto the Luer adapter and tightened securely.
		●	Opened the gauze packet.
		●	Positioned the evacuated tubes in the correct order of draw.
		●	Tapped evacuated tubes with a powdered additive below the stopper.
		▷	Stated the purpose for tapping the tube.
		●	Placed the first tube loosely in the plastic holder.
			Prepared the patient:
		●	Explained the procedure to the patient and reassured patient.
		●	Performed a preliminary assessment of both arms.
		●	Correctly applied the tourniquet.

Trial 1	Trial 2	Point Value	Performance Standards
		●	Asked patient to clench fist.
		▷	Stated the purpose of the tourniquet and clenched fist.
		●	Assessed the veins of both arms.
		●	Determined the best vein to use.
		●	Positioned the patient's arm correctly.
		●	Thoroughly palpated the selected vein.
		●	Did not leave the tourniquet on for more than 1 minute.
		▷	Explained why the tourniquet should not be left on for more than 1 minute.
		●	Removed tourniquet and cleansed the puncture site.
		●	Allowed puncture site to air dry.
		▷	Explained why the site should be allowed to air-dry.
		●	Did not touch the site after cleansing.
		●	Placed supplies within comfortable reach of the nondominant hand.
		●	Reapplied tourniquet and applied gloves.
			Performed the venipuncture:
		●	Correctly positioned safety shield and removed cap from the needle.
		●	Properly held the venipuncture setup (bevel up) with the dominant hand.
		●	Positioned the tube with the label facing downward.
		▷	Explained why the label should face downward.
		●	Grasped the patient's arm and anchored the vein correctly.
		●	Positioned the venipuncture setup at a 15-degree angle to the arm, with the needle pointing in the same direction as the vein to be entered.
		●	Positioned the needle approximately ⅛-inch below the place where the vein is to be entered.
		●	Told the patient that a small stick will be felt.
		●	With one continuous motion, entered the skin and then the vein.
		●	Stabilized the vacuum tube setup.
		▷	Stated why the vacuum tube setup should be stabilized.
		●	Pushed the tube forward slowly to the end of the holder using the flange.
		●	Allowed evacuated tube to fill to the exhaustion of the vacuum.
		▷	Explained why the tube should be allowed to fill to the exhaustion of the vacuum.
		●	Removed the tube from the plastic holder using the flange.
		●	Immediately and gently inverted tube 8 to 10 times if it contained an additive.
		●	Inserted the next tube into the holder using the flange.
		●	Continued until the last tube was filled.
		✳	Removed the tourniquet and asked the patient to unclench fist.
		●	Removed the last tube from the holder.
		▷	Stated why the last tube should be removed.

Trial 1	Trial 2	Point Value	Performance Standards
		●	Placed gauze pad slightly above puncture site and withdrew the needle slowly and at the same angle as that for penetration.
		●	Immediately moved gauze over puncture site and applied pressure.
		●	Pushed safety shield forward with thumb until audible click was heard.
		●	Properly disposed of the venipuncture needle in a biohazard sharps container.
		●	Instructed patient to apply pressure with the gauze pad for 1 to 2 minutes.
		▷	Stated why pressure should be applied.
		●	Applied adhesive bandage to puncture site.
		●	Removed gloves and sanitized hands.
		●	Charted the procedure correctly.
		●	Tested specimen or prepared specimen for transport according to medical office policy.
		✱	Completed the procedure within 10 minutes.
			TOTALS

CHART	
Date	

Evaluation of Student Performance

EVALUATION CRITERIA			COMMENTS
Symbol	Category	Point Value	
✱	Critical Step	16 points	
●	Essential Step	6 points	
▷	Theory Question	2 points	
Score calculation: 100 points			
−_____ points missed			
_____ Score			
Satisfactory score: 85 or above			

CAAHEP Competencies Achieved:

Psychomotor (Skills)
☑ I. 2. Perform venipuncture.

Affective (Behavior)
☑ I. 1. Apply critical thinking skills in performing patient assessment and care.
☑ IV. 1. Demonstrate empathy in communicating with patients, family, and staff.

ABHES Competencies Achieved:

☑ 8. bb. Are impartial and show empathy when dealing with patients.
☑ 10. c. Dispose of biohazardous materials.
☑ 10. d. Collect, label, and process specimens: (1) Perform venipuncture.

Notes

EVALUATION OF COMPETENCY

Procedure 31-2: Venipuncture—Butterfly Method

Name: _____   Date: _____

Evaluated By: _____   Score: _____

Performance Objective

Outcome:	Perform a venipuncture using the butterfly method.
Conditions:	Given the following: disposable gloves, tourniquet, antiseptic wipe, winged infusion set, plastic holder, evacuated tubes with labels, gauze pad, adhesive bandage, biohazard sharps container.
Standards:	Time: 10 minutes. Student completed procedure in ____ minutes.
	Accuracy: Satisfactory score on the Performance Evaluation Checklist.

Performance Evaluation Checklist

Trial 1	Trial 2	Point Value	Performance Standards
		●	Sanitized hands.
		●	Greeted the patient and introduced yourself.
		●	Identified patient.
		▷	Stated why the patient must be correctly identified.
		●	Asked patient if he or she prepared properly.
		▷	Explained why it is important for the patient to prepare properly.
			Prepared the equipment:
		●	Assembled equipment.
		●	Selected the proper evacuated tubes.
		●	Checked the expiration date of the tubes.
		●	Labeled the evacuated tubes.
		●	Completed a laboratory request form, if necessary.
		●	Removed the winged infusion set from its package.
		●	Extended the tubing to its full length and stretched it.
		▷	Explained why the tubing should be extended and stretched.
		●	Screwed the plastic holder onto the Luer adapter and tightened it securely.
		●	Opened the gauze packet.
		●	Positioned the evacuated tubes in the correct order of draw.
		●	Tapped evacuated tubes with a powdered additive below the stopper.
		▷	Stated why tubes with powdered additives must be tapped.
		●	Placed the first tube loosely in the plastic holder with the label facing downward.
		▷	Explained why the label should be facing downward.

Trial 1	Trial 2	Point Value	Performance Standards
			Prepared the patient:
		●	Explained the procedure to the patient and reassured patient.
		●	Performed a preliminary assessment of both arms.
		●	Correctly applied the tourniquet and asked patient to clench fist.
		●	Assessed the veins of both arms.
		●	Determined the best vein to use.
		●	Positioned the patient's arm correctly.
		▷	Stated why arm must be positioned correctly.
		●	Thoroughly palpated the selected vein.
		▷	Stated the purpose of palpating the vein.
		●	Did not leave the tourniquet on for more than 1 minute.
		●	Removed tourniquet and cleansed puncture site.
		●	Allowed puncture site to air-dry.
		●	Did not touch the site after cleansing.
		●	Placed supplies within comfortable reach.
		●	Reapplied tourniquet and applied gloves.
			Performed the venipuncture:
		●	Grasped the winged infusion set correctly.
		●	Removed the protective shield.
		●	Positioned the needle with the bevel up.
		▷	Explained why the bevel should be up.
		●	Grasped patient's arm and anchored the vein correctly.
		●	Positioned the needle at a 15-degree angle to arm, with needle pointing in the same direction as the vein to be entered.
		●	Positioned the needle approximately ⅛-inch below the place where the vein is to be entered.
		●	Told the patient that a small stick will be felt.
		●	With one continuous motion, entered the skin and then the vein.
		▷	Explained why a continuous motion should be used.
		●	Decreased the angle of the needle to 5 degrees.
		●	Seated the needle.
		▷	Stated the purpose of seating the needle.
		●	Opended the butterfly wings and rested them flat against the skin.
		●	Kept the tube and holder in a downward position.
		●	Slowly pushed the tube forward to the end of the plastic holder.
		●	Allowed evacuated tube to fill to the exhaustion of the vacuum.
		▷	Explained why the tube should be filled to the exhaustion of the vacuum.
		●	Removed the tube from the plastic holder.

Trial 1	Trial 2	Point Value	Performance Standards
		•	Immediately and gently inverted evacuated tube 8 to 10 times if it contained an additive.
		▷	Explained why a tube with an additive must be inverted immediately.
		•	Inserted the next tube into the holder.
		•	Continued until the last tube was filled.
		✳	Removed the tourniquet and asked the patient to unclench fist.
		▷	Stated why the tourniquet must be removed before the needle.
		•	Removed the last tube from the holder.
		•	Placed gauze pad over puncture site. Grasped the setup just below the wings and withdrew the needle slowly and at the same angle as that for penetration.
		•	Immediately moved gauze over puncture site and applied pressure.
		•	Instructed the patient to apply pressure with the gauze.
		•	Activated the safety shield on the needle.
		•	Properly disposed of the winged infusion set in a biohazard sharps container.
		•	Continued to apply pressure for 1 to 2 minutes.
		•	Applied adhesive bandage.
		•	Removed gloves and sanitized hands.
		•	Charted the procedure correctly.
		•	Tested specimen or prepared specimen for transport according to medical office policy.
		✳	Completed the procedure within 10 minutes.
			TOTALS

CHART	
Date	

Evaluation of Student Performance

EVALUATION CRITERIA			COMMENTS
Symbol	**Category**	**Point Value**	
∗	Critical Step	16 points	
•	Essential Step	6 points	
▷	Theory Question	2 points	

Score calculation: 100 points

− _____ points missed

_____ Score

Satisfactory score: 85 or above

CAAHEP Competencies Achieved:

Psychomotor (Skills)

☑ I. 2. Perform venipuncture.

Affective (Behavior)

☑ I. 1. Apply critical thinking skills in performing patient assessment and care.
☑ IV. 1. Demonstrate empathy in communicating with patients, family, and staff.

ABHES Competencies Achieved:

☑ 8. bb. Are impartial and show empathy when dealing with patients.
☑ 10. c. Dispose of biohazardous materials.
☑ 10. d. Collect, label, and process specimens: (1) Perform venipuncture.

EVALUATION OF COMPETENCY

DVD **Procedure 31-3: Skin Puncture—Disposable Semiautomatic Lancet Device**

Name: _____   Date: _____

Evaluated By: _____   Score: _____

Performance Objective

Outcome:	Obtain a capillary blood specimen.
Conditions:	Given the following: disposable gloves, antiseptic wipe, Microtainer lancet, gauze pad, and a biohazard sharps container.
Standards:	Time: 5 minutes. Student completed procedure in ____ minutes.
	Accuracy: Satisfactory score on the Performance Evaluation Checklist.

Performance Evaluation Checklist

Trial 1	Trial 2	Point Value	Performance Standards
		•	Sanitized hands.
		•	Greeted the patient and introduced yourself.
		•	Identified the patient.
		•	Asked patient if he or she prepared properly.
		•	Assembled equipment.
		•	Opened sterile gauze packet.
		•	Explained the procedure to the patient and reassured patient.
		•	Seated patient in chair.
		•	Extended the palmar surface of patient's hand facing up.
		•	Selected a puncture site.
		•	Warmed site if needed.
		▷	Explained why the site should be warmed.
		•	Cleansed puncture site and allowed it to air-dry.
		▷	Explained why the site should be allowed to air dry.
		•	Did not touch the site after cleansing.
		•	Applied gloves.
		•	Firmly grasped patient's finger.
		•	Positioned the lancet firmly on the fingertip slightly to the side of center.
		•	Depressed the activation button without moving the lancet or finger.
		▷	Stated why the lancet and finger should not be moved.

Trial 1	Trial 2	Point Value	Performance Standards
		•	Disposed of lancet in biohazard sharps container.
		•	Waited a few seconds to allow blood flow to begin.
		•	Wiped away the first drop of blood with a gauze pad.
		▷	Stated why the first drop of blood should be wiped away.
		•	Allowed a second large, well-rounded drop of blood to form.
		•	Did not squeeze finger to obtain blood.
		•	Collected the blood specimen on a test strip or in the appropriate microcollection device.
		•	Instructed patient to hold a gauze pad over puncture site with pressure.
		•	Remained with patient until bleeding stopped.
		•	Applied an adhesive bandage if needed.
		•	Tested the blood specimen following the manufacturer's instructions.
		•	Removed gloves.
		•	Sanitized hands.
		∗	Completed the procedure within 5 minutes.
			TOTALS

Evaluation of Student Performance

EVALUATION CRITERIA			COMMENTS
Symbol	Category	Point Value	
∗	Critical Step	16 points	
•	Essential Step	6 points	
▷	Theory Question	2 points	

Score calculation: 100 points

− _____ points missed

_____ Score

Satisfactory score: 85 or above

CAAHEP Competencies Achieved:

Psychomotor (Skills)
☑ I. 1. Perform capillary puncture.

Affective (Behavior)
☑ IV. 1. Demonstrate empathy in communicating with patients, family, and staff.

ABHES Competencies Achieved:

☑ 8. bb. Are impartial and show empathy when dealing with patients.
☑ 10. d. Collect, label, and process specimens: (2) Perform capillary puncture.

EVALUATION OF COMPETENCY

Procedure 31-4: Skin Puncture—Reusable Semiautomatic Lancet Device

Name: _____   Date: _____

Evaluated By: _____   Score: _____

Performance Objective

Outcome:	Obtain a capillary blood specimen.
Conditions:	Given the following: disposable gloves, antiseptic wipe, Glucolet II lancet device, sterile lancet/endcap, gauze pad, and a biohazard sharps container.
Standards:	Time: 10 minutes. Student completed procedure in ____ minutes.
	Accuracy: Satisfactory score on the Performance Evaluation Checklist.

Performance Evaluation Checklist

Trial 1	Trial 2	Point Value	Performance Standards
		●	Sanitized hands.
		●	Greeted and identified the patient.
		●	Introduced yourself.
		●	Asked patient if he/she prepared properly.
		●	Assembled equipment.
		●	Pushed the transparent barrel toward the release button until it clicked into place.
		●	Inserted lancet/endcap onto the lancet device.
		●	Opened sterile gauze packet.
		●	Explained the procedure to the patient and reassured patient.
		●	Seated patient in chair.
		●	Extended the palmar surface of patient's hand facing up.
		●	Selected a puncture site.
		●	Warmed site if needed.
		▷	Explained how patient's finger can be warmed.
		●	Cleansed puncture site and allowed it to dry.
		●	Applied gloves.
		●	Twisted off plastic post from the endcap.
		●	Firmly grasped patient's finger.
		●	Placed the endcap firmly on the fingertip slightly to the side of center.
		●	Depressed the activation button without moving the Glucolet or finger.
		●	Wiped away the first drop of blood with a gauze pad.
		●	Allowed a large, well-rounded second drop of blood to form.

Trial 1	Trial 2	Point Value	Performance Standards
		▷	Explained why the finger should not be squeezed.
		•	Collected the blood specimen in the appropriate microcollection device.
		•	Instructed patient to hold a gauze pad over puncture site with pressure.
		•	Remained with patient until bleeding stopped.
		•	Applied an adhesive bandage if needed.
		•	Removed the endcap from the lancet device.
		•	Discarded the endcap in a biohazard waste container.
		•	Tested the blood specimen following the manufacturer's instructions.
		•	Removed gloves.
		•	Sanitized hands.
		•	Sanitized and disinfected the Glucolet.
		•	Stored Glucolet in its resting position.
		✶	Completed the procedure within 5 minutes.
			TOTALS

Evaluation of Student Performance

EVALUATION CRITERIA			COMMENTS
Symbol	Category	Point Value	
✶	Critical Step	16 points	
•	Essential Step	6 points	
▷	Theory Question	2 points	

Score calculation: 100 points

− _____ points missed

_____ Score

Satisfactory score: 85 or above

CAAHEP Competencies Achieved:

Psychomotor (Skills)
☑ I. 1. Perform capillary puncture.

Affective (Behavior)
☑ IV. 1. Demonstrate empathy in communicating with patients, family, and staff.

ABHES Competencies Achieved:

☑ 8. bb. Are impartial and show empathy when dealing with patients.
☑ 10. d. Collect, label, and process specimens: (2) Perform capillary puncture.

32

Hematology

CHAPTER ASSIGNMENTS

√ After Completing	Date Due	Textbook Page(s)	TEXTBOOK ASSIGNMENTS	Possible Points	Points You Earned
		767-779	Read Chapter 32: Hematology		
		771 778	📖 Read Case Study 1 Case Study 1 questions	5	
		774 779	📖 Read Case Study 2 Case Study 2 questions	5	
		776 779	📖 Read Case Study 3 Case Study 3 questions	5	
			TOTAL POINTS		

√ After Completing	Date Due	Study Guide Page(s)	STUDY GUIDE ASSIGNMENTS (CTA: Critical Thinking Activity)	Possible Points	Points You Earned
		817	Pretest	10	
		818	Key Term Assessment	6	
		819-820	Evaluation of Learning questions	12	
		820	CTA A: Diseases	40	
		823	CTA B: Hematocrit	5	
		823	CTA C: Iron Content of Food	10	
		824	CTA D: Iron Deficiency Anemia	20	
		826	CTA E: Dear Gabby	10	
		826-827	CTA F: Hematology Laboratory Report	6	
		827	CTA G: Crossword Puzzle	22	
			CD Activity: Chapter 32 Time for a Test (Record points earned)		
			CD Activity: Chapter 32 Animations	20	

√ After Completing	Date Due	Study Guide Page(s)	STUDY GUIDE ASSIGNMENTS (CTA: Critical Thinking Activity)	Possible Points	Points You Earned
			CD Activity: Chapter 32 Apply Your Knowledge questions (Record points earned)		
		817	Posttest	10	
			ADDITIONAL ASSIGNMENTS		
			TOTAL POINTS		

√ When Assigned by Your Instructor	Study Guide Page(s)	Practices Required	LABORATORY ASSIGNMENTS (Procedure Number and Name)	*Score
	829	3	**DVD** **Practice for Competency** 32-A: Performing a Hemoglobin Determination Textbook reference: p. 768	
	831-832		**Evaluation of Competency** 32-A: Performing a Hemoglobin Determination	*
	829	3	**DVD** **Practice for Competency** 32-1: Hematocrit Determination Textbook reference: pp. 772-774	
	833-835		**Evaluation of Competency** 32-1: Hematocrit Determination	*
	829	10	**DVD** **Practice for Competency** 32-2: Preparation of a Blood Smear for a Differential Cell Count Textbook reference: pp. 776-778	
	837-838		**Evaluation of Competency** 32-2: Preparation of a Blood Smear for a Differential Cell Count	*
			ADDITIONAL ASSIGNMENTS	

Notes

Name _____   Date _____

PRETEST

True or False

_____ 1. The study of blood is known as *serology*.

_____ 2. The function of hemoglobin is to assist in blood clotting.

_____ 3. The normal hemoglobin range for a female is 12 to 16 g/dL.

_____ 4. A low hemoglobin reading occurs with polycythemia.

_____ 5. The normal hematocrit range for a female is 40% to 54%.

_____ 6. Leukocytosis is an abnormal decrease in the number of leukocytes.

_____ 7. Strenuous exercise can result in an increase in the white blood cell count.

_____ 8. Leukemia can cause a decrease in the red blood cell count.

_____ 9. The normal range for a platelet count is 150,000 to 400,000.

_____ 10. The normal range for neutrophils is 50%-70%.

POSTTEST

True or False

_____ 1. Red and white blood counts are included in a CBC.

_____ 2. The normal range for hemoglobin for an adult male is 14 to 18 g/dL.

_____ 3. An increase in the Hgb level occurs with CHF.

_____ 4. The term *hematocrit* means "to separate blood."

_____ 5. The buffy coat consists of red blood cells.

_____ 6. Hematocrit test results should be read at the top of the red blood cell column.

_____ 7. The normal adult range for a white blood cell count is 4500 to 11,000.

_____ 8. Leukopenia occurs when a patient has appendicitis.

_____ 9. The normal range for a red blood cell count for a woman is 4 to 5.5 million.

_____ 10. Two blood smears must be prepared for a differential white blood cell count.

⬦Term **KEY TERM ASSESSMENT**

Directions: Match each medical term with its definition.

_____ 1. Anemia

_____ 2. Hematology

_____ 3. Hemoglobin

_____ 4. Leukocytosis

_____ 5. Leukopenia

_____ 6. Polycythemia

A. An abnormal decrease in the number of white blood cells (below 4,500 per cubic millimeter of blood)
B. A disorder in which there is an increase in the red cell mass
C. A condition in which there is a decrease in the number of erythrocytes or in the amount of hemoglobin in the blood
D. The study of blood and blood-forming tissues
E. An abnormal increase in the number of white blood cells (above 11,000 per cubic millimeter of blood)
F. The iron-containing pigment of erythrocytes that transports oxygen in the body

EVALUATION OF LEARNING

Directions: Fill in each blank with the correct answer.

1. List the tests generally included in a CBC.

   _____

   _____

2. What is the normal range for platelets in an adult?

   _____

3. What is the normal hemoglobin range?

   a. Women: _____

   b. Men: _____

4. List five conditions that cause a decrease in the hemoglobin level.

   _____

   _____

   _____

5. What is the purpose of the hematocrit?

   _____

   _____

6. What is the normal hematocrit range?

   a. Women: _____

   b. Men: _____

7. What is the normal range for the WBC count for an adult?

   _____

8. List examples of conditions that may result in leukocytosis.

   _____

   _____

9. What is the normal range for the RBC count for an adult?

   a. Women: _____

   b. Men: _____

10. List the five types of WBCs and the normal adult range for each.

    _____

    _____

    _____

11. Why must the WBCs be stained when performing a differential cell count?

    _____

    _____

12. List the abbreviation for each of the following tests:

    a. Hematocrit: _____

    b. Hemoglobin: _____

    c. Differential cell count: _____

    d. White blood cell count: _____

    e. Red blood cell count: _____

CRITICAL THINKING ACTIVITIES

A. DISEASES

1. You and your classmates work at a large clinic. It is National Disease Awareness Week. The physicians at your clinic ask you to develop informative, creative, and colorful brochures for patients relating to diseases. Choose a condition from the list and design a brochure using the blank FAQ (Frequently Asked Questions) brochure provided on the following page. Each student in the class should select a different disease. On a separate sheet of paper, write three true/false questions relating to the information in your brochure.

2. Present your brochure to the class. After all the brochures have been presented, each student should ask his or her three questions to the entire class to see how well the class understands the diseases that were presented. (*Note:* You can take notes during the presentations and refer to them when answering the questions.)

Diseases
1. Addison's disease
2. Amyotrophic lateral sclerosis
3. Aplastic anemia
4. Bell's palsy
5. Cirrhosis
6. Crohn's disease
7. Cushing's syndrome
8. Cystic fibrosis
9. Degenerative disc disease
10. Epilepsy
11. Hemolytic anemia
12. Hemophilia
13. Hernia
14. Hodgkin's disease
15. Hyperthyroidism
16. Hypothyroidism
17. Leukemia
18. Lupus erythematosus
19. Multiple sclerosis
20. Muscular dystrophy
21. Parkinson's disease
22. Peptic ulcer
23. Pernicious anemia
24. Polycythemia
25. Sickle cell anemia
26. Ulcerative colitis

FAQ
on:

Q: A:

Q: A:

Q: A:

Q: A:

Q:

A:

Q:

A:

Illustration

Q:

A:

Q:

A:

B. HEMATOCRIT

Label the layers of this microhematocrit capillary tube that has been centrifuged. Place an arrow at the point at which you would take the hematocrit reading.

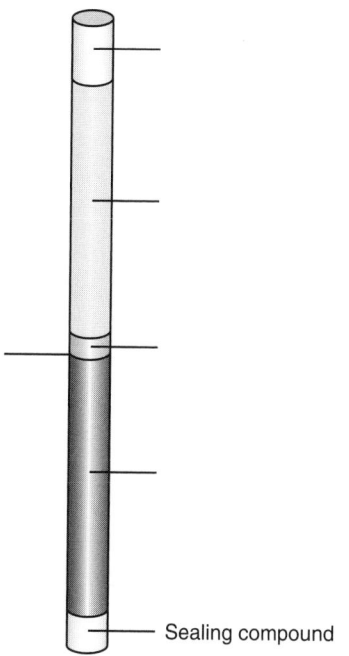

Sealing compound

(From Bonewit-West K: *Study guide for clinical procedures for medical assistants,* ed 7, St. Louis, 2008, Saunders.)

C. IRON CONTENT OF FOOD

Consuming food that is high in iron helps to prevent the development of iron deficiency anemia. To become familiar with foods that are high in iron content and foods that contain little or no iron, plan two meals. One meal should be as high as possible in iron content, and the other meal should not contain any iron at all.

Meal 1

_____

_____

_____

_____

Meal 2

_____

_____

_____

_____

D. IRON DEFICIENCY ANEMIA

Create a profile of a patient who has iron deficiency anemia following these guidelines:

1. Draw a figure of an individual exhibiting iron deficiency anemia using the sheet on the following page and colored pencils, crayons, or markers. Be as creative as possible.

2. Do not use any text on your drawing, other than to label items you have drawn in your picture. (A picture is worth a thousand words!)

3. Try to include all of the symptoms of iron deficiency anemia in your drawing. The Iron Deficiency Anemia Patient Teaching Box in your textbook can be used as a reference source.

4. In the classroom, find a partner and trade drawings. Identify the symptoms of iron deficiency anemia in your partner's drawing. With your partner, discuss what treatment is recommended and what this individual could do to prevent iron-deficiency anemia.

IRON DEFICIENCY ANEMIA

E. DEAR GABBY

Gabby is attending her class reunion and wants you to fill in for her. Respond to the following letter.

Dear Gabby,

I am a housewife with two adorable children, ages 2 and 4. I have been feeling rundown and tired lately, so I bought some iron pills at the drug store. They came individually packaged in foil and plastic. They are hard to open, so I cut each package and transferred the iron pills to a little plastic baggie. When I told my mother about what I thought was a great idea, she got very upset. She told me that I could possibly be putting my children in danger. She said that iron is poisonous to children and that I should not do that. Gabby, my mom has always been overprotective. Is this just another one of her episodes?

Signed,

Curious in Kansas

_____

_____

_____

_____

_____

_____

_____

_____

_____

_____

_____

F. HEMATOLOGY LABORATORY REPORT

The following terms may appear on hematology laboratory reports that describe changes in the shape, size, and staining reaction of erythrocytes. Using a reference source, define each in the space provided.

1. Anisocytosis

_____

_____

_____

2. Macrocyte

_____

_____

_____

3. Microcyte

_____

_____

_____

4. Poikilocyte

_____

_____

_____

5. Hypochromia

_____

_____

_____

6. Hyperchromia

_____

_____

_____

G. CROSSWORD PUZZLE
Hematology
Directions: Complete the crossword puzzle using the clues presented below.

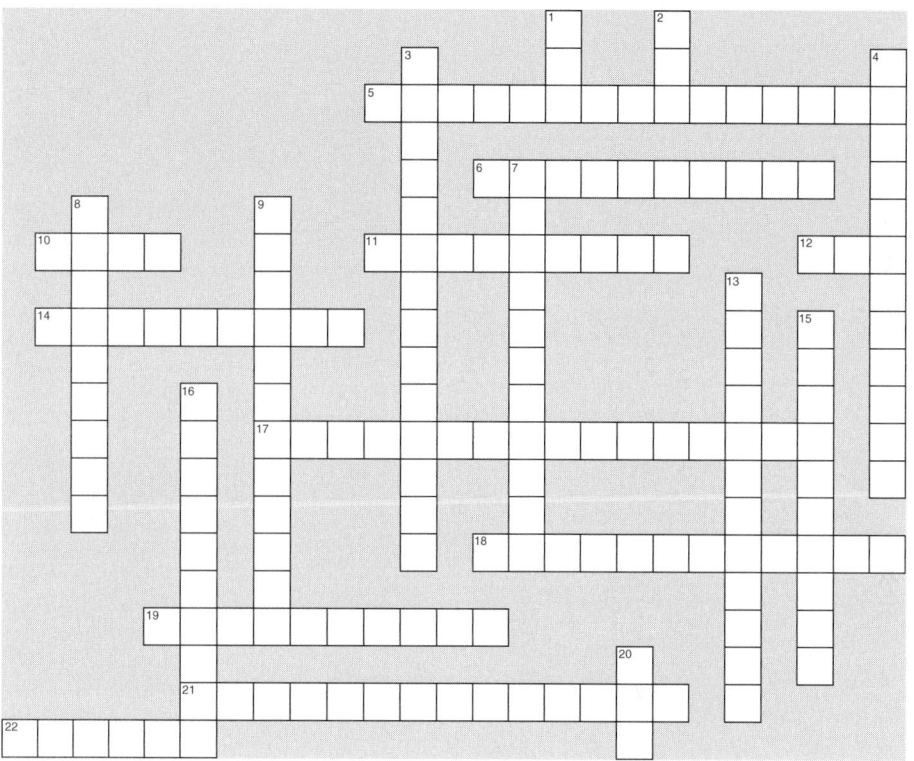

ACROSS
- **5** Screen for coagulation
- **6** Carries oxygen
- **10** Differential WBC count abbreviation
- **11** Platelets and WBCs
- **12** Common hematology test
- **14** WBC
- **17** Decreased platelet count
- **18** Occurs during acute bacterial infections
- **19** To separate blood
- **21** Common cause of anemia
- **22** Liquid part of the blood

DOWN
- **1** Nonspecific test for inflammation
- **2** Hemoglobin abbreviation
- **3** Causes black stool
- **4** Above 11,000 WBCs
- **7** RBC
- **8** Symptom of anemia
- **9** Condition of too many RBCs
- **13** Occurs during allergic conditions
- **15** Study of blood
- **16** Below 4500 WBCs
- **20** Hematocrit abbreviation

Notes

PRACTICE FOR COMPETENCY

Procedure 32-A: Hemoglobin Determination. Perform a hemoglobin determination using an automated blood analyzer and record results in the chart provided. Circle any values falling outside of normal range.

Procedure 32-1: Hematocrit Determination. Perform a hematocrit determination in duplicate and record results in the chart provided. Circle any values falling outside of normal range.

Procedure 32-2: Preparation of a Blood Smear for a Differential Cell Count. Prepare a blood smear for a differential white blood cell count.

CHART	
Date	

	CHART
Date	

EVALUATION OF COMPETENCY

Procedure 32-A: Performing a Hemoglobin Determination

Name: _____   Date: _____

Evaluated By: _____   Score: _____

Performance Objective

Outcome:	Perform a hemoglobin determination.
Conditions:	Using an automated blood analyzer and operating manual.
	Given the following: disposable gloves, antiseptic wipe, lancet, gauze pad, and a biohazard sharps container.
Standards:	Time: 10 minutes. Student completed procedure in ____ minutes.
	Accuracy: Satisfactory score in the Performance Evaluation Checklist.

Performance Evaluation Checklist

Trial 1	Trial 2	Point Value	Performance Standards
		●	Sanitized hands.
		●	Assembled equipment.
		●	Checked expiration date of test cards.
		●	Calibrated the blood analyzer.
		▷	Stated the purpose of calibrating the meter.
		●	Checked expiration date of control solution.
		●	Applied gloves and ran a low and high control.
		▷	Stated the purpose of running controls.
		●	Removed gloves and sanitized hands.
		●	Recorded control results in the quality control log.
		●	Greeted the patient and introduced yourself.
		●	Identified the patient and explained the procedure.
		●	Turned on the hemoglobin meter and checked the code number.
		●	Inserted a test card into the meter.
		●	Opened gauze packet.
		●	Cleansed puncture site and allowed it to air-dry.
		▷	Stated what happens to the blood drop if the site is not dry.
		●	Applied gloves and performed a finger puncture.
		●	Wiped away the first drop of blood.
		●	Collected the blood specimen.
		●	Placed a gauze pad over puncture site and applied pressure.

Trial 1	Trial 2	Point Value	Performance Standards
		•	Applied blood specimen to test card.
		•	Waited while hemoglobin meter analyzed the blood specimen.
		•	Read results on the display screen.
		▷	Stated the normal hemoglobin range for a female (12-16 g/dL) and a male (14-18 g/dL).
		•	Removed test card from meter.
		•	Properly disposed of test card in a biohazard waste container.
		•	Checked puncture site and applied adhesive bandage, if needed.
		•	Removed gloves.
		•	Sanitized hands.
		•	Charted the test results correctly.
		✳	The hemoglobin recording was identical to the reading on the digital display screen.
		✳	Completed the procedure within 10 minutes.
			TOTALS

CHART

Date	

Evaluation of Student Performance

EVALUATION CRITERIA			COMMENTS
Symbol	**Category**	**Point Value**	
✳	Critical Step	16 points	
•	Essential Step	6 points	
▷	Theory Question	2 points	

Score calculation: 100 points

−_____ points missed

_____ Score

Satisfactory score: 85 or above

CAAHEP Competencies Achieved:

Psychomotor (Skills)
☑ I. 11. Perform quality control measures.
☑ I. 12. Perform hematology testing.

Affective (Behavior)
☑ II. 2. Distinguish between normal and abnormal test results.

ABHES Competencies Achieved:

☑ 10. a. Practice quality control.
☑ 10. b. Perform selected CLIA-waived tests that assist with diagnosis and treatment: (2) Hematology testing.

EVALUATION OF COMPETENCY

Procedure 32-1: Hematocrit Determination

Name: _____ Date: _____

Evaluated By: _____ Score: _____

Performance Objective

Outcome:	Perform a hematocrit determination.
Conditions:	Given the following: microhematocrit centrifuge, disposable gloves, lancet, antiseptic wipe, gauze pad, capillary tubes, sealing compound, and a biohazard sharps container.
Standards:	Time: 10 minutes. Student completed procedure in _____ minutes.
	Accuracy: Satisfactory score in the Performance Evaluation Checklist.

Performance Evaluation Checklist

Trial 1	Trial 2	Point Value	Performance Standards
		•	Sanitized hands.
		•	Greeted the patient and introduced yourself.
		•	Identified the patient and explained the procedure.
		•	Assembled equipment.
		•	Opened gauze packet.
		•	Cleansed site with an antiseptic wipe and allowed it to dry.
		•	Applied gloves.
		•	Performed a finger puncture and discarded the lancet in a biohazard sharps container.
		•	Wiped away the first drop of blood.
		•	Massaged finger until large blood drop forms.
		•	Held one end of capillary tube horizontally, but slightly downward next to the free-flowing puncture.
		•	Kept the tip of the pipet in the blood, but did not allow it to press against the skin of the patient's finger.
		▷	Explained why the capillary tube should be kept in the blood specimen.
		•	Filled capillary tube (calibrated tubes filled to the calibration line; uncalibrated tubes filled approximately ¾ full).
		▷	Explained why a tube with air bubbles is unacceptable.
		•	Filled a second capillary tube.
		▷	Stated why 2 capillary tubes must be filled.

Trial 1	Trial 2	Point Value	Performance Standards
		●	Placed gauze pad over puncture site and applied pressure.
		●	Sealed one end of each capillary tube.
		●	Checked puncture site and applied adhesive bandage, if needed.
		●	Placed capillary tubes in the microhematocrit centrifuge with the sealed end facing toward the outside.
		▷	Explained why the sealed end must face toward the outside.
		●	Balanced one tube with the other tube placed opposite it.
		●	Placed the cover on the centrifuge and locked it securely.
		●	Centrifuged blood specimen for 3 to 5 minutes.
		▷	Explained the reason for centrifuging the blood specimen.
		●	Allowed centrifuge to come to a complete stop.
		●	Removed the protective cover from the capillary tubes.
		●	Read the results using the appropriate reading device.
		●	Determined if the results agreed within four percentage points.
		▷	Explained what to do if the results are not within four percentage points.
		●	Averaged the values of the two tubes together to derive the test results.
		✱	The results were within ± 1% of the evaluator's results.
		▷	Stated the normal hematocrit range for a female (37% to 47%) and a male (40% to 54%).
		●	Properly disposed of capillary tubes in a biohazard sharps container.
		●	Removed gloves.
		●	Sanitized hands.
		●	Charted the test results correctly.
		●	Returned equipment.
		✱	Completed the procedure within 10 minutes.
			TOTALS

	CHART
Date	

EVALUATION OF COMPETENCY

Procedure 32-2: Preparation of a Blood Smear for a Differential Cell Count

Name: _____   Date: _____

Evaluated By: _____   Score: _____

Performance Objective

Outcome:	Prepare a blood smear for a differential white blood cell count.
Conditions:	Given the following: disposable gloves, supplies to perform a finger puncture or venipuncture, slides with a frosted edge, slide container, biohazard specimen bag, laboratory request form, and a biohazard sharps container.
Standards:	Time: 10 minutes. Student completed procedure in ____ minutes.
	Accuracy: Satisfactory score in the Performance Evaluation Checklist.

Performance Evaluation Checklist

Trial 1	Trial 2	Point Value	Performance Standards
		●	Sanitized hands.
		●	Greeted the patient and introduced yourself.
		●	Identified the patient and explained the procedure.
		●	Assembled equipment.
		●	Labeled slides.
		●	Cleansed puncture site.
		●	Applied gloves.
		●	Performed a venipuncture or finger puncture.
		●	Placed a drop of blood in the middle of each slide approximately ¼ inch from the frosted edge of the slide.
		●	Held a spreader slide at a 30-degree angle to first slide in front of the drop of blood.
		▷	Stated what occurs if the angle is more than 30 degrees or less than 30 degrees.
		●	Moved the spreader slide until it touched the drop of blood.
		●	Spread the blood thinly and evenly across slide using the spreader slide.
		●	Prepared the second blood smear.
		●	Disposed of the spreader slide in a biohazard sharps container.
		●	Laid the blood smears on a flat surface and allowed them to dry.
		▷	Explained why the blood smears should be dried immediately.
		●	The length of the smear was approximately 1½ inches.
		●	The smear was smooth and even with no ridges, holes, lines, streaks, or clumps.

Trial 1	Trial 2	Point Value	Performance Standards
		•	The smear was not too thick or too thin.
		•	There was a feathered edge at the thin end of the smear.
		•	There was a margin on all sides of the smear.
		•	Placed the slides in a protective slide container.
		•	Prepared blood tube and slides for transport to outside laboratory.
		•	Removed gloves and sanitized hands.
		•	Charted the procedure correctly.
		✻	Completed the procedure within 10 minutes.
			TOTALS

CHART

Date	

Evaluation of Student Performance

EVALUATION CRITERIA			COMMENTS
Symbol	Category	Point Value	
✻	Critical Step	16 points	
•	Essential Step	6 points	
▷	Theory Question	2 points	

Score calculation: 100 points
− _____ points missed
_____ Score

Satisfactory score: 85 or above

CAAHEP Competencies Achieved:

Psychomotor (Skills)
☑ I. 11. Perform quality control measures.

Affective (Behavior)
☑ I. 1. Apply critical thinking skills in performing patient assessment and care.

ABHES Competencies Achieved:

☑ 10. a. Practice quality control.
☑ 10. d. Collect, label, and process specimens.

33

Blood Chemistry and Serology

CHAPTER ASSIGNMENTS

√ After Completing	Date Due	Textbook Page(s)	TEXTBOOK ASSIGNMENTS	Possible Points	Points You Earned
		780-803	Read Chapter 33: Blood Chemistry and Serology		
		789 802	🖉 Read Case Study 1 Case Study 1 questions	5	
		790 802	🖉 Read Case Study 2 Case Study 2 questions	5	
		793 803	🖉 Read Case Study 3 Case Study 3 questions	5	
			TOTAL POINTS		

√ After Completing	Date Due	Study Guide Page(s)	STUDY GUIDE ASSIGNMENTS (CTA: Critical Thinking Activity)	Possible Points	Points You Earned
		843	🗒 Pretest	10	
		844	🔑 Key Term Assessment	11	
		845-848	📑 Evaluation of Learning questions	40	
		848	CTA A: Coronary Heart Disease	20	
		850	CTA B: Cholesterol and Saturated Fat	15	
		850	CTA C: Glucose Tolerance Test	15	
		851	CTA D: Rh Incompatibility	20	
		851	CTA E: Type 2 Diabetes Brochure	40	
			💿 CD Activity: Chapter 33 The Right Chemistry: Blood Chemistry Tests (Record points earned)		
		855	CTA F: Crossword Puzzle	24	
			💿 CD Activity: Chapter 33 It's Serology: Serologic Tests (Record points earned)		

√ After Completing	Date Due	Study Guide Page(s)	STUDY GUIDE ASSIGNMENTS (CTA: Critical Thinking Activity)	Possible Points	Points You Earned
			⊙ CD Activity: Chapter 33 Animations	20	
			⊙ CD Activity: Chapter 33 Apply Your Knowledge questions (Record points earned)		
		843	▤ Posttest	10	
			ADDITIONAL ASSIGNMENTS		
			TOTAL POINTS		

√ When Assigned by Your Instructor	Study Guide Page(s)	Practices Required	LABORATORY ASSIGNMENTS (Procedure Number and Name)	*Score
	857	3	**Practice for Competency** 33-A: Performing a Blood Chemistry Test Textbook reference: pp. 782-788	
	859-860		**Evaluation of Competency** 33-A: Performing a Blood Chemistry Test	*
	857	3	DVD **Practice for Competency** 33-1: Blood Glucose Measurement Using the Accu-Chek Advantage Glucose Meter Textbook reference: pp. 797-799	
	861-863		**Evaluation of Competency** 33-1: Blood Glucose Measurement Using the Accu-Chek Advantage Glucose Meter	*
	857	3	DVD **Practice for Competency** 33-B: Performing a Rapid Mononucleosis Test Textbook reference: p. 801	
	865-866		**Evaluation of Competency** 33-B: Performing a Rapid Mononucleosis Test	*
			ADDITIONAL ASSIGNMENTS	

Notes

Name _____   Date _____

? PRETEST

True or False

_____ 1. Most of the cholesterol found in the blood comes from the intake of dietary cholesterol.

_____ 2. The primary use of the cholesterol test is to screen for the presence of coronary heart disease.

_____ 3. LDL picks up cholesterol from ingested fats and the liver and carries it to the cells.

_____ 4. The function of glucose in the body is to build and repair tissue.

_____ 5. Insulin is required for normal utilization of glucose in the body.

_____ 6. An abnormally low level of glucose in the body is known as *hypoglycemia*.

_____ 7. The hemoglobin A_{1C} test measures the average amount of blood glucose over a 3-month period.

_____ 8. An antibody is a substance that is capable of combining with an antigen.

_____ 9. Mononucleosis is transmitted through coughing and sneezing.

_____ 10. Symptoms of infectious mononucleosis include severe fatigue, fever, and sore throat.

? POSTTEST

True or False

_____ 1. Serum is required for most blood chemistry tests.

_____ 2. The buildup of plaque (due to high cholesterol) on the walls of arteries is known as *thrombophlebitis*.

_____ 3. An HDL cholesterol level greater than 50 mg/dL is a risk factor for coronary heart disease.

_____ 4. The triglyceride test requires that the patient not eat or drink for 12 hours before the test.

_____ 5. The normal range for a fasting blood sugar is 120 to 160 mg/dL.

_____ 6. The glucose tolerance test is used to assist in the diagnosis of diabetes mellitus.

_____ 7. Before meals, it is recommended that the blood glucose level for a diabetic patient fall between 60 and 80 mg/dL.

_____ 8. The recommended A_{1C} level for an individual with diabetes is 4% to 6%.

_____ 9. The RPR test is a screening test for syphilis.

_____ 10. The varicella virus causes infectious mononucleosis.

KEY TERM ASSESSMENT

Directions: Match each medical term with its definition.

_____ 1. Agglutination

_____ 2. Antibody

_____ 3. Antigen

_____ 4. Glycogen

_____ 5. Glycosylation

_____ 6. HDL cholesterol

_____ 7. Hemoglobin A_{1C}

_____ 8. Hyperglycemia

_____ 9. Hypoglycemia

_____ 10. LDL cholesterol

_____ 11. Lipoprotein

A. An abnormally high level of glucose in the blood
B. A complex molecule consisting of protein and a lipid fraction such as cholesterol
C. The form in which carbohydrate is stored in the body
D. A lipoprotein consisting of protein and cholesterol that removes excess cholesterol from the cells
E. An abnormally low level of glucose in the blood
F. A lipoprotein, consisting of protein and cholesterol, that picks up cholesterol and delivers it to the cells
G. A substance that is capable of combining with an antigen resulting in an antigen-antibody reaction
H. A substance capable of stimulating the formation of antibodies
I. Clumping of blood cells
J. The process of glucose attaching to hemoglobin
K. Compound formed when glucose attaches or glycosylates to the protein in hemoglobin

EVALUATION OF LEARNING

Directions: Fill in each blank with the correct answer.

1. What type of specimen is required for most blood chemistry tests?

   _____

2. What is the purpose of quality control?

   _____

   _____

3. What is the purpose of calibrating a blood chemistry analyzer?

   _____

   _____

4. List two reasons why a control may not fall within its normal range.

   _____

   _____

5. What is cholesterol?

   _____

   _____

6. List the two main sources of cholesterol in the blood.

   _____

   _____

7. What is atherosclerosis, and why is it a health risk?

   _____

   _____

8. Why is LDL cholesterol referred to as "bad cholesterol" and HDL referred to as "good cholesterol"?

   _____

   _____

9. What does a total cholesterol test measure?

   _____

   _____

10. List the ranges for each of the following cholesterol categories:
    a. Desirable cholesterol level: _____
    b. Borderline cholesterol level: _____
    c. High cholesterol level: _____

11. At what level is HDL cholesterol considered a risk factor for coronary heart disease?

    _____

    _____

12. What type of patient preparation is required for a triglyceride test?

_____

_____

13. What is the primary use of the cholesterol test?

_____

_____

14. What is the purpose of performing a BUN?

_____

_____

15. What is the function of glucose in the body?

_____

_____

16. Explain the function of insulin in the body.

_____

_____

17. List the abbreviation for each of the following tests:

    a. Fasting blood sugar: _____

    b. 2-hour postprandial blood sugar: _____

    c. Glucose tolerance test: _____

18. What type of patient preparation is required for a fasting blood sugar?

_____

_____

19. What is the normal range for a fasting blood sugar?

_____

20. List two reasons for performing a fasting blood sugar.

_____

21. What type of patient preparation is required for a 2-hour postprandial glucose test?

_____

_____

22. Describe the procedure for performing a 2-hour postprandial glucose test.

_____

_____

23. What is the purpose of the glucose tolerance test?

_____

_____

24. What type of patient preparation is required for the glucose tolerance test?

_____

_____

25. Describe the procedure for a glucose tolerance test.

_____

_____

26. Define hypoglycemia, and list three conditions that may cause it to occur.

_____

_____

27. Why is it important for an insulin-dependent diabetic to perform SMBG?

_____

_____

28. What is the ideal insulin testing schedule for SMBG?

_____

_____

29. What type of damage can occur to the body from prolonged high blood glucose levels?

_____

_____

30. List three advantages of blood glucose monitoring at home.

_____

_____

_____

31. What is the recommended blood glucose level for a diabetic during the following times of the day?
    a. Before meals: _____
    b. 1 to 2 hours after meals: _____
    c. At bedtime: _____

32. What information is provided by a hemoglobin A_{1C} test?

_____

_____

33. What is the normal A_{1C} range for an individual without diabetes?

_____

34. What is the recommended A_{1C} percentage for an individual with diabetes?

_____

_____

35. What are the storage requirements for blood glucose reagent strips?

_____

_____

36. What is the definition of serology?

_____

_____

_____

37. List three examples of antigens.

_____

_____

38. What is the purpose of performing each of the following serologic tests?

   a. Rheumatoid factor

   _____

   _____

   b. Antistreptolysin test

   _____

   _____

   c. C-reactive protein

   _____

   _____

   d. ABO and Rh blood typing

   _____

   _____

39. How is infectious mononucleosis transmitted?

   _____

   _____

40. What are the symptoms of infectious mononucleosis?

   _____

   _____

CRITICAL THINKING ACTIVITIES

A. CORONARY HEART DISEASE

   Create a profile of an individual who is at risk for developing coronary heart disease (CHD) following these guidelines:

   1. Using colored pencils, crayons, or markers, draw a figure of an individual exhibiting risk factors for CHD. Be as creative as possible.

   2. Do not use any text on your drawing, other than to label items you have drawn in your picture. (A picture is worth a thousand words!)

   3. Try to include at least eight risk factors for CHD in your drawing. The *Highlight on Coronary Heart Disease* box in your textbook can be used as a reference source.

   4. In the classroom, find a partner and trade drawings. Identify the risk factors for CHD in your partner's drawing. With your partner, discuss what this person could do to reduce his or her chances of developing coronary artery disease.

AT RISK FOR CHD

B. CHOLESTEROL AND SATURATED FAT

Using a reference source, complete the following activities:

1. Create a dinner meal that is as high as possible in saturated fat and cholesterol.

_____

_____

_____

_____

_____

2. Create a dinner meal that is as low as possible in saturated fat and cholesterol.

_____

_____

_____

_____

_____

3. Choose a fast-food restaurant, and plan a meal that is as low as possible in saturated fat and cholesterol.

_____

_____

_____

_____

_____

C. GLUCOSE TOLERANCE TEST

Marty Wolf has arrived at your office for a glucose tolerance test. What should you tell her regarding the following? Explain the reason for each answer.

1. Consumption of food and fluid

_____

_____

2. Water consumption

_____

_____

3. Smoking

_____

_____

4. Leaving the test site

_____

_____

5. Activity

_____

_____

D. Rh INCOMPATIBILITY

Erythroblastosis fetalis is a blood disorder of the newborn that is usually due to incompatibility between the infant's blood and the mother's blood. Using a reference source, answer the following questions regarding this condition.

1. Explain how an Rh incompatibility between the mother and infant can cause this condition to occur.

   _____

   _____

   _____

   _____

2. Name the symptoms associated with erythroblastosis fetalis.

   _____

   _____

   _____

3. Explain the treatment used for this condition.

   _____

   _____

   _____

4. How can this condition be prevented?

   _____

   _____

   _____

E. TYPE 2 DIABETES BROCHURE

You are working for a physician specializing in internal medicine. Your physician is concerned about the increase in the number of patients developing type 2 diabetes mellitus. He asks you to design a colorful, creative, and informative brochure on type 2 diabetes using the brochure provided on the following page. This brochure will be published and placed in the waiting room to provide patients with education on type 2 diabetes. The diabetes Internet sites listed under **On the Web** in your textbook can be used to complete this activity.

Notes

FAQ on:

Q:　　　　A:

Q:　　　　A:

Q:　　　　A:

Q:　　　　A:

Q:

A:

Q:

A:

Illustration

Q:

A:

Q:

A:

F. CROSSWORD PUZZLE
Blood Chemistry and Serology
Directions: Complete the crossword puzzle using the clues presented below.

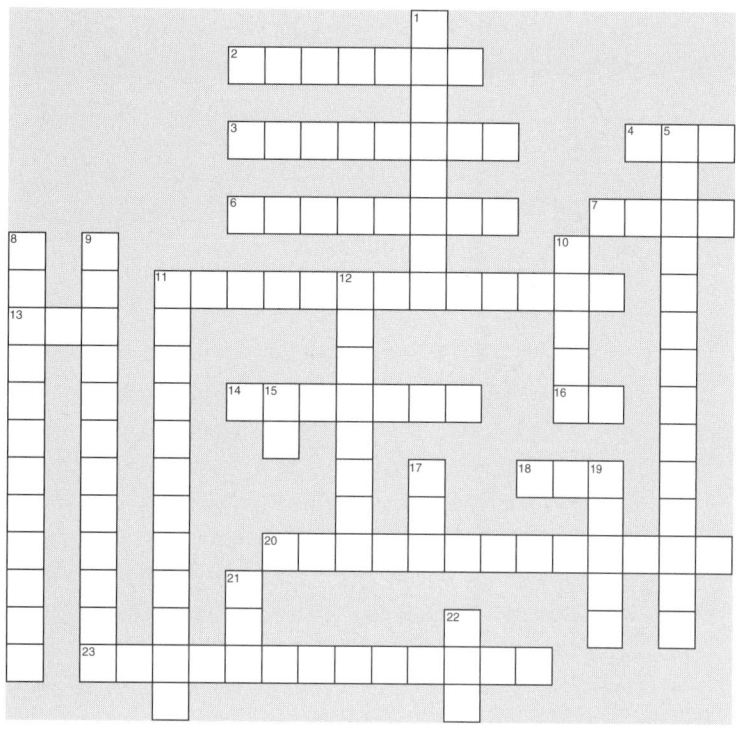

ACROSS
2 Increases risk of CHD
3 Increases HDL cholesterol
4 70-110 mg/dL
6 Unsaturated fat (example)
7 Syphilis test
11 High blood sugar
13 Detects liver disease
14 Provides energy for body
16 Rheumatoid arthritis test
18 Series of glucose tests
20 Kissing disease
23 Normal: <150 mg/dL

DOWN
1 Combines with an antigen
5 Cholesterol: 200-239
8 #1 killer in United States
9 Increases cholesterol
10 Makes cholesterol
11 Low blood sugar
12 Stored glucose
15 Assists in confirming a myocardial infarction
17 Detects renal disease
19 Thyroid functioning test
21 Bad cholesterol
22 Good cholesterol

Notes

PRACTICE FOR COMPETENCY

Procedure 33-A: Blood Chemistry Test. Perform a blood chemistry test, and record results in the chart provided. Examples of blood chemistry tests: cholesterol, triglycerides, hemoglobin A_{1C}, BUN.

Procedure 33-1: Blood Glucose Measurement. Perform a fasting blood sugar, and record results in the chart provided.

Procedure 33-B: Rapid Mononucleosis Test. Perform a rapid mononucleosis test, and record results in the chart provided.

CHART	
Date	

CHART	
Date	

📝 EVALUATION OF COMPETENCY

Procedure 33-A: Performing a Blood Chemistry Test

Name: _____   Date: _____

Evaluated By: _____   Score: _____

Performance Objective

Outcome:	Perform a blood chemistry test.
Conditions:	Given the following: personal protective equipment (including disposable gloves), an antiseptic wipe, a lancet, gauze pads, and a biohazard sharps container. Using an automated blood chemistry analyzer and operating manual.
Standards:	Time: 10 minutes. Student completed procedure in _____ minutes.
	Accuracy: Satisfactory score in the Performance Evaluation Checklist.

Performance Evaluation Checklist

Trial 1	Trial 2	Point Value	*Performance Standards*
		●	Sanitized hands.
		●	Assembled equipment.
		●	Calibrated the blood chemistry analyzer.
		●	Applied gloves and ran controls.
		●	Recorded results in the quality control log.
		●	Sanitized hands. Greeted the patient and introduced yourself.
		●	Identified the patient and explained the procedure.
		●	Applied gloves.
		●	Performed a finger puncture.
		●	Collected the specimen according to manufacturer's instructions.
		●	Placed a gauze pad over the puncture site and applied pressure.
		●	Inserted the specimen into blood chemistry analyzer according to manufacturer's instructions.
		●	Operated the blood chemistry analyzer according to manufacturer's instructions.
		●	Read the results on digital display screen.
		●	Properly disposed of used materials.
		●	Checked puncture site and applied adhesive bandage if needed.
		●	Removed gloves.
		●	Sanitized hands.
		●	Charted the test results correctly.
		✱	The recording was identical to the reading on the digital display screen.
		✱	Completed the procedure within 10 minutes.
		TOTALS	

CHART	
Date	

Evaluation of Student Performance

EVALUATION CRITERIA			COMMENTS
Symbol	Category	Point Value	
*	Critical Step	16 points	
●	Essential Step	6 points	
▷	Theory Question	2 points	

Score calculation: 100 points

−_____ points missed

_____ Score

Satisfactory score: 85 or above

CAAHEP Competencies Achieved:

Psychomotor (Skills)
☑ I. 11. Perform quality control measures.
☑ I. 12. Perform chemistry testing.
☑ II. 2. Maintain laboratory test results using flow sheets.

Affective (Behavior)
☑ II. 2. Distinguish between normal and abnormal test results.

ABHES Competencies Achieved:

☑ 10. a. Practice quality control.
☑ 10. b. Perform selected CLIA-waived tests that assist with diagnosis and treatment: (3) Chemistry testing.

EVALUATION OF COMPETENCY

Procedure 33-1: Bood Glucose Measurement Using the Accu-Chek Advantage Glucose Meter

Name: _____   Date: _____

Evaluated By: _____   Score: _____

Performance Objective

Outcome:	Perform a fasting blood sugar.
Conditions:	Given the following: personal equipment (including disposable gloves), Accu-Chek Advantage glucose monitor, reagent strips, check strip, code key, control solutions, lancet, antiseptic wipe, gauze pad, and a biohazard sharps container.
Standards:	Time: 10 minutes. Student completed procedure in _____ minutes.
	Accuracy: Satisfactory score in the Performance Evaluation Checklist.

Performance Evaluation Checklist

Trial 1	Trial 2	Point Value	Performance Standards
		●	Sanitized hands.
		●	Assembled equipment.
		●	Checked the expiration date on container of reagent strips.
		●	Calibrated the monitor using the code key.
		▷	Stated the purpose of calibrating the meter.
		●	Ran a low and high control.
		▷	Stated the purpose for running controls.
		●	Recorded results in the quality control log.
		●	Sanitized hands. Greeted the patient and introduced yourself.
		●	Identified the patient and explained the procedure.
		●	Asked the patient if he or she prepared properly.
		▷	Stated the preparation required for a fasting blood sugar.
		●	Removed a test strip from the container.
		●	Immediately replaced the lid of the container.
		▷	Explained why the lid should be replaced immediately.
		●	Gently inserted the test strip into the test strip guide.
		●	The yellow target area was facing up.
		●	Turned on the meter (if the meter does not turn on automatically).
		●	Checked the code number.
		●	Opened gauze packet.
		●	Cleansed the puncture site with an antiseptic wipe and allowed it to dry.
		●	Applied gloves.

Trial 1	Trial 2	Point Value	Performance Standards
		●	Performed a finger puncture.
		●	Disposed of the lancet in the biohazard sharps container.
		●	Wiped away the first drop of blood with a gauze pad.
		▷	Explained why the first drop of blood should be wiped away.
		●	Placed the patient's hand in a dependent position and gently squeezed finger until a large drop of blood formed.
		●	Applied the drop of blood to the yellow target area of the test strip.
		●	Completely covered the yellow target area of the test strip.
		▷	Explained what to do if the yellow area is not completely covered.
		●	Placed a gauze pad over puncture site and applied pressure.
		●	Observed the digital display of the test results.
		▷	Stated the normal range for a fasting blood glucose (70 to 110 mg/dL).
		●	Removed the test strip from the meter and discarded it in a biohazard waste container.
		●	Turned off the meter.
		●	Checked puncture site and applied adhesive bandage, if needed.
		●	Removed gloves and sanitized hands.
		●	Charted the test results correctly.
		✶	The recording was identical to the reading on the digital display screen.
		●	Properly stored the glucose monitor.
		✶	Completed the procedure within 10 minutes.
			TOTALS

CHART	
Date	

Evaluation of Student Performance

EVALUATION CRITERIA			COMMENTS
Symbol	**Category**	**Point Value**	
∗	Critical Step	16 points	
•	Essential Step	6 points	
▷	Theory Question	2 points	

Score calculation: 100 points

−_____ points missed

_____ Score

Satisfactory score: 85 or above

CAAHEP Competencies Achieved:

Psychomotor (Skills)
☑ I. 11. Perform quality control measures.
☑ I. 12. Perform chemistry testing.
☑ II. 2. Maintain laboratory test results using flow sheets.

Affective (Behavior)
☑ II. 2. Distinguish between normal and abnormal test results.

ABHES Competencies Achieved:

☑ 10. a. Practice quality control.
☑ 10. b. Perform selected CLIA-waived tests that assist with diagnosis and treatment: (3) Chemistry testing.

Notes

EVALUATION OF COMPETENCY

Procedure 33-B: Performing a Rapid Mononucleosis Test (QuickVue + Mono Test)

Name: _____   Date: _____

Evaluated By: _____   Score: _____

Performance Objective

Outcome:	Perform a rapid mononucleosis test.
Conditions:	Given the following: personal protective equipment including gloves, the supplies needed to perform a finger puncture, a mononucleosis testing kit, and a biohazard waste container.
Standards:	Time: 10 minutes. Student completed procedure in ____ minutes.
	Accuracy: Satisfactory score in the Performance Evaluation Checklist.

Performance Evaluation Checklist

Trial 1	Trial 2	Point Value	Performance Standards
		•	Sanitized hands.
		•	Assembled equipment.
		•	Checked the expiration date on the testing kit.
		•	Applied gloves and ran a positive and a negative control, if necessary.
		•	Removed gloves and recorded results in the quality control log.
		•	Greeted the patient and introduced yourself.
		•	Identified the patient and explained the procedure.
		•	Cleansed the puncture site and allowed it to air dry.
		•	Applied gloves.
		•	Performed a finger puncture.
		•	Disposed of the lancet in a biohazard sharps container.
		•	Wiped away the first drop of blood.
		•	Collected the blood specimen with a capillary tube.
		•	Placed a gauze pad over puncture site and applied pressure.
		•	Dispensed the blood specimen into the add well on the test cassette.
		•	Added five drops of developing solution to the add well.
		•	Waited 5 minutes and read the results.
		▷	Described the appearance of a positive and negative test result.
		•	Disposed of the test cassette in a biohazard waste container.
		•	Checked puncture site and applied adhesive bandage, if needed.
		•	Removed gloves.

Trial 1	Trial 2	Point Value	Performance Standards
		●	Sanitized hands.
		●	Charted the results correctly.
		✷	The results were identical to the evaluator's results.
		✷	Completed the procedure within 10 minutes.
			TOTALS

CHART

Date	

Evaluation of Student Performance

EVALUATION CRITERIA			COMMENTS
Symbol	Category	Point Value	
✷	Critical Step	16 points	
●	Essential Step	6 points	
▷	Theory Question	2 points	

Score calculation: 100 points

−_____ points missed

_____ Score

Satisfactory score: 85 or above

CAAHEP Competencies Achieved:

Psychomotor (Skills)
☑ I. 11. Perform quality control measures.
☑ I. 15. Perform immunology testing.

Affective (Behavior)
☑ II. 2. Distinguish between normal and abnormal test results.

ABHES Competencies Achieved:

☑ 10. a. Practice quality control.
☑ 10. b. Perform selected CLIA-waived tests that assist with diagnosis and treatment: (4) Immunology testing.

34

Medical Microbiology

CHAPTER ASSIGNMENTS

√ After Completing	Date Due	Textbook Page(s)	TEXTBOOK ASSIGNMENTS	Possible Points	Points You Earned
		804-824	Read Chapter 34: Medical Microbiology		
		809 822	📖 Read Case Study 1 Case Study 1 questions	5	
		816 822-823	📖 Read Case Study 2 Case Study 2 questions	5	
		821 823	📖 Read Case Study 3 Case Study 3 questions	5	
			TOTAL POINTS		
√ After Completing	Date Due	Study Guide Page(s)	STUDY GUIDE ASSIGNMENTS (CTA: Critical Thinking Activity)	Possible Points	Points You Earned
		871	Pretest	10	
		872	Key Term Assessment	15	
		873-875	Evaluation of Learning questions	22	
		876	CTA A: Stages of an Infectious Disease	20	
			CD Activity: Chapter 34 Under the Microscope (Record points earned)		
		879	CTA B: Choose-a-Clue Game (Record points earned)		
		885	CTA C: Disease and Infection Control	10	
		885	CTA D: Sensitivity Testing	12	
		886	CTA E: Crossword Puzzle	21	
			CD Activity: Chapter 34 Animations	20	

√ After Completing	Date Due	Study Guide Page(s)	STUDY GUIDE ASSIGNMENTS (CTA: Critical Thinking Activity)	Possible Points	Points You Earned
			CD Activity: Chapter 34 Apply Your Knowledge questions (Record points earned)		
		871	Posttest	10	
			ADDITIONAL ASSIGNMENTS		
			TOTAL POINTS		

√ When Assigned by Your Instructor	Study Guide Page(s)	Practices Required	LABORATORY ASSIGNMENTS (Procedure Number and Name)	*Score
	887	3	**Practice for Competency** 34-1: Using the Microscope Textbook reference: pp. 811-814	
	889-891		**Evaluation of Competency** 34-1: Using the Microscope	*
	887	3	(DVD) **Practice for Competency** 34-2: Collecting a Specimen for a Throat Culture Textbook reference: pp. 816-817	
	893-895		**Evaluation of Competency** 34-2: Collecting a Specimen for a Throat Culture	*
	887	3	(DVD) **Practice for Competency** 34-A: Rapid Strep Testing Textbook reference: p. 818	
	897-898		**Evaluation of Competency** 34-A: Rapid Strep Testing	*
	887	3	**Practice for Competency** 34-3: Preparing a Smear Textbook reference: pp. 821-822	
	899-900		**Evaluation of Competency** 34-3: Preparing a Smear	*
			ADDITIONAL ASSIGNMENTS	

Notes

Name _____   Date _____

PRETEST

True or False

_____   1. Microbiology is the scientific study of microorganisms and their activities.

_____   2. A disease that can be spread from one person to another is known as an *infectious disease.*

_____   3. Droplet infection is the transfer of pathogens from a fine spray emitted from a person already infected with the disease.

_____   4. Streptococci are round bacteria that grow in pairs.

_____   5. Chickenpox is caused by a virus.

_____   6. The course adjustment on a microscope is used to obtain precise focusing of an object.

_____   7. The purpose of transport media is to provide nutrients for the multiplication of the specimen.

_____   8. A throat specimen should be collected from the tonsillar area and posterior pharynx.

_____   9. A wet mount is used to examine microorganisms in the living state.

_____   10. A smear is material spread on a slide for microscopic examination.

POSTTEST

True or False

_____   1. Microorganisms that reside in the body but do not cause disease are known as *transient flora.*

_____   2. The invasion of the body by a pathogenic microorganism is known as *infection.*

_____   3. The interval of time between the invasion by a pathogen and the first symptoms of disease is known as the *prodromal period.*

_____   4. Staphylococcal infections usually result in pus formation.

_____   5. *E. coli* normally reside in the urinary tract.

_____   6. The high-power objective has a magnification of 40 ×.

_____   7. Examination of urine sediment requires the use of the oil immersion objective.

_____   8. A sequela to streptococcal sore throat is rheumatic fever.

_____   9. The purpose of sensitivity testing is to identify the type of microorganism present.

_____   10. When viewed under a microscope, gram-positive bacteria appear pink or red in color.

KEY TERM ASSESSMENT

Directions: Match each medical term with its definition.

_____ 1. Bacilli

_____ 2. Cocci

_____ 3. Contagious

_____ 4. Culture

_____ 5. Culture medium

_____ 6. Incubate

_____ 7. Incubation period

_____ 8. Infectious disease

_____ 9. Inoculate

_____ 10. Microbiology

_____ 11. Normal flora

_____ 12. Sequelae

_____ 13. Smear

_____ 14. Specimen

_____ 15. Spirilla

A. A disease caused by a pathogen that produces harmful effects on its host

B. Capable of being transmitted directly or indirectly from one person to another

C. To introduce microorganisms into a culture medium for growth and multiplication

D. Round bacteria

E. The scientific study of microorganisms and their activities

F. Material spread on a slide for microscopic examination

G. A morbid (secondary) condition occurring as a result of a less serious primary infection

H. A mixture of nutrients in which microorganisms are grown in the laboratory

I. The interval of time between invasion by a pathogenic microorganism and the appearance of the first symptoms of the disease

J. Bacteria that have a spiral or curved shape

K. Harmless, nonpathogenic microorganisms that normally reside in many parts of the body

L. Rod-shaped bacteria

M. The propagation of a mass of microorganisms in a laboratory culture medium

N. In microbiology, the act of placing a culture in a chamber that provides optimal growth requirements for the multiplication of the organisms, such as the proper temperature, humidity, and darkness

O. A small sample taken from the body to show the nature of the whole

EVALUATION OF LEARNING

Directions: Fill in each blank with the correct answer.

1. Explain what happens when a pathogen invades the body.

   _____

   _____

2. How does droplet infection contribute to the transmission of infectious disease?

   _____

   _____

3. What is the prodromal period of an infectious disease?

   _____

   _____

4. List three infectious diseases caused by *Staphylococcus aureus*.

   _____

   _____

5. List three infectious diseases caused by different types of streptococci.

   _____

   _____

6. List three infectious diseases caused by different types of bacilli.

   _____

   _____

7. In what part of the body do *E. coli* normally reside?

   _____

8. List four infectious diseases caused by different types of viruses.

   _____

   _____

9. Explain the purpose of each of the following parts of a microscope:

   Stage

   _____

   _____

   Substage condenser

   _____

   _____

Iris diaphragm

_____

_____

Coarse adjustment

_____

_____

Fine adjustment

_____

_____

Ocular lens

_____

_____

10. Describe the function of each of the following objective lenses:

Low-power

_____

_____

High-power

_____

_____

Oil-immersion

_____

_____

11. What is the purpose of using oil with the oil-immersion objective?

_____

_____

12. List five guidelines that should be followed for proper care of the microscope.

_____

_____

_____

_____

_____

13. List five common areas of the body from which a microbiologic specimen may be obtained.

_____

_____

14. List two ways to prevent contaminating a specimen with extraneous microorganisms.

_____

_____

15. List two precautions the MA should take to prevent infecting herself or himself with a microbiologic specimen.

_____

_____

16. Why should a specimen be processed as soon as possible after collecting it?

_____

17. Why is it important to diagnose streptococcal pharyngitis as early as possible?

_____

_____

18. What type of reaction is used to identify streptococcus with the direct antigen rapid streptococcus test?

_____

19. What is the purpose of performing a sensitivity test on a bacterial culture?

_____

20. List two reasons for examining a microorganism in the living state.

_____

_____

21. What is the purpose of staining a smear?

_____

_____

22. What color do gram-positive bacteria exhibit in a gram-stained smear?

_____

CRITICAL THINKING ACTIVITIES

A. STAGES OF AN INFECTIOUS DISEASE

Your physician wants you to design a poster to hang in the office outlining the stages of an infectious disease. Complete this project using the following diagram in your study guide.

STAGES OF INFECTIOUS DISEASE

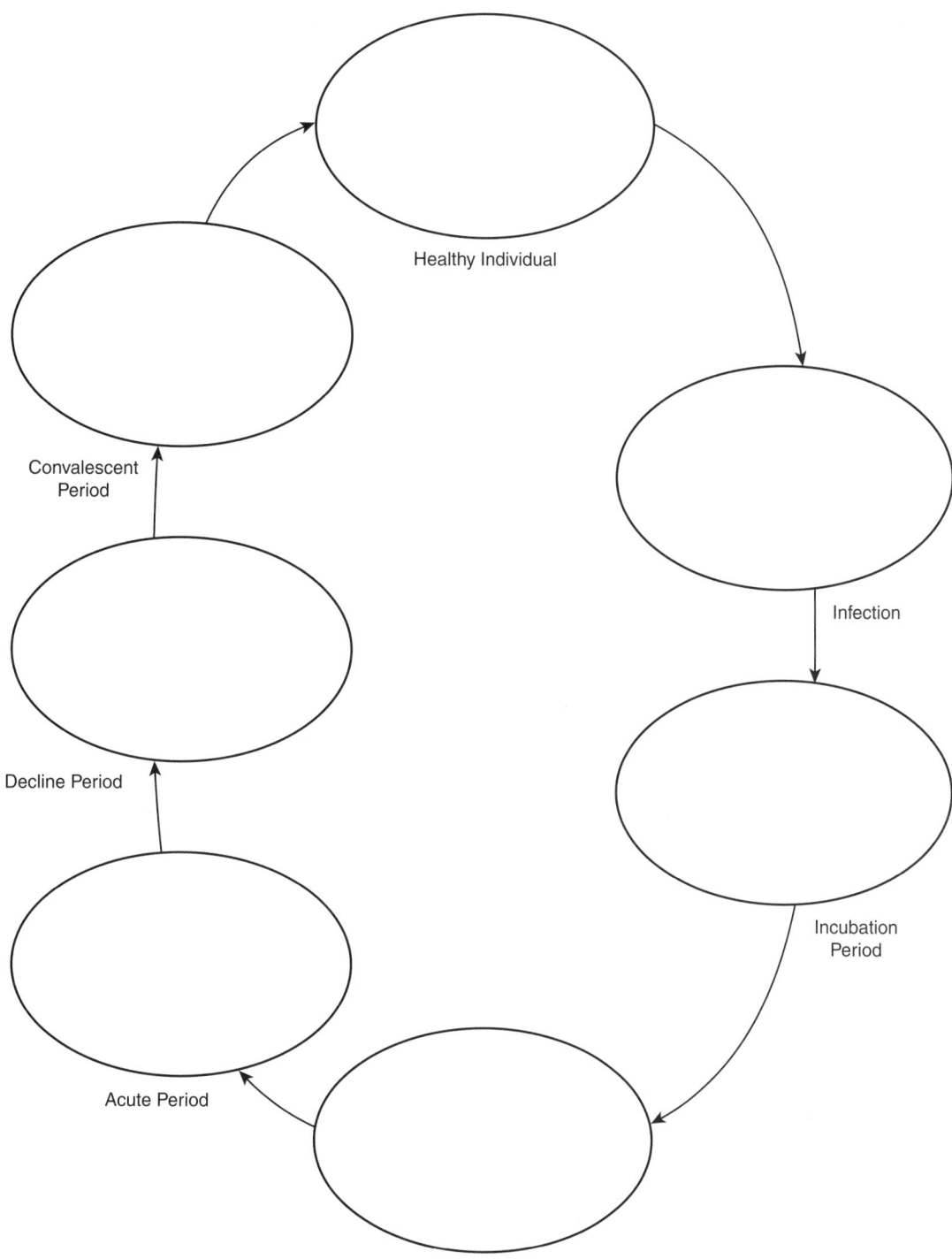

Healthy Individual

Convalescent
Period

Decline Period

Acute Period

Prodromal Period

Infection

Incubation
Period

(From Bonewit-West K: *Clinical procedures for medical assistants,* ed 7, St Louis, 2008, Saunders.)

Notes

B. CHOOSE-A-CLUE GAME

Object: To become familiar with infectious diseases

Directions:
1. Cut out the game cards on the following pages.
2. List three clues for each condition specified on the reverse of the card. Your clues should include information such as symptoms, prevention, and treatment. The name of the disease must not be written on this side of the card.
3. Use the game cards as flash cards to study the diseases.
4. Get into a group of three students.
5. Place your game cards on the table in front of you with the clues facing up.
6. One of the players should name the first disease on the following list.
7. Each player places the appropriate game card in the middle of the table with the clues facing upward.
8. When all players have placed a card on the table, turn the cards over.
9. Award yourself 5 points if you have correctly determined the disease.
10. Review the information each player listed on his or her game card.
11. Keep track of your points on the score card provided.

Good Internet reference sources to help you find clues include www.merck.com and www.kidshealth.org.

Conditions:
1. Botulism
2. Chronic fatigue syndrome
3. Common cold
4. Diphtheria
5. Gonorrhea
6. Infectious mononucleosis
7. Poliomyelitis
8. Rabies
9. Rheumatic fever
10. Rubella
11. Rubeola
12. Salmonella food poisoning
13. Smallpox
14. Staphylococcal food poisoning
15. Syphilis
16. Tetanus

CHOOSE-A-CLUE SCORE CARD

Name: _____

Recording Points:
Cross off a number each time you properly identify a disease (starting with 5 and continuing in sequence). Your total points will be equal to the last number you crossed off. Record this number in the space provided, and determine the knowledge level you attained.

Points:	
5	75
10	80
15	85
20	90
25	95
30	100
35	105
40	110
45	115
50	120
55	125
60	130
65	135
70	140

TOTAL POINTS: _____

LEVEL: _____

☐ 75 points and above: **Free from Infection**
☐ 65 to 70 points: **Putting Up a Good Fight**
☐ 55 to 60 points: **Susceptible**
☐ 50 points and under: **Infected**

Botulism

Chronic fatigue syndrome

Common cold

Diphtheria

Gonorrhea

Infectious mononucleosis

Poliomyelitis

Rabies

Sym:

_____
_____

Prev:

_____
_____

Tx:

_____
_____

Sym:

_____
_____

Prev:

_____
_____

Tx:

_____
_____

Sym:

_____
_____

Prev:

_____
_____

Tx:

_____
_____

Sym:

_____
_____

Prev:

_____
_____

Tx:

_____
_____

Sym:

_____
_____

Prev:

_____
_____

Tx:

_____
_____

Sym:

_____
_____

Prev:

_____
_____

Tx:

_____
_____

Sym:

_____
_____

Prev:

_____
_____

Tx:

_____
_____

Sym:

_____
_____

Prev:

_____
_____

Tx:

_____
_____

Rheumatic fever	**Rubella**
Rubeola	**Salmonella food poisoning**
Smallpox	**Staphylococcal food poisoning**
Syphilis	**Tetanus**

Sym:

_____
_____

Prev:

_____
_____

Tx:

_____
_____

Sym:

_____
_____

Prev:

_____
_____

Tx:

_____
_____

Sym:

_____
_____

Prev:

_____
_____

Tx:

_____
_____

Sym:

_____
_____

Prev:

_____
_____

Tx:

_____
_____

Sym:

_____
_____

Prev:

_____
_____

Tx:

_____
_____

Sym:

_____
_____

Prev:

_____
_____

Tx:

_____
_____

Sym:

_____
_____

Prev:

_____
_____

Tx:

_____
_____

Sym:

_____
_____

Prev:

_____
_____

Tx:

_____
_____

C. DISEASE AND INFECTION CONTROL

Obtain a current article on disease and infection control. The Internet sites under **On the Web** in your textbook at the end of Chapter 34 can be used to locate an article. List the important parts of your article.

_____

_____

_____

_____

_____

_____

_____

_____

_____

_____

_____

_____

D. SENSITIVITY TESTING

Refer to Figure 34-7 in your textbook. Place a check mark next to each antibiotic that is effective against the pathogen growing on the culture medium in the Petri plate.

_____   1. azithromycin

_____   2. cephalothin

_____   3. ciprofloxacin

_____   4. cefprozil

_____   5. clarithromycin

_____   6. doxycycline

_____   7. erythromycin

_____   8. nitrofurantoin

_____   9. norflaxin

_____   10. penicillin

_____   11. sulfisoxazole

_____   12. tetracycline

E. CROSSWORD PUZZLE
Medical Microbiology
Directions: Complete the crossword puzzle using the clues presented below.

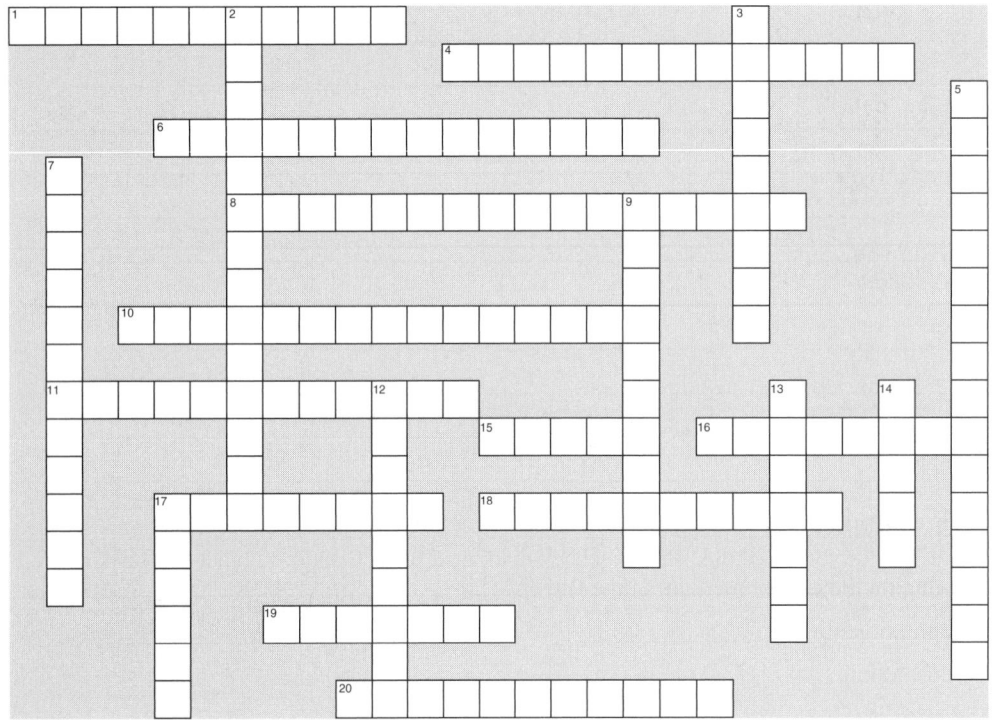

ACROSS

1 Harmless microorganisms residing in body
4 Not really present
6 Sequela to strep throat
8 Way to transmit pathogens
10 Which antibiotic?
11 Body's protective response
15 Round bacteria
16 Sample of the body
17 Disease-producing microorganism
18 It's everywhere!
19 Rod-shaped bacteria
20 Treatment for strep throat

DOWN

2 For precise focusing
3 Magnifies 40 ×
5 Between invasion and first symptoms
7 Study of microorganisms
9 Can catch it!
12 Invasion by pathogens
13 Secondary condition
14 Material spread on a slide
17 Color of gram-positive bacteria

PRACTICE FOR COMPETENCY

Procedure 34-1: Using the Microscope. Practice using a microscope.

Procedure 34-2: Collecting a Specimen for a Throat Culture. Obtain a specimen for a throat culture using a sterile cotton swab and/or a collection and transport system. Record the procedure in the chart provided.

Procedure 34-A: Rapid Strep Testing. Perform a strep test using a rapid strep testing kit and record results in the chart provided.

Procedure 34-3: Preparing a Smear. Prepare a microbiologic smear.

CHART	
Date	

☑ EVALUATION OF COMPETENCY

Procedure 34-1: Using the Microscope

Name: _____ Date: _____

Evaluated By: _____ Score: _____

Performance Objective

Outcome:	Use a microscope.
Conditions:	Given a microscope, lens paper, specimen slide, tissue or gauze, immersion oil, xylene, and a soft cloth.
Standards:	Time: 15 minutes. Student completed procedure in ____ minutes.
	Accuracy: Satisfactory score on the Performance Evaluation Checklist.

Performance Evaluation Checklist

Trial 1	Trial 2	Point Value	Performance Standards
		●	Cleaned the ocular and objective lenses with lens paper.
		●	Turned on the light source.
		●	Rotated the nosepiece to the low-power objective.
		●	Used the coarse adjustment to provide sufficient working space for placing the slide on the stage.
		●	Placed the slide on the stage specimen side up and secured it.
		●	Positioned the low-power objective until it almost touched the slide using the coarse adjustment.
		●	Observed this step.
		▷	Explained why this step should be observed.
		●	Looked through the ocular lens.
		●	Brought the specimen into coarse focus using the coarse adjustment knob.
		●	Observed the specimen until it came into coarse focus.
		●	Used the fine adjustment knob to bring the specimen into a sharp, clear focus.
		●	Adjusted the light as needed using the iris diaphragm.
		●	Rotated the nosepiece to the high-power objective.
		●	Used the fine adjustment knob to bring the specimen into a precise focus.
		●	Did not use the coarse adjustment to focus the high-power objective.
		▷	Explained why the coarse adjustment should not be used for focusing at this point.
		●	Examined the specimen as required by the test or procedure being performed.
		●	Turned off the light after use.

Trial 1	Trial 2	Point Value	Performance Standards
		●	Removed the slide from the stage.
		●	Cleaned the stage with a tissue or gauze.
		●	Properly cared for and stored the microscope.
			Using the oil-immersion objective:
		●	Rotated the nosepiece to the oil-immersion objective.
		●	Placed the objective to one side.
		●	Placed a drop of immersion oil on the slide directly over the center opening in the stage.
		●	Moved the oil-immersion objective into place.
		●	Made sure the objective did not touch the stage or slide.
		●	Used the coarse adjustment to position the oil-immersion objective.
		●	Brought the objective down until the lens touched the oil but did not come in contact with the slide.
		●	Looked through the eyepiece.
		●	Focused slowly using the coarse objective until the object was visible.
		●	Used the fine adjustment to bring the object into sharp focus.
		●	Adjusted the light as needed using the iris diaphragm.
		●	Examined the specimen as required by the test or procedure being performed.
		●	Turned off the light after use.
		●	Removed the slide from the stage.
		●	Cleaned the oil-immersion objective with lens paper.
		▷	Explained why the lens must be cleaned immediately.
		●	Cleaned the oil from the slide by immersing it in xylene and wiping it with a soft cloth.
		✳	Completed the procedure within 15 minutes.
			TOTALS

Evaluation of Student Performance

EVALUATION CRITERIA			COMMENTS
Symbol	Category	Point Value	
✳	Critical Step	16 points	
●	Essential Step	6 points	
▷	Theory Question	2 points	

Score calculation: 100 points

− _____ points missed

_____ Score

Satisfactory score: 85 or above

CAAHEP Competencies Achieved:

Psychomotor (Skills)

☑ I. 10. Assist physician with patient care.

ABHES Competencies Achieved:

☑ 9. m. Assist physician with routine and specialty examinations and treatments.

Notes

EVALUATION OF COMPETENCY

Procedure 34-2: Collecting a Specimen for a Throat Culture

Name: _____   Date: _____

Evaluated By: _____   Score: _____

Performance Objective

Outcome:	Collect a specimen for a throat culture.
Conditions:	Given the following: disposable gloves, tongue depressor, sterile swab, and a waste container.
Standards:	Time: 5 minutes. Student completed procedure in _____ minutes.
	Accuracy: Satisfactory score on the Performance Evaluation Checklist.

Performance Evaluation Checklist

Trial 1	Trial 2	Point Value	*Performance Standards*
			Throat Specimen—Sterile Swab for Strep Testing in Medical Office
		●	Sanitized hands.
		●	Assembled equipment.
		●	Greeted the patient and introduced yourself.
		●	Identified the patient and explained the procedure.
		●	Positioned patient and adjusted light.
		●	Applied gloves.
		●	Removed the sterile swab from its peel-apart package, being careful not to contaminate it.
		●	Depressed patient's tongue with tongue depressor.
		●	Placed swab at the back of patient's throat and firmly rubbed it over lesions or white or inflamed areas of mucous membranes of the tonsillar region and posterior pharynx.
		▷	Explained why swab should be rubbed over these types of areas.
		●	Constantly rotated swab as the specimen was being obtained.
		▷	Described why a rotating motion should be used.
		●	Did not allow swab to touch any area other than throat.
		▷	Explained why swab should not be allowed to touch any areas other than throat.
		●	Kept patient's tongue depressed and withdrew swab and removed tongue depressor.
		●	Disposed of the tongue depressor.
		●	Performed the rapid strep test according to the directions accompanying the rapid strep testing kit.
		●	Removed gloves and sanitized hands.

Trial 1	Trial 2	Point Value	Performance Standards
		•	Charted the test results correctly.
		▷	Completed the procedure within 5 minutes.
			Throat Specimen—Collection and Transport System
		•	Sanitized hands.
		•	Greeted the patient and introduced yourself.
		•	Identified the patient and explained the procedure.
		•	Positioned patient and adjusted light.
		•	Applied gloves.
		•	Checked the expiration date on the peel-apart envelope.
		•	Peeled open the envelope and removed the cap from the collection tube.
		•	Removed the cab/swab unit from the peel-apart package.
		•	Depressed the patient's tongue with tongue depressor.
		•	Placed swab at the back of patient's throat and firmly rubbed it over lesions or white or inflamed areas of the tonsillar area and posterior pharynx.
		•	Constantly rotated swab as the specimen was being obtained.
		•	Did not allow swab to touch any area other than the collection site.
		•	Kept patient's tongue depressed and withdrew swab and removed tongue depressor.
		•	Disposed of the tongue depressor.
		•	Inserted swab into the collection tube.
		•	Pushed cap/swab in as far as it will go.
		•	Made sure the cap was tightly in place.
		•	Removed gloves and sanitized hands.
		•	Labeled tube.
		•	Completed a laboratory request form.
		•	Placed tube in a biohazard specimen transport bag.
		•	Placed laboratory request in outside pocket of bag.
		•	Charted the procedure.
		•	Transported specimen to the laboratory within 24 hours.
		▷	Explained why the specimen must be transported within 24 hours.
		✶	Completed the procedure within 5 minutes.
			TOTALS
			CHART
	Date		

Evaluation of Student Performance

EVALUATION CRITERIA			COMMENTS
Symbol	Category	Point Value	
✳	Critical Step	16 points	
●	Essential Step	6 points	
▷	Theory Question	2 points	

Score calculation: 100 points

         − _____ points missed

         ____ Score

Satisfactory score: 85 or above

CAAHEP Competencies Achieved:

Psychomotor (Skills)

☑ III. 7. Obtain specimens for microbiological testing.

Affective (Behavior)

☑ III. 1. Display sensitivity to patient rights and feelings in collecting specimens.

☑ III. 2. Explain the rationale for performance of a procedure to the patient.

☑ III. 3. Show awareness of patients' concerns regarding their perceptions related to the procedure being performed.

ABHES Competencies Achieved:

☑ 8. cc. Communicate on the recipient's level of comprehension.

☑ 10. d. Collect, label, and process specimens: (4) Obtain throat specimens for microbiologic testing.

Notes

EVALUATION OF COMPETENCY

Procedure 34-A: Rapid Strep Testing

Name: _____   Date: _____

Evaluated By: _____   Score: _____

Performance Objective

Outcome:	Perform a rapid strep test.
Conditions:	Given the following: disposable gloves, tongue blade, a rapid strep testing kit, and the manufacturer's instructions.
Standards:	Time: 10 minutes. Student completed procedure in _____ minutes.
	Accuracy: Satisfactory score on the Performance Evaluation Checklist.

Performance Evaluation Checklist

Trial 1	Trial 2	Point Value	Performance Standards
		•	Sanitized hands.
		•	Assembled equipment.
		•	Checked the expiration date on the testing kit.
		•	Applied gloves and ran a positive and negative control, if needed.
		▷	Stated when controls should be run.
		•	Disposed of test cassettes and swabs in a biohazard waste container.
		•	Removed gloves and sanitized hands.
		•	Recorded results in the quality control log.
		•	Greeted the patient and introduced yourself.
		•	Identified the patient and explained the procedure.
		•	Positioned patient and adjusted light.
		•	Sanitized hands and applied gloves.
		•	Removed test cassette from its foil pouch and placed it on a clean, dry, level surface.
		•	Removed the sterile swab from its peel-apart package.
		•	Depressed patient's tongue with tongue depressor.
		•	Placed swab at the back of patient's head and firmly rubbed it over lesions or white or inflamed areas of the tonsillar area and posterior pharynx.
		•	Constantly rotated swab as the specimen was being obtained.
		•	Did not allow swab to touch any area other than throat.
		•	Kept patient's tongue depressed and withdrew swab.
		•	Removed tongue depressor and discarded it.
		•	Inserted the swab completely into the swab chamber.

Trial 1	Trial 2	Point Value	Performance Standards
		•	Squeezed the extraction bottle once to break the glass ampule.
		•	Vigorously shook the extraction bottle 5 times.
		•	Filled the swab chamber to the rim. Started the timer.
		•	Waited 5 minutes and read the results.
		▷	Described the appearance of a positive and negative result.
		▷	Described the appearance of an invalid result,
		▷	Explained what to do if an invalid result occurs.
		∗	The results were identical to the evaluator's results.
		•	Disposed of the test cassette and swab in a biohazard waste container.
		•	Removed gloves and sanitized hands.
		•	Recorded results in patient's chart.
		∗	Completed the procedure within 10 minutes.
			TOTALS

CHART

Date	

Evaluation of Student Performance

EVALUATION CRITERIA			COMMENTS
Symbol	**Category**	**Point Value**	
∗	Critical Step	16 points	
•	Essential Step	6 points	
▷	Theory Question	2 points	

Score calculation: 100 points
− _____ points missed
_____ Score
Satisfactory score: 85 or above

CAAHEP Competencies Achieved:

Psychomotor (Skills)
☑ I. 11. Perform quality control measures.
☑ III. 7. Obtain specimens for microbiological testing.
☑ III. 8. Perform CLIA-waived microbiology testing.

Affective (Behavior)
☑ II. 2. Distinguish between normal and abnormal test results.
☑ III. 1. Display sensitivity to patient rights and feelings in collecting specimens.
☑ III. 3. Show awareness of patients' concerns regarding their perceptions related to the procedure being performed.

ABHES Competencies Achieved:

☑ 10. a. Practice quality control.
☑ 10. b. Perform selected CLIA-waived tests that assist with diagnosis and treatment: (2) Microbiology testing, (6) Kit testing, (b) Quick Strep.
☑ 10. c. Dispose of biohazardous materials.

☑ EVALUATION OF COMPETENCY

Procedure 34-3: Preparing a Smear

Name: _____   Date: _____

Evaluated By: _____   Score: _____

Performance Objective

Outcome:	Prepare a microbiologic smear.
Conditions:	Given the following: disposable gloves, Bunsen burner, clean glass slide, microbiologic specimen, slide forceps, sterile swab, and a biohazard waste container.
Standards:	Time: 15 minutes. Student completed procedure in ____ minutes.
	Accuracy: Satisfactory score on the Performance Evaluation Checklist.

Performance Evaluation Checklist

Trial 1	Trial 2	Point Value	Performance Standards
		●	Sanitized hands.
		●	Assembled equipment.
		●	Labeled slide.
		●	Applied gloves and held the edge of slide between thumb and index finger.
		●	Started at the right side of slide, used a rolling motion, and gently and evenly spread the material from the specimen over slide.
		▷	Explained why the material should not be rubbed over slide.
		●	Allowed the smear to air dry.
		▷	Explained why heat should not be applied at this point.
		●	Held slide with slide forceps and heat-fixed the smear.
		●	Stated the purpose of heat-fixing the smear.
		●	Allowed the slide to cool completely.
		●	Prepared the slide for examination by the physician under the microscope.
		✳	Completed the procedure within 15 minutes.
			TOTALS

Evaluation of Student Performance

EVALUATION CRITERIA			COMMENTS
Symbol	Category	Point Value	
∗	Critical Step	16 points	
●	Essential Step	6 points	
▷	Theory Question	2 points	

Score calculation: 100 points

−_____ points missed

_____ Score

Satisfactory score: 85 or above

CAAHEP Competencies Achieved:

Psychomotor (Skills)

☑ III. 7. Obtain specimens for microbiological testing.

ABHES Competencies Achieved:

☑ 10. d. Collect, label, and process specimens.

35

Emergency Medical Procedures

CHAPTER ASSIGNMENTS

√ After Completing	Date Due	Textbook Page(s)	TEXTBOOK ASSIGNMENTS	Possible Points	Points You Earned
		825-851	Read Chapter 35: Emergency Medical Procedures		
		844 850	Read Case Study 1 Case Study 1 questions	5	
		845 850	Read Case Study 2 Case Study 2 questions	5	
		847 850	Read Case Study 3 Case Study 3 questions	5	
			TOTAL POINTS		
√ After Completing	Date Due	Study Guide Page(s)	STUDY GUIDE ASSIGNMENTS (CTA: Critical Thinking Activity)	Possible Points	Points You Earned
		903	Pretest	10	
		904	Key Term Assessment	16	
		905-909	Evaluation of Learning questions	27	
		909	CTA A: First Aid Kit	10	
		909	CTA B: EMD Information	5	
		909-910	CTA C: Emergency Care (2 points each)	6	
		910-911	CTA D: Emergency Situations (5 points each)	55	
			CD Activity: Chapter 35 Apply Your Knowledge questions (Record points earned)		
		903	Posttest	10	

√ After Completing	Date Due	Study Guide Page(s)	STUDY GUIDE ASSIGNMENTS (CTA: Critical Thinking Activity)	Possible Points	Points You Earned
			ADDITIONAL ASSIGNMENTS		
			TOTAL POINTS		

Name _____   Date _____

PRETEST

True or False

_____ 1. A specially equipped cart for holding and transporting medications, equipment, and supplies needed in an emergency is known as a *crash cart*.

_____ 2. Symptoms of an asthmatic attack include dyspnea and wheezing.

_____ 3. Symptoms of a heart attack include sudden weakness on one side of the body.

_____ 4. Another name for a stroke is a coronary occlusion.

_____ 5. Arterial bleeding is characterized by a slow and steady flow of blood that is dark red in color.

_____ 6. A laceration is an example of a closed wound.

_____ 7. Symptoms of a fracture include pain, swelling, deformity, and loss of function.

_____ 8. A sprain is a tearing of ligaments at a joint.

_____ 9. Heat stroke is a life-threatening emergency.

_____ 10. Insulin enables glucose to enter the body's cells and be converted to energy.

POSTTEST

True or False

_____ 1. When providing emergency care, you should make sure to obtain information as to what happened from bystanders.

_____ 2. Emphysema is a progressive lung disorder in which there is a loss of elasticity of the alveoli of the lungs.

_____ 3. Symptoms that may occur with hyperventilation include rapid and deep respirations and tachycardia.

_____ 4. The first priority for hypovolemic shock is to control bleeding.

_____ 5. Status asthmaticus is the type of shock caused by a reaction of the body to a substance to which an individual is highly allergic.

_____ 6. Another name for a nosebleed is epistaxis.

_____ 7. The type of fracture in which the broken ends of the bone are forcefully jammed together is a greenstick fracture.

_____ 8. The type of seizure in which the abnormal electrical activity is localized into very specific areas of the brain is a tonic-clonic seizure.

_____ 9. Chipmunks have a high incidence of rabies.

_____ 10. Emergency care for insulin shock is to give the patient sugar immediately.

\textit{Term} KEY TERM ASSESSMENT

Directions: Match each medical term with its definition.

_____ 1. Burn

_____ 2. Crash cart

_____ 3. Crepitus

_____ 4. Dislocation

_____ 5. Emergency medical services

_____ 6. First aid

_____ 7. Fracture

_____ 8. Hypothermia

_____ 9. Poison

_____ 10. Pressure point

_____ 11. Seizure

_____ 12. Shock

_____ 13. Splint

_____ 14. Sprain

_____ 15. Strain

_____ 16. Wound

A. A network of community resources, equipment, and personnel that provides care to victims of injury or sudden illness

B. Any substance that causes illness, injury, or death if it enters the body

C. An injury to the tissues caused by exposure to thermal, chemical, electrical, or radioactive agents

D. An orthopedic device used to immobilize, restrain, or support a part of the body

E. A grating sensation caused by fractured bone fragments rubbing against each other

F. A sudden episode of involuntary muscular contractions and relaxation, often accompanied by a change in sensation, behavior, and level of consciousness

G. A stretching or tearing of muscles or tendons caused by trauma

H. The immediate care that is administered to an individual who is injured or suddenly becomes ill before complete medical care can be obtained

I. A break in the continuity of an external or internal surface caused by physical means

J. A specially equipped cart for holding and transporting medications, equipment, and supplies needed for performing lifesaving procedures in an emergency

K. Any break in a bone

L. The failure of the cardiovascular system to deliver enough blood to all the vital organs of the body

M. An injury in which one end of a bone making up a joint is separated or displaced from its normal anatomic position

N. A life-threatening condition in which the temperature of the entire body falls to a dangerously low level

O. A site on the body where an artery lies close to the surface of the skin and can be compressed against an underlying bone to control bleeding

P. Trauma to a joint that causes tearing of ligaments

EVALUATION OF LEARNING

Directions: Fill in each blank with the correct answer.

1. What are the purposes of first aid?

   _____

   _____

   _____

   _____

2. What is the purpose of the office crash cart?

   _____

   _____

   _____

   _____

3. What is the difference between an EMT-basic and an EMT-paramedic?

   _____

   _____

   _____

4. What are the responsibilities of an emergency medical dispatcher?

   _____

   _____

   _____

5. List five OSHA standards that should be followed when administering first aid.

   _____

   _____

   _____

   _____

   _____

6. What is the reason for performing each of the following during an emergency situation?

   a. Remaining calm and speaking in a normal tone of voice

   _____

   _____

   b. Making sure it is safe before approaching the patient

   _____

   _____

   c. Following the OSHA standard when providing emergency care

   _____

   _____

   d. Activating the emergency medical services

_____

_____

   e. Not moving the patient unnecessarily

_____

_____

   f. Checking the patient for a medical alert tag

_____

_____

7. What are the symptoms of asthma?

_____

_____

8. What is emphysema?

_____

_____

9. What are the symptoms of hyperventilation?

_____

_____

10. What are the symptoms of a heart attack?

_____

_____

11. What are the symptoms of a stroke?

_____

_____

12. What is the cause of the following types of shock?

   a. Hypovolemic

_____

_____

   b. Cardiogenic

_____

_____

   c. Neurogenic

_____

_____

   d. Anaphylactic

_____

_____

    e. Psychogenic

_____

_____

13. What are the characteristics of each of the following types of external bleeding?

    a. Capillary

_____

_____

    b. Venous

_____

_____

    c. Arterial

_____

_____

14. What is the difference between an open wound and a closed wound?

_____

_____

15. What are the signs and symptoms of a fracture?

_____

_____

16. What are the characteristics of each of the following types of fractures?

    a. Impacted

_____

_____

    b. Greenstick

_____

_____

    c. Transverse

_____

_____

    d. Oblique

_____

_____

    e. Comminuted

_____

_____

    f. Spiral

_____

_____

17. What are the characteristics of each of the following types of burns?

   a. Superficial

   _____

   _____

   b. Partial thickness

   _____

   _____

   c. Full thickness

   _____

   _____

18. What is the difference between a partial seizure and a generalized seizure?

   _____

   _____

19. List two examples of each of the following types of poisoning:

   a. Ingested

   _____

   _____

   b. Inhaled

   _____

   _____

   c. Absorbed

   _____

   _____

   d. Injected

   _____

   _____

20. What spiders (found in the United States) have bites that can result in serious or life-threatening reactions?

   _____

   _____

21. What species of snakes (found in the United States) are poisonous?

   _____

   _____

22. What animals tend to have a high incidence of rabies?

   _____

   _____

23. What factors place an individual at higher risk for developing heat-related and cold-related injuries?

   _____

   _____

24. What areas of the body are most susceptible to frostbite?

_____

_____

25. What is the difference between type 1 diabetes and type 2 diabetes?

_____

_____

26. What is insulin shock, and what causes it to occur?

_____

_____

27. What is diabetic coma, and what causes it to occur?

_____

_____

CRITICAL THINKING ACTIVITIES

A. FIRST AID KIT

You are assembling a first aid kit. What supplies should be included in your kit? Identify one use for each of the supplies you list.

_____

_____

_____

_____

_____

_____

_____

_____

_____

_____

B. EMD INFORMATION

Jeff Stickler suddenly develops weakness of his left arm and leg, has difficulty speaking, and has a severe headache and dizziness. You immediately call the EMS. What information should you be prepared to relay to the emergency medical dispatcher?

_____

_____

_____

_____

C. EMERGENCY CARE

In which of the following emergency situations would you be legally permitted to administer first aid? Explain your answers.

1. A patient is unconscious and bleeding profusely.

_____

_____

2. You identify yourself and state your level of training and what you plan to do. You ask the patient if it is alright to administer emergency care. The patient responds by saying, "Yes, please help me."

_____

_____

3. You ask the patient if you can administer emergency care, but the patient refuses your help.

_____

_____

D. EMERGENCY SITUATIONS

Explain what you would do in each of the following situations.

1. Holly Murphy falls while roller skating. She comes down hard on her left arm, which begins to swell and discolor. Holly guards her arm and complains of intense pain.

_____

_____

_____

_____

2. John Phillips is mowing the grass and mows over a yellow jacket nest. He is stung twice and soon afterward starts complaining of intense itching and exhibits erythema and hives on his arms, torso, and face.

_____

_____

_____

_____

3. Steve Williams complains of severe indigestion and squeezing pain in the chest. He is short of breath and perspiring profusely.

_____

_____

_____

4. Clara Miller is playing basketball and is hit in the face with the ball. Her nose begins bleeding profusely.

_____

_____

_____

5. Debbie Carter, age 4, finds some children's chewable vitamins that have been left open on a table. She eats about 10 of them.

_____

_____

_____

6. Rita Preston accidentally cuts her finger with a knife while preparing dinner. Her finger begins bleeding profusely.

_____

_____

_____

_____

7. Jose Perez is jogging on a cinder track. He falls and scrapes his left knee on the cinders.

_____

_____

_____

8. Charlotte Lambert is getting ready to perform a piano recital for her entire church congregation. Suddenly she starts breathing rapidly and deeply and complains that she feels lightheaded and dizzy.

_____

_____

_____

9. Bruce Jones is a diabetic. He is in a hurry and forgets to eat breakfast. He begins exhibiting behavior similar to that of someone who is intoxicated.

_____

_____

_____

_____

10. Debra Murray is delivering newspapers and is bitten by a strange dog. The bite causes several puncture marks and slight bleeding.

_____

_____

_____

11. Tanya Howe is playing tennis on a hot and humid day and begins to feel weak and nauseous. Her skin feels cold and clammy, and she is sweating profusely and complains of dizziness.

_____

_____

_____

_____

36

The Medical Record

CHAPTER ASSIGNMENTS

√ After Completing	Date Due	Textbook Page(s)	TEXTBOOK ASSIGNMENTS	Possible Points	Points You Earned
		852-896	Read Chapter 36: The Medical Record		
		856 895	Read Case Study 1 Case Study 1 questions	5	
		875 895	Read Case Study 2 Case Study 2 questions	5	
		881 895	Read Case Study 3 Case Study 3 questions	5	
			TOTAL POINTS		

√ After Completing	Date Due	Study Guide Page(s)	STUDY GUIDE ASSIGNMENTS (CTA: Critical Thinking Activity)	Possible Points	Points You Earned
		917	Pretest	10	
		918	Key Term Assessment	20	
		919-923	Evaluation of Learning questions	48	
		923	CTA A: Medication Administration Record	4	
		923	CTA B: Consultation Report	4	
		924	CTA C: Radiology Report	3	
		924	CTA D: Diagnostic Imaging Report	4	
		924	CTA E: Discharge Summary Report	5	
		924-925	CTA F: Release of Medical Information	4	
		925	CTA G: Chief Complaint	6	
		926	CTA H: Crossword Puzzle	23	
			CD Activity: Chapter 36 Road to Recovery Game: Medical Abbreviations (Record points earned)		

√ After Completing	Date Due	Study Guide Page(s)	STUDY GUIDE ASSIGNMENTS (CTA: Critical Thinking Activity)	Possible Points	Points You Earned
		942-948	Taking Patient Symptoms: Supplemental Education for Chapter 36 (10 points for each problem)	50	
			CD Activity: Chapter 36 Apply Your Knowledge questions (Record points earned)		
		917	Posttest	10	
			ADDITIONAL ASSIGNMENTS		
			TOTAL POINTS		

√ When Assigned by Your Instructor	Study Guide Page(s)	Practices Required	LABORATORY ASSIGNMENTS (Procedure Number and Name)	*Score
	927-929	1	**Practice for Competency** Health History Form Textbook reference: pp. 883-885	
	930	1	**Practice for Competency** 36-1: Completion of a Consent to Treatment Form Textbook reference: p. 873	
	933-934		**Evaluation of Competency** 36-1: Completion of a Consent to Treatment Form	*
	931	1	**Practice for Competency** 36-2: Release of Medical Information Textbook reference: p. 874	
	935-936		**Evaluation of Competency** 36-2: Release of Medical Information	*
	931	2	**Practice for Competency** 36-3: Preparing a Medical Record Textbook reference: pp. 880-881	
	937-938		**Evaluation of Competency** 36-3: Preparing a Medical Record	*
	931	5	**Practice for Competency** 36-4: Obtaining and Recording Patient Symptoms Textbook reference: p. 892	
	939-941		**Evaluation of Competency** 36-4: Obtaining and Recording Patient Symptoms	*
			ADDITIONAL ASSIGNMENTS	

Notes

Name _____   Date _____

PRETEST

True or False

_____ 1. The medical record serves as a legal document.

_____ 2. The purpose of progress notes is to update the medical record with new information.

_____ 3. The patient registration record consists of a list of the problems associated with the patient's illness.

_____ 4. All OTC medications taken by the patient should be charted on the medication record form.

_____ 5. A consultation report is a narrative report of a clinical opinion about a patient's condition by a practitioner other than the primary physician.

_____ 6. A report of the analysis of body specimens is known as a *diagnostic report*.

_____ 7. Medical impressions are conclusions drawn from an interpretation of data.

_____ 8. A consent to treatment form is required for tuberculin skin testing.

_____ 9. Diabetes mellitus is an example of a familial disease.

_____ 10. Pain is an example of an objective symptom.

POSTTEST

True or False

_____ 1. The purpose of HIPAA is to provide patients with more control over the use and disclosure of their health information.

_____ 2. The health history provides subjective data about a patient to assist the physician in arriving at a diagnosis.

_____ 3. Physical therapy helps a patient with a disability learn new skills to perform the activities of daily living.

_____ 4. A copy of the patient's emergency department report is sent to the patient's family physician.

_____ 5. When an MA witnesses a patient's signature on a form, it means that the MA is verifying that the patient understands the information on the form.

_____ 6. SOAP is the acronym for the format used to organize POR progress notes.

_____ 7. The chief complaint is the symptom causing the patient the most trouble.

_____ 8. The social history includes information on the patient's lifestyle, such as health habits and living environment.

_____ 9. The patient's name must be included at the beginning of each entry charted in the patient's medical record.

_____ 10. A decrease in the amount of water in the body is known as *edema*.

Term KEY TERM ASSESSMENT

Directions: Match each medical term with its definition.

_____ 1. Attending physician

_____ 2. Charting

_____ 3. Consultation report

_____ 4. Diagnosis

_____ 5. Diagnostic procedure

_____ 6. Discharge summary report

_____ 7. Electronic medical record

_____ 8. Familial

_____ 9. Health history report

_____ 10. Informed consent

_____ 11. Inpatient

_____ 12. Medical impressions

_____ 13. Medical record

_____ 14. Objective symptom

_____ 15. Patient

_____ 16. Physical examination report

_____ 17. Problem

_____ 18. Prognosis

_____ 19. Subjective symptom

_____ 20. Symptom

A. A collection of subjective data about a patient

B. A narrative report of an opinion about a patient's condition by a practitioner other than the attending physician

C. Any condition that requires further observation, diagnosis, management, or patient education

D. A symptom felt by the patient but not observed by an examiner

E. The process of making written entries about a patient in the medical record

F. The consent given by a patient for a medical procedure after being informed of the procedure

G. Any change in the body or its functioning indicative that a disease is present

H. The conclusions reached by the physician from an interpretation of data

I. A medical record that is stored on a computer

J. A brief summary of the significant events of a patient's hospitalization

K. A written record of the important information regarding a patient

L. A symptom that can be observed by an examiner

M. The probable course and outcome of a disease and the prospect for recovery

N. The scientific method of determining and identifying a patient's condition

O. A report of the objective findings from the physician's assessment of each body system

P. Occurring or affecting members of a family more frequently than would be expected by chance

Q. The physician responsible for the care of a hospitalized patient

R. A procedure performed to assist in the diagnosis, management, or treatment of a patient's condition

S. A patient who has been admitted to the hospital for at least one overnight stay

T. An individual receiving medical care

EVALUATION OF LEARNING

Directions: Fill in each blank with the correct answer.

1. List three functions of the medical record.

   _____

   _____

   _____

2. What is the meaning of the acronym HIPAA?

   _____

3. What is the purpose of the HIPAA Privacy Rule?

   _____

   _____

4. Who must comply with HIPAA?

   _____

5. What is a Notice of Privacy Practices?

   _____

   _____

6. List examples of when HIPAA does not require written consent for the use or disclosure of a patient's health information in the following categories:

   a. Treatment: _____

   b. Payment: _____

   c. Health care operations: _____

7. What two general categories of information are included on a patient registration record?

   _____

8. List three uses of the health history.

   _____

   _____

   _____

9. What is the purpose of the physical examination?

   _____

   _____

10. What is the purpose of progress notes?

   _____

   _____

11. List three categories of medication that may be included in a medication record.

   _____

   _____

12. What is the purpose of home health care?

_____

_____

13. List five examples of home health services.

_____

_____

_____

_____

_____

14. What is the purpose of a laboratory report?

_____

_____

15. List five examples of diagnostic procedure reports.

_____

_____

16. What is the purpose of a therapeutic service report?

_____

_____

17. What is the difference between physical therapy and occupational therapy?

_____

_____

_____

18. List examples of physical agents used in physical therapy.

_____

_____

19. What is speech therapy?

_____

_____

20. What is the purpose of an operative report?

_____

_____

21. What is the purpose of the discharge summary report?

_____

_____

22. What is included in a pathology report?

_____

_____

23. Why is a copy of an emergency department report sent to the patient's physician?

_____

_____

24. When is a consent to treatment form required?

_____

_____

25. What is the purpose of a consent to treatment form?

_____

26. What information must the patient receive before signing a consent to treatment form?

_____

_____

27. What does "witnessing a signature" mean? What does it not mean?

_____

_____

_____

28. When must a patient complete a release of medical information form?

_____

_____

29. When does a release of medical information form not have to be completed?

_____

_____

30. What is the difference between a PPR and an EMR?

_____

31. How are documents organized in a source-oriented medical record?

_____

_____

32. What is reverse chronological order?

_____

33. How are documents organized in a problem-oriented medical record (POR)?

_____

_____

34. List and describe the four parts of a POR.

_____

_____

_____

_____

35. List and describe the format used to organize progress notes in a POR.

_____

36. What are the seven parts of the health history?

_____

_____

_____

_____

37. What is a chief complaint?

_____

38. What guidelines should be followed in recording the chief complaint?

_____

_____

_____

39. What is the present illness, and how is it obtained?

_____

40. List five examples of information included in the past history.

_____

_____

_____

41. List three examples of familial diseases.

_____

_____

42. Explain the importance of the social history.

_____

_____

43. What is the purpose of the review of systems (ROS)?

_____

_____

44. List the guidelines that should be followed to ensure accurate and concise charting.

_____

_____

_____

_____

45. List four examples of subjective symptoms.

_____

_____

_____

46. List three examples of objective symptoms.

_____

_____

_____

47. What is the difference between a productive and a nonproductive cough?

_____

_____

48. Why should the following be charted in the patient's medical record?

   a. Procedures performed on the patient

_____

_____

   b. Specimens collected from the patient

_____

_____

   c. Laboratory tests ordered on the patient

_____

_____

   d. Instructions given to the patient regarding medical care

_____

_____

CRITICAL THINKING ACTIVITIES

A. MEDICATION ADMINISTRATION RECORD
Refer to the medication administration record (Figure 36-2) in your textbook, and answer the following questions.

1. Does Kristen Antle have any allergies?

_____

2. How much Rocephin was administered to Kristen?

_____

3. What was the route of administration of the Rocephin injection, and where was it administered?

_____

_____

4. What is the name of the company that manufactures Rocephin?

_____

B. CONSULTATION REPORT
Refer to the consultation report (Figure 36-3) in your textbook, and identify the following information using the corresponding number (1, 2, 3, or 4).

1. Documentation that the consultant reviewed the patient's health history.

2. Documentation that the consultant examined the patient.

3. A report of the consultant's impressions.

4. A report of the consultant's recommendations.

C. RADIOLOGY REPORT

Refer to the radiology report (Figure 36-5) in your textbook, and answer the following questions.

1. What type of radiologic examination was performed on Rose Baker?

_____

2. Were the lungs clear?

_____

3. Were any abnormal masses noted in the abdomen?

_____

D. DIAGNOSTIC IMAGING REPORT

Refer to the diagnostic imaging report (Figure 36-6) in your textbook, and answer the following questions.

1. What type of diagnostic imaging procedure was performed on Vera Ruth?

_____

2. Which vertebrae of the spine were scanned?

_____

3. What problem may be present with L4-5?

_____

4. What additional tests might be scheduled for Vera Ruth?

_____

_____

E. DISCHARGE SUMMARY REPORT

Refer to the discharge summary report (Figure 36-10) in your textbook, and answer the following questions.

1. How long was Susan Brennan hospitalized?

_____

2. What was her hemoglobin level at admission?

_____

3. What was the reason for the hospitalization?

_____

4. Was Susan pregnant?

_____

5. What was her discharge diagnosis?

_____

F. RELEASE OF MEDICAL INFORMATION

Refer to the release of medical information form (Figure 36-14) in your textbook, and answer the following questions.

1. What medical information is protected by law and cannot be released unless specifically authorized by the patient?

_____

_____

2. List three reasons why a patient may authorize the release of his or her medical information.

_____

_____

_____

3. After this form is completed and signed, how long is it valid before it expires?

_____

4. What must the patient do if he or she wants to revoke the authorization?

_____

_____

G. CHIEF COMPLAINT

Indicate whether each of the following statements is an incorrect *(I)* or correct *(C)* example of recording a chief complaint. If the example is incorrect, explain which recording guideline is not being followed.

_____1. CC: Low back pain.

_____

_____2. CC: Sore throat and fever for the past 2 days.

_____

_____3. CC: Dyspnea, paleness, and fatigue similar to that associated with anemia, which has lasted for 2 weeks.

_____

_____4. CC: Poor health for the past several months.

_____

_____5. CC: Weakness and fatigue related to poor eating habits and lack of exercise.

_____

_____6. CC: Heart palpitations occurring after drinking coffee in the morning before work.

_____

H. CROSSWORD PUZZLE
Symptoms
Directions: Complete the crossword puzzle using the terms presented below.

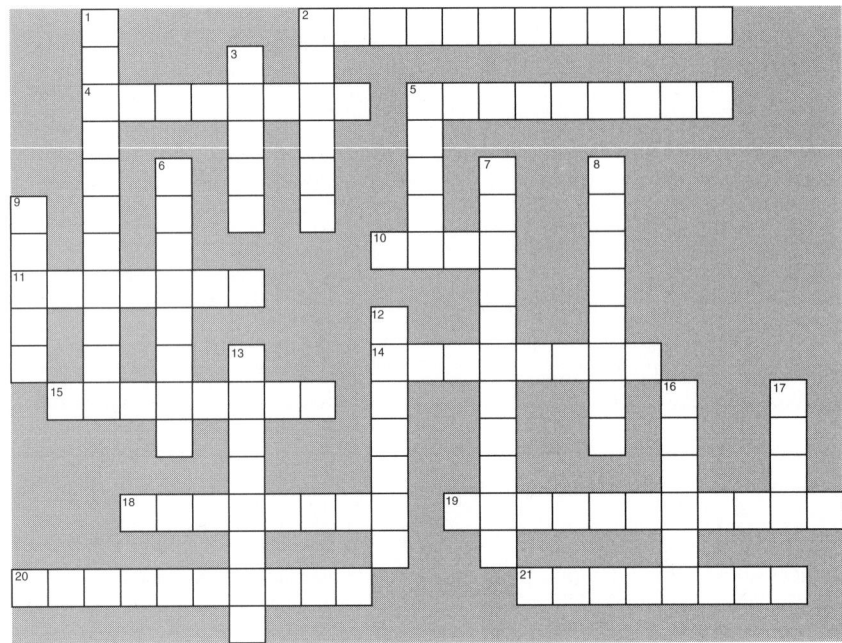

(From Bonewit-West K: *Study guide for clinical procedures for medical assistants,* ed 7, St. Louis, 2008, Saunders.)

ACROSS
2 Stool is hard and dry
4 Blue skin due to lack of O_2
5 Nosebleed
10 Skin eruption
11 Dizziness
14 No appetite
15 Yellow skin
18 Severe itching
19 Involuntary contractions of muscles
20 Gas
21 Head pain

DOWN
1 Fast pulse rate
2 Shivering
3 May be productive or nonproductive
5 Fluid retention
6 Ejection of stomach contents
7 Decreased H_2O levels in the body
8 Red face
9 Elevated temperature
12 Bad all over
13 Loose, watery stools
16 Sensation of stomach discomfort
17 Feeling of distress or suffering

PRACTICE FOR COMPETENCY

Health History Form. Complete the health history form (pages 927-929) using yourself as the patient.

PATIENT HEALTH HISTORY

A **IDENTIFICATION DATA**   Please print the following information.

Today's date _____

Name _____

___ Male ___ Female

Address _____

___ Married ___ Separated ___ Divorced ___ Widowed ___ Single

_____

Date of Birth _____

Telephone _____ _____

B **PAST HISTORY**

Have you ever had the following: (Circle "no" or "yes", leave blank if uncertain)

Measles ____ no yes	Heart Disease ____ no yes	Diabetes ____ no yes	Hemorrhoids ____ no yes
Mumps ____ no yes	Arthritis ____ no yes	Cancer ____ no yes	Asthma ____ no yes
Chickenpox ____ no yes	Sexually Transmitted _ no yes Disease	Polio ____ no yes	Allergies ____ no yes
Whooping Cough ___ no yes	Anemia ____ no yes	Glaucoma ____ no yes	Eczema ____ no yes
Scarlet Fever ____ no yes	Bladder Infections ___ no yes	Hernia ____ no yes	AIDS or HIV+ ____ no yes
Diphtheria ____ no yes	Epilepsy ____ no yes	Blood or Plasma ___ no yes Transfusions	Infectious Mono ____ no yes
Pneumonia ____ no yes	Migraine Headaches _ no yes	Back Trouble ____ no yes	Bronchitis ____ no yes
Rheumatic Fever ___ no yes	Tuberculosis ____ no yes	High Blood ____ no yes Pressure	Mitral Valve Prolapse no yes
Stroke ____ no yes	Ulcer ____ no yes	Thyroid Disease ___ no yes	Any other disease ___ no yes
Hepatitis. ____ no yes	Kidney Disease ____ no yes	Bleeding Tendency _ no yes	Please list: _____ _____

MAJOR HOSPITALIZATIONS: If you have ever been hospitalized for any major medical illness or operation, write in your most recent hospitalizations below.

Hospitalizations	Year	Operation or illness	Name of hospital	City and state
1st Hospitalization				
2nd Hospitalization				
3rd Hospitalization				
4th Hospitalization				

TESTS AND IMMUNIZATIONS: Mark an X next to those that you have had.

Tests: Immunizations:

☐ TB Test   ☐ Electrocardiogram   ☐ Influenza

☐ Rectal/Hemoccult   ☐ Chest X-ray   ☐ Hepatitis B

☐ Sigmoidoscopy   ☐ Mammogram   ☐ Tetanus

☐ Colonoscopy   ☐ Pap Test   ☐ MMR

☐ Polio

CURRENT MEDICATIONS: List the following that you are currently taking: Prescription medications, over-the-counter (OTC) medications, vitamin supplements, and herbal supplements.   ☐ None

Medication	Frequency
_____	_____
_____	_____
_____	_____
_____	_____

ALLERGIES: List all allergies (foods, drugs, environment). ☐ None

_____

_____

_____

_____

ACCIDENTS/ INJURIES: Describe all serious accidents, severe injuries, head injury, or fractures. Include the date each occurred. ☐ None

Accident/Injury: Date:

_____

_____

_____

(From Bonewit-West K: *Study guide for clinical procedures for medical assistants*, ed 7, St. Louis, 2008, Saunders.)

C **FAMILY HISTORY**

For each member of your family, follow the purple or blue line across the page and check boxes for:
1. Their present state of health
2. Any illnesses they have had

	Good Health	Poor Health	Deceased	If deceased, write in age and cause of death.	Allergies or Asthma	Diabetes	Heart Disease	Stroke	Cancer	High Blood Pressure	Glaucoma	Arthritis	Ulcer	Kidney Disease	Mental Health Problems	Alcohol/Drug Abuse	Obesity	High Cholesterol	Thyroid Disease
Father:																			
Mother:																			
Brothers/Sisters:																			

D **SOCIAL HISTORY**

EDUCATION _____ High school _____ College _____ Post graduate

Occupation _____ Years _____

Previous occupations _____ Years _____

_____ Years _____

Have you ever been exposed to any of the following in your environment?

☐ Excess dust (coal, lime, rock)   ☐ Cleaning fluids/solvents   ☐ Radiation   ☐ Other toxic materials

☐ Sand   ☐ Hair spray   ☐ Insecticides

☐ Chemicals   ☐ Smoke or auto exhaust fumes   ☐ Paints

Please answer the following questions by placing an X in the box in front of the word Yes or No, except where you are asked for specific information. This information is obviously highly confidential and will be released to other health professionals or insurance carriers ONLY with your consent.

DIET:
Do you eat a good breakfast? ☐ Yes ☐ No

Do you snack between meals (soft drinks, chips, candy bars)? ☐ Yes ☐ No

Do you eat fresh fruits and vegetables each day? ☐ Yes ☐ No

Do you eat whole grain breads and cereals? ☐ Yes ☐ No

Is your diet high in fat content? ☐ Yes ☐ No

Is your diet high in cholesterol content? ☐ Yes ☐ No

Is your diet high in salt content? ☐ Yes ☐ No

Are you allergic to any foods? ☐ Yes ☐ No

How many glasses of water do you drink each day? _____

How would you describe your overall eating habits? ☐ Excellent ☐ Good ☐ Fair ☐ Poor

PERSONAL HISTORY:
Do you find it hard to make decisions? ☐ Yes ☐ No

Do you find it hard to concentrate or remember? ☐ Yes ☐ No

Do you feel depressed? ☐ Yes ☐ No

Do you have difficulty relaxing? ☐ Yes ☐ No

Do you have a tendency to worry a lot? ☐ Yes ☐ No

Have you gained or lost much weight recently? ☐ Yes ☐ No

Do you lose your temper often? ☐ Yes ☐ No

Are you disturbed by any work or family problems? ☐ Yes ☐ No

Are you having sexual difficulties? ☐ Yes ☐ No

Have you ever considered committing suicide? ☐ Yes ☐ No

Have you ever desired or sought psychiatric help? ☐ Yes ☐ No

EXERCISE:
Do you exercise on a regular basis? ☐ Yes ☐ No

Does your job require strenuous, sustained physical work? ☐ Yes ☐ No

SLEEP PATTERNS:
Do you seem to feel exhausted or fatigued most of the time? ☐ Yes ☐ No

Do you have difficulty either falling asleep or staying asleep? ☐ Yes ☐ No

USE OF TOBACCO/ALCOHOL/CAFFEINE/DRUGS: Amt:
How much do you smoke per day? ☐ Cigarettes ___
☐ Don't smoke   ☐ Cigars/pipes ___

Do you take two or more alcoholic drinks per day? ☐ Yes ☐ No

Do you drink six or more cups of coffee or tea per day? ☐ Yes ☐ No

Are you a regular user of sleeping pills, marijuana, tranquilizers, pain killers, etc? ☐ Yes ☐ No

Have you ever used heroin, cocaine, LSD, PCP, etc? ☐ Yes ☐ No

List any country outside the USA you have visited in the past six months? _____

When did you have your last physical examination? _____

(From Bonewit-West K: *Study guide for clinical procedures for medical assistants,* ed 7, St. Louis, 2008, Saunders.)

Patient's Name _____

E | **REVIEW OF SYSTEMS**

HEAD AND NECK
——— Frequent headaches
——— Neck pain
——— Neck lumps or swelling

EYES
——— Wears glasses
——— Blurry vision
——— Eyesight worsening
——— Sees double
——— Sees halo
——— Eye pain or itching
——— Watering eyes
——— Eye trouble

EARS
——— Hearing difficulties
——— Earaches
——— Running ears
——— Buzzing in ears
——— Motion sickness

MOUTH
——— Dental problems
——— Swellings on gums or jaws
——— Sore tongue
——— Taste changes

NOSE AND THROAT
——— Congested nose
——— Running nose
——— Sneezing spells
——— Headcolds
——— Nose bleeds
——— Sore throat
——— Enlarged tonsils
——— Hoarse voice

RESPIRATORY
——— Wheezes or gasps
——— Coughing spells
——— Coughs up phlegm
——— Coughed up blood
——— Chest colds
——— Excessive sweating, night sweats

CARDIOVASCULAR
——— High blood pressure
——— Racing heart
——— Chest pains
——— Dizzy spells
——— Shortness of breath
——— Shortness of breath at night
——— More pillows to breathe
——— Swollen feet or ankles
——— Leg cramps
——— Heart murmur

DIGESTIVE
——— Heartburn
——— Bloated stomach
——— Belching
——— Stomach pains
——— Nausea
——— Vomited blood
——— Difficulty swallowing
——— Constipation
——— Loose bowels
——— Black stools
——— Grey stools
——— Pain in rectum
——— Rectal bleeding

URINARY
——— Night frequency
——— Day frequency
——— Wets pants or bed
——— Burning on urination
——— Brown, black, or bloody urine
——— Difficulty starting urine
——— Urgency

MALE GENITAL
——— Weak urine stream
——— Prostate trouble
——— Burning or discharge
——— Lumps on testicles
——— Painful testicles

FEMALE GENITAL
__/__/__ Last menstrual period
__/__/__ Last Pap test
——— Post-menopausal or hysterectomy
——— Noticed vaginal bleeding
——— Abnormal LMP
——— Heavy bleeding during periods
——— Bleeding between periods
——— Bleeding after intercourse
——— Recent vaginal itching/ discharge
——— No monthly breast exam
——— Lump or pain in breasts
——— Complications with birth control

OBSTETRIC HISTORY
——— Gravida
——— Para
——— Pre-term
——— Miscarriages
——— Still births
——— Has had an abortion

MUSCULOSKELETAL
——— Aching muscles
——— Swollen joints
——— Back or shoulder pains
——— Painful feet
——— Disability

SKIN
——— Skin problems
——— Itching or burning skin
——— Bleeds easily
——— Bruises easily

NEUROLOGICAL
——— Faintness
——— Numbness
——— Convulsions
——— Change in handwriting
——— Trembles

F | **PROGRESS NOTES**

Date	

(From Bonewit-West K: *Study guide for clinical procedures for medical assistants,* ed 7, St. Louis, 2008, Saunders.)

Procedure 36-1: Consent to Treatment Form. Complete the consent to treatment form (below) using a classmate as the patient.

(attach label or complete blanks)

First name: _____ Last name: _____

Date of Birth: _____ Month _____ Day _____ Year

Account Number: _____

Procedure Consent Form

I, _____, hereby consent to have

Dr. _____, perform _____.

I have been fully informed of the following by my physician:

1. The nature of my condition.
2. The nature and purpose of the procedure.
3. An explanation of risks involved with the procedure.
4. Alternative treatments or procedures available.
5. The likely results of the procedure.
6. The risks involved with declining or delaying the procedure.

My physician has offered to answer all questions concerning the proposed procedure.

I am aware that the practice of medicine and surgery is not an exact science, and I acknowledge that no guarantees have been made to me about the results of the procedure.

Patient _____ Date _____
      (or guardian and relationship)

Witnessed _____ Date _____

(From Bonewit-West K: *Study guide for clinical procedures for medical assistants,* ed 7, St. Louis, 2008, Saunders.)

Procedure 36-2: Release of Medical Information. Complete the release of medical information form (below) using a classmate as the patient.

RELEASE OF MEDICAL INFORMATION

All information contained in the medical record is confidential and the release of information is closely controlled. A properly completed and signed authorization is required for the release of the following information.

PATIENT INFORMATION

Patient Name _____

Address _____   Social Security # _____

City _____ State _____ ZIP _____   Birthdate ____/____/____

Phone (Home) _____ Work _____

RELEASE FROM:

Name _____

Address _____

City _____ State _____ ZIP _____

RELEASE TO:

Name _____

Address _____

City _____ State _____ ZIP _____

INFORMATION TO BE RELEASED:

1. GENERAL RELEASE:

____ Entire Medical Record (excluding protected information)

____ Hospital Records only (specify) _____

____ Lab Results only (specify) _____

____ X-ray Reports only (specify) _____

____ Other Records (specify) _____

2. INFORMATION PROTECTED BY STATE/FEDERAL LAW:
If indicated below, I hereby authorize the disclosure and release of information regarding:

____ Drug Abuse Diagnosis/Treatment

____ Alcoholism Diagnosis/Treatment

____ Mental Health Diagnosis/Treatment

____ Sexually Transmitted Disease

PURPOSE/NEED FOR INFORMATION:

____ Taking records to another doctor

____ Moving

____ Legal purposes

____ Insurance purposes

____ Workman's Compensation

____ Other/Explain: _____

METHOD OF RELEASE:

____ US Mail

____ Fax

____ Telephone

____ To Patient

PATIENT AUTHORIZATION TO RELEASE INFORMATION:

Authorization is valid for 60 days only from the date of my signature. I reserve the right to revoke this authorization at any time prior to 60 days (except for action that has already been taken) by notifying the medical office in writing.

I understand that my records are protected under HIPAA (Health Insurance Portability and Accountability Act) Standards for Privacy of Individually Identifiable Information (45 CFR Parts 160 and 164) unless otherwise permitted by federal law. Any information released or received shall not be further relayed to any other facility or person without my written authorization. I also understand that such information will not be given, sold, transferred or in any way relayed to any other person or party not specified above without my further written authorization.

I hereby grant authorization to release the information listed above. I certify that this request has been made voluntarily and that the information given above is accurate to the best of my knowledge.

_____   _____

Signature of Patient/Legally Responsible Party   Date

_____   _____

Witness Signature   Date

OFFICE USE ONLY

Information indicated above released on _____
Date

Explanation of information released: _____

_____

Signature and credentials of individual releasing information: _____

(From Bonewit-West K: *Study guide for clinical procedures for medical assistants,* ed 7, St. Louis, 2008, Saunders.)

Procedure 36-3: Preparing a Medical Record. Prepare a medical record.

Procedure 36-4: Obtaining and Recording Patient Symptoms. Practice obtaining patient symptoms by completing Taking Patient Symptoms: Supplemental Education for Chapter 36 (pages 942-948 in this study guide).

Notes

EVALUATION OF COMPETENCY

Procedure 36-1: Completion of a Consent to Treatment Form

Name: _____   Date: _____

Evaluated By: _____   Score: _____

Performance Objective

Outcome:	Complete a consent to treatment form.
Conditions:	Given a consent to treatment form.
Standards:	Time: 10 minutes. Student completed procedure in _____ minutes.
	Accuracy: Satisfactory score on the Performance Evaluation Checklist.

Performance Evaluation Checklist

Trial 1	Trial 2	Point Value	Performance Standards
		●	Typed or printed required information on the consent to treatment form.
		●	Confirmed that the physician discussed the procedure with the patient.
		▷	Explained why the procedure should be discussed with the patient before the form is signed.
		●	Greeted the patient and introduced yourself.
		●	Explained the purpose of the form to the patient.
		●	Gave the consent form to the patient to read.
		●	Asked if the patient had any questions.
		●	Asked the patient to sign the form.
		●	Witnessed the patient's signature.
		▷	Explained what "witnessing a signature" means.
		●	Provided the patient with a copy of the completed form.
		✶	Filed the original form in the patient's medical record.
		▷	Explained why the form must be filed in the medical record.
		✶	Completed the procedure within 10 minutes.
			TOTALS

Evaluation of Student Performance

EVALUATION CRITERIA			COMMENTS
Symbol	**Category**	**Point Value**	
∗	Critical Step	16 points	
•	Essential Step	6 points	
▷	Theory Question	2 points	

Score calculation: 100 points

− _____ points missed

_____ Score

Satisfactory score: 85 or above

CAAHEP Competencies Achieved:

Psychomotor (Skills)
☑ IV. 2. Report relevant information to others succinctly and accurately.
☑ IX. 7. Document accurately in the patient record.

Affective (Behavior)
☑ IV. 2. Apply active listening skills.
☑ IV. 7. Demonstrate recognition of the patient's level of understanding in communications.
☑ IV. 8. Analyze communications in providing appropriate responses/feedback.

ABHES Competencies Achieved:

☑ 4.a. Document accurately.
☑ 8. aa. Are attentive, listen, and learn.
☑ 8. cc. Communicate on the recipient's level of comprehension.
☑ 8.dd. Serve as liaison between physician and others.

✅ EVALUATION OF COMPETENCY

📀 Procedure 36-2: Release of Medical Information

Name: _____   Date: _____

Evaluated By: _____   Score: _____

Performance Objective

Outcome:	1. Assist a patient in the completion of a release of medical information form. 2. Release medical information according to a completed release of information form.
Conditions:	Given a release of medical information form.
Standards:	Time: 15 minutes. Student completed procedure in _____ minutes. Accuracy: Satisfactory score on the Performance Evaluation Checklist.

Performance Evaluation Checklist

Trial 1	Trial 2	Point Value	Performance Standards
			Completion of a Release Form
		●	Greeted the patient.
		●	Introduced yourself and explained the purpose of the form to the patient.
		▷	Explained the procedure to follow if you do not recognize the patient.
		●	Provided the patient with a release form.
		●	Asked the patient to complete the form.
		●	Provided assistance if needed.
		●	Checked to make sure all information was completed.
		●	Asked the patient to sign the form.
		●	Witnessed the patient's signature and dated the form.
		●	Provided the patient with a copy of the completed form.
		●	Copied the medical information requested on the form.
		●	Released only the information requested.
		●	Included a copy of the completed form with the medical information.
		●	Documented what information was released along with the date of the release.
		●	Signed the document with your name and credentials.
		✱	Filed the original document and the release form in the patient's medical record.
		▷	Explained the reason for filing the form.
		●	Sent the medical information according to the medical office policy.
			Mailed or Faxed Requests
		●	Checked the expiration date on the release of medical information form.
		▷	Explained the procedure to follow if the form is expired.

Trial 1	Trial 2	Point Value	Performance Standards
		•	Verified the signature on the form.
		▷	Stated what to do if in doubt regarding the authenticity of the signature.
		•	Copied the information requested on the form.
		•	Released only the information requested.
		•	Documented what information was released along with the date of release.
		•	Signed the document with your name and credentials.
		•	Filed the original document and the release form in the patient's medical record.
		•	Sent the medical information according to the medical office policy.
		∗	Completed the procedure within 15 minutes.
			TOTALS

Evaluation of Student Performance

EVALUATION CRITERIA			COMMENTS
Symbol	Category	Point Value	
∗	Critical Step	16 points	
•	Essential Step	6 points	
▷	Theory Question	2 points	

Score calculation: 100 points

− _____ points missed

_____ Score

Satisfactory score: 85 or above

CAAHEP Competencies Achieved:

Psychomotor (Skills)
☑ IV. 2. Report relevant information to others succinctly and accurately.
☑ IV. 4. Explain general office policies.
☑ IX. 1. Respond to issues of confidentiality.
☑ IX. 2. Perform within scope of practice.
☑ IX 3. Apply HIPAA rules in regard to privacy/release of information.
☑ IX. 7. Document accurately in the patient record.
☑ IX.8. Apply local, state, and federal health care legislation and regulation appropriate to the medical assisting practice setting.

Affective (Behavior)
☑ IX. 1. Demonstrate sensitivity to patient rights.
☑ IX. 3. Recognize the importance of local, state, and federal legislation and regulations in the practice setting.

ABHES Competencies Achieved:

☑ 4. a. Document accurately.
☑ 4. b. Institute federal and state guidelines when releasing medical records or information.
☑ 4. f.. Comply with federal, state, and local health laws and regulations.
☑ 8. dd. Serve as liaison between physician and others.
☑ 8. hh. Receive, organize, prioritize, and transmit information expediently.
☑ 9. p. Advise patients of office policies and procedures.

EVALUATION OF COMPETENCY

Procedure 36-3: Preparing a Medical Record

Name: _____   Date: _____

Evaluated By: _____   Score: _____

Performance Objective

Outcome:	Prepare a medical record.
Conditions:	Given the following: patient registration form, Notice of Privacy Practices (NPP) and acknowledgment form, file folder, metal fasteners, name labels, alphabetic labels, miscellaneous chart labels, chart dividers, preprinted forms, and a two-hole punch.
Standards:	Time: 10 minutes. Student completed procedure in ____ minutes.
	Accuracy: Satisfactory score on the Performance Evaluation Checklist.

Performance Evaluation Checklist

Trial 1	Trial 2	Point Value	Performance Standards
		●	Greeted the patient and introduced yourself.
		●	Identified the patient and verified that the patient was a new patient.
		●	Asked the patient to complete a patient registration form, read an NPP, and sign an acknowledgment form.
		●	Offered to answer questions.
		●	Checked the registration form for accuracy and legibility.
		●	Copied the patient's insurance card.
		▷	Stated the purpose of copying the card.
		●	Entered the data on the completed registration form into the computer.
		●	Assembled supplies needed to prepare the medical record.
			Typed the Patient's Full Name on the Name Label
		●	The patient's name was in transposed order.
		●	The name was typed using correct spacing.
		●	The patient's name was spelled correctly.
		●	Attached appropriate color-coded labels to the side tab.
		●	Attached the labels using the indentations on the tab.
		●	Attached the name label immediately above the alphabetical label.
		●	Attached additional labels to the folder as required.
		●	Inserted chart divider onto the metal fasteners.
		●	Placed the original registration form in front of the medical record.
		●	Placed the signed NPP acknowledgement form in the record.
		●	Placed the insurance card (copy) in the appropriate section of the record.

Trial 1	Trial 2	Point Value	Performance Standards
		•	Labeled preprinted forms with required information.
		▷	Stated examples of preprinted forms included in the medical record.
		•	Punched holes into the forms if required.
		•	Inserted each form under its proper chart divider.
		•	Checked the medical record to make sure it was prepared properly.
		✳	Completed the procedure within 10 minutes.
			TOTALS

Evaluation of Student Performance

EVALUATION CRITERIA			COMMENTS
Symbol	Category	Point Value	
✳	Critical Step	16 points	
•	Essential Step	6 points	
▷	Theory Question	2 points	

Score calculation: 100 points

− _____ points missed

_____ Score

Satisfactory score: 85 or above

CAAHEP Competencies Achieved:

Psychomotor (Skills)
☑ IV. 2. Report relevant information to others succinctly and accurately.
☑ IV. 4. Explain general office policies.
☑ V. 3. Organize a patient's medical record.
☑ V. 5. Execute data management using electronic health care records such as the EMR.
☑ V. 6. Use office hardware and software to maintain office systems.
☑ V. 8. Maintain organization by filing.
☑ IX 3. Apply HIPAA rules in regard to privacy/release of information.
☑ IX.8. Apply local, state, and federal health care legislation and regulation appropriate to the medical assisting practice setting.

Affective (Behavior)
☑ IV. 2. Apply active listening skills.
☑ IV. 8. Analyze communications in providing appropriate responses/feedback.
☑ IV. 9. Recognize and protect personal boundaries in communicating with others.
☑ IX. 3. Recognize the importance of local, state, and federal legislation and regulations in the practice setting.

ABHES Competencies Achieved:

☑ 4. a. Document accurately.
☑ 4. b. Institute federal and state guidelines when releasing medical records or information.
☑ 4. c. Follow established policies when initiating or terminating medical treatment.
☑ 4. f. Comply with federal, state, and local health laws and regulations.
☑ 8. b. Prepare and maintain medical records.
☑ 8. aa. Are attentive, listen and learn.
☑ 8. ll. Apply electronic technology.

☑ EVALUATION OF COMPETENCY

Procedure 36-4: Obtaining and Recording Patient Symptoms

Name: _____   Date: _____

Evaluated By: _____   Score: _____

Performance Objective

Outcome:	Obtain and record patient symptoms.
Conditions:	Given the following: medical record of the patient ot be interviewed and a black ink pen.
Standards:	Time: 10 minutes. Student completed procedure in _____ minutes.
	Accuracy: Satisfactory score on the Performance Evaluation Checklist.

Performance Evaluation Checklist

Trial 1	Trial 2	Point Value	Performance Standards
		●	Assembled equipment.
		●	Made sure the correct patient record was obtained.
		●	Went to the waiting room and asked the patient to come back.
		●	Escorted the patient to a quiet room.
		●	In a calm and friendly manner, greeted the patient and introduced yourself.
		●	Identified the patient by full name and date of birth.
		●	Asked the patient to be seated.
		●	Seated yourself facing the patient at a distance of 3 to 4 feet.
		▷	Explained the purpose of this seating arrangement.
			Used Good Communication Skills
		●	Used the patient's name of choice.
		●	Demonstrated genuine interest and concern for the patient.
		●	Maintained appropriate eye contact.
		●	Used terminology the patient could understand.
		●	Listened carefully and attentively to the patient.
		●	Paid attention to the patient's nonverbal messages.
		●	Avoided judgmental comments.
		●	Avoided rushing the patient.
		●	Located the progress note sheet in the medical record.
		●	Charted the date, time, and CC abbreviation.
		●	Used an open-ended question to obtain the chief complaint.
		▷	Explained why an open-ended question should be used.

Trial 1	Trial 2	Point Value	Performance Standards
			Charted the Chief Complaint
		•	Limited the CC to one or two symptoms.
		•	Referred to a specific rather than a vague symptom.
		•	Charted concisely and briefly.
		•	Used the patient's own words as much as possible.
		•	Included the duration of the symptom.
		•	Avoided using names of diseases.
		•	Obtained additional information regarding the chief complaint using what, when, and where questions.
		•	Thanked the patient and proceeded to the next step in the patient workup.
		•	Informed the patient that the physician would be in soon.
		•	Placed the medical record in the appropriate location for review by the physician.
		*	Completed the procedure within 10 minutes.
			TOTALS

	C**HART**
Date	

Evaluation of Student Performance

EVALUATION CRITERIA			COMMENTS
Symbol	Category	Point Value	
*	Critical Step	16 points	
•	Essential Step	6 points	
▷	Theory Question	2 points	

Score calculation: 100 points

−_____ points missed

_____ Score

Satisfactory score: 85 or above

CAAHEP Competencies Achieved:

Psychomotor (Skills)

☑ IV.1. Use reflection, restatement, and clarification techniques to obtain a patient history.
☑ IV. 3. Use medical terminology, pronouncing medical terms correctly, to communicate information, patient history, data, and observations.
☑ IV. 7. Demonstrate telephone techniques.
☑ IV. 11. Respond to nonverbal communication.
☑ IX. 7. Document accurately in the patient record.
☑ X.2. Develop a plan for separation of personal and professional ethics.

Affective (Behavior)

☑ IV. 2. Apply active listening skills.
☑ IV. 3. Use appropriate body language and other nonverbal skills in communicating with parents, family, and staff.
☑ IV. 4. Demonstrate awareness of the territorial boundaries of the person with whom communicating.
☑ IV. 9. Recognize and protect personal boundaries in communicating with others.
☑ IV. 10. Demonstrate respect for individual diversity, incorporating awareness of one's own biases in areas including gender, race, religion, age, and economic status.

ABHES Competencies Achieved:

☑ 3. d. Recognize and identify acceptable medical abbreviations.
☑ 4. a. Document accurately.
☑ 5. b. Identify and respond appropriately when working/caring for patients with special needs.
☑ 8. aa. Are attentive, listen, and learn.
☑ 8. bb. Are impartial and show empathy when dealing with patients.
☑ 8. cc. Communicate on the recipient's level of comprehension.
☑ 8. ee. Use proper telephone techniques.
☑ 8. ff. Interview effectively.
☑ 8. gg. Use pertinent medical terminology.
☑ 8. ii. Recognize and respond to verbal and non-verbal communication.
☑ 8. kk. Adapt to individualized needs.
☑ 9. a. Obtain chief complaint, recording patient history.

TAKING PATIENT SYMPTOMS: SUPPLEMENTAL EDUCATION FOR CHAPTER 36

Taking patient symptoms is a frequent and important responsibility of the medical assistant. Because of this, the medical assistant must have a thorough knowledge of symptoms and related terminology. A **symptom** is defined as any change in the body or its functioning that indicates the presence of disease. The medical assistant will be able to observe objective symptoms presented by the patient, such as coughing, a rash, and swelling. On the other hand, the medical assistant must rely on information relayed by the patient in order to obtain data on **subjective** symptoms. Examples of subjective symptoms include pain, pruritus, and vertigo.

This section is designed as supplemental education for Chapter 36 (The Medical Record) in your textbook. Completion of the exercises in this section will assist you in recording patient symptoms effectively and thoroughly, which is essential to an accurate diagnosis by the physician.

Learning Objectives

After completing this chapter, you should be able to do the following:
1. Explain the purpose of analyzing a symptom.
2. State the seven basic types of information that must be obtained to analyze a symptom.
3. Analyze a symptom by using direct questions.

Analysis of a Symptom

Before a symptom can be analyzed, the chief complaint must first be identified. The chief complaint (CC) is the patient's reason for seeking care, or the symptom causing the patient the most trouble. An open-ended question should be used to elicit the chief complaint from the patient, and it should be charted following the charting guidelines presented in your textbook (pages 886 and 890). The next step is to analyze the chief complaint in detail from the time of its onset. The purpose of this is to provide a complete description of the current status of the chief complaint.

Analyzing the chief complaint requires a combination of good listening and writing skills. The medical assistant must also know what information should be recorded for each symptom as well as the questions to ask the patient to obtain this information. A list and explanation of the information required for each symptom, along with examples of questions to ask the patient, are presented below.

Type of Information Required

The following information is needed for each symptom to provide a full description of the current status of the chief complaint:

1. **Location of the Symptom**. This refers to the specific area of the body where the symptom is located. Locating the symptom is the first step in determining the cause of the patient's disease. The patient may refer to the location in general terms, for example, the head, arm, stomach, or back. It is important that the medical assistant be more specific than this, however, and determine the exact location using descriptions such as "occurs in the lower back" or "occurs under the sternum." Questions that assist in accomplishing this are as follows:

   > - Where exactly does it hurt?
   > - Can you show me where it hurts?
   > - Do you feel it anywhere else?

2. **Quality of the Symptom**. The quality of the symptom includes a complete and concise description of the symptom. The medical assistant should use informative terms to describe the character of each symptom. For example, if the patient complains of pain, the character of the pain must be included. Terms that can be used to describe pain include:

   - Burning
   - Aching
   - Sharp
   - Dull
   - Throbbing
   - Cramplike
   - Squeezing

If the patient has vomited, the medical assistant will need to indicate the color, odor, and consistency of the vomitus. If the patient has a cough, the medical assistant will need to indicate if it is productive or nonproductive and whether or not blood is present. Refer to the table of terms on page 948 of this manual, which will assist you in describing symptoms. Specific examples of questions that are helpful in determining the quality of the symptom are as follows:

> * Describe it (the symptom) to me as fully as possible.
> * What is it (the symptom) like?

3. Severity of the Symptom. The severity refers to the quantitative aspect of the symptom. It includes the following:

> * Intensity of the symptom (e.g., mild, moderate, severe)
> * Number (e.g., of convulsions, of nosebleeds)
> * Volume (e.g., of vomitus, of blood, of mucus)
> * Size or extent (e.g., of the rash, edema, lumps, or masses)

This information assists the physician in determining the extensiveness or seriousness of the illness. Questions to determine severity are often specific to that symptom. For example, if the patient has a productive cough, the medical assistant will need to determine how much phlegm is being coughed up (e.g., a teaspoon, half a cup). At first, this area may appear difficult. As you practice taking symptoms, however, you will learn what questions to ask the patient, and eventually it will become automatic. The examples at the end of this section as well as the student practice problems provide guidance in developing skill in this area. Some examples of general questions that can be used to determine the severity of a symptom are as follows:

> * How bad is it (the symptom)?
> * Does it (the symptom) limit your normal activities?

4. Chronology and Timing of the Symptom. Chronology and timing include a sequential account of the symptom up to the time the patient came to the medical office for treatment. This information is important in determining the duration of the symptom and change in it since it first occurred. Chronology and timing include the following four areas:

a. Date of Onset: The date of onset of the symptom should be indicated, if possible, as a calendar date and clock time. Because of this, the patient may need some time to recall this information. Examples of questions that help obtain this information are as follows:

> * When did you experience this (the symptom) for the first time?
> * Exactly when did this begin?

b. Duration: The duration of the symptom refers to how long the symptom lasts after it occurs, for example: 10 minutes, 2 hours, continuously. Examples of questions to obtain this information are as follows:

> * How long does it last after occurring?
> * For what length of time do you experience this symptom?

c. Frequency: The frequency of the symptom refers to how often the symptom occurs, for example: twice a day, a single attack every 2 weeks. Examples of questions to obtain this information are as follows:

> * How often does it occur?
> * How often has the symptom recurred?

d. **Change over Time:** This area refers to any change in the symptom since it first occurred. A change in a symptom reflects the nature of the underlying disease, which, in turn, assists the physician in making a diagnosis. Examples of questions to obtain this information are as follows:

> - Has the symptom changed since it first occurred?
> - Is it (the symptom) getting better, worse, or staying the same?

5. **Manner of Onset**. The manner of onset refers to what the patient was doing when the symptom first occurred and exactly what was experienced by the patient when the symptom began. These data help provide information on the pathologic process responsible for the symptom. For example, the patient may have been lifting a heavy object before experiencing low back pain. As is evident, this information helps the physician in making an accurate diagnosis. Examples of questions that are helpful in determining the manner of onset are as follows:

> - What exactly did you experience when it (the symptom) first occurred?
> - What was the first thing you noticed?
> - Did it (the symptom) come on suddenly or gradually?
> - What were you doing when it (the symptom) began?
> - Where were you when this happened?
> - How were you feeling before it (the symptom) began?

6. **Modifying Factors**. Symptoms are often influenced by activities or physiological processes such as physical exercise, changes in the weather, bodily functions (e.g., bowel movements, eating, coughing), pregnancy, emotional states, and fatigue. Some activities may aggravate the symptom while others may alleviate it. These influences may help to determine what is causing the problem. For example, pain that becomes worse after the patient eats but is relieved after taking an antacid assists the physician in focusing on gastrointestinal disorders. Questions to assist in determining modifying factors are as follows:

> - Does anything make it (the symptom) better?
> - Does anything make it worse?
> - What have you done to make it better?
> - What did you do to help it?
> - Are you taking any medication for it? Did it help?

7. **Associated Symptoms**. There is usually more than one symptom present with a disease process. Determining these additional symptoms gives the physician a complete picture of the illness. Examples of questions that help to identify the presence of additional symptoms are as follows:

> - Are you having any other symptoms?
> - What other problems have you noticed since you became ill?

Examples

The following examples illustrate how to analyze a symptom. The chief complaint is listed first, followed by questions to ask the patient from the seven basic categories of information.

> *Example: Chief Complaint: Headaches that began 2 months ago.*

1. Using your finger, point to the location of the headache.
2. Describe the pain. Is it sharp, dull, throbbing?
3. Are you able to carry on with normal activities when you have a headache?
4. Is it sometimes more severe than usual?
5. When exactly did your headaches begin?

6. How long does your headache last when it occurs?
7. How often do you get a headache?
8. Since your headaches began, have they gotten better or worse, or have they stayed the same?
9. What were you doing the first time you experienced a headache?
10. What was your health status before your headaches began?
11. Do you get a headache before, during, or after a particular activity, such as reading or watching TV?
12. Does anything make your headache better?
13. Are you taking any medication for your headache? Does it help?
14. Have you had any other problems since your headaches began, such as nausea, vomiting, dizziness, or problems with vision?

> **Example:** *Chief Complaint: The patient has been coughing for the past 3 days.*

1. Does it hurt when you cough? Where? Show me with one of your fingers.
2. What is the cough like?
3. Can you cough for me?
4. Do you bring up any phlegm when you cough? What color is it? Is blood present?
5. Describe the pain. Is it sharp, dull, squeezing?
6. Do you become exhausted when you cough?
7. How much phlegm do you bring up? A teaspoon? Half a cup?
8. How much blood is present in the phlegm?
9. When did your cough first begin?
10. Does it seem like an attack? How long does the attack last?
11. How often do you get a coughing attack?
12. Does your cough seem to be getting better or worse?
13. What was the first thing you noticed when you became ill?
14. How were you feeling before your symptoms began?
15. Is there anything that makes your cough better?
16. Is there anything that makes your cough worse?
17. Do you cough more at night or during the day?
18. Are you taking any medication for it? Does it help?
19. Are you having any other problems?

PRACTICE PROBLEMS

In the space provided, indicate examples of direct questions to ask the patient to obtain the necessary information for the symptom(s) presented in the chief complaint.

Problem 1

> *Chief Complaint: Earache and fever for the past 2 days.*

Questions:

_____

_____

_____

_____

_____

_____

_____

_____

_____

_____

Problem 2

> *Chief Complaint: Rash with itching that began 3 days ago.*

Questions:

_____

_____

_____

_____

_____

_____

_____

_____

_____

_____

_____

Problem 3

> *Chief Complaint: Pain during urination that began yesterday.*

Questions:

_____

_____

_____

_____

_____

_____

_____

_____

_____

_____

Problem 4

Chief Complaint: *Low back pain for the past 3 days.*

Questions:

_____

_____

_____

_____

_____

_____

_____

_____

_____

Problem 5

Chief Complaint: *Sore throat and fever for the past 24 hours.*

Questions:

_____

_____

_____

_____

_____

_____

_____

_____

Problem 6

Chief Complaint: *Chest pain that occurred this morning.*

Questions:

_____

_____

_____

_____

_____

_____

_____

_____

_____

_____

Terms for Describing Symptoms

PAIN

Burning, aching, sharp, dull, throbbing, cramping, squeezing
Radiating, transient, constant
Localized, superficial, deep

RRESPIRATIONS

Rapid, irregular, shallow, deep, labored, gasping, noisy, wheezing
Apnea, dyspnea, orthopnea
Discomfort, pain, cyanosis, cough

COUGH

Nonproductive, productive
Persistent, dry, hacking, barking, spasmodic
Phlegm: color, consistency, presence or absence of blood
Exhausting or painful

CARDIOVASCULAR

Pain, palpitations
Sharp, radiating
Dyspnea, orthopnea
Cyanosis

GASTROINTESTINAL

Abdomen: flaccid, rigid, distended
Appetite: anorexia, intolerance to foods
Heartburn, pain after eating, belching, nausea, vomiting, flatulence, change in bowel habits, constipation, diarrhea, black stools

URINE/STOOL

Abnormality: color, odor, consistency, frequency
Contents: sediment, mucus, blood
Elimination: urgency, nocturia, pain, burning

SKIN

Rash: pruritus, red, swelling, distribution
Lesions: color, character, distribution
Pallor, flushing, jaundice, warm, dry, cold, clammy
Ecchymosis, petechiae, cyanosis, edema
Pruritus, sweating, change in color, bruises easily

EARS

Pain, loss of hearing, tinnitus, vertigo
Discharge, infection

EYES

Itching, burning, blurry vision, seeing double, photophobia
Discharge, watering, infection

37

Patient Reception

√ After Completing	Date Due	Textbook Page(s)	TEXTBOOK ASSIGNMENTS	Possible Points	Points You Earned
		897-910	Read Chapter 37: Patient Reception		
		903 908	Read Case Study 1 Case Study 1 questions	5	
		905 909	Read Case Study 2 Case Study 2 questions	5	
		907 909	Read Case Study 3 Case Study 3 questions	5	
			TOTAL POINTS		
√ After Completing	Date Due	Study Guide Page(s)	STUDY GUIDE ASSIGNMENTS (CTA: Critical Thinking Activity)	Possible Points	Points You Earned
		951	Pretest	10	
		952	Key Term Assessment	5	
		953-954	Evaluation of Learning questions	18	
		954-955	CTA A: Privacy Practices	5	
		955	CTA B: Verifying Insurance and Referrals	8	
		955	CTA C: Patient Information Brochure	20	
			CD Activity: Chapter 37 Apply Your Knowledge questions (Record points earned)		
		951	Posttest	10	
			ADDITIONAL ASSIGNMENTS		
			TOTAL POINTS		

√ When Assigned by Your Instructor	Study Guide Page(s)	Practices Required	LABORATORY ASSIGNMENTS (Procedure Number and Name)	*Score
	957	3	**Practice for Competency** 37-1: Opening the Medical Office Textbook reference: p. 900	
	963-964		**Evaluation of Competency** 37-1: Opening the Medical Office	*
	957	3	**Practice for Competency** 37-2: Closing the Medical Office Textbook reference: pp. 900-901	
	965-966		**Evaluation of Competency** 37-2: Closing the Medical Office	*
	961	3	**DVD Practice for Competency** 37-3: Obtaining New Patient Information Textbook reference: p. 906	
	967-968		**Evaluation of Competency** 37-3: Obtaining New Patient Information	*
	961	3	**Practice for Competency** 37-4: Explaining Office Policies and Procedures Textbook reference: pp. 907-908	
	969-970		**Evaluation of Competency** 37-4: Explaining Office Policies and Procedures	*
			ADDITIONAL ASSIGNMENTS	

Name _____   Date_____

? PRETEST

True or False

_____ 1. The first thing the medical assistant does when opening the office is to unlock the file cabinets, medical record files, and medicine cabinets.

_____ 2. After opening the office, the medical assistant should be sure that the telephones are switched to the day message or call the answering service.

_____ 3. An electronic task system consists of a folder for each month and a folder for each day.

_____ 4. Medical records are usually pulled the evening before the appointment.

_____ 5. A radio, CD player, television, or DVD player is usually turned on in the morning before patients arrive.

_____ 6. The autoclave is often run just before closing the medical office so that instruments can dry overnight.

_____ 7. Only one person should be permitted to stand at the reception desk at a time.

_____ 8. A new patient must sign a form acknowledging receipt of HIPAA privacy practices.

_____ 9. Only the top side of the insurance card must be photocopied.

_____ 10. If a patient has managed care insurance, a referral form may be required to see a physician other than the primary care provider.

? POSTTEST

True or False

_____ 1. As soon as the medical assistant has opened the office, he or she usually runs the autoclave.

_____ 2. After opening the office, the medical assistant should check the fax machine for faxes that may have arrived overnight.

_____ 3. A tickler file is used to remind the medical assistant of tasks to be done on a specific day.

_____ 4. The first major task for the medical assistant in the morning is to pull the medical records for all patients to be seen that day.

_____ 5. Holders for patient information brochures are often located in the waiting room.

_____ 6. The medical assistant turns off all equipment as the last thing when closing the office.

_____ 7. A sliding glass window between the waiting room and reception desk helps maintain patient confidentiality.

_____ 8. A new patient must sign a form providing consent for treatment and release of information.

_____ 9. Insurance companies usually require authorization every time the patient sees the primary care physician.

_____ 10. If the patient has a copayment, it is usually collected before the patient sees the physician.

✏️Term **KEY TERM ASSESSMENT**

Directions: Match each medical term with its definition.

_____ 1. Assignment of benefits

_____ 2. Call-in times

_____ 3. Copayment

_____ 4. Medicaid

_____ 5. Tickler file

A. A fixed amount of money that the patient is responsible to pay at each visit

B. A chronological file containing reminders of things to be done

C. Authorization given by the patient to allow the insurance company to make payments directly to the health care provider

D. Blocks of time when a physician accepts telephone calls from patients

E. A federal and state insurance program for low-income patients

EVALUATION OF LEARNING

Directions: Fill in each blank with the correct answer.

1. List five activities that the MA must perform to open the office.

_____

_____

2. How does the MA prepare the telephone system for patient calls at the beginning of the day?

_____

_____

3. How should the MA prepare for the day's activities in the medical office?

_____

_____

4. If an office uses paper medical records, how are they prepared before patients arrive?

_____

_____

_____

5. What should the MA do to be sure the waiting room is ready for patients?

_____

_____

6. What might the MA need to do to check equipment and prepare supplies at the beginning of the day?

_____

_____

_____

7. List seven tasks that the MA should perform when closing the medical office.

_____

_____

_____

8. How does the medical office identify which patients have arrived for appointments?

_____

_____

9. What is the function of a sliding glass window between the reception desk and the patient waiting area?

_____

10. Identify at least three statements or forms that a new patient must sign before being examined by the physician.

_____

_____

11. What is required by the HIPAA legislation related to notifying patients about privacy practices?

_____

_____

12. How does the MA verify a patient's insurance information?

_____

_____

_____

_____

13. When does a patient need a written referral form?

_____

14. What information is included in a written referral form?

_____

_____

15. What information must be obtained from an established patient who is checking in?

_____

_____

16. What is a copayment, and when is a copayment usually collected?

_____

17. What are at least eight pieces of information that should be included in a brochure for new patients?

_____

_____

_____

_____

_____

18. What are three reasons that a physician might not be accepting new patients?

_____

_____

CRITICAL THINKING ACTIVITIES

A. PRIVACY PRACTICES

Obtain a printed sample Notice of Privacy Practices from a medical office either from your own physician or from the Internet. Many organizations post their privacy statements on their websites. Using the copy of the privacy practices statement, highlight the sections where the following required content is included. Then write a brief statement stating whether your example contains all required information or not.

1. How the medical office may use and disclose protected health information about an individual.

2. The individual's rights with respect to the information and how the individual may exercise these rights, including how the individual may complain to the medical office.

3. The medical office's legal duties with respect to the information, including a statement that the medical office is required by law to maintain the privacy of protected health information.

4. How individuals can obtain further information about the medical office's privacy policies.

5. The effective date of the Notice of Privacy Practices.

B. VERIFYING INSURANCE AND REFERRALS

Based on information in the chapter, choose the following methods necessary to verify that the patient's insurance will cover charges and that the patient has a completed referral form if necessary. Enter the letter(s) of the correct step(s) the MA must take when a patient checks in. Some situations require more than one answer.

   a. Ask to see the patient's insurance card (or card of the insured party).

   b. Ask to see *and* make a photocopy of the patient's insurance card (or card of the insured party).

   c. Check that the patient has current insurance using a card reader, fax, or telephone call.

   d. Call the insurance company to verify insurance coverage and/or obtain preauthorization.

   e. Check to see that there is a completed referral form.

1. An established patient has an appointment with his primary care physician. _____

2. A new patient has an appointment with a primary care physician. _____

3. A new patient with managed care insurance has an appointment with a cardiologist. _____

4. An established patient with Medicaid has an appointment for a blood pressure check. _____

5. An established patient tells the MA that she has changed insurance since the last visit. _____

6. A new patient with managed care insurance visits a dermatologist for a minor surgical procedure. _____

7. A mother brings an infant to the pediatrician for his first well-baby checkup. _____

8. An established patient is being scheduled for a cosmetic laser procedure. _____

C. PATIENT INFORMATION BROCHURE

1. Create a patient information brochure or booklet for a physician in private practice. Assume that the location of the office is at the same address as your medical assisting school. Include the following information:

   • Physician's name, credentials, and specialty

   • Brief statement of the physician's philosophy of patient care

   • Directions to the office, parking, and access to public transportation, if any

   • General statement that most insurance is accepted and that copayments are expected at the time of the visit

   • Policy regarding cancellation of appointments

   • Name of a local hospital that the physician is affiliated with

   • Description of how medication refills are handled

2. Compare your patient information booklet with the booklets of at least two of your classmates and discuss how these booklets could be used by the medical office.

Notes

PRACTICE FOR COMPETENCY

Procedure 37-1: Opening the Medical Office. Practice opening the office.

A. Make a list of tasks to open the office:

_____

_____

_____

_____

_____

_____

Procedure 37-2: Closing the Medical Office. Practice closing the office.

A. Make a list of tasks to close the office:

_____

_____

_____

_____

_____

_____

New Patient Information Form. Complete the new patient information form using yourself as the patient. Use the form to practice Procedure 37-3.

REGISTRATION
(PLEASE PRINT)

Home Phone: _____   Today's Date: _____

PATIENT INFORMATION

Name _____   Soc. Sec.# _____
           Last Name   First Name   Initial

Address _____

City _____ State _____ Zip _____

Single ___ Married ___ Widowed ___ Separated ___ Divorced ___ Sex M___ F___ Age ___ Birthdate _____

Patient Employed by _____ Occupation _____

Business Address _____ Business Phone _____

By whom were you referred? _____

In case of emergency who should be notified? _____ Phone _____
                                          Last Name   Relationship to Patient

PRIMARY INSURANCE

Person Responsible for Account _____
                                    Last Name   First Name   Initial

Relation to Patient _____ Birthdate _____ Soc. Sec.# _____

Address (if different from patient's) _____ Phone _____

City _____ State _____ Zip _____

Person Responsible Employed by _____ Occupation _____

Business Address _____ Business Phone _____

Insurance Company _____

Contract # _____ Group # _____ Subscriber # _____

Name of other dependents covered under this plan _____

ADDITIONAL INSURANCE

Is patient covered by additional insurance?   ___ Yes ___ No

Subscriber Name _____ Relationship to Patient _____ Birthdate _____

Address (if different from patient's) _____ Phone _____

City _____ State _____ Zip _____

Subscriber Employed by _____ Business Phone _____

Insurance Company _____

Contract # _____ Group # _____ Subscriber # _____

Name of other dependents covered under this plan _____

ASSIGNMENT AND RELEASE

I, the undersigned, certify that I (or my dependent) have insurance coverage with _____
                                                                          Name of Insurance Company(ies)
and assign directly to Dr. _____ insurance benefits, if any, otherwise payable to me for services rendered. I
understand that I am financially responsible for all charges whether or not paid by insurance. I hereby authorize the doctor to release
all information necessary to secure the payment of benefits. I authorize the use of this signature on all insurance submissions.

_____   _____   _____
   Responsible Party Signature   Relationship   Date

ORDER# 58-8426 • © 1996 BIBBERO SYSTEMS, INC. • PETALUMA, CALIFORNIA • TO REORDER CALL TOLL FREE: (800) 242-9330

(Courtesy Bibbero Systems, Inc., Petaluma, Calif, [800] 242-2376; Fax [800] 242-9330; www.bibbero.com.)

Acknowledgement of Receipt of Notice of HIPAA Privacy Practices Form. Complete the Acknowledgement of Receipt of Notice of HIPAA Privacy Practices Form using yourself as the patient. Use the form to practice Procedure 37-3.

Acknowledgement of Receipt of the Notice of Privacy Practices

Please Review Carefully

The Notice of Privacy Practices tells you how **[Practice Name]** uses and discloses information about you. Not all situations will be described. We are required to give you a notice of our privacy practices for the information we collect and keep about you. We reserve the right to revise this notice, and you can obtain a copy of any revision upon written request.

I, _____ , have been given a copy of the **Notice of**

Privacy Practices.

_____   _____   _____
Patient or Legal Guardian's Signature   Date   Relationship to Patient

_____   _____
Print Patient's Name   Print Name of Legal Guardian (if any)

_____   _____
Signature of Witness (If signed with an "X" or mark)   Date

Effective Date: April 14, 2003

Procedure 37-3: Obtaining New Patient Information. Practice obtaining new patient information from classmates using the forms they completed above.

Procedure 37-4: Explaining Office Policies and Procedures. Using the patient information brochure prepared for Critical Thinking Activity C, practice orienting classmates (as simulated new patients) to office policies and procedures.

EVALUATION OF COMPETENCY

Procedure 37-1: Opening the Medical Office

Name: _____   Date: _____

Evaluated By: _____   Score: _____

Performance Objective

Outcome:	Open the medical office.
Conditions:	In a medical office.
Standards:	Time: 15 minutes. Student completed procedure in _____ minutes.
	Accuracy: Satisfactory score on the Performance Evaluation Checklist.

Performance Evaluation Checklist

Trial 1	Trial 2	Point Value	Performance Standards
		●	Entered the office and disarmed any alarm system.
		●	Turned on the lights.
		●	Adjusted heat or air conditioning to a comfortable setting.
		●	Unlocked the door for patients and visitors to enter.
		●	Turned on computers, printers, copier, and/or other machines.
		●	Called answering service for messages or listened to messages from voice mail or office answering machine.
		●	Wrote down complete message information on message forms.
		●	Arranged messages in order of importance.
		●	Dealt with urgent messages or calls.
		●	Pulled medical records for routine messages about patients.
		●	Clipped each message about a patient to the correct medical record.
		●	Placed routine messages in appropriate location(s) for office staff to review.
		●	Reviewed the day's activities and noted any special tasks.
		●	Checked the office for safety hazards.
		●	Straightened up the waiting room and turned on radio, television, or DVD player.
		●	Refilled holder of patient information brochures as needed.
		●	Printed appointment lists as needed.
		●	Pulled medical records as needed for the day's appointments.
		●	Arranged patient medical records in order of appointments.
		●	Printed or stamped the date on progress notes of medical records as needed.
		●	Prepared charge slips and clipped to patient records if office policy.

Trial 1	Trial 2		*Performance Standards*
		•	Checked biohazard waste containers and changed or discarded properly.
		•	Ran or emptied the autoclave as needed.
		*	Completed the procedure within 15 minutes.
			TOTALS

Evaluation of Student Performance

EVALUATION CRITERIA			COMMENTS
Symbol	**Category**	**Point Value**	
*	Critical Step	16 points	
•	Essential Step	6 points	
▷	Theory Question	2 points	

Score calculation: 100 points

− _____ points missed

_____ Score

Satisfactory score: 85 or above

CAAHEP Competencies Achieved:

Psychomotor (Skills)
☑ V. 9. Perform routine maintenance of office equipment with documentation.
☑ XI. 2. Evaluate the work environment to identify safe vs. unsafe working conditions.

Affective (Behavior)
☑ V. 2. Implement time management principles to maintain effective office function.

ABHES Competencies Achieved:

☑ 8. x. Maintain medical facility.
☑ 8. y. Perform routine maintenance of administrative and clinical equipment.
☑ 9. k. Prepare and maintain examination and treatment areas.

EVALUATION OF COMPETENCY

Procedure 37-2: Closing the Medical Office

Name: _____   Date: _____

Evaluated By: _____   Score: _____

Performance Objective

Outcome:	Close a medical office.
Conditions:	In a medical office.
Standards:	Time: 15 minutes. Student completed procedure in _____ minutes.
	Accuracy: Satisfactory score on the Performance Evaluation Checklist.

Performance Evaluation Checklist

Trial 1	Trial 2	Point Value	Performance Standards
		•	Made sure examination rooms were clean and contained all necessary supplies.
		•	Ran the autoclave if needed.
		•	Printed a patient schedule for the next day.
		•	Pulled medical records for the next day.
		•	Printed charge slips and clipped to the medical records if office policy.
		•	Made sure cabinets or rooms containing medical records were locked.
		•	Placed any money in the office safe or took to bank to be deposited.
		•	Activated the night telephone system by switching telephone message or calling the answering service.
		•	Turned off office machines including computers, printers, and photocopier.
		•	Unplugged coffee pot, toaster, or other machines that might pose a fire hazard.
		•	Locked door used for patients and visitors.
		•	Turned heat or air conditioning to night setting.
		•	Turned off the lights.
		•	Armed the security system.
		•	Made sure that staff exit door was locked securely.
		∗	Completed the procedure within 15 minutes.
			TOTALS

Evaluation of Student Performance

EVALUATION CRITERIA			COMMENTS
Symbol	Category	Point Value	
∗	Critical Step	16 points	
•	Essential Step	6 points	
▷	Theory Question	2 points	

Score calculation: 100 points

− _____ points missed

_____ Score

Satisfactory score: 85 or above

CAAHEP Competencies Achieved:

Psychomotor (Skills)
☑ III. 6. Perform sterilization procedures.

Affective (Behavior)
☑ V. 2. Implement time management principles to maintain effective office function.

ABHES Competencies Achieved:

☑ 8. x. Maintain medical facility.
☑ 9. o. (4) Perform sterilization techniques.

EVALUATION OF COMPETENCY

Procedure 37-3: Obtaining New Patient Information

Name: _____   Date: _____

Evaluated By: _____   Score: _____

Performance Objective

Outcome:	Obtain new patient information, obtain consents, and validate insurance coverage.
Conditions:	Given the following: clipboard, pen, new patient information form, notice of privacy practices form, receipt of privacy practices form, consent for release of protected health information (optional), photocopier, insurance card reader (optional), telephone, medical record, computer, scanner.
Standards:	Time: 10 minutes. Student completed procedure in _____ minutes. Accuracy: Satisfactory score on the Performance Evaluation Checklist.

Performance Evaluation Checklist

Trial 1	Trial 2	Point Value	Performance Standards
		●	Placed a new patient information form on a clipboard with a pen.
		●	Asked a new patient to complete the form and return it.
		●	Verified that the form was complete and signed by the patient or authorized representative.
		●	Asked to see the insurance card of the patient or insured individual.
		●	Photocopied both sides of the insurance card.
		●	Placed the photocopy of the insurance card in the patient's medical record.
		●	Confirmed patient eligibility for insurance as needed using a card reader or by a telephone call to the insurance company.
		●	Verified that there was a completed referral form as needed.
		●	Discussed the patient's financial responsibility, if the visit would not be completely covered by insurance, in a private area.
		●	Pulled medical records for routine messages about patients.
		●	Gave the patient a copy of the notice of privacy practices or made it available for the patient to read.
		＊	Asked the patient to sign the receipt of privacy practices form.
		●	Signed the receipt of privacy practices form as a witness.
		●	Asked the patient to read and sign any consent for release of personal health information used by the office.
		●	Inserted new forms into the medical record.
		●	Placed the medical record and charge slip to indicate that the patient has been checked in.

Trial 1	Trial 2	Point Value	Performance Standards
		•	Ask the patient to have a seat and indicate the probable wait time.
		•	Enter new patient information into the computer or validate patient information.
		•	Scan patient forms according to office policy (if the office uses an electronic medical record).
		*	Completed the procedure within 10 minutes.
			TOTALS

Evaluation of Student Performance

EVALUATION CRITERIA			COMMENTS
Symbol	Category	Point Value	
*	Critical Step	16 points	
•	Essential Step	6 points	
▷	Theory Question	2 points	

Score calculation: 100 points

− _____ points missed

_____ Score

Satisfactory score: 85 or above

CAAHEP Competencies Achieved:

Psychomotor (Skills)

☑ VII. 1. Apply both managed care policies and procedures.
☑ VII. 2. Apply third party guidelines.
☑ VII. 6. Verify eligibility for managed care services
☑ IX. 1. Respond to issues of confidentiality.
☑ IX. 8. Apply local, state and federal health care legislation and regulation appropriate to the medical assisting practice setting.

Affective (Behavior)

☑ IV. 2. Apply active listening skills.
☑ IX. 1. Demonstrate sensitivity to patient rights.
☑ IX. 3. Recognize the importance of local, state and federal legislation and regulations in the practice setting.

ABHES Competencies Achieved:

☑ 4. c. Follow established policies when initiating or terminating medical treatment.
☑ 4. f. Comply with federal, state and local health laws and regulations.
☑ 8. r. Apply third party guidelines.
☑ 8. y. Perform routine maintenance of administrative and clinical equipment.
☑ 8. ff. Interview effectively.

✒ EVALUATION OF COMPETENCY

Procedure 37-4: Explaining Office Policies and Procedures

Name: _____   Date: _____

Evaluated By: _____   Score: _____

Performance Objective

Outcome:	Orient a new patient to the medical office.
Conditions:	Given the following: patient information booklet, map, list of points to cover.
Standards:	Time: 10 minutes. Student completed procedure in ____ minutes.
	Accuracy: Satisfactory score on the Performance Evaluation Checklist.

Performance Evaluation Checklist

Trial 1	Trial 2	Point Value	Performance Standards
		•	Offered to give or send a patient information booklet if one is available.
		•	Identified the name, credentials, and specialty of each physician who would accept new patients.
		•	Offered information as required about languages spoken in the office and any additional services that would be available.
		•	Identified the location of the office, gave directions, and discussed parking as needed.
		•	Told the patient if the office accepted his or her medical insurance plan.
		•	Discussed expectations for payment of the patient's bill..
		•	Described how far in advance to make and/or cancel appointments.
		•	Told the patient how to contact the office.
		•	Informed the patient if the physician had specific call-in times.
		•	Explained how prescription refills would be handled.
		•	Identified hospital affiliation(s) of the office physician(s).
		•	Asked if there were other questions and responded appropriately.
		*	Completed the procedure within 10 minutes.
			TOTALS

Evaluation of Student Performance

EVALUATION CRITERIA			COMMENTS
Symbol	Category	Point Value	
✳	Critical Step	16 points	
●	Essential Step	6 points	
▷	Theory Question	2 points	

Score calculation: 100 points

− _____ points missed

_____ Score

Satisfactory score: 85 or above

CAAHEP Competencies Achieved:

Psychomotor (Skills)
☑ IV. 4. Explain general office policies.

Affective (Behavior)
☑ IV. 2. Apply active listening skills.
☑ IV. 7. Demonstrate recognition of the patient's level of understanding in communication.
☑ VII. 3. Communicate in language the patient can understand regarding managed care and insurance plans.

ABHES Competencies Achieved:

☑ 8. cc. Communicate on the recipient's level of understanding.
☑ 8. ii. Recognize and respond to verbal and non-verbal communication.

38

Medical Office Computerization

CHAPTER ASSIGNMENTS

√ After Completing	Date Due	Textbook Page(s)	TEXTBOOK ASSIGNMENTS	Possible Points	Points You Earned
		911-938	Read Chapter 38: Medical Office Computerization		
		930 936	Read Case Study 1 Case Study 1 questions	5	
		931 936	Read Case Study 2 Case Study 2 questions	5	
		935 937	Read Case Study 3 Case Study 3 questions	5	
			TOTAL POINTS		

√ After Completing	Date Due	Study Guide Page(s)	STUDY GUIDE ASSIGNMENTS (CTA: Critical Thinking Activity)	Possible Points	Points You Earned
		973	Pretest	10	
		974-975	Term Key Term Assessment	30	
		976-984	Evaluation of Learning questions	108	
		984	CTA A: Computer System	7	
		985	CTA B: Computer Monitor	6	
		985-986	CTA C: Medical Practice Management Program	22	
		987	CTA D: Crossword Puzzle	29	
			CD Activity: Chapter 38 Road to Recovery Game: Computer Terminology (Record points earned)		

√ After Completing	Date Due	Study Guide Page(s)	STUDY GUIDE ASSIGNMENTS (CTA: Critical Thinking Activity)	Possible Points	Points You Earned
			CD CD Activity: Chapter 38 Apply Your Knowledge questions (Record points earned)		
		973	? Posttest	10	
			ADDITIONAL ASSIGNMENTS		
			TOTAL POINTS		

Name _____   Date_____

PRETEST

True or False

_____ 1. Computers that are linked together are known as a *network*.

_____ 2. The transfer of data to the computer for processing is known as *input*.

_____ 3. Spreadsheet software consists of an electronic ledger designed to perform mathematical calculations quickly.

_____ 4. The CPU consists of the control unit and RAM.

_____ 5. Monitor resolution is measured in millimeters.

_____ 6. A microfiber cloth can be used to clean the screen of a monitor.

_____ 7. Printed output from a computer is known as *hardcopy*.

_____ 8. A USB flash drive stores information in the form of magnetized particles.

_____ 9. The posting transactions system is used to post patient charges and payments.

_____ 10. Paper documents are entered into a patient's EMR by scanning them into the computer.

POSTTEST

True or False

_____ 1. A program consists of raw, unorganized facts about subject matter presented to the computer for processing.

_____ 2. An operating system assists the computer in carrying out its tasks.

_____ 3. The mainboard directs the step-by-step operation of all the processing functions.

_____ 4. One gigabyte is equal to 1000 MB.

_____ 5. The visual display of information on the screen of a monitor is termed *softcopy*.

_____ 6. The contrast control is used to adjust the intensity of the images on the screen of a monitor.

_____ 7. Grime can be removed from a computer keyboard using a can of compressed inert gas.

_____ 8. The transfer of information from RAM to a hard disk is known as *write*.

_____ 9. The reports system allows the user to customize a medical management program to meet the specific requirements of a medical office.

_____ 10. Software designed to penetrate a computer or network without consent is known as a *computer virus*.

✏️Term KEY TERM ASSESSMENT

Directions: Match each computer term with its definition.

_____ 1. Computer

_____ 2. Computer system

_____ 3. CPU (central processing unit)

_____ 4. Data

_____ 5. Data processing

_____ 6. Documentation

_____ 7. Electronic medical record (EMR)

_____ 8. Firewall

_____ 9. Hard disk

_____ 10. Hardcopy

_____ 11. Hardware

_____ 12. Input

_____ 13. Input device

_____ 14. Medical practice management program

_____ 15. Microcomputer

_____ 16. Operating system

_____ 17. Optical disc

_____ 18. Optical drive

_____ 19. Output

A. A circuit board connected to the mainboard that converts computer video output into electronic signals

B. A computerized record of the important health information regarding a patient including the care of that individual and the progress of the patient's condition

C. A device for entering data into the computer (e.g., keyboard, mouse, scanner)

D. A device installed in a drive bay on the main computer unit that uses a laser to read an optical disc or write onto (burn) an optical disc

E. A device that permanently stores information for later retrieval by the computer

F. A device that transfers processed data to the user (e.g., computer monitor and printer)

G. A general term for the programs or instructions that tell a computer what to do

H. A program that provides instructions to the computer for performing medical practice management procedures

I. A set of instructions organized in a logical step-by-step sequence, which tells the computer how to perform a specific function

J. A small general purpose computer that relies on a tiny microprocessor chip to perform its processing functions

K. A storage device consisting of a flat, round, portable disk that stores data using laser technology

L. A storage device consisting of one or more rigid, nonflexible platters coated with a magnetically sensitive material and encased in a permanently sealed, air-tight container

M. A system that protects a computer network from unauthorized access by users on its own network or another network, such as the Internet

N. A type of system software that performs tasks required by the computer to operate itself

_____ 20. Output device

_____ 21. Printing speed

_____ 22. Processing

_____ 23. Program

_____ 24. RAM (random-access memory)

_____ 25. Softcopy

_____ 26. Software

_____ 27. Storage capacity

_____ 28. Storage device

_____ 29. User

_____ 30. Video card

O. A written set of instructions accompanying an application program, designed to assist the user in understanding how to operate the program

P. All of the hardware and software components making up the computer

Q. An electronic machine that has the ability to process data according to a program in order to produce a desired result

R. Printed output from a computer

S. Raw, unorganized facts about subject matter presented to the computer for processing.

T. The "brain" of the computer housed in the main unit that interprets and executes the instructions that operate the computer

U. The changing of raw facts or data into usable information following a three-part sequence: input, processing, output

V. The individual using the computer

W. The main computer memory of a microcomputer, which is used to temporarily store items until needed by the computer for processing

X. The manipulation and reorganization of data according to the instructions in a program

Y. The maximum amount of information that a device can hold, measured in bytes

Z. The number of pages per minute (ppm) generated by a printer

AA. The physical devices making up a computer system (e.g., main computer unit, keyboard, monitor, printer)

BB. The transfer of data to the computer for processing

CC. The transfer of processed data back to the user

DD. The visual display of information on the display screen of a computer monitor

EVALUATION OF LEARNING

Directions: Fill in each blank with the correct answer.

Computer Concepts

1. What is a computer?

   _____

   _____

2. What are the principal advantages of using a computer to perform administrative procedures in the medical office?

   _____

   _____

3. What type of computer is used most often in a private practice medical office?

   _____

4. What is a computer network?

   _____

5. What are the three phases included in the data processing sequence?

   _____

6. Why must data be converted into an electronic code before being processed by the computer?

   _____

7. What are four examples of input devices?

   _____

8. List five types of processing functions performed on data by the computer.

   _____

   _____

9. List two examples of output devices.

   _____

10. What is the difference between system software and application software?

    _____

    _____

11. What is the function of an operating system?

    _____

    _____

12. What is an example of an operating system?

    _____

13. List the four types of application software that make up a practice management program.

    _____

    _____

14. What are the functions performed by a word processing program?

_____

15. What tasks are performed by the word processing program included in a medical practice management program?

_____

16. What is spreadsheet software?

_____

_____

17. What is the function of the spreadsheet software included in a practice management program?

_____

18. What are the functions of the telecommunications software included in a practice management program?

_____

19. What is database management?

_____

20. List examples of information included in a medical practice database.

_____

_____

21. What functions can be performed by database management software?

_____

_____

22. What are examples of documentation?

_____

23. What computer hardware is necessary to perform administrative procedures in the medical office?

_____

_____

24. What are the eight major components of a main computer unit?

_____

_____

25. What is the function of the mainboard?

_____

_____

26. What is the meaning of the following abbreviation: CPU?

_____

27. What is the function of the CPU?

_____

28. What is the difference in processing speed between a CPU with a 3-GHz chip and one with a 1.5-GHz chip?

_____

29. What two parts make up the CPU?

_____

30. What is the function of the control unit?

_____

31. What is the function of the ALU?

_____

_____

32. What is the function of main memory (RAM)?

_____

_____

33. What items are commonly held in RAM?

_____

_____

34. What is the difference between random access and sequential access?

_____

_____

35. What happens to items in RAM when a computer is turned off?

_____

36. One byte is equivalent to how many characters?

_____

37. How many bytes are in a kilobyte (KB)?

_____

38. How many megabytes are in a gigabyte?

_____

39. Explain how to prevent overheating of the computer.

_____

_____

40. What is the primary cause of improper functioning of the computer?

_____

41. How should the casing of the main unit be cleaned?

_____

42. What can happen if a liquid spills into the main computer unit?

_____

43. What is the function of the computer monitor?

_____

44. What does the abbreviation CRT mean?

_____

45. What are the advantages and disadvantages of an LCD flat panel monitor?

_____

_____

46. How is the screen size of a computer monitor measured?

_____

47. What type of image is displayed on a high-resolution monitor?

_____

48. Monitor resolution is measured in what type of units?

_____

49. What is dot pitch?

_____

50. Explain the function of each of the following monitor controls:
    a. Brightness control

    _____

    b. Contrast control

    _____

51. How should the monitor be positioned to prevent back and neck tension?

_____

52. What can be done to prevent eye strain when working with a computer monitor?

_____

_____

53. How should the screen of a monitor be cleaned?

_____

_____

54. What can cause a monitor to overheat?

_____

55. What happens when a key is pressed on the computer keyboard?

_____

56. What is the function of special keys?

_____

_____

57. What is the function and examples of the following special keys?

a. Modifier keys

_____

_____

b. Lock keys

_____

_____

c. Navigation keys

_____

_____

58. How should the computer keyboard be positioned to prevent muscle fatigue?

_____

59. How should the following parts of a keyboard be cleaned?

a. Surface of the keyboard: _____

b. Interior of the keyboard: _____

60. What should be done if water spills into the keyboard?

_____

_____

_____

61. What is a printer?

_____

62. What types of printers are most commonly used in the medical office?

_____

63. How does an inkjet printer produce images on paper?

_____

64. What is the printing speed range for an inkjet printer?

_____

65. What are the advantages and disadvantages of an inkjet printer?

_____

_____

66. What are the advantages and disadvantages of a laser printer?

_____

_____

67. What is the printing speed range of a laser printer?

_____

68. How should the outside casing of a computer be cleaned?

_____

69. Where should you look to find information on cleaning the inside of the printer?

_____

70. List examples of storage devices used with a microcomputer.

_____

71. What method or organization is used to store and retrieve information from a hard disk?

_____

72. What occurs during the formatting process?

_____

73. What is the function of a hard disk drive?

_____

74. What is the function of the read/write head?

_____

_____

75. Explain the difference between read and write.

_____

_____

76. What is the storage capacity range for a hard disk?

_____

77. What are the advantages and disadvantages of a floppy disk?

_____

78. How does an optical disk store data?

_____

79. How much information can a CD-ROM hold?

_____

80. What is the difference between a CD-ROM and a CD-RW?

_____

_____

81. How much information can a DVD store in comparison with a CD-ROM?

_____

82. What makes up a USB flash drive?

_____

83. What is the storage capacity range of a USB flash drive?

_____

Medial Office Computerization

1. Why should the MA acquire a computer concepts base before working with microcomputers?

   _____

   _____

2. What are the advantages of medical office computerization?

   _____

   _____

   _____

3. What is an audit trail?

   _____

4. What are the disadvantages of computerization of the medical office?

   _____

   _____

5. What can cause a computer system to malfunction?

   _____

6. What measures should be taken to promote the efficient running of a computerized medical office?

   _____

   _____

7. What is the function of each of the following systems included in a medical practice management program?

   a. Patient registration system: _____

   b. Appointment system: _____

   c. Posting transactions system: _____

   d. Patient billing system: _____

   e. Insurance billing system: _____

   f. Reports system: _____

   g. File maintenance system: _____

8. Information entered into the patient registration system is used to perform what types of procedures?

   _____

   _____

9. What are examples of start-up tasks?

   _____

   _____

10. What functions can be performed by an EMR program?

    _____

    _____

11. What are advantages of the electronic medical record?

_____

_____

12. How are paper documents entered into a patient's EMR?

_____

13. How can a health history be entered into the EMR?

_____

_____

14. How does an EMR alleviate the need for medical transcription?

_____

_____

15. What is provided by the program for entering data into an EMR?

_____

16. What functions are performed by an EMR prescription program?

_____

_____

_____

17. How can an EMR program send a prescription to the pharmacy?

_____

18. What laboratory functions can be performed by an EMR program?

_____

_____

19. What are the advantages of having a diagnostic image available as a digital image?

_____

20. What procedures typically are performed by an MA using an EMR?

_____

_____

_____

21. Describe the following measures that maintain security of the EMR.

a. Authentification: _____

_____

b. Levels of authorization: _____

_____

c. Automatic logoff: _____

_____

d. Audit controls: _____

_____

e. Antiviral software: _____

_____

f. Firewall: _____

_____

22. List two ways in which backups are performed in the medical office.

_____

_____

23. Why is it important to periodically perform a disk cleanup?

_____

24. What occurs during disk defragmentation?

_____

_____

25. What type of service agreements might a medical office have related to its computer system?

_____

_____

CRITICAL THINKING ACTIVITIES

A. COMPUTER SYSTEM

Observe a computer system, and complete the following questions.

1. What is the brand name of the computer?

_____

2. What hardware is included with this computer system?

_____

_____

3. What application software is installed on this computer system?

_____

_____

4. What operating system is being used with this computer?

_____

5. What input devices are included with this computer system?

_____

6. What output devices are included with this computer system?

_____

7. How many optical drives does this computer have?

_____

B. COMPUTER MONITOR

Observe a computer monitor, and complete the following questions.

1. Is this a CRT monitor or an LCD flat panel monitor?

_____

2. What is the screen size (in inches) of this monitor?

_____

3. Where are the ventilation slots of this monitor located?

_____

4. Where are the following controls located?

   a. On/off button:_____

   b. Brightness control:_____

   c. Contrast control:_____

5. Position the monitor correctly to prevent back and neck tension. Explain what steps you took to do this.

_____

_____

6. Adjust the brightness and contrast control to determine the setting that works best for your viewing comfort. Explain what you did to accomplish this.

_____

_____

_____

C. MEDICAL PRACTICE MANAGEMENT PROGRAM

Indicate which system you would use to perform the following using a medical practice management program.

A. Patient registration system

B. Appointments system

C. Posting transactions system

D. Patient billing system

E. Insurance billing system

F. Reports system

G. File maintenance system

_____ 1. Assign a user password

_____ 2. Change a patient's address

_____ 3. Reschedule a patient's appointment

_____ 4. Change a patient's insurance carrier and policy number

_____ 5. Electronically submit insurance claims

_____ 6. Enter a new insurance carrier

_____ 7. Enter demographic and insurance information for a new patient

_____ 8. Make an appointment

_____ 9. Post a charge for an allergy injection

_____ 10. Look up a patient's telephone number

_____ 11. Post an insurance payment

_____ 12. Prepare and print out a practice analysis report

_____ 13. Prepare bills for processing

_____ 14. Prepare insurance forms

_____ 15. Print billing statements

_____ 16. Print out a patient receipt

_____ 17. Print out a patient reminder card

_____ 18. Enter a new referring physician

_____ 19. Print out an appointment log

_____ 20. Change a patient's last name

_____ 21. Enter a new diagnosis code

_____ 22. Post a copayment made by a patient

39

Telephone Techniques

CHAPTER ASSIGNMENTS

√ After Completing	Date Due	Textbook Page(s)	TEXTBOOK ASSIGNMENTS	Possible Points	Points You Earned
		939-955	Read Chapter 39: Telephone Techniques		
		945 954	Read Case Study 1 Case Study 1 questions	5	
		946 954	Read Case Study 2 Case Study 2 questions	5	
		952 954	Read Case Study 3 Case Study 3 questions	5	
			TOTAL POINTS		

√ After Completing	Date Due	Study Guide Page(s)	STUDY GUIDE ASSIGNMENTS (CTA: Critical Thinking Activity)	Possible Points	Points You Earned
		993	Pretest	10	
		994	Key Term Assessment	6	
		995-997	Evaluation of Learning questions	28	
		997-998	CTA A: Screening Telephone Calls	8	
		998	CTA B: Follow-up Questions	5	
		999	CTA C: Telephone Messages When the Office Is Closed	10	
		999	CTA D: Outgoing Calls	4	
			CD Activity: Chapter 39 Taking a Telephone Message	10	
			CD Activity: Chapter 39 Apply Your Knowledge questions (Record points earned)		
		993	Posttest	10	

√ After Completing	Date Due	Study Guide Page(s)	STUDY GUIDE ASSIGNMENTS (CTA: Critical Thinking Activity)	Possible Points	Points You Earned
			ADDITIONAL ASSIGNMENTS		
			TOTAL POINTS		

√ When Assigned by Your Instructor	Study Guide Page(s)	Practices Required	LABORATORY ASSIGNMENTS (Procedure Number and Name)	*Score
	1001	3	**Practice for Competency** 39-1: Performing Telephone Screening Textbook reference: pp. 948-949	
	1005-1006		**Evaluation of Competency** 39-1: Performing Telephone Screening	*
	1001	3	**DVD** **Practice for Competency** 39-2: Taking a Telephone Message Textbook reference: pp. 949-950	
	1007-1008		**Evaluation of Competency** 39-2: Taking a Telephone Message	*
	1001	3	**Practice for Competency** 39-3: Taking Requests for Medication or Prescription Refills Textbook reference: pp. 950-951	
	1009-1010		**Evaluation of Competency** 39-3: Taking Requests for Medication or Prescription Refills	*
	1004	3	**Practice for Competency** 39-4: Telephoning a Patient for Follow-Up Textbook reference: p. 953	
	1011-1012		**Evaluation of Competency** 39-4: Telephoning a Patient for Follow-Up	*
			ADDITIONAL ASSIGNMENTS	

Notes

Name _____   Date_____

PRETEST

True or False

_____ 1. The medical assistant should obtain a caller's name before placing the caller on hold.

_____ 2. A caller will not be able to pick up nonverbal cues during a telephone call with the medical office.

_____ 3. Call forwarding sends telephone calls to a different extension or telephone number.

_____ 4. Most medical offices rely only on voicemail during the night and weekends.

_____ 5. Patient insurance information may be sent electronically using telephone lines.

_____ 6. Physicians should not be contacted when out of the office using cell phones or pagers.

_____ 7. A telephone electronic routing system avoids placing incoming calls on hold.

_____ 8. A physician will accept a call from another physician, even if it interrupts a patient examination.

_____ 9. The medical assistant may not take a message from a laboratory that includes the results of diagnostic tests.

_____ 10. If a patient requests a prescription refill, the medical assistant should ask for the pharmacy name and telephone number.

POSTTEST

True or False

_____ 1. If a call is on hold, the medical assistant should check back with the caller at least every 30 seconds.

_____ 2. When answering the telephone, the medical assistant should first identify the practice and himself or herself.

_____ 3. Call park places a call on hold so that it can be retrieved from a different telephone.

_____ 4. Voice mail mailboxes each have a separate extension.

_____ 5. Confidential information should never be transmitted via a fax machine.

_____ 6. Physicians may have access to e-mail using their smartphones.

_____ 7. A telephone electronic routing system saves the expense of designating one person to answer incoming telephone calls.

_____ 8. Most physicians take calls from patients while they are seeing other patients.

_____ 9. Medical assistants routinely give patients the results of normal diagnostic tests over the telephone.

_____ 10. The medical assistant may take a message if a patient wants a referral or a diagnostic test.

⟋Term KEY TERM ASSESSMENT

Directions: Match each medical term with its definition.

_____ 1. DSL (digital subscriber line)

_____ 2. Enunciation

_____ 3. Pager

_____ 4. PDA (personal digital assistant)

_____ 5. Smartphone

_____ 6. SSL (Secure Sockets Layer)

_____ 7. Voice mail

A. A portable handheld computing device with access to various reference tools
B. Technology that allows digital signals to be transmitted over telephone lines at high speed
C. A method for delivery, storage, and retrieval of telephone messages that is built into the telephone system
D. An electronic device that notifies the recipient to receive a message or return a telephone call
E. The act of speaking clearly and concisely
F. A protocol for managing secure transmission of data over the Internet by means of encryption
G. A cell phone with computer capabilities

✎ EVALUATION OF LEARNING

Directions: Fill in each blank with the correct answer.

1. Give examples of three ways the MA can display courtesy when answering the telephone in the medical office.

   _____

   _____

2. How can the MA project a pleasing telephone personality when talking to callers in the medical office?

   _____

   _____

3. How should the MA answer the office telephone?

   _____

   _____

4. Identify three ways to maintain proper body mechanics and avoid muscle strain when spending several minutes on the telephone.

   _____

   _____

   _____

5. How does the MA handle a second call when speaking to a caller on a multiline telephone?

   _____

   _____

   _____

6. Identify and describe four features of most telephone systems.

   _____

   _____

   _____

7. How is voice mail used in the medical office?

   _____

   _____

   _____

8. How can patients get assistance for an urgent situation that occurs when the office is closed?

   _____

   _____

9. How should the MA maintain patient confidentiality when sending sensitive information using a fax machine?

   _____

   _____

   _____

10. What type of information does the medical office send electronically using telephone lines or a cable modem?

_____

_____

11. What should the MA remember about privacy of e-mail transmissions?

_____

_____

12. What are two devices that may be used to maintain contact with the physician when he or she is not in the medical office?

_____

13. What is an electronic routing system for incoming telephone calls?

_____

_____

14. When answering incoming calls, what three types of calls take priority over other telephone calls?

_____

_____

15. Identify four types of calls that are usually handled by the MA.

_____

_____

_____

16. List nine pieces of information that should be included if the MA takes a telephone message.

_____

_____

_____

_____

_____

17. How should the MA handle a telephone call requesting test results?

_____

_____

_____

18. If a patient or pharmacy calls with a request to have a prescription refilled or renewed, what specific information should the MA record on a telephone message?

_____

_____

_____

19. How should the MA handle a call if the caller has a medical question?

_____

_____

20. How should the MA handle a call from another physician?

_____

_____

21. How should the MA handle a telephone call about a serious emergency?

_____

_____

_____

22. If a telephone call concerns a possible case of poisoning, where should the caller be referred?

_____

_____

23. What should the MA do if a caller's condition does not seem to be a serious emergency, but the MA is not sure how urgent the problem is?

_____

_____

24. How should the MA handle a call if the caller asks for the physician but will not identify himself or herself?

_____

_____

_____

25. How should the MA handle a call if the caller has a complaint about service received in the medical office?

_____

_____

26. What guidelines should the MA follow when calling a patient?

_____

_____

27. What guidelines should the MA follow related to his or her own personal telephone calls?

_____

_____

28. How can the MA set up a conference call for a physician or other office staff member?

_____

_____

_____

CRITICAL THINKING ACTIVITIES

A. SCREENING TELEPHONE CALLS

For each of the following telephone calls, choose the best action for the MA from the following options. Assume that Dr. Warner is in the office seeing patients and a registered nurse is also in the office.

a. Transfer the call to Dr. Warner

b. Transfer the call to a licensed professional, such as one of the physicians or a nurse

c. Handle the call

d. Tell the caller that Dr. Warner is seeing patients, and offer to take a message

_____ 1. The caller identifies himself as Dr. Stephen Miller and asks to speak to Dr. Warner.

_____ 2. The caller asks for Dr. Warner and states that she wants the results of an MRI done last week.

_____ 3. The caller says that she has a question about her bill.

_____ 4. The caller asks for an appointment because the practice has been recommended to her.

_____ 5. The caller says that her daughter, a patient of Dr. Warner, fell off a swing and screams when anyone touches her left arm.

_____ 6. The caller identifies herself as a pharmacist and asks for Dr. Warner.

_____ 7. The caller says that she is calling to get results of a blood test done that morning.

_____ 8. The caller asks for an appointment because she has a sore throat and fever of 101°F.

B. FOLLOW-UP QUESTIONS

If you were the MA taking a message in each of the following examples, identify two questions you would ask the patient to complete the message.

1. Maria Reyes, a 38-year-old patient of Dr. Gomez, is calling because she wants to know the results of blood tests that were done for her 6-year-old daughter the previous week. She tells you her daughter's date of birth. She tells you that she is at work, and the best time to call is after 2:00 PM.

_____

_____

2. John Dalton, a 24-year-old patient of Dr. Hughes, is calling to get a refill of his cholesterol medication. He takes Lipitor 20 mg every morning. He tells you his date of birth. He only has two tablets left. He gives you his home telephone number and says that it is his day off.

_____

_____

3. A nurse calls from the hospital and says that she would like to obtain an order for a stronger pain medication for Angela White, a hospitalized patient. She tells you the patient's date of birth and gives you the telephone number of the nurse's station. She will be available until the end of the shift at 4:00 PM.

_____

_____

4. Melissa Sanders calls about her daughter who fell at school and twisted her ankle. Mrs. Sanders picked her daughter up from school, and she would like to discuss the injury with Dr. Warner. She gives you her home telephone number and cell phone number and says she will be available at any time.

_____

_____

5. A caller identifies himself as Robert Warner. He says that Dr. Gomez contacted him to obtain information about purchasing new examination tables. He gives you his office telephone number and cell phone number.

_____

_____

C. TELEPHONE MESSAGE WHEN THE OFFICE IS CLOSED

Create a telephone message for Western Medical Center to be used when the office is closed. The message should include instructions for an emergency, instructions if the caller needs medical advice, and instructions to leave a nonurgent message. If the caller wants a prescription refill, he or she should be referred to a different specific number to leave a detailed message.

_____

_____

_____

_____

_____

_____

D. OUTGOING CALLS

Explain the procedure for each of the following:

1. Calling a patient for an appointment reminder

_____

_____

2. Calling a pharmacy with a prescription refill

_____

_____

3. Placing a telephone call from a physician in the office to another physician

_____

_____

4. Arranging a conference call using an 800 number

_____

_____

Notes

PRACTICE FOR COMPETENCY

Procedure 39-1: Performing Telephone Screening. Practice the procedure with a classmate as if you are an MA at Western Medical Center. When you are the caller, choose one of the scenarios below without preparing your classmate ahead of time.

1. Pretend to be another physician calling to speak to Dr. Warner.
2. Pretend to be a patient calling for results of a laboratory or diagnostic test for your husband or mother.
3. Pretend to be a patient who wants directions to the office or who has questions about public transportation to the office.
4. Pretend to be a relative of Dr. Warner who wants to speak to the physician.
5. Pretend to be a patient experiencing severe chest pain or bleeding.

Procedure 39-2: Taking a Telephone Message. Practice the procedure with a classmate as if you are an MA at Western Medical Center. When you are the caller, choose one of the scenarios below without telling your classmate ahead of time. One person should choose the scenarios for Dr. Gomez, and the other should choose the scenarios for Dr. Warner. When you are the MA, complete a telephone message form making sure to ask for all necessary information.

1. You are calling from the Admitting Department at Memorial Hospital to get admitting orders from Dr. Warner for Diane Walters, DOB 1/22/1972. The patient is in the admitting department.
2. You are calling from the Nuclear Medicine Department at Memorial Hospital. You want to speak to Dr. Gomez about a test you just did on John Perkins. You are concerned about the test because the results seem to be very abnormal.
3. You are calling to find out the results of an upper GI x-ray that you had at Memorial Hospital yesterday. Your physician is Dr. Warner.
4. You are calling to find out the results of a complete blood count and chemistry screen that was done at the laboratory two days ago. Your physician is Dr. Gomez.
5. You cut your left hand with a knife, and you are a patient of Dr. Warner. It's a deep cut, about ¾ inch long. It doesn't bleed if you put pressure on it, but it does start to bleed again if you take the gauze square off. You want to know if you should come to the office or go to the emergency room.
6. A neighbor's child told you she saw your 3-year-old daughter eat several berries from a plant in the yard. The child does not seem ill, but you want to ask her doctor, Dr. Gomez, what to do. Should you bring her to the office or take her to the emergency room? Can the doctor call you back?

Procedure 39-3: Taking Requests for Medication or Prescription Refills. Practice this procedure with a classmate. Use information from the following simulated prescription labels to call for prescription refills. If the medication is an antibiotic or analgesic, ask for symptoms that require the refill. Document in the medical record.

Furosemide 20 mg Tab
Generic equivalent for: Lasix
Take 1 Tablet Daily
Rx: 9822122   Call: (490) 555-2211
                        West Street Pharmacy
	Indomethacin 25 mg Cap
	Take 1-2 capsules with food up to
	three times daily for moderate to severe pain
	Rx: 9332211 Call (490) 555-6155
	                        Best Pharmacy

Tetracycline 250 mg Cap
Take 1 Capsule Twice Daily
Rx: 9032811   Call (490) 555-8719
                        Twelve Oaks Pharmacy
	Lipitor 20 mg Tab
	Take 1 Tablet Every Day
	Rx: 9211554 Call (490) 555-1981
	                        Wide River Pharmacy

Crestor 10 mg Tab
Take 1 Tablet by Mouth Every Day
Rx: 228112   Call (490) 555-6155
                        Best Pharmacy
	Atenolol 50 mg Tab
	Take 1 Tablet by Mouth Daily
	Rx: 4483112 Call (490) 555-2211
	                        West Street Pharmacy

MESSAGE FROM

For Dr.	Name of Caller	Ref. to pt.	Patient	Pt. Age	Pt. Temp.	Message Date	Message Time	Urgent
						/ /	AM PM	☐ Yes ☐ No

Message: Allergies

Respond to Phone #	Best Time to Call AM PM	Pharmacy Name / #	Patient's Chart Attached ☐ Yes ☐ No	Patient's chart #	Initials

DOCTOR - STAFF RESPONSE

Doctor's / Staff Orders / Follow-up Action

	Call Back ☐ Yes ☐ No	Chart. Mes. ☐ Yes ☐ No	Follow-up Date / /	Follow-up Completed-Date/Time / / AM PM	Response By:

Product # 78-9156-Pkg, #78-9157-Pads, Bibbero Systems, Inc., Petaluma, CA. To order, call toll free 800-BIBBERO (800 242-2376) OR FAX 800-242-9330.

MESSAGE FROM

For Dr.	Name of Caller	Ref. to pt.	Patient	Pt. Age	Pt. Temp.	Message Date	Message Time	Urgent
						/ /	AM PM	☐ Yes ☐ No

Message: Allergies

Respond to Phone #	Best Time to Call AM PM	Pharmacy Name / #	Patient's Chart Attached ☐ Yes ☐ No	Patient's chart #	Initials

DOCTOR - STAFF RESPONSE

Doctor's / Staff Orders / Follow-up Action

	Call Back ☐ Yes ☐ No	Chart. Mes. ☐ Yes ☐ No	Follow-up Date / /	Follow-up Completed-Date/Time / / AM PM	Response By:

Product # 78-9156-Pkg, #78-9157-Pads, Bibbero Systems, Inc., Petaluma, CA. To order, call toll free 800-BIBBERO (800 242-2376) OR FAX 800-242-9330.

MESSAGE FROM

For Dr.	Name of Caller	Ref. to pt.	Patient	Pt. Age	Pt. Temp.	Message Date	Message Time	Urgent
						/ /	AM PM	☐ Yes ☐ No

Message: Allergies

Respond to Phone #	Best Time to Call AM PM	Pharmacy Name / #	Patient's Chart Attached ☐ Yes ☐ No	Patient's chart #	Initials

DOCTOR - STAFF RESPONSE

Doctor's / Staff Orders / Follow-up Action

	Call Back ☐ Yes ☐ No	Chart. Mes. ☐ Yes ☐ No	Follow-up Date / /	Follow-up Completed-Date/Time / / AM PM	Response By:

Product # 78-9156-Pkg, #78-9157-Pads, Bibbero Systems, Inc., Petaluma, CA. To order, call toll free 800-BIBBERO (800 242-2376) OR FAX 800-242-9330.

(Courtesy Bibbero Systems, Inc., Petaluma, Calif, [800] 242-2376; Fax [800] 242-9330; www.bibbero.com.)

MESSAGE FROM

For Dr.	Name of Caller	Ref. to pt.	Patient	Pt. Age	Pt. Temp.	Message Date / /	Message Time AM PM	Urgent ❏ Yes ❏ No

Message: _____   Allergies _____

Respond to Phone #	Best Time to Call AM PM	Pharmacy Name / #	Patient's Chart Attached ❏ Yes ❏ No	Patient's chart #	Initials

DOCTOR - STAFF RESPONSE

Doctor's / Staff Orders / Follow-up Action

Call Back ❏ Yes ❏ No	Chart. Mes. ❏ Yes ❏ No	Follow-up Date / /	Follow-up Completed-Date/Time / /	AM PM	Response By:

Product # 78-9156-Pkg, #78-9157-Pads, Bibbero Systems, Inc., Petaluma, CA. To order, call toll free 800-BIBBERO (800 242-2376) OR FAX 800-242-9330.

MESSAGE FROM

For Dr.	Name of Caller	Ref. to pt.	Patient	Pt. Age	Pt. Temp.	Message Date / /	Message Time AM PM	Urgent ❏ Yes ❏ No

Message: _____   Allergies _____

Respond to Phone #	Best Time to Call AM PM	Pharmacy Name / #	Patient's Chart Attached ❏ Yes ❏ No	Patient's chart #	Initials

DOCTOR - STAFF RESPONSE

Doctor's / Staff Orders / Follow-up Action

Call Back ❏ Yes ❏ No	Chart. Mes. ❏ Yes ❏ No	Follow-up Date / /	Follow-up Completed-Date/Time / /	AM PM	Response By:

Product # 78-9156-Pkg, #78-9157-Pads, Bibbero Systems, Inc., Petaluma, CA. To order, call toll free 800-BIBBERO (800 242-2376) OR FAX 800-242-9330.

MESSAGE FROM

For Dr.	Name of Caller	Ref. to pt.	Patient	Pt. Age	Pt. Temp.	Message Date / /	Message Time AM PM	Urgent ❏ Yes ❏ No

Message: _____   Allergies _____

Respond to Phone #	Best Time to Call AM PM	Pharmacy Name / #	Patient's Chart Attached ❏ Yes ❏ No	Patient's chart #	Initials

DOCTOR - STAFF RESPONSE

Doctor's / Staff Orders / Follow-up Action

Call Back ❏ Yes ❏ No	Chart. Mes. ❏ Yes ❏ No	Follow-up Date / /	Follow-up Completed-Date/Time / /	AM PM	Response By:

Product # 78-9156-Pkg, #78-9157-Pads, Bibbero Systems, Inc., Petaluma, CA. To order, call toll free 800-BIBBERO (800 242-2376) OR FAX 800-242-9330.

(Courtesy Bibbero Systems, Inc., Petaluma, Calif, [800] 242-2376; Fax [800] 242-9330; www.bibbero.com.)

Record medication refills or prescriptions in the medical record below.

Chart	
Date	

Procedure 39-4: Telephoning a Patient for Follow-Up. Practice the procedure with a classmate as if you are an MA at Western Medical Center. When you are the caller, choose one of the scenarios below without telling your classmate ahead of time. One person should choose the scenarios for Dr. Gomez, and the other should choose the scenarios for Dr. Warner.

1. Dr. Warner has asked you to call the patient above who had an upper GI to schedule an appointment to discuss the test results. Give the patient an appointment this week.
2. Dr. Gomez has asked you to call the patient who had a complete blood count and chemistry screen above and instruct the patient to repeat the blood tests in a week. The patient should also make an appointment with Dr. Gomez next week.
3. Dr. Warner has asked you to call the patient who had a knife cut and instruct her to come to the office to be seen. Ask how long it will take her to get to the office, and give her that appointment time.
4. Dr. Gomez has asked you to call the patient whose child was seen eating berries. Ask the mother to get a sample of the plant leaves and berries if possible and call Poison Control. Give her the telephone number of the local Poison Control center.
5. Dr. Warner has asked you to call a patient and tell her that her throat culture is positive for strep, and that he has prescribed an antibiotic. Instruct the patient to pick up the medication at her usual pharmacy.
6. Dr. Gomez has asked you to call a patient and tell him that he is prescribing a new medication for his cholesterol based on his recent blood test. The patient should pick up the medication at the pharmacy and make an appointment to follow up after 3 months.

EVALUATION OF COMPETENCY

Procedure 39-1: Performing Telephone Screening

Name: _____   Date: _____

Evaluated By: _____   Score: _____

Performance Objective

Outcome:	Screen telephone calls.
Conditions:	Given the following: telephone, message pad, pen or pencil, appointment book or computer, and clock or watch.
Standards:	Time: 10 minutes. Student completed procedure in ____ minutes.
	Accuracy: Satisfactory score in the Performance Evaluation Checklist.

Performance Evaluation Checklist

Trial 1	Trial 2	Point Value	*Performance Standards*
		•	Answered the telephone within the first three rings.
		•	Identified the medical office and gave name.
		•	Listened as the caller identified the reason for the call.
		•	Decided promptly if it was a call that should be transferred.
		•	Asked for the caller's name if not given by the caller.
		•	Took a message if appropriate (see Procedure 39-2: Taking a Telephone Message).
		•	If necessary to transfer the call, placed the caller on hold.
		•	Told the person to whom the call would be transferred the caller's name and extension (if necessary).
		•	Asked questions to assess any problem requiring immediate care.
		•	Transferred an urgent call to a physician or licensed professional if possible or followed office guidelines.
		•	Instructed a caller whose health was at risk to call 911.
		•	Monitored calls on hold and returned to a caller on hold within 30-45 seconds if a transferred call was not picked up.
		•	Asked a caller for permission before placing on hold to take a new call.
		•	Gave a second caller the option to be placed on hold or have the call returned before returning to a previous call.
		•	Repeated important information before ending a call.
		•	Ended the call politely.
		✲	Completed the procedure within 10 minutes.
			TOTALS

Evaluation of Student Performance

EVALUATION CRITERIA			COMMENTS
Symbol	Category	Point Value	
✳	Critical Step	16 points	
●	Essential Step	6 points	
▷	Theory Question	2 points	

Score calculation: 100 points

−_____ points missed

_____ Score

Satisfactory score: 85 or above

CAAHEP Competencies Achieved:

Psychomotor (Skills)
☑ IV. 7. Demonstrate telephone techniques.

Affective (Behavior)
☑ IV. 2. Apply active listening skills.
☑ IV. 7. Demonstrate recognition of the patient's level of understanding in communication.

ABHES Competencies Achieved:

☑ 8. cc. Communicate on the recipient's level of comprehension.
☑ 8. ee. Use proper telephone techniques.

EVALUATION OF COMPETENCY

Procedure 39-2: Taking a Telephone Message

Name: _____   Date: _____

Evaluated By: _____   Score: _____

Performance Objective

Outcome:	Take a telephone message.
Conditions:	Given the following: telephone, message pad, pen or pencil, and clock or watch.
Standards:	Time: 5 minutes. Student completed procedure in ____ minutes.
	Accuracy: Satisfactory score in the Performance Evaluation Checklist.

Performance Evaluation Checklist

Trial 1	Trial 2	Point Value	*Performance Standards*
		•	Determined that the person being called was not available.
		•	Offered to take a message.
		•	Gave the caller a reason why the person could not take the call.
		•	Filled in complete information legibly on the telephone message pad.
		•	Wrote down the name of the caller.
		•	Wrote down the business affiliation of the caller if appropriate.
		•	Wrote down the date and time of the call.
		•	Wrote down the telephone number of the caller including area code.
		•	Wrote down the reason for the call and information the caller included in the message.
		•	Initialed the message form.
		•	Left any response section blank for the intended recipient to complete.
		•	Verified information.
		•	Gave caller a time when the call might be returned or told caller that the message would be given to the intended recipient.
		•	Ended the call politely.
		•	Clipped a message related to a patient to the patient's medical record.
		•	Placed the message where the intended recipient would expect to find it.
		★	Completed the procedure within 5 minutes.
			TOTALS

Evaluation of Student Performance

EVALUATION CRITERIA			COMMENTS
Symbol	Category	Point Value	
✳	Critical Step	16 points	
●	Essential Step	6 points	
▷	Theory Question	2 points	

Score calculation: 100 points

     − _____ points missed

     _____ Score

Satisfactory score: 85 or above

CAAHEP Competencies Achieved:

Psychomotor (Skills)
☑ IV. 7. Demonstrate telephone techniques.

Affective (Behavior)
☑ IV. 2. Apply active listening skills.
☑ IV. 7. Demonstrate recognition of the patient's level of understanding in communication.

ABHES Competencies Achieved:

☑ 8. cc. Communicate on the recipient's level of comprehension.
☑ 8. ee. Use proper telephone techniques.

EVALUATION OF COMPETENCY

Procedure 39-3: Taking Requests for Medication or Prescription Refills

Name: _____   Date: _____

Evaluated By: _____   Score: _____

Performance Objective

Outcome:	Take a message requesting medication or a prescription refill.
Conditions:	Given the following: Telephone, message pad, pen or pencil, medical record, and clock or watch.
Standards:	Time: 5 minutes. Student completed procedure in _____ minutes.
	Accuracy: Satisfactory score in the Performance Evaluation Checklist.

Performance Evaluation Checklist

Trial 1	Trial 2	Point Value	Performance Standards
		•	Identified the caller and telephone number.
		•	Identified if the caller was a patient or a pharmacy.
		•	Wrote complete information on the message pad legibly.
		•	Included the name of the medication, dose, and number of times taken daily.
		•	Included the patient's name and telephone number (if the patient was the caller).
		•	Included pharmacy name and telephone number.
		•	If the caller was the pharmacy, gave a time when the physician would be likely to approve the refill.
		•	Ended the call politely.
		•	Clipped the message to the patient's medical record.
		•	Placed the message for review by the physician.
		•	If the physician was available to take the call, pulled the patient medical record before transferring it.
		•	If instructed by the physician, called the pharmacy with the new medication order.
		•	Read the information exactly as written by the physician.
		•	Documented the refill or prescription in the patient's medical record or filed the message as documentation.
		∗	Completed the procedure within 5 minutes.
			TOTALS

CHART	
Date	

Evaluation of Student Performance

EVALUATION CRITERIA			COMMENTS
Symbol	Category	Point Value	
*	Critical Step	16 points	
•	Essential Step	6 points	
▷	Theory Question	2 points	

Score calculation: 100 points
– _____ points missed
_____ Score
Satisfactory score: 85 or above

CAAHEP Competencies Achieved:

Psychomotor (Skills)
☑ IV. 7. Demonstrate telephone techniques.

Affective (Behavior)
☑ IV. 2. Apply active listening skills.
☑ IV. 7. Demonstrate recognition of the patient's level of understanding in communication.

ABHES Competencies Achieved:

☑ 8. cc. Communicate on the recipient's level of comprehension.
☑ 8. ee. Use proper telephone techniques.

EVALUATION OF COMPETENCY

Procedure 39-4: Telephoning a Patient for Follow-Up

Name: _____   Date: _____

Evaluated By: _____   Score: _____

Performance Objective

Outcome:	Telephone a patient for follow-up.
Conditions:	Given the following: telephone, scratch paper, pen or pencil, telephone book or instructions from the physician, and patient medical record as needed.
Standards:	Time: 5 minutes. Student completed procedure in _____ minutes.
	Accuracy: Satisfactory score in the Performance Evaluation Checklist.

Performance Evaluation Checklist

Trial 1	Trial 2	Point Value	Performance Standards
		•	Organized information that might be necessary during the telephone call.
		•	Wrote down telephone number including area code and country code as needed.
		•	Placed the telephone call.
		•	Asked for the patient or correct individual.
		•	Identified the medical practice and self.
		•	If call was not answered, left message on voice mail or answering machine including name of medical office, own name, and telephone number.
		•	When speaking to the patient, gave information as instructed by the physician.
		•	Did not give the patient other information than what was authorized by the physician.
		•	Repeated instructions if any were given.
		•	Ended call professionally and said "goodbye."
		✶	Completed the procedure within 5 minutes.
			TOTALS

Evaluation of Student Performance

EVALUATION CRITERIA			COMMENTS
Symbol	Category	Point Value	
✳	Critical Step	16 points	
●	Essential Step	6 points	
▷	Theory Question	2 points	

Score calculation: 100 points

  − _____ points missed

  _____ Score

Satisfactory score: 85 or above

CAAHEP Competencies Achieved:

Psychomotor (Skills)
☑ IV. 7. Demonstrate telephone techniques.

Affective (Behavior)
☑ IV. 2. Apply active listening skills.
☑ IV. 7. Demonstrate recognition of the patient's level of understanding in communication.

ABHES Competencies Achieved:

☑ 8. cc. Communicate on the recipient's level of comprehension.
☑ 8. ee. Use proper telephone techniques.

40

Scheduling Appointments

CHAPTER ASSIGNMENTS

√ After Completing	Date Due	Textbook Page(s)	TEXTBOOK ASSIGNMENTS	Possible Points	Points You Earned
		956-977	Read Chapter 40: Scheduling Appointments		
		964 975-976	Read Case Study 1 Case Study 1 questions	5	
		965 976	Read Case Study 2 Case Study 2 questions	5	
		970 976	Read Case Study 3 Case Study 3 questions	5	
			TOTAL POINTS		
√ After Completing	Date Due	Study Guide Page(s)	STUDY GUIDE ASSIGNMENTS (CTA: Critical Thinking Activity)	Possible Points	Points You Earned
		1017	Pretest	10	
		1018	Key Term Assessment	15	
		1019-1021	Evaluation of Learning questions	20	
		1021	CTA A: Computer-Generated Appointment Schedule	5	
		1021	CTA B: Methods of Scheduling	5	
		1022	CTA C: Appointment Matrix	5	
		1022	CTA D: Setting Priorities for Appointments	4	
		1023	CTA E: Scheduling Diagnostic Tests and Procedures	5	
			CD Activity: Chapter 40 Preparing and Maintaining the Appointment Book	10	
			CD Activity Chapter 40 Scheduling a New Patient	10	

√ After Completing	Date Due	Study Guide Page(s)	STUDY GUIDE ASSIGNMENTS (CTA: Critical Thinking Activity)	Possible Points	Points You Earned
			⊙ CD Activity: Chapter 40 Scheduling an Outpatient Diagnostic Test	10	
			⊙ CD Activity: Chapter 40 Scheduling an Inpatient Admission and an Inpatient Surgical Procedure	10	
			⊙ CD Activity: Chapter 40 Apply Your Knowledge questions (Record points earned)		
		1017	▤ Posttest	10	
			ADDITIONAL ASSIGNMENTS		
			TOTAL POINTS		

√ When Assigned by Your Instructor	Study Guide Page(s)	Practices Required	LABORATORY ASSIGNMENTS (Procedure Number and Name)	*Score
	1025	3	**Practice for Competency** 40-1: Setting Up the Appointment Matrix Textbook reference: p. 962	
	1037-1038		**Evaluation of Competency** 40-1: Setting Up the Appointment Matrix	*
	1029	3	**Practice for Competency** 40-2: Making an Appointment Textbook reference: p. 966	
	1039-1040		**Evaluation of Competency** 40-2: Making an Appointment	*
	1029	1	**Practice for Competency** 40-3: Managing the Appointment Schedule Textbook reference: pp. 968-969	
	1041-1042		**Evaluation of Competency** 40-3: Managing the Appointment Schedule	*
	1031	1	**Practice for Competency** 40-4: Completing a Referral Form for Managed Care Textbook reference: pp. 972-973	
	1043-1044		**Evaluation of Competency** 40-4: Completing a Referral Form for Managed Care	*
	1033	1	**Practice for Competency** 40-5: Scheduling Inpatient or Outpatient Diagnostic Tests or Procedures Textbook reference: pp. 973-974	
	1045-1046		**Evaluation of Competency** 40-5: Scheduling Inpatient or Outpatient Diagnostic Tests or Procedures	*
	1035	1	**Practice for Competency** 40-6: Scheduling Inpatient or Outpatient Admissions Textbook reference: pp. 974-975	
	1047-1048		**Evaluation of Competency** 40-6: Scheduling Inpatient or Outpatient Admissions	*
			ADDITIONAL ASSIGNMENTS	

Notes

Name _____   Date _____

PRETEST

True or False

_____ 1. For legal purposes, a daily schedule is usually the official record of appointments.

_____ 2. Corrections or changes to the official daily schedule are usually made in pencil.

_____ 3. Most medical offices use some type of time-specified appointment system.

_____ 4. In the stream method of appointment scheduling, each patient is given a different appointment time.

_____ 5. An example of clustering patient appointments is making appointments for new patients.

_____ 6. In the appointment matrix, times when physicians are available to see patients are blocked.

_____ 7. Demographic data for new patients are usually obtained when scheduling the first appointment.

_____ 8. Many medical offices call patients a few days before an appointment as a reminder.

_____ 9. The physician can usually admit a patient to the hospital without insurance preauthorization.

_____ 10. Patients usually call the hospital to schedule their own surgery.

POSTTEST

True or False

_____ 1. A written appointment book must be kept to provide a legal record of appointments.

_____ 2. If a patient fails to call or keep an appointment, the appointment is crossed out in red on the official daily schedule.

_____ 3. In wave scheduling, several patients are given the same appointment time.

_____ 4. The method of scheduling appointments with the least waiting time for patients is open hours.

_____ 5. *Categorization* refers to the practice of scheduling patients with similar problems back to back.

_____ 6. Most medical offices set up the appointment matrix for only the next 2-3 months.

_____ 7. If a patient makes an appointment while in the office, he or she should be given a written appointment reminder card.

_____ 8. The primary care physician must always obtain insurance preauthorization before providing a referral for a patient.

_____ 9. If a medical assistant schedules a diagnostic test for a patient, he or she should also provide any written instructions about preparation for the test.

_____ 10. A patient must almost always be scheduled to have an ECG and blood work before he or she can have inpatient or outpatient surgery.

KEY TERM ASSESSMENT

Directions: Match each medical term with its definition.

_____ 1. Blocked

_____ 2. Clustering

_____ 3. Double booking

_____ 4. Established patient

_____ 5. Hospice

_____ 6. Matrix

_____ 7. Modified wave scheduling

_____ 8. New patient

_____ 9. No-show

_____ 10. Preadmission testing (PAT)

_____ 11. Preauthorization

_____ 12. Referral

_____ 13. Stream scheduling (single booking)

_____ 14. Triage

_____ 15. Wave scheduling

A. Grouping patients with similar problems or conditions on certain days or at certain times of the day

B. The process of sorting patients according to their need for care

C. Times that are crossed out of the appointment schedule (not available for appointments)

D. A patient who has never been seen by the physician or for billing purposes has not been seen within the past three years

E. A scheduling method that uses both fixed appointments and more than one patient scheduled for the same appointment time

F. In managed care, written authorization by the primary care physician for a patient to receive additional services

G. Booking two people into a single time slot

H. Scheduling three or four patients every half hour, who are seen in the order in which they arrive

I. A patient who has been seen by one of the physicians in the practice within the past three years

J. A form or arrangement for information, such as appointments

K. An appointment scheduling method where each patient is given a specific appointment time

L. Diagnostic tests that are performed before the patient is admitted for surgery or a diagnostic procedure

M. A person who does not appear for his or her appointment

N. A program or facility that provides care to terminally ill patients

O. Permission from a patient's insurance company for a test, procedure, or surgery

EVALUATION OF LEARNING

Directions: Fill in each blank with the correct answer.

1. Identify seven guidelines to follow when making appointments.

   _____

   _____

   _____

   _____

   _____

2. Identify two methods of scheduling appointments.

   _____

   _____

3. Why must the daily appointment sheet record any changes in the schedule and/or patients who miss appointments in ink? How is it handled to preserve patient confidentiality?

   _____

   _____

   _____

4. Identify and describe each of the following types of appointment scheduling.

   a. Time-specified (stream) scheduling (single booking)

   _____

   b. Wave scheduling

   _____

   c. Modified wave scheduling

   _____

   d. Double booking

   _____

   e. Open booking

   _____

   f. Categorization (clustering)

   _____

5. What factors must be considered when setting up the appointment matrix?

   _____

   _____

   _____

6. How are new patients treated differently from established patients when making appointments?

   _____

   _____

7. Identify eight types of medical problems for which patients would usually be given a same-day appointment.

_____

_____

_____

_____

8. Identify four categories of medical problems that are usually referred to an emergency department.

_____

_____

_____

9. How should the medical assistant (MA) handle a patient who comes to the office without an appointment?

_____

_____

10. What should an MA do if an appointment needs to be changed?

_____

_____

11. What should the MA do if a patient who has an appointment does not keep the appointment or call to cancel the appointment?

_____

_____

_____

12. Identify three common methods to help patients remember appointments.

_____

_____

_____

13. What is the difference between a referral and a preauthorization?

_____

_____

14. Why is it usually necessary to obtain preauthorization before surgery, certain diagnostic tests, and some kinds of therapy?

_____

_____

15. What are three common reasons for a referral?

_____

_____

16. How does an MA schedule a diagnostic test at a facility like the hospital x-ray department?

_____

_____

_____

17. What should the MA document in the patient's medical record after scheduling a diagnostic test for the patient?

_____

_____

18. How should the MA arrange for a patient to be admitted to the hospital?

_____

_____

_____

_____

19. Where will preadmission testing be performed before surgery?

_____

_____

20. If a patient will have inpatient surgery, how should the MA schedule it?

_____

_____

CRITICAL THINKING ACTIVITIES

A. COMPUTER-GENERATED APPOINTMENT SCHEDULE
Refer to the computer-generated appointment schedule in your textbook, and answer the following questions.

1. How many minutes is an appointment of Dr. Gomez for a well-child visit? _____

2. How many minutes is an appointment of Dr. Gomez for a physical examination? _____

3. What times are blocked in the schedule? _____

4. When is the first open appointment with Dr. Gomez? _____

5. What time could be offered to a new patient who needs a physical examination in this schedule?

_____

B. METHODS OF SCHEDULING
Refer to the comparison of single booking, wave scheduling, and modified wave scheduling (Figure 40-3) in your textbook, and answer the following questions.

1. In which method are all patients in the same hour given the same appointment time? _____

2. In which method is each patient given a different appointment time? _____

3. Which method makes it most likely that there will always be a patient waiting even if some patients are delayed or cancel? _____

4. Which method(s) make it easier to work patients in while other patients undress or have diagnostic tests?

_____

5. Which method decreases waiting time for the patient? _____

C. APPOINTMENT MATRIX
Refer to the manual and computerized appointment matrix (Figure 40-4) in your textbook, and answer the following questions.

1. What is the first available time for patients to have appointments with Dr. Gomez after lunch

   (computer schedule)? _____

2. What is the advantage of using color to create the matrix with a computer system? _____

   _____

3. How much time has been allowed for lunch (appointment book)? _____

4. If appointments are at least 29 minutes long, what is the last available time for an appointment in Dr. Hughes'

   schedule (appointment book)? _____

5. From the matrix, what do you assume about scheduling for the satellite clinic? _____

   _____

D. SETTING PRIORITIES FOR APPOINTMENTS
Consider the following four patients who call the office on a day where there are no open appointments. Which patients should be worked into the schedule today, and which patients can be given appointments tomorrow? Give a reason for your answer.

1. Edna Willis, a 64-year-old woman, reports that she has a fever of 100°F and she also has had nausea and diarrhea during the previous night.

   _____

   _____

2. Daniel Jordan, a 32-year-old man, reports that he fell at work that morning, injuring his right arm and shoulder. He can move his right arm and shoulder, but the pain is severe and seems to be becoming worse.

   _____

   _____

3. Mary Anderson, a patient of Dr. Hughes, calls about her father, Lawrence Sheehan, a 72-year-old man who is visiting from out of town. Mr. Sheehan has had angina pectoris for several years, but for the past 2 days he has been having more frequent and more severe episodes of chest pain. He has had one episode that morning that was relieved by rest and his usual medication.

   _____

   _____

4. Linda Jones, a 25-year-old woman, calls complaining of generally feeling tired and without energy for the past 3 weeks. She is concerned because she expected to start feeling better before this.

   _____

   _____

E. SCHEDULING DIAGNOSTIC TESTS AND PROCEDURES

Using yourself as a patient, answer the following questions that you might be asked when calling to schedule a diagnostic test or procedure:

1. What is the patient's name? _____

2. What is the patient's date of birth? _____

3. What is the patient's address and telephone number? _____

4. What type of insurance does the patient have? _____

    Insurance ID number? _____

5. Who is the patient's employer? _____

Notes

PRACTICE FOR COMPETENCY

Procedure 40-1: Setting Up the Appointment Matrix. Using one of the blank appointment matrix forms, set up the appointment matrix for Blackburn Primary Care Associates.

1. Monday, October 12, 20XX: Dr. Lawler and Dr. Hughes are scheduled for hospital rounds early in the morning and will begin appointments at 9:00 AM. They will take their lunch break at 12:00 noon. Their first afternoon appointment is at 1:00 PM. Dr. Lawler has a regular Monday meeting from 4:00 PM to 5:00 PM at the hospital. He will not return to the office. Dr. Lopez is scheduled at the satellite office in the morning. His first scheduled appointment will be at 10:30 AM. He will take lunch at 12:30 PM and begin seeing patients again at 1:00 PM. The appointment times from 3:20 PM through 3:30 PM are blocked out for Dr. Hughes and Dr. Lopez as catch-up time.

2. Wednesday, October 14, 20XX: Dr. Lawler, Dr. Hughes, and Dr. Lopez are scheduled for hospital rounds early in the morning and will begin appointments at 9:00 AM. Dr. Lawler and Dr. Lopez will take their lunch break at 12:00 noon and will see patients in the afternoon from 1:00 PM to 3:00 PM. Dr. Hughes will leave the office at 12:30 PM to attend a conference that will last all afternoon.

3. Friday, October 16, 20XX: Dr. Lawler, Dr. Hughes, and Dr. Lopez are scheduled for hospital rounds early in the morning and will begin appointments at 9:00 AM. They will take their lunch break at 12:00 noon. They will begin afternoon appointments at 1:00 PM. The appointment times from 2:00 PM to 2:10 PM should be blocked as catch-up time. No appointments should be scheduled after 4:30 PM.

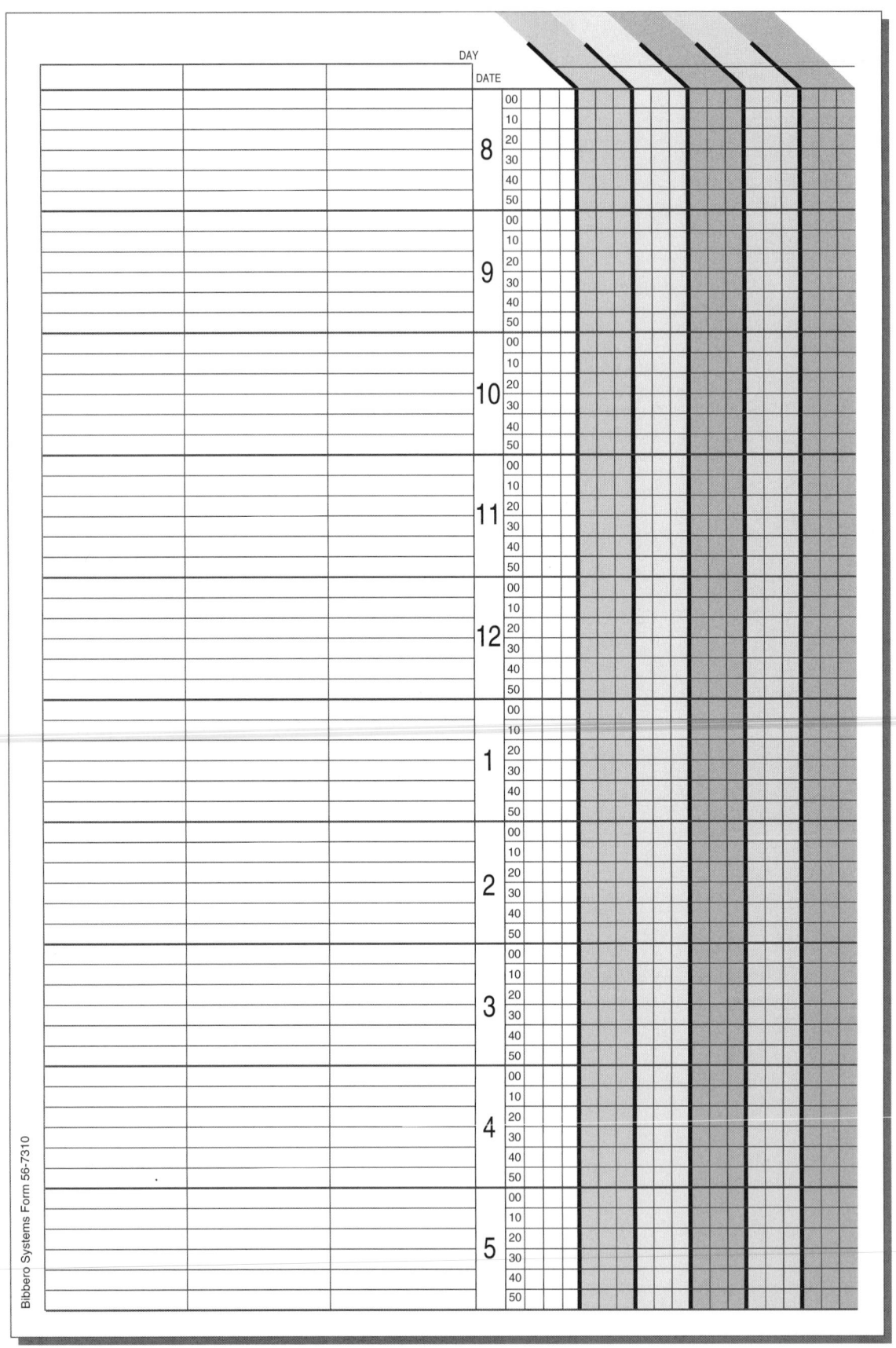

Bibbero Systems Form 56-7310

(Courtesy Bibbero Systems, Inc., Petaluma, Calif, [800] 242-2376; Fax [800] 242-9330; www.bibbero.com.)

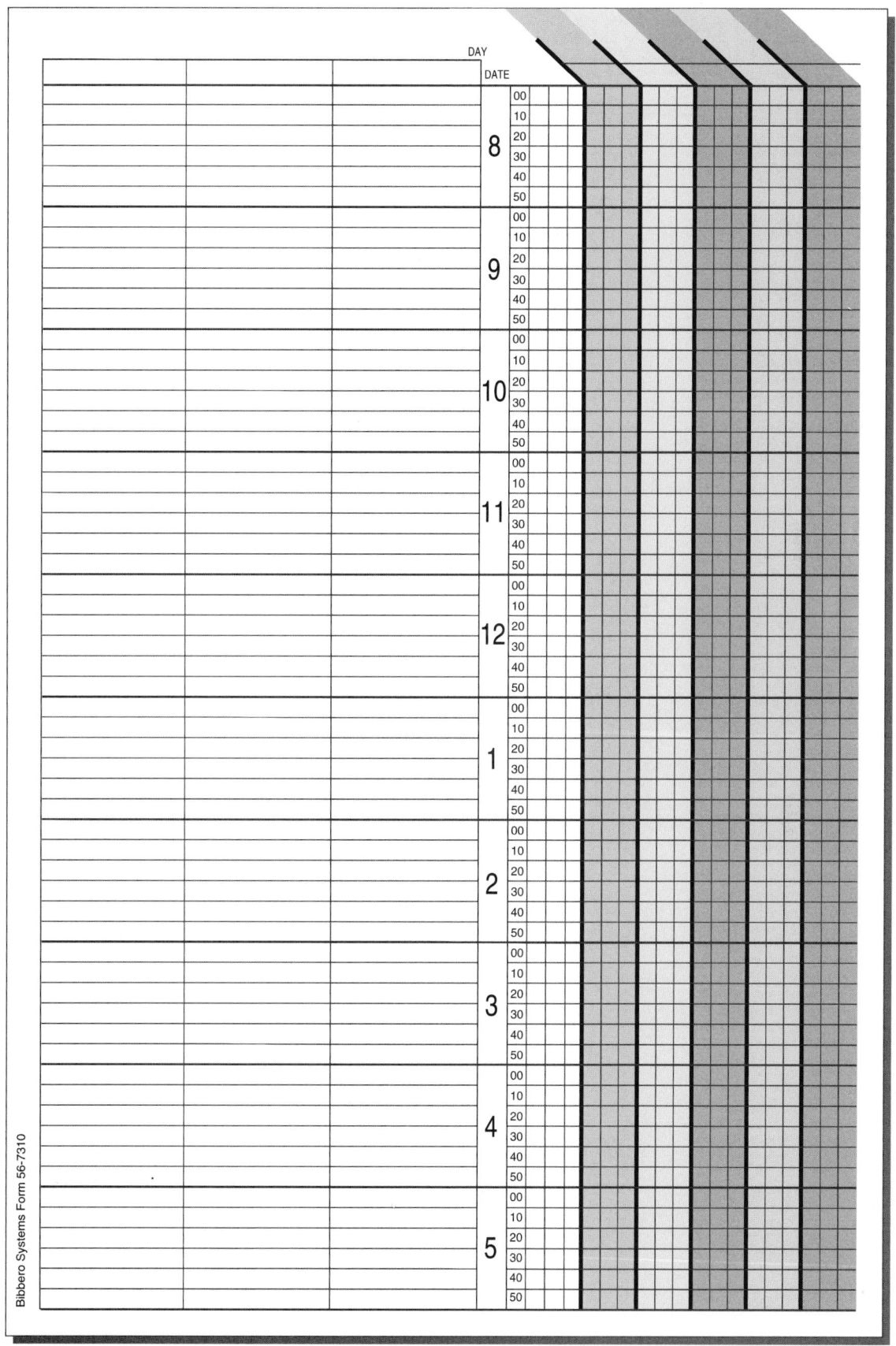

(Courtesy Bibbero Systems, Inc., Petaluma, Calif, [800] 242-2376; Fax [800] 242-9330; www.bibbero.com.)

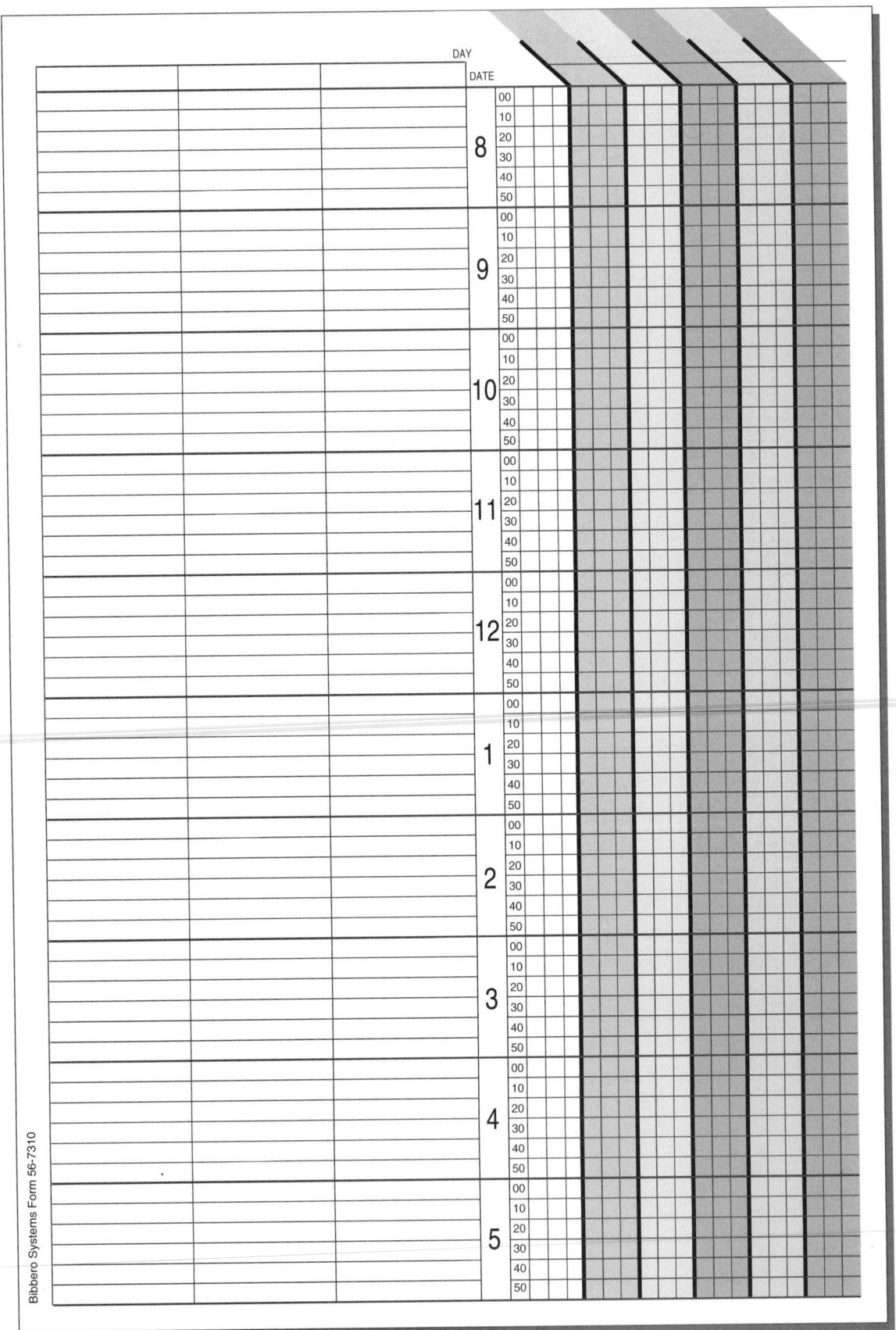

Bibbero Systems Form 56-7310

(Courtesy Bibbero Systems, Inc., Petaluma, Calif, [800] 242-2376; Fax [800] 242-9330; www.bibbero.com.)

Procedure 40-2: Making an Appointment. Schedule appointments for the following patients using the first appointment matrix you created for Procedure 40-1. Assume that established patients will be given 20-minute appointments and new patients will be given 30-minute appointments (except for Dr. Lawler, whose new patients are seen for 40 minutes). Use the abbreviation *PE* for examinations and the abbreviation *re* √ for patients who are returning for follow-up. Include the patient's day telephone number. All telephone numbers are in area code (555). Make appointments back to back to avoid 10-minute gaps in the schedule. Make appointments in the order that patients call.

1. June St. Cyr, an established patient, calls for an appointment with Dr. Hughes. She is working and wants to come as late as possible. Her telephone number is 648-3333.

2. William Reardon makes an appointment for follow-up. He is retired, and his telephone number is 648-9292. He is to see Dr. Lopez as early in the day as possible.

3. Diana Starr telephones for an appointment for an examination. She is a new patient who has recently moved to the area. Her home telephone has not yet been connected, but her work telephone number is 731-1998. She asks to see Dr. Hughes and requests a late afternoon appointment. She works until 5:00 PM.

4. Douglas Wright telephones for an appointment because he has been having dizziness and feeling weak. He has never had an appointment with Dr. Lawler before, but a friend told him that Dr. Lawler is very experienced. He would prefer to come before lunch or as early in the day as possible. His telephone number is 731-8282.

5. Angela Newton needs an appointment for follow-up with Dr. Lopez. She is in high school and cannot arrive before 3:00. Her home telephone number is 452-2001.

Procedure 40-3: Managing the Appointment Schedule. Use the computer-generated appointment schedule below to manage appointments for May 30, 20XX. Note that the appointment schedule is full because stars denote times that are booked for the patient whose name appears above. New patients with physical examinations are scheduled for 40 minutes, physical examinations for established patients are 30 minutes, and other visits for established patients are scheduled for 20 minutes. Assume that any patient will need 30 minutes to get to the office. Be sure to mark any cancellations who do not reschedule or any no-shows in red. If a patient cancels, you can give his or her appointment to another patient. Double book any patient with an urgent problem who must be seen today.

1. Robert Ricigliano calls at 8:00 AM to cancel his appointment at 9:00 AM. He doesn't want to reschedule at this time.

2. Douglas Wright telephones at 8:15 AM because he has been running a fever of 102°F since yesterday and has been off work. He would like to come as early as possible. His home telephone number is 648-9010. He is a patient of Dr. Warner.

3. Lucille Morena calls at 9:00 AM and to reschedule her appointment for next week. She is a new patient.

4. Peter Williams calls at 9:30 AM. He hurt his finger after slamming it in his car door this morning. He has gone to work, but it is hurting more now. It has swollen up, and he can't bend it. He would like to come in to see Dr. Gomez. His work telephone number is 932-6554.

5. Maria Santos calls at 10:00 AM to say that she has car trouble and won't be able to arrive by 11:00 AM. She asks there is any way she could come after lunch.

Western Medical Center

Richard Warner, MD
Schedule for May 30, 20XX

Time	Name	Reason	Home Phone	Work Phone
9:00 AM	ROBERT RICIGLIANO	Physical exam	(490) 459-2811	(490) 459-6217
9:10 AM	*			
9:20 AM	*			
9:30 AM	JUNE ST. JAMES	BP & ECG	(490) 459-5807	(490) 459-9222
9:40 AM	*			
9:50 AM	DARLA SISSLE	Influenza vaccine	(490) 220-1156	
10:00 AM	Catch-up			
10:10 AM	*			
10:20 AM	LLOYD RIDLON	Recheck	(490) 459-4242	(490) 459-0419
10:30 AM	ESTELLE JORDAN	New patient	(490) 459-8249	(490) 459-1062
10:40 AM	*			
10:50 AM	*			
11:00 AM	MARIA SANTOS	Physical exam	(490) 459-0022	
11:10 AM	*			
11:20 AM	THOMAS MAXWELL	Recheck	(490) 459-4123	(490) 459-9201
11:30 AM	*			
11:40 AM	ROBIN SOTO	Well baby	(490) 459-1349	
11:50 AM	*			
12:00 PM	LUNCH			
12:10 PM	*			
12:20 PM	*			
12:30 PM	*			
12:40 PM	*			
12:50 PM	*			
1:00 PM	LUCILLE MORENA	Chem screen	(490) 459-6677	(490) 459-1566
1:10 PM	*			
1:20 PM	*			
1:30 PM	*			

Record the information about the cancelled appointment for Robert Ricigliano in the chart provided.

CHART	
Date	

Procedure 40-4: Completing a Referral Form for Managed Care. Complete the following referral form for Dr. Gomez to sign. The patient's name is Agnes Mitchell. She is being referred by Maria Gomez, MD. 6000 Pine Circle, Western, OH 44770 to see Dr. Winston Gray, a cardiologist whose address is 662 North Central Street, Western, OH 44770. Her insurance number is 2452687 and the suffix is -02. Her date of birth is 6/13/1945. She is being referred for a consultative opinion and necessary diagnostic studies (not to exceed three visits). Her diagnosis is cardiac arrhythmia and dyspnea on exertion.

Health Plan
Referral Form

REFERRAL NUMBER: A06

WRITTEN REFERRALS ARE REQUIRED FOR ALL SERVICES, EXCEPT FOR ROUTINE YEARLY EYE EXAMS, ORAL SURGERY, LAB, DIAGNOSTIC & RADIOLOGICAL SERVICES.

(1) Patient Name: _____

Date of
(2) Referral: _____ / _____ / _____

(3) Patient Identification Number: _____ (4) [SUFFIX # REQUIRED]

(5) Date of Birth: _____ / _____ / _____

(6) Referred From: _____
NAME OF PERSONAL CARE PHYSICIAN   Provider ID #

(7) I.P.A. No. [ ][ ]

(8) _____
ADDRESS OF PERSONAL CARE PHYSICIAN

Referred To: _____
NAME OFSPECIALTY CARE PHYSICIAN/PROVIDER/EMERGENCY   Provider ID #

(10) _____
ADDRESS OF SPECIALTY CARE PHYSICIAN/PROVIDER/EMERGENCY

REFERRAL STATUS:
(CHECK ONE)

In I.P.A.
☐   ☐   ☐   ☐

REASON FOR REFERRAL (STATE DIAGNOSIS): _____

SERVICES REQUESTED (CHECK ONE)

REFERRAL VALID FOR TWELVE MONTHS FROM DATE OF REFERRAL.

☐ Consultative OPINION. (One (1) visit only) CONTACT PCP PRIOR TO INITIATING TREATMENT.

☐ SECOND SURGICAL OPINION ONLY (Surgery is not to be performed by this provider)

☐ Consultative OPINION and NECESSARY DIAGNOSTIC STUDIES. (Not to exceed three (3) visits)

☐ Consultative OPINION and NECESSARY DIAGNOSTIC STUDY AND TREATMENT. **Indicate number of visits** [ ]

☐ Mental Health EVALUATION: Circle one (1) or two (2) visits only. (FOR PCP USE ONLY)

☐ Substance Abuse Outpatient EVALUATION: Circle one (1) or two (2) visits only. (FOR PCP USE ONLY)

☐ Mental Health/Substance Abuse Treatment (PSYCHIATRIC REVIEWER USE ONLY) subsequent visits, indicate number [ ]

AUTHORIZATION FOR MENTAL HEALTH OR SUBSTANCE ABUSE OUTPATIENT SERVICES DOES NOT OVERRIDE BENEFIT MAXIMUMS.

☐ Therapies (type of therapy: _____). **Indicate number of visits** [ ] (PT not to exceed six (6) visits per referral)

☐ Obstetrical Treatment. Designate duration of care: _____

☐ Emergency Room Treatment. Date of service: _____ / _____ / _____
SEPARATE REFERRAL FORM REQUIRED FOR EACH EMERGENCY ROOM DATE OF SERVICE

Note: Only those services included in the Health Plan Description of Benefits will be covered. If you have any questions contact your Professional Relations Coordinator.

I have enclosed a clinical document summary, have performed the followingt diagnostic studies and arm supplying the information to assist you.

DIAGNOSTIC PROCEDURES	DATE OF SERVICE	RESULTS

INSTRUCTIONS

PCP:
- Complete Form
- Send Health Plan Copy and Specialist Copy to Specialist
- Retain PCP Copy for your file

SPECIALIST:
- For Referrals to another Specialist Consult W/ PCP
- Send Health Plan Copy to Appropriate Address (see above)

ER AUTHORIZATION
- Send Health Plan Copy to Appropriate Address (see above)
- Retain Copy for your file
- Be sure to notify

X _____
SIGNATURE OF PERSONAL CARE PHYSICIUAN

_____ / _____ / _____
AUTHORIZATION DATE

X _____
SIGNATURE OF PHYSICIUAN REVIEWER*

_____ / _____ / _____
AUTHORIZATION DATE

*ALL OUT OF PLAN REFERRALS REQUIRE PHYSICIAN REVIEWER SIGNATURE

(Courtesy Bibbero Systems, Inc., Petaluma, Calif, [800] 242-2376; Fax [800] 242-9330; www.bibbero.com.)

Procedure 40-5: Scheduling Inpatient or Outpatient Diagnostic Tests or Procedures. Working with a classmate, call the ultrasound department of Memorial Hospital. One student should schedule the diagnostic test, and the other student should ask the questions and record information. Use the New Patient Information sheets for patient information.

Student 1: Schedule the first available time for a CT scan of the head with contrast for Charles Latham. The patient has never had a procedure done at Memorial Hospital.

Diagnosis:	Severe frontal headaches for one month. No known allergies.
Preparation for this test:	No preparation
Questions to ask:	Allergy to iodine or shellfish; ask female if she is pregnant

Student 2: Schedule the first available time for a barium swallow (x-ray) for Darlene Jordan. The patient has never had a procedure done at Memorial Hospital.

Diagnosis:	Epigastric pain for two weeks. No known allergies.
Preparation for this test:	NPO after midnight
Questions to ask:	Ask female if she is pregnant

Record the information about the diagnostic test and instructions given to the patient below.

CHART	
Date	

Questions to ask when scheduling an x-ray or CT scan:

1. What is the test to be scheduled? _____
2. What date and time would the patient prefer? _____
3. What is the patient's name?   _____
4. What is the patient's birth date? _____
5. What is the patient's address? _____
6. What city and zip? _____
7. What is the patient's telephone number? _____
8. What is the physician's name? _____
9. What insurance does the patient have? _____
10. Who is the insured? _____
11. What is the group (policy) number? _____
12. What is the ID (subscriber) number? _____

13. What is the diagnosis? _____

14. If female, could the patient be pregnant? _____

15. Does the patient have any allergies to medication or iodine? _____

New Patient Information

(Please Print)   Physician: *Richard Warner, MD*
Home Phone: *(490) 555-3319*   Date: *9/14/2010*

PATIENT INFORMATION

Last Name _____*LATHAM*_____ First _____*CHARLES*_____ Initial _*R*_

Address _____*10971 CLARKWELL ROAD*_____

City _____*WESTERN*_____ State ___*OH*___ Zip __44770__

Single ___ Married _*X*_ Widowed ___ Separated ___ Divorced _____

Sex M _*X*_ F ___ Age _*49*_ Birth date _____*7/19/1961*_____

Employer _____*LATHAM PLUMBING*_____

Occupation _____*PLUMBER*_____

In an emergency, who should be notified?

___*ANNA LATHAM*___ (wife) _____ Phone _____*(490) 555-3319*_____

    Name   Relationship

PRIMARY INSURANCE

Name of insured _____*CHARLES LATHAM*_____ Responsible Party Yes _*X*_ No _____

Relation to Patient _*SELF*_ Birth date _*7/19/1961*_

Address (if different from patient)

_____ Phone_____

City _____ State _____ Zip _____

Insured employed by _____*LATHAM PLUMBING*_____

Occupation _____*PLUMBER*_____

Business Address _*10971 CLARKWELL ROAD, WESTERN, OH 44770*_

Business Phone ___*(490) 555-3320*___

Insurance Company _*STANDARD HEALTH INDEMNITY*_ ID # _*665514281*_

Policy (Group) # ___*544281*___

I the undersigned assign directly to Blackburn Primary Care Associates insurance benefits, if any, otherwise payable to me for services rendered. I understand that I am financially responsible for all charges whether or not paid by insurance. I hereby authorize the doctor to release all information necessary to secure the payment of benefits. I authorize the use of this signature on all insurance submissions.

*Charles Latham*   _*self*_   _*10/25/2010*_
Responsible party Signature   Relationship   Date

New Patient Information

(Please Print)
Home Phone: _(490) 555-4810_

Physician: _Richard Warner, MD_
Date: _9/14/2010_

PATIENT INFORMATION

Last Name _____ _JORDAN_ _____ First _____ _DARLENE_ _____ Initial _L_

Address _____ _617 HILLSIDE ROAD_ _____

City _____ _WESTERN_ _____ State ___ _OH_ ___ Zip ___ _44770_ ___

Single ___ Married _X_ Widowed ____ Separated ___ Divorced _____

Sex M _____ F _X_ Age _30_ Birth date ___ _4/19/1980_ ___

Employer _____ _BEST SUPERMARKET_ _____

Occupation _____ _CASHIER_ _____

In an emergency, who should be notified?

_____ _EDWARD JORDAN_ _____ (husband) _____ Phone _____ _(490) 555-4810_ _____

Name _____ Relationship

PRIMARY INSURANCE

Name of insured _____ _EDWARD JORDAN_ Responsible Party Yes _X_ No _____

Relation to Patient ___ _HUSBAND_ _____ Birth date ___ _2/24/1978_ ___

Address (if different from patient)

_____ Phone_____

City _____ State _____ Zip _____

Insured employed by _____ _MEYERS PHARMACY_ _____

Occupation _____ _PHARMACIST_ _____

Business Address ___ _428 MAIN STREET, WESTERN, OH 44770_ ___

Business Phone ___ _(490) 555-6192_ ___

Insurance Company _STANDARD HEALTH HMO_ ID # ___ _28621954_ ___

Policy (Group) # ___ _86190_ ___

I the undersigned assign directly to Blackburn Primary Care Associates insurance
benefits, if any, otherwise payable to me for services rendered. I understand that
I am financially responsible for all charges whether or not paid by insurance.
I hereby authorize the doctor to release all information necessary to secure the
payment of benefits. I authorize the use of this signature on all insurance
submissions.

___ _Darlene Jordan_ _____ _self_ _____ _9/14/2010_ ___

Responsible party Signature ____ Relationship _____ Date

Procedure 40-6: Scheduling an Inpatient Admission. Working with a classmate, call Memorial Hospital to schedule an admission for a patient.

Student 1: Schedule an admission for Charles Latham. The patient will be admitted this afternoon, and admission orders will be faxed from the office. His wife will bring him to the hospital. Use the patient information form in Procedure 40-5.

Diagnosis: Pneumococcal pneumonia.

Insurance precertification number: M 200068AC

Student 2: Schedule an admission for Darlene Jordan. The patient will be arriving at the hospital by ambulance from home. Admission orders will be faxed from the office. Use the patient information form in Procedure 40-5.

Diagnosis: Hematemesis; R/O acute peptic ulcer with hemorrhage.

Insurance precertification number: 0011582

Record the information about the hospital admission below.

CHART	
Date	

Questions to ask when the MA is calling for hospital admission (answer telephone as Memorial Hospital Admitting Department):

1. What is the patient's name and address? _____

    _____

    _____

2. What is the patient's birth date? _____

3. What is the patient's admission diagnosis? _____

4. What type of insurance does the patient have? _____

5. What is/are the patient's insurance number(s)? _____

6. What is the physician's name? _____

7. How is the patient being transported? _____

8. When will the patient be admitted? _____

9. How will the physician's orders be provided? _____

EVALUATION OF COMPETENCY

Procedure 40-1: Setting Up the Appointment Matrix

Name: _____   Date: _____

Evaluated By: _____   Score: _____

Performance Objective

Outcome:	Set up an appointment matrix.
Conditions:	Given the following: appointment book or computer scheduling program, physician schedule, pen, and office calendar.
Standards:	Time: 10 minutes. Student completed procedure in ____ minutes.
	Accuracy: Satisfactory score on the Performance Evaluation Checklist.

Performance Evaluation Checklist

Trial 1	Trial 2	Point Value	Performance Standards
		•	Blocked times when the office would not be open.
		•	Blocked times when each individual physician would NOT be available to see patients including lunch and hospital rounds.
		•	Blocked days or parts of days when individual physicians would be away from the office for vacation, conferences, or other scheduled events.
		•	For each physician, marked times scheduled for certain types of examinations or procedures.
		•	Blocked time for same-day appointments, catch-up time, and unexpected needs. If using an appointment book, used pencil so that these times could be changed as needed.
		*	Completed an accurate appointment matrix.
		*	Completed the procedure within 10 minutes.
		TOTALS	

Evaluation of Student Performance

EVALUATION CRITERIA			COMMENTS
Symbol	**Category**	**Point Value**	
*	Critical Step	16 points	
•	Essential Step	6 points	
▷	Theory Question	2 points	
Score calculation: 100 points			
−_____ points missed			
_____ Score			
Satisfactory score: 85 or above			

CAAHEP Competencies Achieved:

Psychomotor (Skills)
☑ V. 1. Manage appointment schedule, using established priorities.

Affective (Behavior)
☑ V. 2. Implement time management principles to maintain effective office function.

ABHES Competencies Achieved:

☑ 8. c. Schedule and manage appointments.

EVALUATION OF COMPETENCY

Procedure 40-2: Making an Appointment

Name: _____   Date: _____

Evaluated By: _____   Score: _____

Performance Objective

Outcome:	Make an appointment for a patient.
Conditions:	Given the following: appointment book or computer program, and pencil.
Standards:	Time: 5 minutes. Student completed procedure in _____ minutes.
	Accuracy: Satisfactory score on the Performance Evaluation Checklist.

Performance Evaluation Checklist

Trial 1	Trial 2	Point Value	Performance Standards
		●	Obtained physician name and scheduling preference from the patient.
		●	Found an open appointment of the correct length of time.
		●	Offered the patient a date and time for the appointment.
		●	Kept locating appointments until an acceptable date and time was found.
		●	Entered demographic data into computer for a new patient.
		●	Discussed cost of the visit with a new patient without insurance.
		●	Informed a new patient if a written referral form would be necessary.
		●	Recorded patient name, date of birth, reason for the visit, and daytime telephone number for an established patient or a new patient.
		●	Blocked out correct amount of time based on the reason for the visit. (Used pencil in a manual appointment book.)
		●	Repeated the information to the patient before ending the call.
		●	Offered a new patient directions to the office.
		✳	Completed the procedure within 5 minutes.
			TOTALS

Evaluation of Student Performance

EVALUATION CRITERIA			COMMENTS
Symbol	Category	Point Value	
✴	Critical Step	16 points	
●	Essential Step	6 points	
▷	Theory Question	2 points	

Score calculation: 100 points
      −_____ points missed
      _____ Score

Satisfactory score: 85 or above

CAAHEP Competencies Achieved:

Psychomotor (Skills)
☑ V. 1. Manage appointment schedule, using established priorities.

Affective (Behavior)
☑ V. 2. Implement time management principles to maintain effective office function.

ABHES Competencies Achieved:

☑ 8. c. Schedule and manage appointments.

✔ EVALUATION OF COMPETENCY

Procedure 40-3: Managing the Appointment Schedule

Name: _____   Date: _____

Evaluated By: _____   Score: _____

Performance Objective

Outcome:	Review the appointment schedule, cancel an appointment, change an appointment, indicate a missed appointment, and document cancellations and missed appointments.
Conditions:	Given the following: Appointment book or computer scheduling program, printed appointment schedule, and red pen.
Standards:	Time: 10 minutes. Student completed procedure in _____ minutes.
	Accuracy: Satisfactory score on the Performance Evaluation Checklist.

Performance Evaluation Checklist

Trial 1	Trial 2	Point Value	Performance Standards
		•	Using the appointment schedule, made sure all medical records and necessary paperwork were prepared.
		•	Checked patients in on the official schedule as they arrived.
		•	Canceled an appointment on the day it was scheduled by drawing a line through the appointment in red on the official schedule.
		•	Deleted appointment in computer scheduling program or erased in appointment book.
		•	Offered to make another appointment when a patient cancelled an appointment.
		•	If a patient declined to make another appointment after canceling, documented in the patient's medical record.
		•	If a patient wanted to reschedule, found a new appointment time.
		•	Entered the patient's name and contact information in the new appointment time.
		•	Repeated the new date and time to the patient if using the telephone or filled out an appointment card for a patient in the office.
		•	If the patient missed an appointment without canceling, draw a red line through the appointment on the daily schedule and labeled the appointment "No Show."
		•	Telephoned the patient to offer another appointment if office policy.
		•	Documented the missed appointment in the medical record with any information available.
		✱	Completed the procedure within 10 minutes.
			TOTALS

CHART	
Date	

Evaluation of Student Performance

EVALUATION CRITERIA			COMMENTS
Symbol	Category	Point Value	
*	Critical Step	16 points	
●	Essential Step	6 points	
▷	Theory Question	2 points	

Score calculation: 100 points

−_____ points missed

_____ Score

Satisfactory score: 85 or above

CAAHEP Competencies Achieved:

Psychomotor (Skills)
☑ V. 1. Manage appointment schedule, using established priorities.

Affective (Behavior)
☑ V. 2. Implement time management principles to maintain effective office function.

ABHES Competencies Achieved:

☑ 8. c. Schedule and manage appointments.

EVALUATION OF COMPETENCY

Procedure 40-4: Completing a Referral Form for Managed Care

Name: _____   Date: _____

Evaluated By: _____   Score: _____

Performance Objective

Outcome:	Complete a referral form for managed care.
Conditions:	Given the following: medical record, patient insurance information, physician's directions about service to be provided, referral form, and a telephone.
Standards:	Time: 10 minutes. Student completed procedure in ____ minutes.
	Accuracy: Satisfactory score on the Performance Evaluation Checklist.

Performance Evaluation Checklist

Trial 1	Trial 2	Point Value	Performance Standards
		●	Assembled information to complete the referral form.
		●	Determined the service for the referral from the medical record or physician's directions.
		●	Obtained preauthorization from the patient's insurance if necessary.
		●	Described the service requested, reason for the referral, and number of visits if necessary to obtain preauthorization.
		●	Filled out a referral form.
		●	Included the information about the patient, referring physician, and specialist or facility to which the patient was being referred on the referral form.
		●	Included the reason for the referral, preauthorization number (if any), and amount of service authorized on the referral form.
		✳	Included all necessary information and completed form accurately.
		●	Submitted a copy of the referral form to the patient's insurance if required for preauthorization.
		●	Retained a copy of the referral in the patient's medical record.
		●	Sent a copy of the referral form to the specialist or facility to whom the patient was referred or gave the form to the patient to bring to the appointment.
		●	Made the appointment for the patient or instructed the patient how to make the appointment.
		●	Filed the referral form in the patient's medical record.
		✳	Completed the procedure within 10 minutes.
			TOTALS

Evaluation of Student Performance

EVALUATION CRITERIA			COMMENTS
Symbol	Category	Point Value	
＊	Critical Step	16 points	
●	Essential Step	6 points	
▷	Theory Question	2 points	

Score calculation: 100 points

− _____ points missed

_____ Score

Satisfactory score: 85 or above

CAAHEP Competencies Achieved:

Psychomotor (Skills)
☑ VII. 1. Apply both managed care policies and procedures.
☑ VII. 6. Verify eligibility for managed care services.

Affective (Behavior)
☑ VII. 1. Demonstrate assertive communication with managed care and/or insurance providers.

ABHES Competencies Achieved:

☑ 8. s. Obtain managed care referrals and pre-certification.

EVALUATION OF COMPETENCY

Procedure 40-5: Scheduling Inpatient or Outpatient Diagnostic Tests or Procedures

Name: _____   Date: _____

Evaluated By: _____   Score: _____

Performance Objective

Outcome:	Schedule an inpatient or outpatient diagnostic test or procedure.
Conditions:	Given the following: patient medical record and insurance information, name of test or procedure to be scheduled, telephone, and telephone number of facility and department to schedule the test or procedure.
Standards:	Time: 5 minutes. Student completed procedure in ____ minutes.
	Accuracy: Satisfactory score on the Performance Evaluation Checklist.

Performance Evaluation Checklist

Trial 1	Trial 2	Point Value	Performance Standards
		•	Assembled necessary information about the patient.
		•	Determined the facility and department to call for scheduling using the medical record or a diagnostic test or procedure requisition.
		•	Determined the time frame for scheduling from the physician order.
		•	Asked the patient about preferred days and times for scheduling.
		•	Obtained preauthorization from the patient's insurance if necessary.
		•	Placed a telephone call to the department where the test or procedure would be scheduled and identified the test to be scheduled.
		•	Provided the patient's name and demographic information as needed.
		•	Provided patient insurance information and preauthorization number as needed.
		•	Set up a specific day and time for the procedure.
		•	Informed the patient of the date and time for the test or procedure.
		•	Provided verbal and written instructions about preparation for the test or procedure.
		•	Sent an electronic or paper requisition to the facility or gave a paper requisition to the patient to take to the test.
		•	Documented the scheduled diagnostic test or procedure in the patient's medical record.
		•	Included patient instructions in the documentation.
		★	Completed the procedure within 5 minutes.
			TOTALS

CHART	
Date	

Evaluation of Student Performance

EVALUATION CRITERIA			COMMENTS
Symbol	**Category**	**Point Value**	
∗	Critical Step	16 points	
●	Essential Step	6 points	
▷	Theory Question	2 points	

Score calculation: 100 points

− _____ points missed

_____ Score

Satisfactory score: 85 or above

CAAHEP Competencies Achieved:

Psychomotor (Skills)
☑ V. 2. Schedule patient admissions and/or procedures.
☑ VII. 4. Obtain precertification, including documentation.
☑ VII. 5. Obtain preauthorization, including documentation.

ABHES Competencies Achieved:

☑ 8. c. Schedule and manage appointments.
☑ 8. s. Obtain managed care referrals and pre-certification.

EVALUATION OF COMPETENCY

Procedure 40-6: Scheduling Inpatient or Outpatient Admissions

Name: _____   Date: _____

Evaluated By: _____   Score: _____

Performance Objective

Outcome:	Schedule an inpatient or outpatient admission for a patient
Conditions:	Given the following: patient's medical record and insurance information, reason for admission, telephone, and telephone number of the facility and admitting department.
Standards:	Time: 10 minutes. Student completed procedure in ____ minutes.
	Accuracy: Satisfactory score on the Performance Evaluation Checklist.

Performance Evaluation Checklist

Trial 1	Trial 2	Point Value	Performance Standards
		•	Assembled patient demographic and insurance information.
		•	Determined the reason for the outpatient or inpatient admission.
		•	Determined the time frame for the admission from the physician's orders.
		•	Discussed preferred days and times with the patient.
		•	Obtained preauthorization from the patient's insurance company.
		•	Called the admissions department to schedule the admission.
		•	Provided the patient's name and demographic information as needed.
		•	Provided patient insurance information and preauthorization number.
		•	Provided the patient diagnosis or reason for the admission.
		•	Set up a specific day and time for the admission.
		•	Provided admitting orders as needed and faxed to the admitting department or nursing floor.
		•	If patient was to be admitted directly from the office, arranged transport and prepared a patient transfer form.
		•	If the patient was to be admitted at a future date, informed the patient of the date and time and provided written instructions for any preoperative needs or procedure.
		•	Documented the admission and instructions given to the patient in the patient's medical record.
		•	For a direct admission from the office, identified any documents sent with the patient.
		∗	Completed the procedure within 10 minutes.
		TOTALS	

CHART	
Date	

Evaluation of Student Performance

EVALUATION CRITERIA			COMMENTS
Symbol	Category	Point Value	
✳	Critical Step	16 points	
●	Essential Step	6 points	
▷	Theory Question	2 points	

Score calculation: 100 points

− _____ points missed

_____ Score

Satisfactory score: 85 or above

CAAHEP Competencies Achieved:

Psychomotor (Skills)
☑ V. 2. Schedule patient admissions and/or procedures.
☑ VII. 4. Obtain precertification, including documentation.
☑ VII. 5. Obtain preauthorization, including documentation.

ABHES Competencies Achieved:

☑ 8. f. Schedule inpatient and outpatient admissions.
☑ 8. s. Obtain managed care referrals and pre-certification.

41

Medical Records Management

CHAPTER ASSIGNMENTS

√ After Completing	Date Due	Textbook Page(s)	TEXTBOOK ASSIGNMENTS	Possible Points	Points You Earned
		978-991	Read Chapter 41: Medical Records Management		
		982 990	🖎 Read Case Study 1 Case Study 1 questions	5	
		984 990	🖎 Read Case Study 2 Case Study 2 questions	5	
		987 991	🖎 Read Case Study 3 Case Study 3 questions	5	
			TOTAL POINTS		

√ After Completing	Date Due	Study Guide Page(s)	STUDY GUIDE ASSIGNMENTS (CTA: Critical Thinking Activity)	Possible Points	Points You Earned
		1053	? Pretest	10	
		1054	Term Key Term Assessment	13	
		1055-1057	Evaluation of Learning questions	27	
		1058	CTA A: Filing Units: Alphabetic	10	
		1058	CTA B: Alphabetic Filing	8	
		1058	CTA C: Filing Units: Terminal Digit	8	
		1059	CTA D: Numeric Filing	8	
		1059	CTA E: Filing Reports and Correspondence	8	
			CD CD Activity: Chapter 41 Filing Records Using the Alphabetic Filing System (Record points earned)		

√ After Completing	Date Due	Study Guide Page(s)	STUDY GUIDE ASSIGNMENTS (CTA: Critical Thinking Activity)	Possible Points	Points You Earned
			⊙CD⊙ CD Activity: Chapter 41 Filing Records Using the Terminal Digit Filing System (Record points earned)		
			⊙CD⊙ CD Activity: Chapter 41 Adding Supplementary Items to Established Patient File	10	
			⊙CD⊙ CD Activity: Chapter 41 Apply Your Knowledge questions (Record points earned)		
		1053	🗒 Posttest	10	
			ADDITIONAL ASSIGNMENTS		
			TOTAL POINTS		

√ When Assigned by Your Instructor	Study Guide Page(s)	Practices Required	LABORATORY ASSIGNMENTS (Procedure Number and Name)	*Score
	1061	3	🔘 **Practice for Competency** 41-1: Filing Patient Records—Alphabetic Textbook reference: p. 985	
	1063-1064		📋 **Evaluation of Competency** 41-1: Filing Patient Records—Alphabetic	*
	1061	3	🔘 **Practice for Competency** 41-2: Filing Patient Records—Numeric Textbook reference: p. 985	
	1065-1066		📋 **Evaluation of Competency** 41-2: Filing Patient Records—Numeric	*
	1061	3	🔘 **Practice for Competency** 41-3: Filing Reports Textbook reference: pp. 987-988	
	1067-1068		📋 **Evaluation of Competency** 41-3: Filing Reports	*
			ADDITIONAL ASSIGNMENTS	

Notes

Name _____ Date_____

PRETEST

True or False

_____   1. The patient owns the original medical record.

_____   2. The main way to enter information into an electronic medical record is to use a scanner.

_____   3. Medical record files or filing rooms should always be locked when the office is closed.

_____   4. Color-coded labels are used for alphabetic filing but not for numeric file systems.

_____   5. Out guides are placed where a paper medical record has been removed from the filing shelves.

_____   6. If a numeric medical record system is used, the filing system is indirect.

_____   7. In an alphabetic filing system, prefixes such as van, von, and de are the third filing unit.

_____   8. The medical record of a married woman is filed under her last name and her husband's first name.

_____   9. In a terminal digit numeric filing system, the last group of two digits is the first filing unit.

_____   10. The length of time that medical records must be retained can vary depending on the age of the patient.

POSTTEST

True or False

_____   1. The patient controls the information in the medical record and access to it.

_____   2. An electronic medical record system is less expensive to initiate than a paper record system.

_____   3. If shelving units are used to store paper medical records, folders with side tabs should be used.

_____   4. Use of a current year label helps identify inactive paper medical records.

_____   5. An out guide is placed in the individual medical record when removing papers to file new reports.

_____   6. In an alphabetic medical record filing system the patient's surname is the first filing unit.

_____   7. If a business name includes an acronym, it is filed as if it were spelled out in full.

_____   8. Hyphenated names are indexed as one filing unit in an alphabetic filing system.

_____   9. A numeric terminal digit filing system is commonly used in hospitals and large clinics.

_____   10. Medical records for minors can be destroyed seven years after the record becomes inactive.

Term KEY TERM ASSESSMENT

Directions: Match each medical term with its definition.

_____ 1. Acronym

_____ 2. Active record

_____ 3. Cross-index

_____ 4. Electronic medical record (electronic health record)

_____ 5. Filing system

_____ 6. Inactive record

_____ 7. Indexing units

_____ 8. Medical records management

_____ 9. Out guide

_____ 10. Sorter

_____ 11. Surname

_____ 12. Tab

_____ 13. Terminal digit filing

A. A device that facilitates putting papers or records in alphabetic or numeric order

B. To file under one unit and use a guide or card filed under another unit that refers to the primary filing location

C. Pieces of information used to identify a correct filing location

D. The way in which records are arranged such as alphabetically or numerically

E. A cardboard or plastic card to insert in a file when a medical record is removed

F. A word formed from the first letters in a name

G. An individual patient's health record in digital format

H. The medical record of a patient who has not been seen within the past 2 to 3 years, or some other time frame specified by a given medical office

I. A projection of a folder that extends beyond the top or side of the folder

J. Activities related to the creation, management, use, and disposition of patient medical records

K. The medical record of a patient who has been seen within a time frame specified by the office (usually 2 to 3 years)

L. Last name or family name of an individual

M. Record-keeping method in which the last digits are used as the first filing unit

EVALUATION OF LEARNING

Directions: Fill in each blank with the correct answer.

1. Discuss the ownership of a paper medical record.

   _____

   _____

2. If an electronic medical record is used, how is new information entered into the record? Information from a previous paper medical record?

   _____

   _____

   _____

3. Identify five advantages to using an electronic medical record.

   _____

   _____

   _____

4. What are three challenges when a medical office changes from a paper medical record to an electronic medical record?

   _____

   _____

5. What equipment is used for storage of paper medical records?

   _____

   _____

6. What is the advantage of using color-coded labels on medical record file folders?

   _____

   _____

7. List seven common categories for chart dividers.

   _____

   _____

8. How is an out guide used when filing medical records?

   _____

   _____

9. What is the difference between a direct filing system and an indirect filing system?

   _____

   _____

10. What is the first indexing unit if an alphabetic filing system is used?

   _____

11. How are names with prefixes filed if an alphabetic filing system is used?

_____

12. How are hyphenated names filed if an alphabetic filing system is used?

_____

13. What is the second filing unit if the patient's name is Mary Johnson White?

_____

14. How is the medical record of a married woman filed if an alphabetic filing system is used?

_____

15. What are two advantages of a numeric filing system for paper medical records?

_____

_____

16. Compare and contrast a terminal digit filing system with a consecutive filing system.

_____

_____

17. What are three types of documents that might be filed using a subject filing system?

_____

18. Identify two ways that documents might be arranged within a subject category.

_____

19. Describe the form and function of a tickler file.

_____

_____

20. Before returning medical records to the files, what are three things the medical assistant should do to condition the records?

_____

_____

21. How are reports and letters filed into existing medical records?

_____

_____

_____

22. What are three measures to prevent misplaced records?

_____

_____

_____

23. What conditions should be present in the storage area for active or inactive medical records?

_____

_____

_____

24. How are medical records selected to be moved to the location of inactive records?

_____

_____

25. How long should the medical records of minors be retained? Why?

_____

_____

_____

26. How long should the records of adult patients be retained? Why?

_____

_____

27. How should computerized records be stored?

_____

_____

CRITICAL THINKING ACTIVITIES

A. FILING UNITS: ALPHABETIC
Identify the filing units in the following list of names:

Name	Unit 1	Unit 2	Unit 3	Unit 4
Diane Riel				
George A. Ricker, Jr.				
Marie A. von Hayden				
Mrs. Carolyn Richenburg				
Robert T. Van Wilder				
Maria Rivera Santos				
G. A. Rickers				
James D. Smith-Richards				
The Blackburn Daily Times				
Uptown Management Corp.				

B. ALPHABETIC FILING
Arrange the names in the column on the left in correct filing order in the spaces on the right.

Diane Riel

George A. Ricker, Jr.

Marie A. von Hayden

Mrs. Carolyn Richenburg

Robert T. Van Wilder

Maria Rivera Santos

G. A. Rickers

James D. Smith-Richards

1. _____
2. _____
3. _____
4. _____
5. _____
6. _____
7. _____
8. _____

C. FILING UNITS: TERMINAL DIGIT
Identify the filing units in the following numbers assuming that a terminal digit system is used with two digits in each group.

Number	Unit 1	Unit 2	Unit 3
01-23-52			
22-19-08			
62-41-33			
00-82-99			
15-66-18			
21-19-44			
66-01-11			
21-18-08			

D. NUMERIC FILING

Arrange the following numbers in the column on the left in correct filing order in the spaces on the right.

01-23-52	1. _____
22-19-08	2. _____
62-41-33	3. _____
00-82-99	4. _____
15-66-18	5. _____
21-19-44	6. _____
66-01-11	7. _____
21-18-08	8. _____

E. FILING REPORTS AND CORRESPONDENCE

Indicate which section of the medical record each of the following reports would be filed in by writing the name of the report in the correct section of the table below.

1. Report of shoulder x-ray

2. Report of complete blood count

3. Report of laparoscopic cholecystectomy

4. Discharge summary from hospitalization

5. History and physical examination report

6. Progress note dictated at the most recent patient visit

7. Letter from consulting physician regarding a consultation visit by the patient

8. Report of MRI scan of left knee

Section of Medical Record	Location of Reports to Be Filed
Progress notes	
History and physical examination	
Laboratory reports	
Diagnostic testing	
Hospital reports	
Immunizations/medications	
Correspondence	

Notes

PRACTICE FOR COMPETENCY

Procedure 41-1: Filing Patient Records—Alphabetic. File medical records using the alphabetic system.

Procedure 41-2: Filing Medical Records—Numeric. File medical records using the terminal digit system.

Procedure 41-3: Filing Reports. File reports and correspondence in medical records.

Notes

📖 **EVALUATION OF COMPETENCY**

📀 **Procedure 41-1: Filing Medical Records—Alphabetic**

Name: _____   Date: _____

Evaluated By: _____   Date: _____

Performance Objective

Outcome:	File patient records using an alphabetic filing system.
Conditions:	Given the following: patient records with patient names, alphabetic sorter, file cabinet or shelves, out guides, and index cards.
Standards:	Time: 10 minutes. Student completed procedure in ____ minutes.
	Accuracy: Satisfactory score on the Performance Evaluation Checklist.

Performance Evaluation Checklist

Trial 1	Trial 2	Point Value	*Performance Standards*
		•	Gathered the records and removed any elastic bands or paper clips.
		•	Secured any loose sheets of paper.
		•	Sorted the records alphabetically by last name.
		∗	Found the correct location in the file for each record.
		•	Slid the record in front of the out guide and removed the out guide from the shelf or drawer.
		•	Stored the out guide with other unused out guides.
		•	Removed any index card from the out guide and discarded or stored according to office policy.
		•	Filed each record until all records were filed.
		∗	Completed the procedure within 10 minutes.
			TOTALS

Evaluation of Student Performance

EVALUATION CRITERIA			COMMENTS
Symbol	Category	Point Value	
∗	Critical Step	16 points	
•	Essential Step	6 points	
▷	Theory Question	2 points	
Score calculation: 100 points			
−_____ points missed			
_____ Score			
Satisfactory score: 85 or above			

CAAHEP Competencies Achieved:

Psychomotor (Skills)
☑ V. 4. File medical records.
☑ V. 8. Maintain organization by filing.

Affective (Behavior)
☑ V. 1. Consider staff needs and limitations in establishment of a filing system.

ABHES Competencies Achieved:

☑ 8. b. Prepare and maintain medical records.

EVALUATION OF COMPETENCY

Procedure 41-2: Filing Patient Records—Numeric

Name: _____   Date: _____

Evaluated By: _____   Date: _____

Performance Objective

Outcome:	File patient records using a terminal digit filing system.
Conditions:	Given the following: Patient records with terminal digit labels, file cabinet or shelves, numeric sorter, out guides, and index cards.
Standards:	Time: 10 minutes. Student completed procedure in ____ minutes.
	Accuracy: Satisfactory score on the Performance Evaluation Checklist.

Performance Evaluation Checklist

Trial 1	Trial 2	Point Value	Performance Standards
		•	Gathered the records and removed any elastic bands or paper clips.
		•	Secured any loose sheets of paper.
		•	Sorted the records according to the terminal digit indexing units.
		∗	Found the correct location in the file for each record based on the final group of numbers.
		∗	Refined search based on the middle group of numbers and then the first group of numbers.
		•	Slid the record in front of the out guide and removed the out guide from the shelf or drawer.
		•	Stored the out guide with other unused out guides.
		•	Removed any index card from the out guide and discarded or stored according to office policy.
		•	Filed each record until all records were filed.
		∗	Completed the procedure within 10 minutes.
			TOTALS

Evaluation of Student Performance

EVALUATION CRITERIA			COMMENTS
Symbol	Category	Point Value	
∗	Critical Step	16 points	
•	Essential Step	6 points	
▷	Theory Question	2 points	

Score calculation: 100 points

−_____ points missed

_____ Score

Satisfactory score: 85 or above

CAAHEP Competencies Achieved:

Psychomotor (Skills)
☑ V. 4. File medical records.
☑ V. 8. Maintain organization by filing.

Affective (Behavior)
☑ V. 1. Consider staff needs and limitations in establishment of a filing system.

ABHES Competencies Achieved:

☑ 8. b. Prepare and maintain medical records.

EVALUATION OF COMPETENCY

Procedure 41-3: Filing Reports

Name: _____   Date: _____

Evaluated By: _____   Date: _____

Performance Objective

Outcome:	File patient records using a terminal digit filing system.
Conditions:	Given the following: Medical records, assorted reports, letters or other material to be filed, hole punch, tape, stapler, and sorter.
Standards:	Time: 10 minutes. Student completed procedure in _____ minutes.
	Accuracy: Satisfactory score on the Performance Evaluation Checklist.

Performance Evaluation Checklist

Trial 1	Trial 2	Point Value	Performance Standards
		•	Assembled materials to be filed and necessary supplies.
		•	Removed paper clips, pins, or other extraneous materials from records or materials to be filed.
		•	Mended any tears with tape.
		•	Stapled related pages together.
		•	Punched holes as needed.
		•	Verified that each report was initialed by the physician.
		•	Set aside any report without initials to be returned for physician review.
		•	Sorted reports alphabetically or numerically depending on the office filing system.
		•	Assembled all reports for a particular patient.
		•	Located the patient's medical record.
		✱	Inserted the reports into the medical record in the correct location in reverse chronological order.
		•	Inserted dividers into the medical record if necessary.
		•	Put the record back together as needed.
		•	Replaced the record in the file.
		•	Repeated until all the reports for all patients were filed.
		•	If the record could not be located in the file, placed the report back in sorter or in the pocket of the out guide according to office policy.
		✱	Completed the procedure within 10 minutes.
			TOTALS

Evaluation of Student Performance

EVALUATION CRITERIA			COMMENTS
Symbol	Category	Point Value	
∗	Critical Step	16 points	
•	Essential Step	6 points	
▷	Theory Question	2 points	

Score calculation: 100 points

− _____ points missed

_____ Score

Satisfactory score: 85 or above

CAAHEP Competencies Achieved:

Psychomotor (Skills)
☑ V. 4. File medical records.
☑ V. 8. Maintain organization by filing.

ABHES Competencies Achieved:

☑ 8. b. Prepare and maintain medical records.

42

Written Communications

CHAPTER ASSIGNMENTS

√ After Completing	Date Due	Textbook Page(s)	TEXTBOOK ASSIGNMENTS	Possible Points	Points You Earned
		992-1011	Read Chapter 42: Written Communications		
		1000 1010	Read Case Study 1 Case Study 1 questions	5	
		1004 1010	Read Case Study 2 Case Study 2 questions	5	
		1007 1010-1011	Read Case Study 3 Case Study 3 questions	5	
			TOTAL POINTS		
√ After Completing	Date Due	Study Guide Page(s)	STUDY GUIDE ASSIGNMENTS (CTA: Critical Thinking Activities)	Possible Points	Points You Earned
		1073	Pretest	10	
		1074	Key Term Assessment	15	
		1075-1076	Evaluation of Learning questions	25	
		1077	CTA A: Parts of a Letter	6	
		1077	CTA B: Letter Styles	6	
		1077	CTA C: Parts of Speech	16	
		1077-1078	CTA D: Proofreading	10	
			CD Activity: Chapter 42 Quiz Show (Record points earned)		
			CD Activity: Chapter 42 Comma Exercise (Record points earned)		

√ After Completing	Date Due	Study Guide Page(s)	STUDY GUIDE ASSIGNMENTS (CTA: Critical Thinking Activities)	Possible Points	Points You Earned
			📀 CD Activity: Chapter 42 Hyphen Exercise (Record points earned)		
			📀 CD Activity: Chapter 42 Proofreading Written Correspondence	10	
			📀 CD Activity: Chapter 42 Dictation	15	
			📀 CD Activity: Chapter 42 Apply Your Knowledge questions (Record points earned)		
		1073	📄 Posttest	10	
			ADDITIONAL ASSIGNMENTS		
			TOTAL POINTS		

√ When Assigned by Your Instructor	Study Guide Page(s)	Practices Required	LABORATORY ASSIGNMENTS (Procedure Number and Name)	*Score
	1079	3	**Practice for Competency** 42-1: Composing a Business Letter Textbook reference: pp. 998-999	
	1083-1084		**Evaluation of Competency** 42-1: Composing a Business Letter	*
	1079	3	**Practice for Competency** 42-2: Responding to Written Communication Textbook reference: p. 1002	
	1085-1086		**Evaluation of Competency** 42-2: Responding to Written Communication	*
	1079	3	**Practice for Competency** 42-3: Transcribing a Dictated Letter or Report Textbook reference: p. 1006	
	1087-1088		**Evaluation of Competency** 42-3: Transcribing a Dictated Letter or Report	*
	1079	3	**Practice for Competency** 42-4: Sending a Fax Textbook reference: pp. 1007-1008	
	1089-1090		**Evaluation of Competency** 42-4: Sending a Fax	*
	1079	3	**Practice for Competency** 42-5: Preparing Copies of Multiple-Page Documents Textbook reference: p. 1009	
	1091-1092		**Evaluation of Competency** 42-5: Preparing Copies of Multiple-Page Documents	*
			ADDITIONAL ASSIGNMENTS	

Notes

Name _____ Date _____

? PRETEST

True or False

_____ 1. Business letters are more formal than personal correspondence in form and content.

_____ 2. The body of a business letter is double spaced.

_____ 3. The name of the individual sending a business letter should always be printed below the handwritten signature.

_____ 4. If additional forms or printed material is included with a letter, this should be indicated in an end notation.

_____ 5. In the semiblock letter style, all lines of the letter are left justified.

_____ 6. An adverb modifies a verb, adjective, or other adverb.

_____ 7. Sentence fragments and comma splices are errors that should always be corrected in a business letter.

_____ 8. A comma should be used to separate two sentences that are not joined by a conjunction or separated by a period.

_____ 9. The common headings for a memo are: TO, FROM, SUBJECT, and DATE.

_____ 10. Because e-mail and fax transmissions are considered secure, they are a good way to transmit confidential information about patients.

? POSTTEST

True or False

_____ 1. All business letters sent from the medical office are dictated by the physician and prepared by office staff.

_____ 2. The inside address of a business letter is placed two lines below the date line.

_____ 3. The standard closing of a business letter is "Sincerely yours."

_____ 4. If a letter has been dictated by the physician and prepared by the medical assistant, a reference line should be included below the typed signature.

_____ 5. In the modified block letter style, the date line, complimentary close, and printed signature may be lined up at the center of the letter.

_____ 6. A conjunction joins words, phrases, or clauses in a sentence.

_____ 7. When two sentences are connected without punctuation, it is called a *comma splice*.

_____ 8. A comma should be used to set off information that could be omitted from a sentence without changing the meaning.

_____ 9. Progress notes dictated by a physician are often set up in SOAP format.

_____ 10. Most office photocopy machines will collate and staple documents, as well as copy on both sides of a piece of paper.

Term KEY TERM ASSESSMENT

Directions: Match each medical term with its definition.

_____ 1. Collate

_____ 2. Duplex

_____ 3. E-mail

_____ 4. Fax

_____ 5. Full block style

_____ 6. Grammar

_____ 7. Left justified

_____ 8. Letterhead

_____ 9. Memo (memorandum)

_____ 10. Modified block style

_____ 11. Right-justified

_____ 12. Semiblock style

_____ 13. Simplified letter style

_____ 14. Template

_____ 15. Transcription

A. A format for business letters where the date line, complimentary close, and printed signature line are aligned at the center and all other parts of the letter are left justified

B. A letter format in which all elements are left justified, the greeting is replaced by a subject line in all capital letters, and the complimentary close and typed signature are replaced by a typed signature in all capital letters

C. A form of communication within a company that is usually short and limited to one subject

D. A letter format where all parts of the letter begin at the left margin

E. To assemble the pages of a document in numerical order

F. The process of changing verbal dictation to typed or printed form

G. A standard form to which additional information can be added as needed

H. A letter format similar to modified block style, but all paragraphs are indented

I. Type that is aligned with the right margin of a document

J. The exchange of information from one computer to another using telecommunication

K. A sheet of stationery preprinted with information about a business, including name, address, telephone number, and other information.

L. The study of accepted rules used to create meaning in a language

M. To produce double-sided copies by storing images from both sides of the original in the memory of a photocopier

N. Lines of type that begin at the left margin of a document

O. Transmission of scanned, printed material by telephone

EVALUATION OF LEARNING

Directions: Fill in each blank with the correct answer.

1. What is letterhead stationery?

    _____

    _____

2. What is included in the heading of a letter?

    _____

3. Where is the inside address located on a letter?

    _____

4. What is the correct salutation for a business letter to William Masterson, MD, including punctuation?

    _____

5. What spacing is used in the body of a letter?

    _____

6. Give examples of at least two acceptable complimentary closings for a business letter.

    _____

7. How many spaces below the complimentary closing should the typed signature be placed? Why?

    _____

8. What are three examples of end notations for a letter?

    _____

9. Compare and contrast full block letter style with modified block letter style.

    _____

    _____

10. What is the advantage of using the simplified letter style?

    _____

11. Identify the eight parts of speech.

    _____

12. What type of sentence is composed of one independent clause?

    _____

13. What is a compound sentence?

    _____

14. What is a complex sentence?

_____

15. What is a sentence fragment?

_____

16. When does a comma splice occur?

_____

17. Identify at least six occasions when a comma should be used.

_____

_____

_____

_____

18. When does the spell check feature of a word processing program fail to find errors?

_____

19. How does a physician dictate medical reports and correspondence?

_____

_____

20. What is the format of a memo (memorandum)?

_____

_____

21. Identify three types of reports that a physician might dictate in the medical office.

_____

_____

22. Give three examples of individuals that an MA might communicate with via e-mail.

_____

_____

23. Compare the tone of an e-mail to that of a business letter.

_____

24. What features on a photocopier are helpful when photocopying a multiple-page document?

_____

_____

25. What information should be included on the cover sheet for fax transmissions from a medical office?

_____

_____

CRITICAL THINKING ACTIVITIES

A. PARTS OF A LETTER
   Refer to the letter in Chapter 49, Figure 49-5. Identify the following parts of that letter.

   1. Inside address: _____

   2. Salutation: _____

   3. First three words of the body of the letter: _____

   4. Complimentary close: _____

   5. Printed signature: _____

   6. End notation(s): _____

B. LETTER STYLES
   Name the letter style(s) to which each of the following apply:

   1. Date line is left justified: _____

   2. Instead of a salutation, a reference line is included in all caps: _____

   3. The body of the letter is single spaced with two spaces between paragraphs: _____

   _____

   4. Paragraphs are indented: _____

   5. The complimentary close is right justified or at the center: _____

   6. The inside address is left justified: _____

C. PARTS OF SPEECH
   Enter each word in the following sentence into the table below under the heading of the correct part of speech.
   My name is Christine Walters, and I have worked continuously at a nephrology practice for the past 3 years.

Noun(s)	Pronoun(s)	Verb(s)	Adjective(s)	Adverb(s) Article(s)	Preposition(s)	Conjunction(s)

D. PROOFREADING
   Proofread the passage on the left. In the lines on the right, correct each mistake, including spelling, punctuation, and grammar.

   1. Patient instructed in perfromance of range of   1. _____

   2. motion activities, especially for the weak, right   2. _____

   3. lower, extremity. He was instructed to use both   3. _____

   4. hands to assisting in extension of the knee and   4. _____

   5. ankle, flexion of the toes, as well as invershun   5. _____

6. and eversion of the foot. The pateint was able

6. _____

7. to demonstrate all exercises, included those

7. _____

8. done as assistave exercises. The patient could

8. _____

9. verbalized understanding of the need to keep all

9. _____

10. joints mobile.

10. _____

PRACTICE FOR COMPETENCY

Procedure 42-1: Composing a Business Letter. Practice preparing business letters and preparing envelopes using the two letters found under Procedure 42-2 and the dictation for Procedure 42-3.

Procedure 42-2: Responding to Written Communication. Practice responding to written communication using the following situations. Assume you are using letterhead stationery. Your position: medical assistant.

Letter 1:

Content: You received an invoice (bill) from Physicians' Medical Supply Company, 22 Birkwood Street, Western, XY 44770. It includes a charge for three boxes of extra small gloves, but you only received two boxes. The purchase order number was 12345. You need the extra box of gloves.

Format: Full block using letterhead stationery. Use 1-inch margins. Be sure the letter has at least two paragraphs and that the body of the letter is centered on the page. Prepare an envelope to accompany the letter.

Letter 2:

Content: You have received a letter from a patient asking if it is time for her to schedule a physical examination. The patient's name and address are Lucille Freeman, 22 White Circle, Western, XY 44770. When you check the patient's medical record, you notice that the patient has not been seen for 2 years. Mrs. Freeman is a patient of Dr. Warner, who prefers to perform an annual physical examination.

Format: Simplified style using letterhead stationery.

Respond by e-mail:

You receive an e-mail from a pharmaceutical representative named Richard Jensen asking if Friday the 22nd is a convenient day for him to visit the office. He hopes to speak the physician. You can schedule him for 12:15 on that day if that is possible.

Assume that you work at Western Medical Center, 109 River Street, Western, XY 44770.

Procedure 42-3: Transcribing a Dictated Letter or Report. Practice transcribing letters and reports.

Procedure 42-4: Sending a Fax. Practice the procedure to send a fax using the following cover sheets.

Procedure 42-5: Preparing Copies of Multiple-Page Documents. Practice the procedure for preparing copies of multiple-page documents.

WESTERN MEDICAL CENTER
109 RIVER STREET
WESTERN, XY 44770

PHONE: (490) 555-6464
FAX: (490) 668-1414

To: _____

From: _____

Fax: _____

Pages: _____

Phone: _____

Date: _____

Re: _____

CC

☐ URGENT   ☐ FOR REVIEW   ☐ PLEASE COMMENT   ☐ PLEASE REPLY   ☐ PLEASE RECYCLE

CONFIDENTIALITY STATEMENT:
The documents accompanying this transmission may contain confidential information that is protected under the Privacy Act of 1974. It is being faxed to you after appropriate patient authorization or under circumstances that do not require patient authorization. This information is intended only for the use of the intended recipient(s). The authorized recipient(s) of this information is/are prohibited from disclosing this information to any other party unless permitted to do so by law or regulation.

If the reader of this message is not the intended recipient(s) or the employee or agent responsible for delivering the attached information to the intended recipient(s), please note that any dissemination, distribution, or copying of this information is strictly prohibited. **Anyone who receives this information in error should notify the sender immediately and arrange for the return or destruction of the transmitted information.**

MESSAGE:

WESTERN MEDICAL CENTER
109 RIVER STREET
WESTERN, XY 44770

PHONE: (490) 555-6464
FAX: (490) 668-1414

To: _____

From: _____

Fax: _____

Pages: _____

Phone: _____

Date: _____

Re: _____

CC _____

☐ URGENT   ☐ FOR REVIEW   ☐ PLEASE COMMENT   ☐ PLEASE REPLY   ☐ PLEASE RECYCLE

CONFIDENTIALITY STATEMENT:
The documents accompanying this transmission may contain confidential information that is protected under the Privacy Act of 1974. It is being faxed to you after appropriate patient authorization or under circumstances that do not require patient authorization. This information is intended only for the use of the intended recipient(s). The authorized recipient(s) of this information is/are prohibited from disclosing this information to any other party unless permitted to do so by law or regulation.

If the reader of this message is not the intended recipient(s) or the employee or agent responsible for delivering the attached information to the intended recipient(s), please note that any dissemination, distribution, or copying of this information is strictly prohibited. **Anyone who receives this information in error should notify the sender immediately and arrange for the return or destruction of the transmitted information.**

MESSAGE:

WESTERN MEDICAL CENTER
109 RIVER STREET
WESTERN, XY 44770

PHONE: (490) 555-6464
FAX: (490) 668-1414

To: _____

From: _____

Fax: _____

Pages: _____

Phone: _____

Date: _____

Re: _____

CC _____

☐ URGENT   ☐ FOR REVIEW   ☐ PLEASE COMMENT   ☐ PLEASE REPLY   ☐ PLEASE RECYCLE

CONFIDENTIALITY STATEMENT:
The documents accompanying this transmission may contain confidential information that is protected under the Privacy Act of 1974. It is being faxed to you after appropriate patient authorization or under circumstances that do not require patient authorization. This information is intended only for the use of the intended recipient(s). The authorized recipient(s) of this information is/are prohibited from disclosing this information to any other party unless permitted to do so by law or regulation.

If the reader of this message is not the intended recipient(s) or the employee or agent responsible for delivering the attached information to the intended recipient(s), please note that any dissemination, distribution, or copying of this information is strictly prohibited. **Anyone who receives this information in error should notify the sender immediately and arrange for the return or destruction of the transmitted information.**

MESSAGE:

EVALUATION OF COMPETENCY

Procedure 42-1: Composing a Business Letter

Name: _____   Date: _____

Evaluated By: _____   Date: _____

Performance Objective

Outcome:	Compose and key a business letter.
Conditions:	Given the following: letterhead stationery, blank stationery, and typewriter or computer and printer.
Standards:	Time: 10 minutes. Student completed procedure in _____ minutes.
	Accuracy: Satisfactory score on the Performance Evaluation Checklist.

Performance Evaluation Checklist

Trial 1	Trial 2	Point Value	Performance Standards
		•	Assembled materials.
		•	Determined the address of the recipient.
		•	Set up the letter according to selected format.
		•	Listed and organized essential content for the letter.
		•	Inserted the date on the second or third line below the letterhead.
		•	Placed the inside address four to ten lines below the date at the left margin (to center the body the of the letter on the page).
		•	Placed the salutation two lines below the inside address followed by a colon.
		•	Placed a subject line two lines below the salutation, if desired.
		•	Began the body of the letter two lines below the subject line (or salutation if no subject line was used).
		•	Single-spaced the letter with double spacing between paragraphs.
		•	Began paragraphs at the left margin or indented according to the letter style being used.
		•	Summarized the contents or most important ideas in the final paragraph of the letter.
		•	Placed the complimentary close two spaces below the final paragraph of the letter followed by a comma.
		•	Placed the typed signature four lines below the complimentary close with a title on the line below if appropriate.
		•	Added reference line, enclosure notation, and/or distribution notation as needed below the typed signature.
		•	Began a second page one inch from the top including the name of the recipient, the date, and the page number in the top left corner.

Trial 1	Trial 2	Point Value	Performance Standards
		•	Included at least two lines of the body of the letter on the second page, if one was used.
		*	Made sure that there were no errors in the letter using the computer and manual proofreading.
		•	Printed the letter.
		•	Signed the letter or obtained the appropriate signature.
		•	Made one copy of the letter for the file and additional copies for any individuals identified in the distribution notation.
		•	Prepared an envelope (Procedure 43-3: Preparing Envelopes for Mailing).
		•	Inserted the letter in the envelope and placed in the designated area to be mailed.
		•	Filed the copy of the letter according to office policy.
		*	Completed the procedure within 10 minutes.
			TOTALS

Evaluation of Student Performance

EVALUATION CRITERIA			COMMENTS
Symbol	Category	Point Value	
*	Critical Step	16 points	
•	Essential Step	6 points	
▷	Theory Question	2 points	

Score calculation: 100 points

− _____ points missed

_____ Score

Satisfactory score: 85 or above

CAAHEP Competencies Achieved:

Psychomotor (Skills)
☑ IV. 10. Compose professional/business letters.

ABHES Competencies Achieved:

☑ 8. jj. Perform fundamental writing skills including correct grammar, spelling, and formatting techniques when writing prescriptions, documenting medical records, etc.

⬛ **EVALUATION OF COMPETENCY**

Procedure 42-2: Responding to Written Communication

Name: _____   Date: _____

Evaluated By: _____   Date: _____

Performance Objective

Outcome:	Respond to written communication.
Conditions:	Given the following: received correspondence, letterhead stationery, blank stationery, typewriter or computer, and printer.
Standards:	Time: 10 minutes. Student completed procedure in ____ minutes.
	Accuracy: Satisfactory score on the Performance Evaluation Checklist.

Performance Evaluation Checklist

Trial 1	Trial 2	Point Value	Performance Standards
		•	Reviewed correspondence to determine an appropriate response.
		•	Looked up information needed to respond to the received correspondence.
		•	Made notes and/or composed a rough draft for a written response.
		•	Created a business letter or an e-mail as appropriate.
		•	Saved a copy of the letter or e-mail on the computer.
		•	Printed the letter.
		•	Signed the letter or obtained the appropriate signature.
		•	Made a copy of the letter and filed appropriately.
		•	Prepared the letter for mailing or sent the e-mail.
		*	Completed the procedure within 10 minutes.
		TOTALS	

Evaluation of Student Performance

EVALUATION CRITERIA			COMMENTS
Symbol	Category	Point Value	
*	Critical Step	16 points	
•	Essential Step	6 points	
▷	Theory Question	2 points	
Score calculation: 100 points			
− _____ points missed			
_____ Score			
Satisfactory score: 85 or above			

CAAHEP Competencies Achieved:

Psychomotor (Skills)

☑ IV. 3. Use medical terminology, pronouncing medical terms correctly, to communicate information, patient history, data and observations.

☑ IV. 10. Compose professional/business letters.

Affective (Behavior)

☑ IV. 8. Analyze communications in providing appropriate responses/feedback.

ABHES Competencies Achieved:

☑ 8. gg. Use pertinent medical terminology.

☑ 8. hh. Receive, organize, prioritize, and transmit information expediently.

☑ 8. jj. Perform fundamental writing skills including correct grammar, spelling, and formatting techniques when writing prescriptions, documenting medical records, etc.

▣ EVALUATION OF COMPETENCY

Procedure 42-3: Transcribing a Dictated Letter or Report

Name: _____   Date: _____

Evaluated By: _____   Date: _____

Performance Objective

Outcome:	Transcribe a dictated letter or report.
Conditions:	Given the following: letterhead stationery, blank stationery or paper, transcription machine or computer with foot pedal, headphones, dictation tape or file, computer, and printer.
Standards:	Time: 15 minutes. Student completed procedure in _____ minutes.
	Accuracy: Satisfactory score on the Performance Evaluation Checklist.

Performance Evaluation Checklist

Trial 1	Trial 2	Point Value	*Performance Standards*
		●	Assembled materials.
		●	Decided on a format for the letter or report.
		●	Set up the transcription equipment and plugged headphones into the transcriber or computer.
		●	While listening to the dictation, keyed the letter or report.
		●	Used correct format for the letter or report.
		●	Spell-checked the letter or report and printed a copy for proofreading.
		●	Checked for correct grammar and spelling, and overall appearance.
		＊	Made corrections as needed and printed a final copy without errors.
		●	Placed the letter or report in the designated area for physician review and signature.
		＊	Completed the procedure within 15 minutes.
			TOTALS

Evaluation of Student Performance

EVALUATION CRITERIA			COMMENTS
Symbol	Category	Point Value	
＊	Critical Step	16 points	
●	Essential Step	6 points	
▷	Theory Question	2 points	

Score calculation: 100 points

− _____ points missed

_____ Score

Satisfactory score: 85 or above

CAAHEP Competencies Achieved:

Psychomotor (Skills)

☑ IV. 3. Use medical terminology, pronouncing medical terms correctly, to communicate information, patient history, data and observations.

☑ IV. 10. Compose professional/business letters.

ABHES Competencies Achieved:

☑ 8. gg. Use pertinent medical terminology.

☑ 8. jj. Perform fundamental writing skills including correct grammar, spelling, and formatting techniques when writing prescriptions, documenting medical records, etc.

EVALUATION OF COMPETENCY

Procedure 42-4: Sending a Fax

Name: _____   Date: _____

Evaluated By: _____   Date: _____

Performance Objective

Outcome:	Send a fax.
Conditions:	Given the following: fax machine, cover sheet, pen, and document to be faxed.
Standards:	Time: 5 minutes. Student completed procedure in _____ minutes.
	Accuracy: Satisfactory score on the Performance Evaluation Checklist.

Performance Evaluation Checklist

Trial 1	Trial 2	Point Value	Performance Standards
		●	Prepared the cover sheet including name, address, and fax and telephone number of the recipient, telephone number of the sender, and number of pages (including cover sheet).
		●	Placed any message to the sender at the bottom of the cover sheet.
		●	Organized all pages of the fax with the cover sheet first.
		●	Placed pages in the fax machine, face up or face down as required by the machine.
		●	Entered the fax number, including extra digits if required.
		●	Verified that the fax number was correct as it appeared in the window.
		●	Pressed the correct button to send the fax.
		●	Returned to remove the fax and verify that it had been sent.
		●	Filed the original document appropriately.
		∗	Completed the procedure within 5 minutes.
			TOTALS

Evaluation of Student Performance

EVALUATION CRITERIA			COMMENTS
Symbol	**Category**	**Point Value**	
*	Critical Step	16 points	
•	Essential Step	6 points	
▷	Theory Question	2 points	

Score calculation: 100 points

− _____ points missed

_____ Score

Satisfactory score: 85 or above

CAAHEP Competencies Achieved:

Psychomotor (Skills)

☑ IX. 3. Apply HIPAA rules in regard to privacy/release of information.

ABHES Competencies Achieved:

☑ 8. a. Perform basic clerical functions.
☑ 8. ll. Apply electronic technology.

EVALUATION OF COMPETENCY

Procedure 42-5: Preparing Copies of Multiple-Page Documents

Name: _____   Date: _____

Evaluated By: _____   Date: _____

Performance Objective

Outcome:	Copy a document with multiple pages.
Conditions:	Given the following: photocopy machine, paper, document to be copied, stapler, staples, and staple remover.
Standards:	Time: 10 minutes. Student completed procedure in ____ minutes.
	Accuracy: Satisfactory score on the Performance Evaluation Checklist.

Performance Evaluation Checklist

Trial 1	Trial 2	Point Value	Performance Standards
		•	Assembled all pages of the document and removed staples.
		•	Made sure that the copy machine was warmed up.
		•	Placed the originals in the machine according to its directions.
		•	Selected the size, number of copies, and available options to collate and/or staple the copies.
		•	Pressed the "start" button.
		•	Arranged copies in the correct order if needed, and stapled if needed.
		•	Verified number of copies, recorded as needed, and submitted for billing as needed.
		*	Completed the procedure within 10 minutes.
			TOTALS

Evaluation of Student Performance

EVALUATION CRITERIA			COMMENTS
Symbol	Category	Point Value	
*	Critical Step	16 points	
•	Essential Step	6 points	
▷	Theory Question	2 points	
Score calculation: 100 points			
− _____ points missed			
_____ Score			
Satisfactory score: 85 or above			

CAAHEP Competencies Achieved:

Psychomotor (Skills)

☑ IX. 3. Apply HIPAA rules in regard to privacy/release of information.

ABHES Competencies Achieved:

☑ 8. a. Perform basic clerical functions.

43

Mail

CHAPTER ASSIGNMENTS

√ After Completing	Date Due	Textbook Page(s)	TEXTBOOK ASSIGNMENTS	Possible Points	Points You Earned
		1012-1028	Read Chapter 43: Mail		
		1017 1027	📖 Read Case Study 1 Case Study 1 questions	5	
		1018 1027	📖 Read Case Study 2 Case Study 2 questions	5	
		1025 1028	📖 Read Case Study 3 Case Study 3 questions	5	
			TOTAL POINTS		

√ After Completing	Date Due	Study Guide Page(s)	STUDY GUIDE ASSIGNMENTS (CTA: Critical Thinking Activity)	Possible Points	Points You Earned
		1097	📝 Pretest	10	
		1098	🔑 Term Key Term Assessment	7	
		1099-1101	📋 Evaluation of Learning questions	30	
		1101	CTA A: Classifications of Mail	6	
		1101	CTA B: Insurance and Delivery Confirmation Services	6	
		1102	CTA C: Determining Postage	8	
			💿 CD Activity: Chapter 43 Preparing an Envelope (Record points earned)		
			💿 CD Activity: Chapter 43 Apply Your Knowledge questions (Record points earned)		
		1097	📝 Posttest	10	

√ After Completing	Date Due	Study Guide Page(s)	STUDY GUIDE ASSIGNMENTS (CTA: Critical Thinking Activity)	Possible Points	Points You Earned
			ADDITIONAL ASSIGNMENTS		
			TOTAL POINTS		

√ When Assigned by Your Instructor	Study Guide Page(s)	Practices Required	LABORATORY ASSIGNMENTS (Procedure Number and Name)	*Score
	1103	3	🔵 **Practice for Competency** 43-1: Processing Incoming Mail Textbook reference: pp. 1018-1019	
	1105-1106		📋 **Evaluation of Competency** 43-1: Processing Incoming Mail	*
	1103	3	**Practice for Competency** 43-2: Looking Up a ZIP Code Textbook reference: p. 1023	
	1107-1108		📋 **Evaluation of Competency** 43-2: Looking Up a ZIP Code	*
	1103	3	🔵 **Practice for Competency** 43-3: Preparing Envelopes for Mailing Textbook reference: pp. 1025-1026	
	1109-1110		📋 **Evaluation of Competency** 43-3: Preparing Envelopes for Mailing	*
			ADDITIONAL ASSIGNMENTS	

Notes

Name _____

                                                        Date _____

PRETEST

True or False

_____ 1. The ZIP + 4 gives more specific information about the destination of a letter than the 5-digit ZIP code.

_____ 2. The delivery time for Priority Mail is approximately the same as for First-Class Mail.

_____ 3. Standard Mail is used by the medical office to mail packages.

_____ 4. The post office has machines that can read bar codes but not printed addresses.

_____ 5. The attention line of the address is placed directly below the recipient line.

_____ 6. The barcode free area of an envelope is at the lower right side of the envelope.

_____ 7. If the office does not have a typewriter, a label must be prepared to place the address on an envelope.

_____ 8. A letter should be folded first in half and then in thirds to place in a number 6 ¾ envelope.

_____ 9. The medical office may purchase a postage meter for more efficient processing of the mail.

_____ 10. The same postage is required for a large envelope as a standard business envelope of the same weight.

POSTTEST

True or False

_____ 1. A postal bar code is often added to first-class letters by the post office to identify the letter's destination.

_____ 2. The fastest way to send an item through the USPS is Priority Mail.

_____ 3. A Return Receipt is usually combined with Certified Mail for proof of both mailing and receipt.

_____ 4. If the medical assistant opens mail for a physician, each item should be stamped with the date.

_____ 5. The attention line of the address should be placed below and to the left of the city, state, and ZIP line.

_____ 6. The address of an envelope should be printed in uppercase letters for easier optical character recognition.

_____ 7. A letter is folded exactly the same way to place in a window envelope as in a number 6 ¾ envelope.

_____ 8. Postage can be purchased for a postage meter by telephone, through the Internet, or from the post office.

_____ 9. Stamps can be printed in the office using an online postage service.

_____ 10. Postage meters print postage on tapes that are applied to letters but not directly on the envelope.

✦Term KEY TERM ASSESSMENT

Directions: Match each medical term with its definition.

_____ 1. Annotate

_____ 2. Bar code clear zone

_____ 3. Metered mail

_____ 4. Postage meter

_____ 5. Postal bar code

_____ 6. ZIP code

_____ 7. ZIP + 4 code

A. The area on the lower right-hand corner of a card or letter which is left clear for the postal barcode to be printed

B. A more detailed mailing code consisting of the original 5-digit ZIP code followed by a hyphen and four additional digits

C. A 5-digit code that identifies the post office to which a given piece of mail is to be delivered

D. Mail for which the postage has been applied using a postage meter

E. To underline or highlight important words and phrases in correspondence

F. A machine that automatically stamps a piece of mail with the correct postage

G. A series of vertical bars of two lengths, which represent the delivery address of a piece of mail that facilitates automated sorting of mail

EVALUATION OF LEARNING

Directions: Fill in each blank with the correct answer.

1. What is a ZIP + 4 code, and how is it different from a five-digit ZIP code?

    _____

2. How does the USPS use barcodes?

    _____

    _____

3. Describe each of the following classifications of mail:

    Express Mail: _____

    First-Class Mail: _____

    Priority Mail: _____

    Standard Mail: _____

    Parcel Post: _____

    Media Mail: _____

    Bound Printed Matter: _____

4. What is Certified Mail?

    _____

5. Why does the medical office usually use Return Receipt instead of Signature Confirmation to obtain a record of the individual who signed for receipt of a mailed item?

    _____

    _____

6. When is a Certificate of Mailing obtained?

    _____

7. What service limits delivery of an item of mail specifically to the addressee?

    _____

8. What services are included when an item of mail is sent Registered Mail?

    _____

9. What service should be purchased for an item of value sent through the mail?

    _____

10. What are the advantages of using a private delivery service instead of the USPS to deliver packages?

_____

_____

11. What are general guidelines for sorting mail in the medical office?

_____

_____

12. If the MA opens mail for the physician, what should he or she do as soon as each item is opened?

_____

13. How should letters regarding patients be arranged for the physician?

_____

14. Why do some physicians ask the MA to annotate their correspondence?

_____

15. How should the physician's mail be handled when he or she is on vacation?

_____

_____

16. What happens to a piece of mail that has a printed address after it has been mailed?

_____

_____

17. Name three pieces of automated equipment used by the USPS.

_____

18. If an optional attention line is used in an address, where does the USPS recommend that it be placed?

_____

19. What should be included in the bottom line of a delivery address?

_____

20. What is the recommendation regarding punctuation in the address of an envelope?

_____

21. Where should instructions such as *Personal* or *Confidential* be placed on an envelope?

_____

22. Where should instructions for special services such as *Certified* or *Registered* be placed on an envelope?

_____

23. What is the barcode clear zone, and where is it located on an envelope?

_____

24. How does the MA prepare an envelope with the address directly on the envelope?

_____

_____

25. How does the MA prepare envelopes for a mailing of more than 30 envelopes?

_____

_____

26. Describe how to fold a letter for a standard #10 business envelope and for a window envelope.

_____

_____

27. Describe three ways to add postage to envelopes.

_____

_____

28. What are six safety measures to keep in mind when using a postage meter?

_____

_____

_____

29. How can the MA obtain additional postage for a postage meter?

_____

30. What services are offered by online postage services?

_____

_____

CRITICAL THINKING ACTIVITIES

A. CLASSIFICATIONS OF MAIL
Identify the classification of mail you would use to mail each of the following items using the USPS.

1. Patient bill: _____

2. Order form for office supplies: _____

3. Package containing two books (needs to arrive in 2 to 3 days): _____

4. Package containing two books (no rush): _____

5. Specimen for testing (weighs 9 oz): _____

6. Package of office supplies weighing 16 lb: _____

B. INSURANCE AND DELIVERY CONFIRMATION SERVICES
For each of the following items identify whether the item should be insured, if Delivery Confirmation should be obtained, and/or if a Return Receipt should be obtained.

1. X-ray of the hip mailed to another physician: _____

2. Item of jewelry worth $12.00: _____

3. Item of jewelry worth $650.00: _____

4. Letter informing a patient that a physician is retiring: _____

5. Letter informing a patient that he or she must find a new physician for failing to keep appointments: _____

_____

6. Official letter that must be received by a specific deadline: _____

C. DETERMINING POSTAGE

For each of the following, determine the correct postage using the USPS website (www.usps.com).

First Class (rates effective 5/12/08):

1. Letter in a #10 envelope weighing 2 oz from ZIP code 19101 to 60606: _____

2. Letter in a square envelope weighing 1 oz from ZIP code 19101 to 60606: _____

Priority Mail:

3. Package weighing 3 lb 2 oz from ZIP code 19101 to 60606: _____

4. Envelope weighing 14 oz from ZIP code 19101 to 60606: _____

Express Mail:

5. Letter weighing 2 oz (flat rate envelope) from ZIP code 02114 to 90806: _____

6. Letter weighing 2 oz (ordinary envelope) from ZIP code 02114 to 60606: _____

Parcel Post and/or Media Mail:

7. Package of 3 boxes of gloves weighing 3 lb 2 oz from ZIP code 19101 to 60606: _____

8. Package of books weighing 4 lb 8 oz from ZIP code 02114 to 90806: _____

PRACTICE FOR COMPETENCY

Procedure 43-1: Processing Incoming Mail. Process incoming mail.

Procedure 43-2: Looking Up a ZIP Code. Look up ZIP codes to prepare envelopes or mailing labels for Procedure 43-3 using the USPS website (www.usps.com).

Procedure 43-3: Preparing Envelopes for Mailing. Prepare envelopes of various sizes for mailing, weigh, and look up correct postage using the USPS website. Be sure to include ZIP + 4 from Procedure 43-2.

Centers for Disease Control and Prevention
1600 Clifton Road
Atlanta, GA [ZIP + 4]

National Institutes of Health
9000 Rockville Pike
Bethesda, MD [ZIP + 4]

Centers for Medicare and Medicaid Services
7500 Security Boulevard
Baltimore, MD [ZIP + 4]

U.S. Department of Health and Human Services
200 Independence Avenue, S.W.
Washington, DC [ZIP + 4]

Notes

EVALUATION OF COMPETENCY

Procedure 43-1: Processing Incoming Mail

Name: _____   Date: _____

Evaluated By: _____   Date: _____

Performance Objective

Outcome:	Process incoming mail.
Conditions:	Given the following: letter opener, date stamp, stamp pad, paper clips, stapler, pen or highlighter, and transparent tape.
Standards:	Time: 10 minutes. Student completed procedure in ____ minutes.
	Accuracy: Satisfactory score on the Performance Evaluation Checklist.

Performance Evaluation Checklist

Trial 1	Trial 2	Point Value	Performance Standards
		•	Assembled supplies in a work area large enough to make several piles.
		•	Arranged all envelopes so they faced in the same direction.
		•	Placed any envelopes marked "personal" or "confidential" to the side.
		•	Tapped the lower edge of the first envelope on the desk so contents fell to the bottom.
		•	Removed the contents of the envelope.
		•	Checked to make sure the envelope was empty.
		•	Unfolded and flattened contents of the envelope.
		•	Stamped the date on the first page, preferably in the upper right corner.
		•	Checked to be sure the letter contained an inside address.
		•	Discarded the envelope if the letter contained an inside address; if not, stapled the envelope to the letter.
		•	Fastened enclosures to the letter with a paper clip.
		•	If enclosures not found, wrote "no" beside the enclosure notation.
		•	Mended any tears with tape.
		•	Used a highlighter or pen to annotate important points if directed to by the physician.
		•	Attached a sticky note indicating action that should be taken in response to the correspondence as needed.
		•	Opened additional envelopes in the same way until all mail was opened.
		•	Separated mail into piles of urgent mail, letters or reports containing patient information or results, medical journals, advertising, and other categories as needed.
		•	Arranged letters and reports containing patient information in alphabetical order.

Trial 1	Trial 2	Point Value	Performance Standards
		•	Found and used a paper clip to attach the appropriate medical record to each letter or report containing medical information.
		•	Arranged the mail for each recipient from most important on top to least important on the bottom.
		•	Distributed each stack of mail to the appropriate individual.
		*	Completed the procedure within 10 minutes.
			TOTALS

Evaluation of Student Performance

EVALUATION CRITERIA			COMMENTS
Symbol	**Category**	**Point Value**	
*	Critical Step	16 points	
•	Essential Step	6 points	
▷	Theory Question	2 points	
Score calculation: 100 points			
–_____ points missed			
_____ Score			
Satisfactory score: 85 or above			

CAAHEP Competencies Achieved:

Psychomotor (Skills)
☑ IX. 3. Apply HIPAA rules in regard to privacy/release of information.

ABHES Competencies Achieved:

☑ 8. a. Perform basic clerical functions.

☑ EVALUATION OF COMPETENCY

Procedure 43-2: Looking Up a ZIP Code

Name: _____   Date: _____

Evaluated By: _____   Date: _____

Performance Objective

Outcome:	Find the correct ZIP + 4 code for a given address.
Conditions:	Given the following: computer with Internet access, pen and pencil, address with incorrect and/or missing ZIP code.
Standards:	Time: 3 minutes. Student completed procedure in ____ minutes.
	Accuracy: Satisfactory score on the Performance Evaluation Checklist.

Performance Evaluation Checklist

Trial 1	Trial 2	Point Value	Performance Standards
		●	Opened the computer's web browser and entered the web address for the United States Postal Service.
		●	From the USPS home page, selected "Find a ZIP code."
		●	On the "Search by Address" tab, entered the complete delivery address.
		✶	Copied the correct ZIP + 4 code on a piece of paper or used the computer copy function to copy and past into a computer file.
		✶	Completed the procedure within 3 minutes.
			TOTALS

Evaluation of Student Performance

EVALUATION CRITERIA			COMMENTS
Symbol	Category	Point Value	
✶	Critical Step	16 points	
●	Essential Step	6 points	
▷	Theory Question	2 points	
Score calculation: 100 points			
–_____ points missed			
_____ Score			
Satisfactory score: 85 or above			

CAAHEP Competencies Achieved:

Psychomotor (Skills)

☑ V. 7. Use internet to access information related to the medical office.

ABHES Competencies Achieved:

☑ 8. a. Perform basic clerical functions.

EVALUATION OF COMPETENCY

Procedure 43-3: Preparing Envelopes for Mailing

Name: _____   Date: _____

Evaluated By: _____   Date: _____

Performance Objective

Outcome:	Prepare envelopes for mailing.
Conditions:	Given the following: Envelope, other items to be mailed, pen, typewriter, computer and printer, postal scale, postage meter (optional), and/or stamps.
Standards:	Time: 3 minutes. Student completed procedure in _____ minutes.
	Accuracy: Satisfactory score on the Performance Evaluation Checklist.

Performance Evaluation Checklist

Trial 1	Trial 2	Point Value	Performance Standards
		•	Determined the exact address to be used for the envelope.
		•	Selected an envelope of the appropriate size.
		•	Decided on a means to address the envelope (e.g., typewriter, envelope wizard, label template, label program).
		*	Keyed or typed the address correctly according to USPS guidelines including the ZIP + 4 code.
		•	Added any special notations such as "personal" or "confidential" below the return address in the upper left corner of the envelope.
		•	Added any mailing instructions on the right side of the envelope below the postage area.
		•	Folded and placed the letter or item to be mailed in the envelope and sealed it.
		•	Weighed the piece of mail if it contained more than two sheets of paper or if the envelope was larger than 6 ⅛" × 11 ½".
		•	Calculated and applied the correct amount of postage.
		•	If a postage meter was used, processed all envelopes to be mailed that day.
		•	Sorted envelopes and other items to be mailed according to size.
		•	Separated any items with special mailing instructions to be taken to the post office.
		•	Placed items with postage in a mailbox or requested a pick-up from the postal service.
		•	Set special items aside to be taken to the post office.
		*	Completed the procedure within 10 minutes.
			TOTALS

Evaluation of Student Performance

EVALUATION CRITERIA			COMMENTS
Symbol	Category	Point Value	
*	Critical Step	16 points	
•	Essential Step	6 points	
▷	Theory Question	2 points	

Score calculation: 100 points

− _____ points missed

_____ Score

Satisfactory score: 85 or above

CAAHEP Competencies Achieved:

Psychomotor (Skills)
☑ IV. 10. Compose professional/business letters.

ABHES Competencies Achieved:

☑ 8. a. Perform basic clerical functions.

44

Managing Practice Finances

CHAPTER ASSIGNMENTS

√ After Completing	Date Due	Textbook Page(s)	TEXTBOOK ASSIGNMENTS	Possible Points	Points You Earned
		1029-1055	Read Chapter 44: Managing Practice Finances		
		1034 1054	📖 Read Case Study 1 Case Study 1 questions	5	
		1035 1054	📖 Read Case Study 2 Case Study 2 questions	5	
		1047 1054	📖 Read Case Study 3 Case Study 3 questions	5	
			TOTAL POINTS		

√ After Completing	Date Due	Study Guide Page(s)	STUDY GUIDE ASSIGNMENTS (CTA: Critical Thinking Activity)	Possible Points	Points You Earned
		1115	📝 Pretest	10	
		1116	🔑 Key Term Assessment	25	
		1117-1119	📋 Evaluation of Learning questions	28	
		1120	CTA A: The Charge Slip	8	
		1120	CTA B: Posting Transactions	8	
		1120	CTA C: Writing Checks	6	
		1120-1121	CTA D: Endorsing Checks	6	
			💿 CD Activity: Chapter 44 Completing a Charge Slip and Posting Entries on a Day Sheet (Record points earned)		
			💿 CD Activity: Chapter 44 Posting Insurance Payments and Adjustments (Record points earned)		

√ After Completing	Date Due	Study Guide Page(s)	STUDY GUIDE ASSIGNMENTS (CTA: Critical Thinking Activity)	Possible Points	Points You Earned
			CD CD Activity: Chapter 44 Balancing a Day Sheet (Record points earned)		
			CD CD Activity: Chapter 44 Preparing a Bank Deposit	10	
			CD CD Activity: Chapter 44 Reconciling a Bank Statement	10	
			CD CD Activity: Chapter 44 Writing Checks in Payment of Bills	10	
			CD CD Activity: Chapter 44 Apply Your Knowledge questions (Record points earned)		
		1115	Posttest	10	
			ADDITIONAL ASSIGNMENTS		
			TOTAL POINTS		

√ When Assigned by Your Instructor	Study Guide Page(s)	Practices Required	LABORATORY ASSIGNMENTS (Procedure Number and Name)	*Score
	1124	3	📀 **Practice for Competency** 44-1: Completing a Patient Charge Slip Textbook reference: pp. 1037-1038	
	1143-1144		📖 **Evaluation of Competency** 44-1: Completing a Patient Charge Slip	*
	1124	3	**Practice for Competency** 44-2: Posting Charges to the Patient Ledger Textbook reference: p. 1038	
	1145-1146		📖 **Evaluation of Competency** 44-2: Posting Charges to the Patient Ledger	*
	1131	3	**Practice for Competency** 44-3: Posting Payments and/or Adjustments Textbook reference: pp. 1039-1040	
	1147-1148		📖 **Evaluation of Competency** 44-3: Posting Payments and/or Adjustments	*
	1131	3	**Practice for Competency** 44-4: Recording a Patient's Visit on the Day Sheet Textbook reference: pp. 1040-1042	
	1149-1150		📖 **Evaluation of Competency** 44-4: Recording a Patient's Visit on the Day Sheet	*
	1135	1	**Practice for Competency** 44-5: Balancing the Day Sheet Textbook reference: pp. 1042-1043	
	1151-1152		📖 **Evaluation of Competency** 44-5: Balancing the Day Sheet	*
	1135	3	**Practice for Competency** 44-6: Writing a Check Textbook reference: pp. 1050-1051	
	1153-1154		📖 **Evaluation of Competency** 44-6: Writing a Check	*
	1135	1	📀 **Practice for Competency** 44-7: Preparing a Bank Deposit Textbook reference: p. 1051	
	1155-1156		📖 **Evaluation of Competency** 44-7: Preparing a Bank Deposit	*
	1135	1	**Practice for Competency** 44-8: Reconciling a Bank Statement Textbook reference: p. 1052	

√ When Assigned by Your Instructor	Study Guide Page(s)	Practices Required	LABORATORY ASSIGNMENTS (Procedure Number and Name)	*Score
	1157-1158		📖 **Evaluation of Competency** 44-8: Reconciling a Bank Statement	*
			ADDITIONAL ASSIGNMENTS	

Name _____ Date_____

PRETEST

True or False

_____   1. In the cash basis of accounting, income is entered when an item is sold or a service is provided.

_____   2. Money owed to the medical practice by patients makes up accounts receivable.

_____   3. Medical billing programs are usually based on the traditional pegboard system of bookkeeping.

_____   4. A superbill contains a list of procedures commonly performed in the medical office.

_____   5. An adjustment always reduces the balance of a patient's account.

_____   6. If a computer billing program is used, the office will not create a manual day sheet.

_____   7. A money market account usually has features of both a savings account and a checking account.

_____   8. Each bank in the United States has a unique identification number.

_____   9. Business accounting programs can often create and print checks.

_____   10. To replenish the petty cash fund, the medical assistant can use any cash payment by a patient.

POSTTEST

True or False

_____   1. If income is entered when an item is sold, the accrual basis of accounting is being used.

_____   2. Each patient account is one of the accounts payable.

_____   3. A daily journal is a chronological record of charges and payments for each day.

_____   4. A superbill is an itemized charge slip.

_____   5. The patient ledger records the charges and payments for a patient on a specific day.

_____   6. The proof of posting section of a manual day sheet verifies that all columns were totaled correctly.

_____   7. In order to receive interest on a checking account, it is usually necessary to maintain a minimum balance.

_____   8. The MICR line is printed in magnetic ink across the bottom of a check.

_____   9. If the medical assistant makes a mistake on a check, the check should be shredded or destroyed.

_____   10. Every time money is taken from petty cash, a receipt should be completed.

Term **KEY TERM ASSESSMENT**

Directions: Match each medical term with its definition.

_____ 1. ABA routing number

_____ 2. Accounting

_____ 3. Accounts payable

_____ 4. Accounts receivable

_____ 5. Accrual basis of accounting

_____ 6. Adjustment

_____ 7. Assets

_____ 8. Bookkeeping

_____ 9. Cash basis of accounting

_____ 10. Cashier's check

_____ 11. Certified check

_____ 12. Charge slip

_____ 13. Credit

_____ 14. Day sheet

_____ 15. Debit

_____ 16. Disbursements

_____ 17. Fee schedule

_____ 18. Ledger

_____ 19. Liabilities

_____ 20. MICR line

_____ 21. Payee

_____ 22. Petty cash

_____ 23. Proof of posting

_____ 24. Reconciling

_____ 25. Superbill

A. Accounting method where income is entered when payment is received

B. A posting that is subtracted from an account balance

C. Accounting method where income is entered at the time of sale

D. An itemized charge slip usually also containing diagnosis codes and procedure codes

E. A form used to keep track of charges and payments at the time of a patient visit

F. A nine-digit number that identifies an individual bank

G. In accounting, the amount owed by a business to creditors

H. A check on an individual account that a bank assumes responsibility for

I. The person to whom a check is made out

J. A line of numbers across the bottom of a check that are read by a magnetic character reader

K. A cash account kept in a business office to pay for incidentals

L. A change to a patient account that is neither a charge nor a payment

M. List of charges for specific procedures that may be performed in a medical office

N. In accounting, a combination of property owned and money owed to a business

O. The outstanding bills of a business such as a medical office

P. Money paid out

Q. A posting that is added to an account balance

R. Making sure that two financial records agree

S. Systematic recording and reporting of financial transactions

T. A book, card, or computer account used to record financial transactions

U. The process of recording financial transactions and keeping financial records

V. The chronological record of daily transactions

W. A process of calculation to verify that all totals on a day sheet are correct

X. Total amount owed to a business for goods and services

Y. A check drawn on a bank instead of an individual account

EVALUATION OF LEARNING

Directions: Fill in each blank with the correct answer.

1. What is the difference between the cash basis and the accrual basis of accounting?

    _____

    _____

2. What is the origin of income in the medical office?

    _____

    _____

3. If patient charges are recorded manually using a pegboard system, in what three places are these charges usually recorded?

    _____

    _____

4. If patient charges are recorded using a computer billing program, where must the data about the charge be entered? Why is it sufficient to enter the data once?

    _____

    _____

5. Why does a charge slip (superbill) usually contain diagnosis and procedure codes?

    _____

    _____

6. How does the medical assistant (MA) know what to charge a patient for a specific procedure?

    _____

    _____

7. If the office typically charges $30.00 to perform an electrocardiogram, is this the amount paid by all patients? Why or why not?

    _____

    _____

8. How is information arranged in the patient ledger?

    _____

9. What are four ways that payments are made to a patient account?

    _____

    _____

10. What is the difference between a credit adjustment and a debit adjustment? Give one example of each.

_____

_____

11. When an insurance company pays an amount that is lower than the usual charge, how is the patient's balance due returned to zero?

_____

_____

12. What information is recorded on a day sheet?

_____

13. What is the purpose of completing the proof of posting section at the bottom of a day sheet?

_____

_____

14. What does it mean to "close the day," and why is this important for accurate financial record keeping?

_____

_____

15. Describe three types of bank accounts.

_____

_____

_____

16. Describe the services and function of a checking account.

_____

17. What is the advantage of maintaining a savings account or money market account compared with a checking account?

_____

_____

18. Differentiate between a cashier's check and a certified check. Which is used more often?

_____

_____

19. What is the MICR line on a check, and what information does it contain?

_____

_____

20. Identify four ways that checks can be generated or bills can be paid, and describe how information is recorded.

_____

_____

_____

_____

21. What should the MA do if he or she writes a check incorrectly?

_____

_____

22. Who signs the checks to pay bills for a medical practice?

_____

23. What is necessary before a check can be cashed or deposited? How is this handled in a medical office?

_____

_____

24. What is the difference between a special endorsement and a restricted endorsement?

_____

_____

25. Identify five reasons why the monthly bank statement may not agree with the medical office's calculation of the bank balance in a checking account.

_____

_____

_____

26. What steps must be taken to reconcile a bank account?

_____

_____

_____

27. What financial accounts does a medical office usually have, and what do those accounts include?

_____

_____

28. How is a petty cash fund (account) managed?

_____

_____

_____

CRITICAL THINKING ACTIVITIES

A. THE CHARGE SLIP
Refer to the completed charge slip in your textbook (Figure 44-2), and identify the following information.

1. The name of the insured person: _____

2. The patient's insurance ID number: _____

3. The charge for the patient's office visit: _____

4. The patient's telephone number: _____

5. The name of the diagnostic test performed: _____

6. The balance owed by the patient: _____

7. The patient's birth date: _____

8. The patient's physician: _____

B. POSTING TRANSACTIONS
Identify whether each of the following transactions would be posted as a charge, a payment, or an adjustment in the computer billing program or on a pegboard day sheet.

1. Office visit: _____

2. Check from insurance company: _____

3. Tetanus injection: _____

4. Dipstick urinalysis: _____

5. Insurance excluded amount: _____

6. Professional courtesy discount: _____

7. Spirometry test: _____

8. Patient check: _____

C. WRITING CHECKS
Demonstrate how to write the following amounts in words on a check.

1. $76.42 _____ DOLLARS

2. $189.28 _____ DOLLARS

3. $1,020.00 _____ DOLLARS

4. $6.40 _____ DOLLARS

5. $16.04 _____ DOLLARS

6. $382.00 _____ DOLLARS

D. ENDORSING CHECKS
Identify if each of the following is a blank endorsement, restrictive endorsement, or special endorsement:

1. *Maria S. Sanchez* _____

2. Pay to the order of: Robert A. Wilson

   Maria S. Sanchez _____

3. *Robert A. Wilson*

   Acct. # 12345-67890 _____

4. For deposit only

   Robert A. Wilson _____

5. Pay to the order of: Diane M. Casey

Frederick Underwood _____

6. For deposit Acct. # 23456-78901

Edward B. Young _____

Notes

PRACTICE FOR COMPETENCY

Use the following information to practice Procedures 44-1 through 44-5. Use today's date for all work.

FEE SCHEDULE

OFFICE VISIT, NEW PATIENT			OFFICE VISIT, ESTABLISHED PATIENT	
			99211 Nurse/Minimal OV	$ 40.00
99201	Problem Focused OV	$ 55.00	99212 Problem Focused OV	$ 50.00
99202	Exp Problem Focused OV	$ 70.00	99213 Exp Problem Focused OV	$ 65.00
OFFICE PROCEDURES				
36415	Venipuncture Collection	$ 12.00	93000 ECG (Global)	$ 65.00
81002	Urinalysis (Dip only)	$ 15.00	94010 Pulmonary Function (spirometry)	$ 50.00
87880	Strep test (rapid)	$ 30.00	94640 Inhalation Treatment	$ 45.00

PATIENT INFORMATION

June Simmons
16 Winston Terrace
Western, XY 44770
(490) 459-1000
DOB: 2/23/1962
Diagnosis: Hypertension, primary
Procedures: Problem-focused office visit
Previous Balance: $45.00
Payment: $10.00 by patient check on
  bank #242-XX/110

Patient Number: 1010
Established Patient of Dr. Warner
Name of Insured: self
Insurance Plan: Standard Health HMO (490) 459-3344
Insurance ID # 10229876 Group # 45215

Robert Underwood
224 Lakeview Drive
Western, XY 44770
(490) 459-1111
DOB: 1/31/1992
Diagnosis: Streptococcal sore throat
Procedures: Problem-focused office visit,
  Strep test (rapid)
Previous Balance: -0-
Payment: $70.00 by check on
  bank # 02-XX/502
Cash Discount: - $15.00 (credit adjustment)

Patient Number: 5010
New Patient of Dr. Gomez
Name of Insured: N/A
Insurance Plan: None
Policy #: None

James Winston
25 Magnolia Lane
Western, XY 44770
(490) 459-1222
DOB: 12/14/40
Diagnoses: Angina pectoris; Hypertension,
  benign
Procedures: Expanded problem-focused
  office visit, ECG
Previous Balance: $15.00

Patient Number: 1020
Established Patient of Dr. Gomez
Name of Insured: self
Insurance Plan: Medicare (490) 555-2800
Policy # 000-70-7000A

Marie Richards
19 Maple Street
Western, XY 44770
(490) 459-1333
DOB: 8/22/82
Previous Balance:
Insurance Payment for Visit 9/02/XX:
Insurance Excluded Amount:

Patient Number: 3020
Established Patient of Dr. Warner
Name of Insured: John Richards
Insurance Plan: Standard Health HMO

$39.00
$26.00 by check on bank #602-XX/110
$13.00

Procedure 44-1: Completing a Patient Charge Slip. Fill out charge slips for June Simmons, Robert Underwood, and James Winston using today's date and time, using the forms on pages 1125-1129.

Procedure 44-2: Posting Charges to the Patient Ledger. Post charges for June Simmons, Robert Underwood, and James Winston for the information above. Use a separate ledger for each patient. For charges, use the CPT code.

Transaction Entry

Date	Pt #	Patient Name	Provider	Code	Description	Amount

Transaction Entry

Date	Pt #	Patient Name	Provider	Code	Description	Amount

Transaction Entry

Date	Pt #	Patient Name	Provider	Code	Description	Amount

Western Medical Center
109 River Street
Western, XY 44770
(490) 555-6464

Richard Warner, MD   NPI # 23456781XX
Maria Gomez, MD   NPI # 34567891XX
TAX ID 52-XX63777

PATIENT NAME AND ADDRESS	BIRTHDATE	SUBSCRIBER NAME	MD NAME	TODAY'S DATE
	ACCOUNT #	INSURANCE COMPANY	INSURANCE PHONE #	TIME
TELEPHONE NO. ( )		INSURANCE ID #	GROUP/PLAN #	SEX MALE ☐ FEMALE ☐

√	DESCRIPTION	CPT	FEE	√	DESCRIPTION	CPT	FEE	√	DESCRIPTION	CPT	FEE
	OFFICE VISIT				**IMMUNIZATIONS**				**PROCEDURES**		
	NEW PATIENT				Imm. admin, one	90471			EKG w// interpretation	93000	
	Problem Focused	99201			Imm. admin, each add'l	90472			Spirometry	94010	
	Exp. Prob. Focused	99202			Influenza < 3	90657			Inhalation treatment	94640	
	Detailed	99203			Influenza 3 and >	90658			Remove skin tag < 15	11200	
	Comp/ Mod MDM	99204			Medicare code	G0008			Cerumen removal	69210	
	Comp./ High MDM	99205			Varicella	90716			Wart destruction < 14	17110	
	ESTABLISHED PATIENT				DTaP	90700			I & D abscess	10060	
	Minimal / Nurse Visit	99211			Td adult	90718					
	Problem Focused	99212			Rubella	90706					
	Exp. Problem Focused	99213			MMR	90707			**LABORATORY**		
	Detailed	99214			Hep B Child	90744			Blood collection Vein	36415	
	Comprehensive	99215			Hep B Adult	90746			Strep, rapid	87880	
	Post-op Exam	99024	0.00		IPV	90713			UA, dipstick	81000	

DIAGNOSTIC CODES (ICD-9-CM)

☐ 789.0 Abdominal Pain	☐ 562.11 Diverticulitis	☐ 724.2 Low Back Pain	☐ 034.0 Streptococcal Sore Throat
☐ 795.0 Abnormal Pap Smear	☐ 562.10 Diverticulosis	☐ 424.0 Mitral Valve Prolapse	☐ 785.6 Swollen Glands
☐ 706.1 Acne	☐ 782.3 Edema	☐ 715.90 Osteoarthritis, Unspec	☐ 598.0 Urinary Tract Infection
☐ 477.9 Allergic Rhinitis	☐ 492.8 Emphysema	☐ 733.00 Osteoporosis, Unspec	☐ V06.8 Vaccination, Combination
☐ 285.9 Anemia, NOS	☐ V18.0 Family History of Diabetes	☐ 627.1 Postmenopausal Bleeding	☐ V04.8 Vaccination, Influenza
☐ 282.6 Anemia, Sickle Cell	☐ 744.0 Headache	☐ 569.3 Rectal Bleeding	☐ V20.2 Well Child Check
☐ 413.9 Angina Pectoris	☐ 070.1 Hepatits, type A	☐ 714.0 Rheumatoid Arthritis	☐ V70.0 Well Adult
☐ 427.9 Arrhythmia, NOS	☐ 054.9 Herpes Simplex	☐ 706.2 Sebaceous Cyst	☐ ____ _____
☐ 440.9 Arteriosclerosis	☐ 708.9 Hives/Urticaria	☐ 431.9 Sinusitis, Acute, NOS	☐ ____ _____
☐ 414.0 ASHD	☐ 401.1 Hypertension, Benign	☐ 701.9 Skin Tag(s)	☐ ____ _____
☐ 493.9 Asthma, Unspecified	☐ 401.0 Hypertension, Malignant	☐ 707.9 Skin Ulcer	☐ ____ _____
☐ 466.0 Bronchitis, Acute	☐ 244.9 Hypothyroidism, Primary	☐ 845.00 Sprain, Ankle	☐ ____ _____
☐ 491.2 Bronchitis, chronic obstr.	☐ 380.4 Impacted Cerumen	☐ 848.9 Sprain, Muscle, Unspec.	☐ ____ _____
☐ 786.50 Chest Pain	☐ 487.1 Influenza		
☐ 250.01 Diabetes I	☐ 564.1 Irritable Bowel Syndrome		
Uncomplicated	☐ 464.0 Laryngitis, Acute		
☐ 250.00 Diabetes II	☐ Laryngopharyngitis, acute		
Uncomplicated	☐ 454.9 Leg Varicose Veins		

RETURN APPOINTMENT	**BALANCE DUE**	
_____ Days	Total Charge	$
_____ Weeks	Amount Paid	$
_____ Months	Previous Bal	$
_____ PRN	Adjustment	$
	Balance Due	$

Notes

Western Medical Center
109 River Street
Western, XY 44770
(490) 555-6464

Richard Warner, MD   NPI # 23456781XX
Maria Gomez, MD   NPI # 34567891XX
TAX ID 52-XX63777

PATIENT NAME AND ADDRESS	BIRTHDATE	SUBSCRIBER NAME	MD NAME	TODAY'S DATE
	ACCOUNT #	INSURANCE COMPANY	INSURANCE PHONE #	TIME
TELEPHONE NO.		INSURANCE ID #	GROUP/PLAN #	SEX
( )				MALE ☐ FEMALE ☐

√	DESCRIPTION	CPT	FEE	√	DESCRIPTION	CPT	FEE	√	DESCRIPTION	CPT	FEE
	OFFICE VISIT				**IMMUNIZATIONS**				**PROCEDURES**		
	NEW PATIENT				Imm. admin, one	90471			EKG w// interpretation	93000	
	Problem Focused	99201			Imm. admin, each add'l	90472			Spirometry	94010	
	Exp. Prob. Focused	99202			Influenza < 3	90657			Inhalation treatment	94640	
	Detailed	99203			Influenza 3 and >	90658			Remove skin tag < 15	11200	
	Comp/ Mod MDM	99204			Medicare code	G0008			Cerumen removal	69210	
	Comp./ High MDM	99205			Varicella	90716			Wart destruction < 14	17110	
	ESTABLISHED PATIENT				DTaP	90700			I & D abscess	10060	
	Minimal / Nurse Visit	99211			Td adult	90718					
	Problem Focused	99212			Rubella	90706			**LABORATORY**		
	Exp. Problem Focused	99213			MMR	90707			Blood collection Vein	36415	
	Detailed	99214			Hep B Child	90744			Strep, rapid	87880	
	Comprehensive	99215			Hep B Adult	90746			UA, dipstick	81000	
	Post-op Exam	99024	0.00		IPV	90713					

DIAGNOSTIC CODES (ICD-9-CM)			
☐ 789.0 Abdominal Pain	☐ 562.11 Diverticulitis	☐ 724.2 Low Back Pain	☐ 034.0 Streptococcal Sore Throat
☐ 795.0 Abnormal Pap Smear	☐ 562.10 Diverticulosis	☐ 424.0 Mitral Valve Prolapse	☐ 785.6 Swollen Glands
☐ 706.1 Acne	☐ 782.3 Edema	☐ 715.90 Osteoarthritis, Unspec	☐ 598.0 Urinary Tract Infection
☐ 477.9 Allergic Rhinitis	☐ 492.8 Emphysema	☐ 733.00 Osteoporosis, Unspec	☐ V06.8 Vaccination, Combination
☐ 285.9 Anemia, NOS	☐ V18.0 Family History of Diabetes	☐ 627.1 Postmenopausal Bleeding	☐ V04.8 Vaccination, Influenza
☐ 282.6 Anemia, Sickle Cell	☐ 744.0 Headache	☐ 569.3 Rectal Bleeding	☐ V20.2 Well Child Check
☐ 413.9 Angina Pectoris	☐ 070.1 Hepatits, type A	☐ 714.0 Rheumatoid Arthritis	☐ V70.0 Well Adult
☐ 427.9 Arrhythmia, NOS	☐ 054.9 Herpes Simplex	☐ 706.2 Sebaceous Cyst	☐ ____ _____
☐ 440.9 Arteriosclerosis	☐ 708.9 Hives/Urticaria	☐ 431.9 Sinusitis, Acute, NOS	☐ ____ _____
☐ 414.0 ASHD	☐ 401.1 Hypertension, Benign	☐ 701.9 Skin Tag(s)	☐ ____ _____
☐ 493.9 Asthma, Unspecified	☐ 401.0 Hypertension, Malignant	☐ 707.9 Skin Ulcer	☐ ____ _____
☐ 466.0 Bronchitis, Acute	☐ 244.9 Hypothyroidism, Primary	☐ 845.00 Sprain, Ankle	☐ ____ _____
☐ 491.2 Bronchitis, chronic obstr.	☐ 380.4 Impacted Cerumen	☐ 848.9 Sprain, Muscle, Unspec.	☐ ____ _____

☐ 786.50 Chest Pain	☐ 487.1 Influenza	**RETURN APPOINTMENT**	**BALANCE DUE**	
☐ 250.01 Diabetes I	☐ 564.1 Irritable Bowel Syndrome	_____ Days	Total Charge	$
Uncomplicated	☐ 464.0 Laryngitis, Acute	_____ Weeks	Amount Paid	$
☐ 250.00 Diabetes II	☐ Laryngopharyngitis, acute	_____ Months	Previous Bal	$
Uncomplicated	☐ 454.9 Leg Varicose Veins	_____ PRN	Adjustment	$
			Balance Due	$

Notes

Western Medical Center
109 River Street
Western, XY 44770
(490) 555-6464

Richard Warner, MD NPI # 23456781XX
Maria Gomez, MD   NPI # 34567891XX
TAX ID 52-XX63777

PATIENT NAME AND ADDRESS	BIRTHDATE	SUBSCRIBER NAME	MD NAME	TODAY'S DATE
	ACCOUNT #	INSURANCE COMPANY	INSURANCE PHONE #	TIME
TELEPHONE NO.		INSURANCE ID #	GROUP/PLAN #	SEX
( )				MALE ☐ FEMALE ☐

√	DESCRIPTION	CPT	FEE	√	DESCRIPTION	CPT	FEE	√	DESCRIPTION	CPT	FEE
	OFFICE VISIT				**IMMUNIZATIONS**				**PROCEDURES**		
	NEW PATIENT				Imm. admin, one	90471			EKG w/// interpretation	93000	
	Problem Focused	99201			Imm. admin, each add'l	90472			Spirometry	94010	
	Exp. Prob. Focused	99202			Influenza < 3	90657			Inhalation treatment	94640	
	Detailed	99203			Influenza 3 and >	90658			Remove skin tag < 15	11200	
	Comp/ Mod MDM	99204			Medicare code	G0008			Cerumen removal	69210	
	Comp./ High MDM	99205			Varicella	90716			Wart destruction < 14	17110	
	ESTABLISHED PATIENT				DTaP	90700			I & D abscess	10060	
	Minimal / Nurse Visit	99211			Td adult	90718					
	Problem Focused	99212			Rubella	90706					
	Exp. Problem Focused	99213			MMR	90707			**LABORATORY**		
	Detailed	99214			Hep B Child	90744			Blood collection Vein	36415	
	Comprehensive	99215			Hep B Adult	90746			Strep, rapid	87880	
	Post-op Exam	99024	0.00		IPV	90713			UA, dipstick	81000	

DIAGNOSTIC CODES (ICD-9-CM)

☐ 789.0 Abdominal Pain	☐ 562.11 Diverticulitis	☐ 724.2 Low Back Pain	☐ 034.0 Streptococcal Sore Throat
☐ 795.0 Abnormal Pap Smear	☐ 562.10 Diverticulosis	☐ 424.0 Mitral Valve Prolapse	☐ 785.6 Swollen Glands
☐ 706.1 Acne	☐ 782.3 Edema	☐ 715.90 Osteoarthritis, Unspec	☐ 598.0 Urinary Tract Infection
☐ 477.9 Allergic Rhinitis	☐ 492.8 Emphysema	☐ 733.00 Osteoporosis, Unspec	☐ V06.8 Vaccination, Combination
☐ 285.9 Anemia, NOS	☐ V18.0 Family History of Diabetes	☐ 627.1 Postmenopausal Bleeding	☐ V04.8 Vaccination, Influenza
☐ 282.6 Anemia, Sickle Cell	☐ 744.0 Headache	☐ 569.3 Rectal Bleeding	☐ V20.2 Well Child Check
☐ 413.9 Angina Pectoris	☐ 070.1 Hepatits, type A	☐ 714.0 Rheumatoid Arthritis	☐ V70.0 Well Adult
☐ 427.9 Arrhythmia, NOS	☐ 054.9 Herpes Simplex	☐ 706.2 Sebaceous Cyst	☐ ____ _____
☐ 440.9 Arteriosclerosis	☐ 708.9 Hives/Urticaria	☐ 431.9 Sinusitis, Acute, NOS	☐ ____ _____
☐ 414.0 ASHD	☐ 401.1 Hypertension, Benign	☐ 701.9 Skin Tag(s)	☐ ____ _____
☐ 493.9 Asthma, Unspecified	☐ 401.0 Hypertension, Malignant	☐ 707.9 Skin Ulcer	☐ ____ _____
☐ 466.0 Bronchitis, Acute	☐ 244.9 Hypothyroidism, Primary	☐ 845.00 Sprain, Ankle	☐ ____ _____
☐ 491.2 Bronchitis, chronic obstr.	☐ 380.4 Impacted Cerumen	☐ 848.9 Sprain, Muscle, Unspec.	☐ ____ _____
☐ 786.50 Chest Pain	☐ 487.1 Influenza		
☐ 250.01 Diabetes I	☐ 564.1 Irritable Bowel Syndrome		
Uncomplicated	☐ 464.0 Laryngitis, Acute		
☐ 250.00 Diabetes II	☐ Laryngopharyngitis, acute		
Uncomplicated	☐ 454.9 Leg Varicose Veins		

RETURN APPOINTMENT		BALANCE DUE	
_____ Days		Total Charge	$
_____ Weeks		Amount Paid	$
_____ Months		Previous Bal	$
_____ PRN		Adjustment	$
		Balance Due	$

Notes

Procedure 44-3: Posting Payments and/or Adjustments. Post payment (CHECK) for June Simmons. Post payment (CHECK) and credit adjustment (CRADJ) for Robert Richardson. Post insurance payment (INSPAY) and insurance adjustment (INSADJ) for Marie Richards. Use a separate ledger for each payment. The codes are given in parentheses.

Transaction Entry

Date	Pt #	Patient Name	Provider	Code	Description	Amount

Transaction Entry

Date	Pt #	Patient Name	Provider	Code	Description	Amount

Transaction Entry

Date	Pt #	Patient Name	Provider	Code	Description	Amount

Procedure 44-4: Recording a Patient's Visit on the Day Sheet. Record information for June Simmons, Robert Underwood, James Winston, and Marie Richards on the following day sheet.

Notes

PLACE
FIRST PEG
HERE

JOURNAL OF DAILY CHARGES, PAYMENTS & DEPOSITS

	DATE	PROFESSIONAL SERVICE	FEE	PAYMENT	ADJUST-MENT	NEW BALANCE	OLD BALANCE	PATIENT'S NAME	
1									1
2									2
3									3
4									4
5									5
6									6
7									7
8									8
9									9
10									10
11									11
12									12
13									13
14									14
15									15
16									16
17									17
18									18
19									19
20									20
21									21
22									22
23									23
24									24
25									25
26									26
27									27
28									28
29									29
30									30
31								TOTALS THIS PAGE	31
32								TOTALS PREVIOUS PAGE	32
33								TOTALS MONTH TO DATE	33

COLUMN A   COLUMN B   COLUMN C   COLUMN D   COLUMN E

MEMO _____

DAILY-FROM LINE 31	
ARITHMETIC POSTING PROOF	
Column E	
Plus Column A	
Sub-Total	
Minus Column B	
Sub-Total	
Minus Column C	
Equals Column D	

Box 1

MONTH-FROM LINE 31	
ARITHMETIC POSTING PROOF	
Accts. Receivable Previous Day	$
Plus Column A	
Sub-Total	
Minus Column B	
Sub-Total	
Minus Column C	
Accts. Receivable End of Day	

Box 2

(From Hunt SA: *Saunders fundamentals of medical assisting student mastery manual,* St. Louis, 2007, Saunders.)

Notes

Procedure 44-5: Balancing the Day Sheet. Total columns A through E and place the totals in the correct box on line 31 of the day sheet used for Procedure 44-4 in pencil. Complete the daily arithmetic posting proof using the totals from columns A through E. When the day sheet is balanced, rewrite the totals in ink.

Procedure 44-6: Writing a Check. Write checks to pay the following bills beginning with check number 1837 found on page 1137. Use today's date. The beginning balance brought forward is $4,482.21. Complete each check stub.
a. Write a check for $822.00 to Mitchell Associates for rent.
b. Write a check for $329.62 to ABC Pharmacy for medical supplies.
c. Write a check for $219.64 to Holt Office Supply for office supplies.

Procedure 44-7: Preparing a Bank Deposit. Prepare a bank deposit slip for the checks received from June Simmons, Robert Underwood, and Standard Health HMO (for Marie Richards). Use today's date. Place the practice name (Western Medical Center) on the deposit slip found on page 1139.

Procedure 44-8: Reconciling a Bank Deposit. Reconcile a bank statement using the form on page 1141 based on the following information.
    The new balance identified by the bank is $4,179.30. Two deposits are shown in your register but not on this statement, namely $254.00 and $48.91. There are three outstanding checks for $822.00, $329.62, and $219.64.

Notes

1837

DATE _____

TO _____

FOR _____

BALANCE BROUGHT FORWARD		
DEPOSITS		
BALANCE		
AMT THIS CK		
BALANCE CARRIED FORWARD		

BLACKBURN PRIMARY CARE ASSOCIATES, PC
1990 Turquiose Drive
Blackburn, WI 54937
608-459-8857

1837

94-72/1224

DATE _____

PAY TO THE
ORDER OF _____ $ [   ]

_____ *DOLLARS*

DERBYSHIRE SAVINGS Member FDIC
P.O. BOX 8923
Blackburn, WI 54937

FOR _____   _____

⑆055003⑆ 446782011⑆ 678800470

1838

DATE _____

TO _____

FOR _____

BALANCE BROUGHT FORWARD		
DEPOSITS		
BALANCE		
AMT THIS CK		
BALANCE CARRIED FORWARD		

BLACKBURN PRIMARY CARE ASSOCIATES, PC
1990 Turquiose Drive
Blackburn, WI 54937
608-459-8857

1838

94-72/1224

DATE _____

PAY TO THE
ORDER OF _____ $ [   ]

_____ *DOLLARS*

DERBYSHIRE SAVINGS Member FDIC
P.O. BOX 8923
Blackburn, WI 54937

FOR _____   _____

⑆055003⑆ 446782011⑆ 678800470

1839

DATE _____

TO _____

FOR _____

BALANCE BROUGHT FORWARD		
DEPOSITS		
BALANCE		
AMT THIS CK		
BALANCE CARRIED FORWARD		

BLACKBURN PRIMARY CARE ASSOCIATES, PC
1990 Turquiose Drive
Blackburn, WI 54937
608-459-8857

1839

94-72/1224

DATE _____

PAY TO THE
ORDER OF _____ $ [   ]

_____ *DOLLARS*

DERBYSHIRE SAVINGS Member FDIC
P.O. BOX 8923
Blackburn, WI 54937

FOR _____   _____

⑆055003⑆ 446782011⑆ 678800470

(From Hunt SA: *Saunders fundamentals of medical assisting student mastery manual,* St. Louis, 2007, Saunders.)

Notes

BANK DEPOSIT DETAIL

BANK NUMBER	PAYMENTS			CREDIT CARD
	BY CHECK OR PMO	BY COIN OR CURRENCY		
TOTALS				

CURRENCY

COIN

CHECKS

CREDIT CARDS

TOTAL RECEIPTS

LESS CREDIT CARD $

TOTAL DEPOSITS

DEPOSIT DATE: _____ FIRM: _____

(From Hunt SA: *Saunders fundamentals of medical assisting student mastery manual,* St. Louis, 2007, Saunders.)

Notes

THIS WORKSHEET IS PROVIDED TO HELP YOU BALANCE YOUR ACCOUNT

1. Go through your register and mark each check, withdrawal, Express ATM transaction, payment, deposit or other credit listed on this statement. Be sure that your register shows any interest paid into your account, and any service charges, automatic payments, or Express Transfers withdrawn from your account during this statement period.

2. Using the chart below, list any outstanding checks, Express ATM withdrawals, payments or any other withdrawals (including any from previous months) that are listed in your register but are not shown on this statement.

3. Balance your account by filling in the spaces below.

ITEMS OUTSTANDING		
NUMBER	AMOUNT	
TOTAL	$	

ENTER

The NEW BALANCE shown on
this statement_____$

ADD

Any deposits listed in your register $
or transfers into your account $
whichare not shown on this $
statement.   + $ _____

                                    TOTAL

CALCULATE THE SUBTOTAL_____$

SUBTRACT

The total outstanding checks and
withdrawals from the chart at left_____ -$

CALCULATE THE ENDING BALANCE

This amount should be the same
as the current balance shown in
your check register_____$

(From Hunt SA: *Saunders fundamentals of medical assisting student mastery manual,* St. Louis, 2007, Saunders.)

Notes

EVALUATION OF COMPETENCY

Procedure 44-1: Completing a Patient Charge Slip

Name: _____ Date: _____

Evaluated By: _____ Date: _____

Performance Objective

Outcome:	Complete a patient charge slip.
Conditions:	Given the following: blank charge slip, patient information form or computer data, daily patient schedule, calculator, and fee schedule.
Standards:	Time: 5 minutes. Student completed procedure in _____ minutes.
	Accuracy: Satisfactory score on the Performance Evaluation Checklist.

Performance Evaluation Checklist

Trial 1	Trial 2	Point Value	Performance Standards
		•	Completed the top part of a patient charge slip manually, using a computer, or by printing a label from the computer.
		•	Verified that the patient's name, date of birth, insurance, insurance group and ID numbers, and name of the subscriber have been entered or have printed correctly.
		•	Entered the patient's previous balance on the bottom of the charge slip.
		•	Used the fee schedule to fill in the fee in the box beside the code and name of each procedure performed during the office visit.
		•	Completed the bottom of the charge slip by entering the total charges, payments, and any adjustments.
		•	Totaled the new balance at the bottom of the charge slip correctly.
		•	Completed any other information requested on the charge slip.
		*	Completed the entire charge slip accurately.
		*	Completed the procedure within 5 minutes.
			TOTALS

Evaluation of Student Performance

EVALUATION CRITERIA			COMMENTS
Symbol	Category	Point Value	
∗	Critical Step	16 points	
•	Essential Step	6 points	
▷	Theory Question	2 points	

Score calculation: 100 points

− _____ points missed

_____ Score

Satisfactory score: 85 or above

CAAHEP Competencies Achieved:

Psychomotor (Skills)
☑ VI. 2. b. Perform billing procedures.

Affective (Behavior)
☑ VI. 1. Demonstrate sensitivity and professionalism in handling accounts receivable activities with clients.

ABHES Competencies Achieved:

☑ 8. i. Perform billing and collection procedures.
☑ 8. k. Perform accounts receivable procedures.
☑ 8. v. Use physician fee schedule.

EVALUATION OF COMPETENCY

Procedure 44-2: Posting Charges to the Patient Ledger

Name: _____   Date: _____

Evaluated By: _____   Date: _____

Performance Objective

Outcome:	Post charges to the patient ledger.
Conditions:	Given the following: patient charge slip, patient ledger, fee schedule, and pen and/or computer.
Standards:	Time: 5 minutes. Student completed procedure in ____ minutes.
	Accuracy: Satisfactory score on the Performance Evaluation Checklist.

Performance Evaluation Checklist

Trial 1	Trial 2	Point Value	Performance Standards
		•	Posted total charges in the column labeled "charges" of a manual ledger or the first charge on the first line of a transaction entry screen in a computer program.
		•	If using a computer system, posted each additional charge on a new line.
		•	If using a manual system, entered the total charge in the balance column. If using a computer system, saved work after all charges were posted.
		*	Entered the charges and calculated the new balance accurately.
		*	Completed the procedure within 5 minutes.
			TOTALS

Evaluation of Student Performance

EVALUATION CRITERIA			COMMENTS
Symbol	Category	Point Value	
*	Critical Step	16 points	
•	Essential Step	6 points	
▷	Theory Question	2 points	
Score calculation: 100 points			
−_____ points missed			
_____ Score			
Satisfactory score: 85 or above			

CAAHEP Competencies Achieved:

Psychomotor (Skills)

☑ VI. 2. b. Perform billing procedures.
☑ VI. 3. Use computerized office billing systems.

ABHES Competencies Achieved:

☑ 8. i. Perform billing and collection procedures.
☑ 8. k. Perform accounts receivable procedures.
☑ 8. w. Use manual or computerized bookkeeping systems.

EVALUATION OF COMPETENCY

Procedure 44-3: Posting Payments and/or Adjustments

Name: _____ Date: _____

Evaluated By: _____ Date: _____

Performance Objective

Outcome:	Post payments and/or adjustments.
Conditions:	Given the following: Patient ledger card or computer, cash or check from the patient or check from the insurance carrier, calculator, stamp with a restrictive endorsement, stamp pad, and pen.
Standards:	Time: 5 minutes. Student completed procedure in ____ minutes.
	Accuracy: Satisfactory score on the Performance Evaluation Checklist.

Performance Evaluation Checklist

Trial 1	Trial 2	Point Value	Performance Standards
		•	Located the patient account in the computer or selected the patient ledger card.
		•	Posted a payment from a completed patient charge slip to the patient ledger accurately using the same line or screen as the charges for that day.
		•	Included the check number in a manual system or used the correct code for a patient payment in a computer system.
		•	Posted an insurance payment under the date the payment was received.
		•	Used a new line for an insurance payment in a manual system and a new transaction entry screen or a payment screen in a computer system.
		•	Used the correct code or designation for an insurance payment.
		•	Entered the amount excluded by the insurance carrier as a credit adjustment in the adjustment column of a manual system and using the code for insurance write off in a computer system.
		•	Calculated or verified the patient balance and saved work in a computer system.
		∗	Posted payment and adjustment accurately, and calculated correct new patient balance.
		•	Endorsed the check using a stamp with the restrictive endorsement "For deposit only" and the number of the checking account.
		•	Placed the processed check or cash in the designated drawer or money box.
		∗	Completed the procedure within 5 minutes.
			TOTALS

Evaluation of Student Performance

EVALUATION CRITERIA			COMMENTS
Symbol	Category	Point Value	
＊	Critical Step	16 points	
●	Essential Step	6 points	
▷	Theory Question	2 points	

Score calculation: 100 points

−_____ points missed

_____ Score

Satisfactory score: 85 or above

CAAHEP Competencies Achieved:

Psychomotor (Skills)
☑ VI. 2. b. Perform billing procedures.
☑ VI. 2. d. Post adjustments.
☑ VI. 3. Use computerized office billing systems.

ABHES Competencies Achieved:

☑ 8. i. Perform billing and collection procedures.
☑ 8. k. Perform accounts receivable procedures.
☑ 8. m. Post adjustments.
☑ 8. w. Use manual or computerized bookkeeping systems.

EVALUATION OF COMPETENCY

Procedure 44-4: Recording a Patient's Visit on the Day Sheet

Name: _____   Date: _____

Evaluated By: _____   Date: _____

Performance Objective

Outcome:	Post charges and payments on a day sheet.
Conditions:	Given the following: day sheet, day sheet from the previous day, charge slips, ledger cards (optional), checks, and pen.
Standards:	Time: 10 minutes. Student completed procedure in ____ minutes.
	Accuracy: Satisfactory score on the Performance Evaluation Checklist.

Performance Evaluation Checklist

Trial 1	Trial 2	Point Value	Performance Standards
		•	Placed the day sheet on the pegboard and dated the day sheet and deposit itemization.
		•	Copied the previous day's totals from the day sheet of the previous day on the line for "TOTALS PREVIOUS PAGE."
		•	Copied the month to date totals from the day sheet of the previous day into the boxes labeled "TOTALS MONTH TO DATE."
		•	Entered the previous day's total accounts receivable on the first line of the month to date arithmetic posting proof box.
		•	If using pegboard receipts, laid a bank of patient receipts on the pegs so that the top receipt lined up with the first line of the day sheet.
		•	Entered information for a patient appointment on the first blank line in ink including the name of the patient, code for professional services, fee, payment, any adjustment, new balance, and old balance.
		•	Completed columns on the right side of the day sheet according to office policy (such as tracking for individual physicians).
		•	Entered information for the charges for each patient in the order that the patient was seen.
		•	Recorded each payment received in the mail on a separate line on the day sheet and in the patient ledger when the mail was processed.
		•	Recorded insurance write-offs with insurance payments as needed.
		•	Recorded payments made at the time of an office visit and payments received in the mail on the corresponding line of the deposit itemization at the far right of the day sheet.
		∗	Completed all entries on the day sheet accurately.
		∗	Completed the procedure within 10 minutes.
			TOTALS

Evaluation of Student Performance

Symbol	Category	Point Value
∗	Critical Step	16 points
●	Essential Step	6 points
▷	Theory Question	2 points

EVALUATION CRITERIA	COMMENTS

Score calculation: 100 points

    – _____ points missed

    _____ Score

Satisfactory score: 85 or above

CAAHEP Competencies Achieved:

Psychomotor (Skills)

☑ VI. 2. a. Post entries on a day sheet.

ABHES Competencies Achieved:

☑ 8. h. Post entries on a day sheet.
☑ 8. w. Use manual or computerized bookkeeping systems.

EVALUATION OF COMPETENCY

Procedure 44-5: Balancing the Day Sheet

Name: _____   Date: _____

Evaluated By: _____   Date: _____

Performance Objective

Outcome:	Balance the day sheet.
Conditions:	Given the following: day sheet with all transactions for one day, calculator, pencil, and pen.
Standards:	Time: 15 minutes. Student completed procedure in _____ minutes.
	Accuracy: Satisfactory score on the Performance Evaluation Checklist.

Performance Evaluation Checklist

Trial 1	Trial 2	Point Value	Performance Standards
		•	Verified that all entries had been posted for the day by checking patient names against charge slips or the appointment schedule.
		•	Added each column using a calculator and placed the total in pencil in the bottom row labeled "TOTALS THIS PAGE."
		•	Entered the total amount from each column in the correct box of the daily arithmetic posting proof.
		•	Added or subtracted the amounts in the daily posting proof as directed to total the amount in Column D.
		•	If the total was incorrect, recalculated the totals for each column until the error was identified.
		•	Added the totals from the current day to totals from the previous day and entered amounts in the correct column on the line labeled "TOTALS MONTH TO DATE."
		•	Entered amounts from the "MONTH TO DATE" line in the month arithmetic proof box.
		•	Added or subtracted the amounts in the daily posting proof as directed to total the amount in Column D.
		•	If the total was incorrect, recalculated the totals for each column until the error was identified.
		•	If office policy, completed the year to date proof using the month to date totals or compared totals to a computer report.
		•	When the day sheet was balanced, rewrote all totals in pen and made no further alterations in the day sheet.
		✶	Balanced the day sheet accurately.
		✶	Completed the procedure within 15 minutes.
			TOTALS

Evaluation of Student Performance

EVALUATION CRITERIA			COMMENTS
Symbol	**Category**	**Point Value**	
∗	Critical Step	16 points	
•	Essential Step	6 points	
▷	Theory Question	2 points	

Score calculation: 100 points

−_____ points missed

_____ Score

Satisfactory score: 85 or above

CAAHEP Competencies Achieved:

Psychomotor (Skills)
☑ VI. 2. a. Post entries on a day sheet.

ABHES Competencies Achieved:
☑ 8. k. Perform accounts receivable procedures.
☑ 8. w. Use manual or computerized bookkeeping systems.

EVALUATION OF COMPETENCY

Procedure 44-6: Writing a Check

Name: _____   Date: _____

Evaluated By: _____   Date: _____

Performance Objective

Outcome:	Write a check, and record and calculate new account balance.
Conditions:	Given the following: checks, check register or check stubs, bill to be paid, and pen.
Standards:	Time: 5 minutes. Student completed procedure in ____ minutes.
	Accuracy: Satisfactory score on the Performance Evaluation Checklist.

Performance Evaluation Checklist`

Trial 1	Trial 2	Point Value	*Performance Standards*
		•	Selected a bill to be paid.
		•	Using a pen, wrote the date on the date line.
		•	Wrote the name of the payee on the correct line.
		•	Wrote the amount of the check in numbers in the box next to the dollar sign.
		•	Used a decimal between the number of dollars and the number of cents.
		•	Wrote the amount of the check in words on the line below the name of the payee correctly.
		•	Expressed the number of cents as a fraction over 100.
		•	Drew a line from the end of the fraction to the word "dollars."
		•	Wrote the invoice number, account number, and/or purpose of the check on the memo line.
		•	Completed the checkbook stub or register including the date, check number, payee, amount of the check, and reason for the check.
		•	Added any deposits since the previous check and entered the new balance.
		•	Subtracted the amount of the check from the previous balance and entered the balance carried forward.
		•	Drew a single line through a minor mistake, corrected the error, and initialed the correction.
		∗	Wrote the check for the correct amount using the correct format with minor corrections as necessary.
		•	Wrote "void" across the any check with a major mistake and entered "void" on the check stub or in the check register.
		•	Placed a voided check in the folder with accounts payable records.
		•	Prepared an envelope to mail the payment (or used the envelope supplied by the vendor).

Trial 1	Trial 2	Point Value	Performance Standards
		●	Clipped the prepared check to the envelope with the payment slip and placed in the designated place for review and signature by the physician authorized to sign office checks.
		✳	Completed the procedure within 5 minutes.
			TOTALS

Evaluation of Student Performance

EVALUATION CRITERIA			COMMENTS
Symbol	**Category**	**Point Value**	
✳	Critical Step	16 points	
●	Essential Step	6 points	
▷	Theory Question	2 points	

Score calculation: 100 points

       − _____ points missed

           ____ Score

Satisfactory score: 85 or above

CAAHEP Competencies Achieved:

Psychomotor (Skills)
☑ VI. 2. Perform accounts receivable procedures.

ABHES Competencies Achieved:
☑ 8. j. Perform accounts payable procedures.

EVALUATION OF COMPETENCY

Procedure 44-7: Preparing a Bank Deposit

Name: _____   Date: _____

Evaluated By: _____   Date: _____

Performance Objective

Outcome:	Prepare a bank deposit.
Conditions:	Given the following: account deposit slip, deposit itemization record from a day sheet (optional), cash and checks received as payments, calculator, and bank deposit envelope or bag.
Standards:	Time: 10 minutes. Student completed procedure in _____ minutes.
	Accuracy: Satisfactory score on the Performance Evaluation Checklist.

Performance Evaluation Checklist

Trial 1	Trial 2	Point Value	Performance Standards
		•	Obtained an account deposit slip and placed a date on it. If the deposit itemization from a day sheet will be used as a deposit slip, wrote the name of the medical practice and the account number.
		•	Counted any currency and coins and entered the totals on the correct line of the deposit slip.
		•	Stamped each check with a restrictive endorsement (if not already done).
		•	Wrote the amount of each check on a separate line of the bank deposit detail, or verified that each check was entered on the daysheet deposit itemization record.
		•	Used the numerator of the fractional ABA number or other means to identify each check on the itemization.
		•	Totaled all checks and entered the total correctly.
		∗	Totaled the cash and check amounts and entered as the total amount of the bank deposit.
		•	Verified that the total deposit was equal to the amount in the payments column on the day sheet (minus any credit card payments).
		•	Made a copy of the deposit slip and deposit itemization.
		•	Placed the cash, checks, deposit slip, and deposit itemization (if separate) in a bank envelope or bank deposit bag.
		•	Recorded the amount of the deposit in the check register or on the check stub nearest to the date of deposit.
		•	Recorded the amount of the deposit in the accounts payable record according to office policy.
		•	Filed the copy of the bank deposit and bank deposit itemization as well as the bank deposit receipt after the deposit has been made.
		∗	Completed the procedure within 10 minutes.
			TOTALS

Evaluation of Student Performance

EVALUATION CRITERIA			COMMENTS
Symbol	Category	Point Value	
∗	Critical Step	16 points	
●	Essential Step	6 points	
▷	Theory Question	2 points	

Score calculation: 100 points

− _____ points missed

_____ Score

Satisfactory score: 85 or above

CAAHEP Competencies Achieved:

Psychomotor (Skills)

☑ VI. 1. Prepare a bank deposit.

ABHES Competencies Achieved:

☑ 8. g. Prepare and reconcile a bank statement and deposit record.

EVALUATION OF COMPETENCY

Procedure 44-8: Reconciling a Bank Statement

Name: _____   Date: _____

Evaluated By: _____   Date: _____

Performance Objective

Outcome:	Reconcile a bank statement.
Conditions:	Given the following: monthly bank statement, checkbook, check stubs or check register, calculator, and pen.
Standards:	Time: 15 minutes. Student completed procedure in _____ minutes.
	Accuracy: Satisfactory score on the Performance Evaluation Checklist.

Performance Evaluation Checklist

Trial 1	Trial 2	Point Value	Performance Standards
		•	Located the ending balance and the list of checks and deposits on the current bank statement.
		•	Located the same time period in the checkbook register or check stubs.
		•	Checked the checkbook register against the bank statement, placing a check mark against each check and deposit recorded on the bank statement.
		•	Noted any checks or deposits in the check register that did not appear on the bank statement.
		•	Recorded any service charges, ATM charges, or other additional charges on the bank statements in the checkbook register or on a check stub and subtracted it from the account balance.
		•	Entered any credit such as interest in the checkbook register or on a check stub and added it to the account balance.
		•	Used the bank reconciliation to balance the account.
		•	Entered the bank's ending balance.
		•	Added any deposits listed on the check register that were not listed on the bank statement.
		•	Subtracted any outstanding checks from the subtotal.
		•	Compared to the checkbook register or last check stub.
		∗	If the total did not equal the account balance in the checkbook register, recalculated until the error was found.
		∗	Completed the procedure within 15 minutes.
			TOTALS

Evaluation of Student Performance

EVALUATION CRITERIA			COMMENTS
Symbol	Category	Point Value	
✳	Critical Step	16 points	
●	Essential Step	6 points	
▷	Theory Question	2 points	

Score calculation: 100 points

      – _____ points missed

      _____ Score

Satisfactory score: 85 or above

CAAHEP Competencies Achieved:

Psychomotor (Skills)

☑ VI. 1. Prepare a bank deposit.

ABHES Competencies Achieved:

☑ 8. g. Prepare and reconcile a bank statement and deposit record.

45

Medical Coding

CHAPTER ASSIGNMENTS

√ After Completing	Date Due	Textbook Page(s)	TEXTBOOK ASSIGNMENTS	Possible Points	Points You Earned
		1056-1070	Read Chapter 45: Medical Coding		
		1062 1069	Read Case Study 1 Case Study 1 questions	5	
		1064 1069	Read Case Study 2 Case Study 2 questions	5	
		1067 1069-1070	Read Case Study 3 Case Study 3 questions	5	
			TOTAL POINTS		

√ After Completing	Date Due	Study Guide Page(s)	STUDY GUIDE ASSIGNMENTS (CTA: Critical Thinking Activity)	Possible Points	Points You Earned
		1163	Pretest	10	
		1164	Key Term Assessment	7	
		1165-1167	Evaluation of Learning questions	28	
		1168	CTA A: Evaluation and Management Codes	6	
		1168	CTA B: CPT Codes	10	
		1168-1169	CTA C: HCPCS Codes	10	
		1169	CTA D: ICD-9-CM Codes	10	
		1169	CTA E: Code Format	8	
			CD Activity: Chapter 45 Assigning CPT Codes	10	
			CD Activity: Chapter 45 Assigning ICD-9 Codes	10	
			CD Activity: Chapter 45 Apply Your Knowledge questions (Record points earned)		

√ After Completing	Date Due	Study Guide Page(s)	STUDY GUIDE ASSIGNMENTS (CTA: Critical Thinking Activity)	Possible Points	Points You Earned
		1163	Posttest	10	
			ADDITIONAL ASSIGNMENTS		
			TOTAL POINTS		

√ When Assigned by Your Instructor	Study Guide Page(s)	Practices Required	LABORATORY ASSIGNMENTS (Procedure Number and Name)	*Score
	1171	3	**Practice for Competency** 45-1: Looking Up a CPT Code Textbook reference: pp. 1062-1063	
	1173-1174		🗐 **Evaluation of Competency** 45-1: Looking Up a CPT Code	*
	1171	3	**Practice for Competency** 45-2: Looking Up a HCPCS Code Textbook reference: p. 1064	
	1175-1176		🗐 **Evaluation of Competency** 45-2: Looking Up a HCPCS Code	*
	1171	3	**Practice for Competency** 45-3: Looking Up an ICD-9-CM Code Textbook reference: p. 1068	
	1177-1178		🗐 **Evaluation of Competency** 45-3: Looking Up an ICD-9-CM Code	*
			ADDITIONAL ASSIGNMENTS	

Notes

Name _____   Date _____

PRETEST

True or False

_____ 1. The radiology section of the CPT coding manual is the largest and has the most codes.

_____ 2. CPT codes for surgical procedures automatically include all services related to the surgery.

_____ 3. There are different codes for office visits for new patients and established patients.

_____ 4. The type of physical examination is a major factor in determining the correct code for the office visit.

_____ 5. Medical decision making is not taken into account when selecting a CPT code for an office visit.

_____ 6. If an injection is given to a patient with Medicare, a HCPCS Level II code is required for the medication.

_____ 7. The fifth digit of an ICD-9-CM code is always the first digit of the code.

_____ 8. ICD-9-CM codes for patients who are having physical examinations begin with the letter V.

_____ 9. Coding books in the medical office must be updated every 2-3 years.

_____ 10. When the diagnosis includes the words "rule out," it should not receive an ICD-9-CM code.

POSTTEST

True or False

_____ 1. The CPT manual is arranged according to body system.

_____ 2. CPT codes consist of five digits and may also include a two-digit modifier.

_____ 3. In addition to office visits, CPT codes are used for physician visits to patients in nursing homes.

_____ 4. A problem-focused patient history includes information about the patient's family history.

_____ 5. The CPT code should always be chosen from the alphabetic index.

_____ 6. HCPCS Level II codes are arranged alphabetically by letter, then numerically.

_____ 7. Sometimes two codes are required to accurately reflect a patient's diagnosis.

_____ 8. The third volume of the ICD-9-CM manual contains the alphabetic index.

_____ 9. The ICD-9-CM code should always be selected from the tabular list, not the alphabetic index.

_____ 10. All ICD-9-CM codes have two digits after the decimal point.

✎Term KEY TERM ASSESSMENT

Directions: Match each medical term with its definition.

_____ 1. Modifier

_____ 2. Morphology

_____ 3. NEC

_____ 4. Neoplasm

_____ 5. NOS

_____ 6. Panel

_____ 7. Surgical package

A. A diagnosis code that is not otherwise specified

B. A diagnosis code that is not elsewhere classified

C. Surgical services covered by a single procedure code that includes a preoperative visit, postoperative care and local anesthesia

D. Abnormal growth or tumor

E. An addition to a CPT code that indicates unusual circumstances related to the procedure

F. A group of diagnostic tests done in one machine at the same time

G. The study of structure and form

EVALUATION OF LEARNING

Directions: Fill in each blank with the correct answer.

1. What are three reasons for the development of procedure codes?

    _____

    _____

2. How and when were the Current Procedural Terminology and HCPCS coding systems developed?

    _____

    _____

3. What is a modifier, and how is it used?

    _____

4. What are the six sections of the CPT manual?

    _____

    _____

5. What types of services are covered in the Evaluation and Management section of the CPT manual?

    _____

    _____

6. Identify the seven factors that affect the level of service when identifying E/M codes.

    _____

    _____

    _____

    _____

7. What factors must be considered when determining a code in the Evaluation and Management section of the CPT manual?

    _____

    _____

8. Give a general statement that identifies when a code can be chosen that will provide more reimbursement for a patient visit.

    _____

9. Differentiate between a problem-focused medical history and a detailed history.

    _____

10. Differentiate between an expanded problem-focused physical examination and a comprehensive examination.

_____

11. What factors influence the level of medical decision making?

_____

12. How are CPT codes specified in the Anesthesia section of the CPT manual?

_____

_____

13. What is a physical status modifier, and how are physical status modifiers used related to anesthesia services?

_____

_____

14. What services are included in a code for surgical services (surgical package)?

_____

_____

_____

15. What are the four subsections of the Radiology section of the CPT manual?

_____

_____

16. When coding for a cardiac panel, can the coder use a separate code for each test in the panel if all tests were done? Why or why not?

_____

_____

17. How does the medical office code for a blood test for a cardiac panel if the specimen was drawn in the office by the MA and sent out to the hospital laboratory for testing?

_____

18. What types of procedures are included in the Medicine section of the CPT manual?

_____

_____

19. Describe the steps to look up a procedure code properly.

_____

_____

_____

20. What are five pieces of information that may be significant when choosing a code for a procedure?

_____

_____

_____

21. Describe Level I and Level II HCPCS codes.

Level I: _____

Level II: _____

22. Give several examples of services that require HCPCS codes.

_____

_____

23. Describe the process for looking up HCPCS codes.

_____

_____

24. Describe the history of the International Classification of Disease coding system.

_____

_____

_____

25. What is the format of ICD-9-CM codes?

_____

_____

26. How are the numeric codes arranged in the ICD-9-CM code book?

_____

27. Identify what types of diagnosis codes begin with the following letters:

V codes: _____

E codes: _____

M codes: _____

28. Describe the steps to look up a diagnosis code properly.

_____

_____

_____

CRITICAL THINKING ACTIVITIES

A. EVALUATION AND MANAGEMENT CODES

Select the best code for the E/M service for each of the following:

1. New patient seen in the office for gradual onset of joint pain (polyarthralgia), reddened areas on face covering the nose and surrounding cheek area, and decreased circulation to fingers, especially in cold weather. The physician performed a complete history and review of systems and a comprehensive examination of the patient's musculoskeletal, cardiovascular, and integumentary systems. Management of the patient required moderate

   decision making. _____

2. Follow-up visit in the office for a patient with asthma requiring minor adjustment of medication, although the

   patient is generally doing well. _____

3. Office visit for an established patient with arteriosclerotic heart disease who is now complaining of increasing frequency of chest tightness during and after exercise. The cardiovascular history was reviewed and the

   cardiovascular system was examined with referral to a cardiologist. _____

4. An established patient is seen in the office for the second in a series of three hepatitis B injections given by the

   nurse. _____

5. A 30-year-old woman is seen for an initial consultation because of a large and uncomfortable bunion on her right foot. The orthopedic surgeon performs a problem-focused history and problem-focused physical examination and recommends outpatient surgery to remove the bunion at the patient's convenience.

   _____

6. A new patient is seen in the office for a sore throat with fever. The history is problem focused, the examination

   is problem focused, and the decision making is straightforward. _____

B. CPT CODES

Identify the most specific CPT code for the following services.

1. A patient receives a 12-lead electrocardiogram (ECG) with interpretation. _____

2. The physician performs a flexible sigmoidoscopy on a patient in the special procedure room of the office suite.

   No problems are identified. _____

3. The MA performs a dipstick urinalysis. _____

4. The MA performs a rapid strep test (Streptococcus, group A by immunoassay with direct optical observation).

   _____

5. The patient receives a chest x-ray, two views (AP and lateral). _____

6. The patient receives a urine culture and colony count. _____

7. A spun microhematocrit is performed on blood from a capillary puncture. _____

8. The patient has a wart frozen with liquid nitrogen. _____

9. The patient receives an intramuscular injection of antibiotic. _____

10. The patient receives an inhalation (nebulizer) treatment in the office. _____

C. HCPCS CODES

Identify the specific HCPCS code for the following services:

1. The patient receives a pair of wooden underarm crutches: _____

2. Injection of ceftazidime 350 mg: _____

3. The patient receives an electric heat pad, moist: _____

4. Cervical traction equipment for over the door: _____

5. Injection, lincomycin HCl 250 mg: _____

6. Transcutaneous electrical joint stimulation device system: _____

7. Tubular dressing, 1 yard: _____

8. Infusion, albumin (human) 5%, 250 ml: _____

9. Knee orthosis with joints, prefabricated including fitting and adjustment: _____

10. Dynamic adjustable ankle extension/flexion device: _____

D. ICD-9-CM CODES
Identify the following ICD-9-CM codes for the following diagnoses:

1. Portal cirrhosis: _____

2. Hiatal hernia: _____

3. Malignant tumor of the urinary system: _____

4. Vaginitis: _____

5. Tendinitis: _____

6. Long-term (current) use of anticoagulants: _____

7. Carpal tunnel syndrome: _____

8. Breast, fibrocystic disease: _____

9. Congestive heart failure: _____

10. Hypercholesterolemia: _____

E. CODE FORMAT
Choose the letter of the type of code for which each of the following descriptions is true. (Each answer may be used more than once.)

a. ICD-9-CM codes

b. CPT codes

c. HCPCS codes

_____ 1. Consists only of five numbers without a decimal

_____ 2. Used to code the patient's diagnosis

_____ 3. Contains two levels of codes

_____ 4. A two-digit modifier added to the code gives more information

_____ 5. Consists of three digits, often followed by a decimal point and one to two digits

_____ 6. Contains codes describing evaluation and management

_____ 7. Used to bill Medicare for supplies, materials, and injections

_____ 8. E codes are used to classify external causes of injuries and poisoning.

Notes

PRACTICE FOR COMPETENCY

Procedure 45-1: Looking Up a CPT Code. Look up CPT codes for the following:

1. Patient seen in a nursing home by the office physician for initial nursing facility care, detailed history, detailed examination, straightforward medical decision making: _____

2. Urine pregnancy test by visual color comparison method: _____

3. Spinal chiropractic manipulative treatment, one region: _____

Procedure 45-2: Looking Up a HCPCS Code. Look up HCPCS codes for the following:

1. Injection, ceftriaxone sodium 250 mg: _____

2. One foot arch support, removable, premolded, longitudinal: _____

3. Injection, vitamin B-12 cyanocobalamin 500 mcg: _____

Procedure 45-3: Looking Up an ICD-9-CM Code. Look up ICD-9-CM codes for the following diagnoses:

1. Pernicious anemia: _____

2. Hematuria: _____

3. Lumbar disc disorder: _____

Notes

☑ EVALUATION OF COMPETENCY

Procedure 45-1: Looking Up a CPT Code

Name: _____   Date: _____

Evaluated By: _____   Date: _____

Performance Objective

Outcome:	Look up a CPT code.
Conditions:	Given the following: charge slip or procedure to look up code for, medical record, and CPT manual.
Standards:	Time: 5 minutes. Student completed procedure in _____ minutes.
	Accuracy: Satisfactory score on the Performance Evaluation Checklist.

Performance Evaluation Checklist

Trial 1	Trial 2	Point Value	Performance Standards
		●	Found name of procedure to look up from charge slip or other document.
		●	Determined any necessary additional information from the patient's medical record.
		●	For evaluation and management services, identified if the patient is a new patient or an established patient.
		●	For evaluation and management services, identified the location where the patient was seen.
		●	Located the name of the procedure in the index.
		●	From the information in the index, located the correct range of codes in the list of codes.
		▷	Stated the reason for coding from the list of codes instead of the index.
		✲	Selected the correct code from the list of codes
		●	If the service was unusual, decided if a modifier was needed.
		✲	Selected the correct modifier, if one was needed
		●	Entered the correct code on the charge slip, on any other document, and in the computer as needed.
		✲	Completed the procedure within 5 minutes.
			TOTALS

Evaluation of Student Performance

EVALUATION CRITERIA			COMMENTS
Symbol	Category	Point Value	
＊	Critical Step	16 points	
●	Essential Step	6 points	
▷	Theory Question	2 points	

Score calculation: 100 points

     − _____ points missed

     _____ Score

Satisfactory score: 85 or above

CAAHEP Competencies Achieved:

Psychomotor (Skills)
☑ VIII. 1. Perform procedural coding.

ABHES Competencies Achieved:
☑ 8. t. Perform diagnostic and procedure coding.

EVALUATION OF COMPETENCY

Procedure 45-2: Looking Up a HCPCS Code

Name: _____   Date: _____

Evaluated By: _____   Date: _____

Performance Objective

Outcome:	Look up a HCPCS code.
Conditions:	Given the following: charge slip or procedure to look up code for, medical record, and HCPCS manual.
Standards:	Time: 5 minutes. Student completed procedure in _____ minutes.
	Accuracy: Satisfactory score on the Performance Evaluation Checklist.

Performance Evaluation Checklist

Trial 1	Trial 2	Point Value	Performance Standards
		●	Found name of procedure or item to look up from charge slip or other document.
		●	Determined any necessary additional information from the patient's medical record.
		●	Located the name of the procedure or item in the index.
		●	From the information in the index, located the correct range of codes in the list of codes.
		▷	Stated the reason for coding from the list of codes instead of the index.
		✶	Selected the correct code from the list of codes
		●	Validated that the code was appropriate for the patient's insurance.
		●	Entered the correct code on the charge slip, on any other document, and in the computer as needed.
		✶	Completed the procedure within 5 minutes.
			TOTALS

Evaluation of Student Performance

EVALUATION CRITERIA			COMMENTS
Symbol	Category	Point Value	
✶	Critical Step	16 points	
●	Essential Step	6 points	
▷	Theory Question	2 points	

Score calculation: 100 points

  −_____ points missed

  _____ Score

Satisfactory score: 85 or above

CAAHEP Competencies Achieved:

Psychomotor (Skills)
☑ VIII. 1. Perform procedural coding.

ABHES Competencies Achieved:

☑ 8. t. Perform diagnostic and procedure coding.

EVALUATION OF COMPETENCY

Procedure 45-3: Looking Up an ICD-9-CM Code

Name: _____ Date: _____

Evaluated By: _____ Date: _____

Performance Objective

Outcome:	Look up an ICD-9-CM code.
Conditions:	Given the following: charge slip or diagnosis to look up code for, medical record, and an ICD-9-CM manual.
Standards:	Time: 5 minutes. Student completed procedure in _____ minutes.
	Accuracy: Satisfactory score on the Performance Evaluation Checklist.

Performance Evaluation Checklist

Trial 1	Trial 2	Point Value	Performance Standards
		•	Found name of procedure to look up from charge slip or other document.
		•	Determined any necessary additional information from the patient's medical record.
		•	Looked under as many terms as necessary to locate the diagnosis in the index.
		•	From the information in the index, located the correct range of codes in the tabular list.
		▷	Stated the reason for coding from the tabular list instead of the index.
		•	Checked all potential codes against the diagnosis to identify the most specific fourth and fifth digit (if available).
		∗	Selected the correct code from the list of codes.
		•	Entered the correct code on the charge slip, on any other document, and in the computer as needed.
		∗	Completed the procedure within 5 minutes.
			TOTALS

Evaluation of Student Performance

EVALUATION CRITERIA			COMMENTS
Symbol	Category	Point Value	
✷	Critical Step	16 points	
●	Essential Step	6 points	
▷	Theory Question	2 points	

Score calculation: 100 points

      – _____ points missed

      _____ Score

Satisfactory score: 85 or above

CAAHEP Competencies Achieved:

Psychomotor (Skills)
☑ VIII. 2. Perform diagnostic coding.

ABHES Competencies Achieved:

☑ 8. t. Perform diagnostic and procedure coding.

46

Medical Insurance

CHAPTER ASSIGNMENTS

√ After Completing	Date Due	Textbook Page(s)	TEXTBOOK ASSIGNMENTS	Possible Points	Points You Earned
		1071-1091	Read Chapter 46: Medical Insurance		
		1075 1089	📖 Read Case Study 1 Case Study 1 questions	5	
		1082 1089	📖 Read Case Study 2 Case Study 2 questions	5	
		1087 1090	📖 Read Case Study 3 Case Study 3 questions	5	
			TOTAL POINTS		

√ After Completing	Date Due	Study Guide Page(s)	STUDY GUIDE ASSIGNMENTS (CTA: Critical Thinking Activity)	Possible Points	Points You Earned
		1183	❓ Pretest	10	
		1184	🔑Term Key Term Assessment: General Insurance Terms	25	
		1185	🔑Term Key Term Assessment: Insurance Plans and Methods of Reimbursement	10	
		1186-1189	📝 Evaluation of Learning questions	30	
		1189-1190	CTA A: Primary and Secondary Insurance	10	
		1190	CTA B: Managed Care Plans	5	
		1190	CTA C: The Insurance Claim Form	10	
			💿 CD Activity: Chapter 46 Completing a Health Insurance Claim Form	10	
			💿 CD Activity: Chapter 46 Apply Your Knowledge questions (Record points earned)		

√ After Completing	Date Due	Study Guide Page(s)	STUDY GUIDE ASSIGNMENTS (CTA: Critical Thinking Activity)	Possible Points	Points You Earned
		1183	📰 Posttest	10	
			ADDITIONAL ASSIGNMENTS		
			TOTAL POINTS		

√ When Assigned by Your Instructor	Study Guide Page(s)	Practices Required	LABORATORY ASSIGNMENTS (Procedure Number and Name)	*Score
	1191	3	**ᴅᵛᴰ Practice for Competency** 46-1: Completing/Reviewing the CMS-1500 Insurance Claim Form Textbook reference: pp. 1082-1088	
	1193-1195		**Evaluation of Competency** 46-1: Completing/Reviewing the CMS-1500 Insurance Claim Form	*
			ADDITIONAL ASSIGNMENTS	

Notes

Name _____   Date _____

PRETEST

True or False

_____ 1. Capitation is a term meaning that the insurance company pays a specific amount for each service.

_____ 2. If an individual obtains health insurance through employment, it is usually through a group plan.

_____ 3. If a patient's insurance is a Staff Model HMO, the patient must usually pay an annual deductible.

_____ 4. If a patient is covered by more than one health insurance plan, the primary insurance must be billed first.

_____ 5. If a patient is covered by more than one health insurance policy, insurance may pay more than 100% of charges.

_____ 6. Usually the medical office accepts assignment of benefits.

_____ 7. A patient covered by traditional indemnity insurance always requires a written referral to see a specialist.

_____ 8. Precertification by the insurance company is usually required if a patient will be scheduled for surgery.

_____ 9. Patients with Medicare Part B must pay an annual deductible before any other services are covered.

_____ 10. A patient's usual health insurance plan will deny any claim for a work-related injury.

POSTTEST

True or False

_____ 1. Health insurance for the spouses and dependents of active military personnel is called *TRICARE*.

_____ 2. The age for eligibility for Medicare is 65.

_____ 3. The amount of money that is paid to an insurance company for insurance coverage is called a *benefit*.

_____ 4. If a child is covered by insurance plans through both parents, the birthday rule establishes the primary insurance.

_____ 5. Medicare supplemental insurance is always the primary insurance.

_____ 6. If a physician participates in the Medicare plan, he or she must accept assignment of benefits.

_____ 7. In an HMO, the primary care provider controls a patient's access to specialty services and specialists.

_____ 8. PPOs cover in-network and out-of-network services.

_____ 9. Both Medicare and Medicaid usually have different names in different states.

_____ 10. A separate medical record should be established for a patient being seen for a work-related injury.

KEY TERM ASSESSMENT: GENERAL INSURANCE TERMS

Directions: Match each insurance term with its definition.

_____ 1. Assignment of benefits

_____ 2. Authorization

_____ 3. Benefit

_____ 4. Birthday rule

_____ 5. Carrier

_____ 6. Coinsurance

_____ 7. Coordination of benefits

_____ 8. Copayment

_____ 9. Crossover claim

_____ 10. Deductible

_____ 11. Established patient

_____ 12. Explanation of benefits (EOB)

_____ 13. Fee-for-service

_____ 14. Fiscal intermediary

_____ 15. Guarantor

_____ 16. Indemnity

_____ 17. Insured

_____ 18. New patient

_____ 19. Premium

_____ 20. Primary care provider

_____ 21. Primary insurance

_____ 22. Reimbursement

_____ 23. Secondary insurance

_____ 24. Signature on file (SOF)

_____ 25. Subscriber

A. Rules followed by insurance companies so that no claim is reimbursed at more than 100% of the charges

B. An obligation to provide compensation for loss or damage

C. A patient who has been seen by any provider in a medical office within the past three years

D. The insurance company which must be billed first

E. Insurance that an individual has in addition to primary insurance

F. A statement issued by the insurance company explaining reimbursement

G. The amount of money paid for a covered service under a health insurance plan

H. A person with financial responsibility for a bill

I. Official permission

J. The subscriber on an insurance policy

K. A fixed amount of money that the patient must pay for any health care service

L. The signature of the patient is maintained by the medical office to authorize submission of insurance claims

M. For coding and insurance purposes, a patient who has not been seen by any practitioner within the past three years

N. Authorization for insurance reimbursement to be made to the provider of health service

O. The physician chosen by a patient to provide general medical care and also authorize additional medical services

P. An amount of money that an insured person must pay annually before health services are covered

Q. A percentage of the payment for health services that the patient is responsible for

R. An insurance claim that is automatically forwarded from Medicare to Medicaid

S. The rule that determines which insurance is primary for the children of two parents who have a family health plan

T. An insurance company that contracts to review Medicare claims

U. The person named on an insurance certificate

V. The amount paid for a procedure by insurance

W. An amount of money paid in a given period to purchase health insurance

X. An insurance company

Y. Insurance reimbursement that is based on to the services provided and the amount charged

🔑 Term KEY TERM ASSESSMENT: INSURANCE PLANS AND METHODS OF REIMBURSEMENT

Directions: Match each insurance plan with its method of reimbursement.

_____ 1. Capitation

_____ 2. CHAMPVA

_____ 3. Diagnosis-related groups

_____ 4. Managed care

_____ 5. Medicaid

_____ 6. Medicare

_____ 7. Resource-based relative value scale (RBRVS)

_____ 8. TRICARE

_____ 9. Usual, customary, and reasonable (UCR)

_____ 10. Workers' compensation

A. A movement to reduce health care costs while providing quality care

B. Covers lost wages and health care costs of workers injured on the job or who suffer from work-related illnesses

C. Establishes the fee schedule for Medicare Part B based on the service provided and the geographic location of the provider

D. The government insurance program for low-income individuals and families

E. A fixed amount is paid to the provider per member for a specific time period

F. Provides medical care to spouses and dependents of individuals on active duty in the military

G. Provides insurance coverage for the elderly, permanently disabled, and individuals with end-stage kidney disease

H. Covers dependents of military personnel with service-connected disabilities

I. Insurance payment based on a physician's usual charge and the customary charge of other physicians in the same area

J. A system to determine Medicare reimbursement for a hospital stay based on the patient's diagnosis

EVALUATION OF LEARNING

Directions: Fill in each blank with the correct answer.

1. Briefly describe the history of health insurance in the United States.

    _____

    _____

    _____

    _____

2. Identify three ways for individuals and families to obtain health insurance coverage.

    _____

    _____

3. What is the tax advantage to obtaining health insurance through the employer?

    _____

    _____

4. What types of payments must the subscriber make for health care?

    _____

    _____

5. If both parents have health insurance through their employers, what determines which parent's insurance is primary for their children? Is it the same if the parents are divorced?

    _____

    _____

    _____

6. If the patient authorizes assignment of benefits, how does that affect the medical office?

    _____

    _____

    _____

7. What are two ways that fee-for-service insurance plans determine the amount they will pay for services?

    _____

    _____

8. What is meant by managed care?

    _____

    _____

9. What is the function of the primary care provider in a managed care plan?

_____

_____

10. What is the cost to patients if they seek services outside a managed care plan?

_____

_____

11. Describe each of the following managed care plans:

a. Staff model HMO: _____

_____

b. Network model HMO: _____

_____

c. Preferred provider organization (PPO): _____

_____

d. Exclusive provider organization (EPO): _____

_____

e. Independent practice association (IPA): _____

_____

f. Point-of-service (POS) plan: _____

_____

12. Identify three differences between Medicare Part A and Medicare Part B.

_____

_____

13. What are Medicare Part B payments based on, and how is the allowable charge calculated?

_____

_____

14. What part of the bill for services is the patient covered by Medicare Part B responsible for if the physician participates in the Medicare program? If the physician does not participate?

_____

_____

15. If a patient is covered by Medicaid insurance, what portion of the bill is the patient responsible for?

_____

16. What additional services are covered by Medicaid that other health insurance is usually not responsible for?

_____

_____

17. Why do some physicians refuse to accept Medicaid patients?

_____

_____

18. What is a SCHIP?

_____

_____

19. Describe who purchases workers' compensation insurance and when claims must be filed to this program.

_____

_____

20. Why is a separate medical record established for a patient who is being treated for a work-related injury or illness?

_____

_____

21. Describe who receives benefits under the government TRICARE plan, and describe the three levels of service briefly.

_____

_____

_____

22. What group of people is covered by CHAMPVA?

_____

23. What is the CMS-1500 claim form?

_____

_____

24. Identify the three boxes on the CMS-1500 form that require signatures, who must sign, and what each signature authorizes. What can replace the signature for each for most insurance carriers?

_____

_____

25. What are recommendations for completing insurance forms to facilitate optical scanning?

_____

_____

26. Identify three advantages of submitting insurance claims electronically.

_____

_____

_____

27. Describe the two basic types of reimbursement from insurance companies.

_____

_____

_____

28. What is the purpose of an insurance claims register?

_____

_____

29. What information is contained on an explanation of benefits (EOB) form?

_____

_____

30. How should the MA handle an insurance claim that was denied?

_____

_____

CRITICAL THINKING ACTIVITIES

A. PRIMARY AND SECONDARY INSURANCE

In the Swann family, the mother has insurance from her own employment (individual plan) and the father has insurance from his employment (family plan). The mother's birthday is January 31, and her husband's birthday is May 10. Whose insurance is the primary insurance and whose is the secondary insurance (if any) for each of the following family members?

1. mother   primary insurance: _____

               secondary insurance: _____

2. father   primary insurance: _____

               secondary insurance: _____

3. son   primary insurance: _____

               secondary insurance: _____

4. daughter   primary insurance: _____

               secondary insurance: _____

In the McGrath family, the mother has insurance from her own employment (family plan) and the father has insurance from his employment (family plan). The mother's birthday is January 31, and her husband's birthday is May 10. Whose insurance is the primary insurance and whose is the secondary insurance (if any) for each of the following family members?

5. mother   primary insurance: _____

   secondary insurance: _____

6. father   primary insurance: _____

   secondary insurance: _____

7. son   primary insurance: _____

   secondary insurance: _____

8. daughter   primary insurance: _____

   secondary insurance: _____

Eleanor Whitby is 68, and her husband Jeremy Whitby is 69. Eleanor is a retired office worker with Medicare (Part A and Part B) and an individual Medigap insurance policy through her previous employment. Jeremy is covered by Medicare Part A because he is older than 65, but he is still employed full time and has health insurance from his employer (individual policy). Which is the primary and which is the secondary insurance (if any) for each for medical office charges?

9. Eleanor   primary insurance: _____

   secondary insurance: _____

10. Jeremy   primary insurance: _____

   secondary insurance: _____

B. MANAGED CARE PLANS

For each of the following types of managed care plans, choose the letter that describes access to out-of-network services for a subscriber (member).

a. Plan does not pay for out-of-network services (except for emergencies)

b. Out-of-network services are available at a higher cost

1. Staff model HMO: _____

2. Network model HMO: _____

3. Preferred provider organization (PPO): _____

4. Exclusive provider organization (EPO): _____

5. Point-of-service (POS) plan: _____

C. THE INSURANCE CLAIM FORM

Looking at the figure of the CMS-1500 health insurance claim form in Figure 46-3, identify which box should be used for each of the following pieces of information.

1. The patient's address: _____

2. The name of the insured: _____

3. If an outside laboratory was used: _____

4. If the physician accepts assignment of benefits: _____

5. The CPT code of the first procedure: _____

6. The patient's birth date: _____

7. If there is another insurance plan: _____

8. The NPI number of the referring physician: _____

9. The balance owed by the patient: _____

10. The federal tax ID number: _____

PRACTICE FOR COMPETENCY

Procedure 46-1: Completing/Reviewing the CMS-1500 Insurance Claim Form. Using the patient information and charge slips from Chapter 44 (Practice for Competency, Procedure 44-1), complete insurance claim forms for June Simmons and James Winston.

In addition, complete an insurance claim form for the following:

Marie Richards	Patient number: 3020
19 Maple Street	Established patient of Dr. Warner
Western, XY 44770	Name of insured: John Richards (DOB: 6/15/78)
(490) 459-1333	Insurance plan: Standard Health HMO
DOB: 8/22/82	

10/18/10	Expanded problem focused OV (99212)	$65.00
	Venipuncture collection (36415)	$12.00
Diagnoses:	Inflammatory polyarthritis	
	Discoid lupus erythematosus	

Notes

EVALUATION OF COMPETENCY

Procedure 46-1: Completing/Reviewing the CMS-1500 Insurance Claim Form

Name: _____ Date: _____

Evaluated By: _____ Date: _____

Performance Objective

Outcome:	Complete (or review) a CMS-1500 insurance claim form.
Conditions:	Given the following: patient information form or computer screen, patient account or ledger, photocopy of patient's insurance card, insurance claim form, computer with medical billing program, printer, and pen.
Standards:	Time: 15 minutes. Student completed procedure in _____ minutes.
	Accuracy: Satisfactory score on the Performance Evaluation Checklist.

Performance Evaluation Checklist

Trial 1	Trial 2	Point Value	Performance Standards
		●	Assembled information and supplies.
		●	If creating a paper claim, used only capital letters without commas, dollar signs, or other punctuation.
		●	In the carrier section entered or validated the name and address of the insurance company using correct address format.
		●	Entered the type of insurance.
		●	Entered the ID number and group number of the insured individual as shown on photocopy of the insurance card.
		●	Entered patient information accurately.
		●	Identified the patient's relationship to the insured.
		●	If the insured was not the patient, entered the required information about the insured.
		●	Entered the patient's marital status and employment status.
		●	Entered complete information about any secondary insurance as needed.
		●	Entered information related to the cause of the patient's condition(s).
		●	Identified if the patient did or did not have other insurance.
		●	Validated the patient signature on the form to allow insurance billing and assignment of benefits.
		●	Entered SOF or Signature on File in boxes authorizing permission.
		▷	Explained how to obtain signatures if they were not on file.
		✶	Completed the patient and insured information section accurately and completely.
		●	Entered any special information required by a specific insurance carrier as needed.
		●	Entered the name and identifying number of the referring physician, if any.

Trial 1	Trial 2	Point Value	Performance Standards
		●	Entered dates of hospitalization if services were provided in the hospital.
		●	Checked the correct box to identify if outside laboratory services were provided.
		●	Entered up to four ICD-9-CM codes.
		●	Entered reference numbers for a Medicaid resubmission, referral, preauthorization, and/or precertification.
		●	Entered information about the first procedure including date(s) of service, place of service, CPT or HCPCS code and modifiers, number to point to the appropriate diagnosis, charges, number of units, and the NPI number or other ID number.
		●	Entered complete information about each additional procedure.
		●	Entered the tax identification number and checked if the Social Security number or employer identification number was used.
		●	Entered the patient account number, if any.
		●	Checked the correct box to indicate acceptance of assignment of benefits.
		●	Entered the total charges, total amount paid, and total balance due.
		●	Entered SOF, Signature on File, or the physician's legal signature including credentials and date.
		●	Entered the name, address, and telephone number of the billing facility, and the name of the facility where services were provided, if different.
		●	Entered the NPI number or other ID number for the billing facility and facility where services were provided, if different.
		●	Made a copy of a paper claim and filed in an insurance claims file.
		●	Reviewed the claim for accuracy before submission.
		✳	Completed the physician or supplier section accurately and completely.
		✳	Completed the procedure within 15 minutes.
			TOTALS

Evaluation of Student Performance

EVALUATION CRITERIA			COMMENTS
Symbol	Category	Point Value	
∗	Critical Step	16 points	
•	Essential Step	6 points	
▷	Theory Question	2 points	

Score calculation: 100 points

－_____ points missed

_____   Score

Satisfactory score: 85 or above

CAAHEP Competencies Achieved:

Psychomotor (Skills)
☑ VII. 3. Complete insurance claim form.

Affective (Behavior)
☑ VIII. 1. Work with physician to achieve the maximum reimbursement.

ABHES Competencies Achieved:

☑ 8. u. Prepare and submit insurance claims.

Notes

47

Billing and Collections

CHAPTER ASSIGNMENTS

√ After Completing	Date Due	Textbook Page(s)	TEXTBOOK ASSIGNMENTS	Possible Points	Points You Earned
		1092-1108	Read Chapter 47: Billing and Collections		
		1095 1107	📖 Read Case Study 1 Case Study 1 questions	5	
		1099 1107-1108	📖 Read Case Study 2 Case Study 2 questions	5	
		1104 1108	📖 Read Case Study 3 Case Study 3 questions	5	
			TOTAL POINTS		

√ After Completing	Date Due	Study Guide Page(s)	STUDY GUIDE ASSIGNMENTS (CTA: Critical Thinking Activity)	Possible Points	Points You Earned
		1201	Pretest	10	
		1202	Key Term Assessment	9	
		1203-1205	Evaluation of Learning questions	23	
		1205-1206	CTA A: Cycle Billing	10	
		1206	CTA B: Adjustments	8	
		1206	CTA C: Aging Accounts	8	
			CD Activity: Chapter 47 Preparing Monthly Billing Statements	10	
			CD Activity: Chapter 47 Apply Your Knowledge questions (Record points earned)		
		1201	Posttest	10	

√ After Completing	Date Due	Study Guide Page(s)	STUDY GUIDE ASSIGNMENTS (CTA: Critical Thinking Activity)	Possible Points	Points You Earned
			ADDITIONAL ASSIGNMENTS		
			TOTAL POINTS		

√ When Assigned by Your Instructor	Study Guide Page(s)	Practices Required	LABORATORY ASSIGNMENTS (Procedure Number and Name)	*Score
	1207	3	(DVD) **Practice for Competency** 47-1: Processing Patient Bills Textbook reference: p. 1094	
	1223-1224		**Evaluation of Competency** 47-1: Processing Patient Bills	*
	1207	1	**Practice for Competency** 47-2: Posting an NSF Check Textbook reference: pp. 1095-1096	
	1225-1226		**Evaluation of Competency** 47-2: Posting an NSF Check	*
	1213	1	**Practice for Competency** 47-3: Posting an Overpayment Textbook reference: pp. 1096-1097	
	1227-1228		**Evaluation of Competency** 47-3: Posting an Overpayment	*
	1213	1	**Practice for Competency** 47-4: Processing a Refund Textbook reference: pp. 1097-1098	
	1229-1230		**Evaluation of Competency** 47-4: Processing a Refund	*
	1217	1	**Practice for Competency** 47-5: Creating an Accounts Receivable Aging Record Textbook reference: pp. 1099-1100	
	1231-1232		**Evaluation of Competency** 47-5: Creating an Accounts Receivable Aging Record	*
	1221	1	**Practice for Competency** 47-6: Writing a Collection Letter Textbook reference: p. 1105	
	1233-1234		**Evaluation of Competency** 47-6: Writing a Collection Letter	*
	1221	1	**Practice for Competency** 47-7: Posting a Collection Agency Payment Textbook reference: pp. 1105-1106	
	1235-1236		**Evaluation of Competency** 47-7: Posting a Collection Agency Payment	*
			ADDITIONAL ASSIGNMENTS	

Notes

Name _____   Date _____

PRETEST

True or False

_____ 1. The first bill is usually sent to the patient the day after a patient visit.

_____ 2. Almost all medical offices do monthly billing from the office.

_____ 3. Credit agreements with patients must be in writing even if the patient is not charged interest.

_____ 4. A check written on an account that does not have sufficient funds is called an *overdraft*.

_____ 5. When a check is reported lost, the bank should be notified to stop payment on the check.

_____ 6. If a patient overpays his or her account, the office usually issues a refund to the patient.

_____ 7. The medical assistant must create an accounts receivable aging report manually at least once a month.

_____ 8. Overdue accounts older than 120 days are definitely subject to collection activity.

_____ 9. The first time a claim message is used on a patient's bill is when the bill is older than 120 days.

_____ 10. It is illegal to call a patient at his or her place of employment about an overdue bill.

POSTTEST

True or False

_____ 1. Medical offices usually send a bill to patients to collect copayments.

_____ 2. The billing cycle is a term used to describe how long it takes to prepare bills for mailing.

_____ 3. Sending some patient bills every week is usually more efficient than sending all bills monthly.

_____ 4. The bank only charges a fee to the account an NSF check is written on.

_____ 5. An NSF check is entered to the patient's account as a positive adjustment to increase the balance.

_____ 6. If a patient has a credit balance, it means that the office owes the patient money.

_____ 7. Accounts are first considered overdue at 90 days after the date billed.

_____ 8. The medical office can sue patients for overdue accounts in small claims court.

_____ 9. The best time to call a patient about an overdue bill is after 9:00 PM.

_____ 10. A written truth in lending statement is required if the medical office makes an agreement for monthly payments.

✎Term KEY TERM ASSESSMENT

Directions: Match each medical term with its definition.

_____ 1.   Account aging

_____ 2.   Balance due

_____ 3.   Bankruptcy

_____ 4.   Claim message

_____ 5.   Credit balance

_____ 6.   Collection agency

_____ 7.   Overdraft

_____ 8.   Skip

_____ 9.   Truth in lending

A. Money owed by the medical office to a patient, usually due to an overpayment

B. A check (or draft) that exceeds the amount of funds in a bank account

C. Total amount owed

D. A firm that is in the business of collecting overdue accounts

E. The process of finding out how long specific account balances have been outstanding

F. Legal requirement to provide written terms of a loan in language that can be easily understood

G. The legal process by which the debts of an individual or business are resolved if they cannot be paid

H. Messages encouraging payment of a bill, usually attached to or printed on the monthly statement

I. Account for which no billing information is available

EVALUATION OF LEARNING

Directions: Fill in each blank with the correct answer.

1. What is the advantage to the office of weekly cycle billing?

   _____

   _____

2. If the medical office bills every week, how are patient accounts usually divided?

   _____

   _____

3. What are three ways that bills can be produced?

   _____

   _____

4. Give examples of two special situations that may affect billing.

   _____

   _____

5. What is overdraft protection?

   _____

   _____

6. When should the medical office stop payment on a check?

   _____

   _____

7. How should the MA handle a check that is returned for not sufficient funds?

   _____

   _____

8. When does a credit balance occur in a patient account, and how is a credit balance handled?

   _____

   _____

9. When is a patient account considered overdue?

   _____

10. What are the usual categories of overdue accounts when an accounts receivable aging record is created?

_____

_____

11. What is the usual progression in collection activity when a patient's account is overdue?

_____

_____

12. Why is it recommended to place a telephone call regarding an overdue account in addition to placing claim messages on the bill?

_____

_____

13. When does the office need to have a written credit arrangement with a patient?

_____

_____

14. What does a truth in lending statement include, and when should it be sent to a patient?

_____

_____

15. Identify three methods to try to trace a patient whose bill is returned with the notation "address unknown."

_____

_____

16. If the three methods identified in the previous question fail to locate a "skip," what should the medical office do to try to collect a bill?

_____

_____

17. What is the process for sending a patient account to a collection agency?

_____

_____

18. How should a collection agency payment be entered on the patient's ledger card and on the day sheet?

_____

_____

19. What is small claims court, and how might it be used by the medical office?

_____

_____

_____

20. If a patient has died, how and when should the bill for services rendered before death be sent?

_____

_____

21. If the bill of a deceased individual is not paid promptly, how should the MA follow up?

_____

_____

22. What is the status of outstanding medical bills if a person declares bankruptcy under Chapter VII? Under Chapter XIII?

_____

_____

_____

23. Describe briefly how each of the following laws affects credit and collection activities in the medical office:

a.   Equal Credit Opportunity Act: _____

_____

b.   Fair Debt Collection Practices Act: _____

_____

c.   Federal Truth in Lending Act: _____

_____

d.   Fair Credit Reporting Act: _____

_____

e.   Bankruptcy Abuse and Consumer Protection Act of 2005: _____

_____

CRITICAL THINKING ACTIVITIES

A. CYCLE BILLING

Assume that a billing cycle is used where the first week of the month, patients with a last name beginning with the letters A-E are billed; the second week, F-L; the third week, M-S; and the fourth week, T-Z. Identify which week each of the following patients would be billed.

1. John T. Sanders   _____

2. Eileen McDonald   _____

3. Winston A. Robertson   _____

4. Tracy Marie Jordan   _____

5. Julian W. Allen   _____

6. Edward Elliot Hubbard   _____

7. Joanne Mason-Taylor   _____

8. Diane von Bohlen   _____

9. Carolyn Ann Oppenheimer   _____

10. Douglas P. Benson   _____

B. ADJUSTMENTS

For each of the following situations identify whether the MA will post the transaction to the patient account as a credit adjustment (reduces the patient balance), a payment, or a debit adjustment (increases the patient balance).

1. Patient pays $50.00 by check, which is an overpayment of $25.00: _____

2. Patient's check for $25.00 is returned by the bank marked "Not sufficient funds": _____

3. A collection agency payment is received, and the patient balance is zero: _____

4. A check from an insurance company is received for a patient account: _____

5. A patient pays a copayment of $10.00 at the time of the visit: _____

6. A patient is given a discount of $15.00 for paying the bill in cash: _____

7. A check is issued as a refund for a patient overpayment: _____

8. The insurance company identifies $12.00 of the patient charge as an excluded amount: _____

C. AGING ACCOUNTS

Assume that accounts are aged from the date of billing. If you are aging accounts on 10/30/10, select the letter of the correct length of time that each of the following accounts has been outstanding.

a. Current (0-30 days)

b. 31-60 days

c. 61-90 days

d. 91-120 days

e. over 120 days

_____ 1. Service provided on 7/4/XX, billed on 8/1/XX

_____ 2. Service provided on 9/22/XX, billed on 10/3/XX

_____ 3. Service provided on 8/13/XX, billed on 8/22/XX

_____ 4. Service provided on 4/18/XX, billed on 4/25/XX

_____ 5. Service provided on 5/13/XX, billed on 6/6/XX

_____ 6. Service provided on 6/19/XX, billed on 7/12/XX

_____ 7. Service provided on 6/25/XX, billed on 7/18/XX

_____ 8. Service provided on 7/18/XX, billed on 8/15/XX

PRACTICE FOR COMPETENCY

Procedure 47-1: Processing Patient Bills. Using a computer billing program, practice printing selected patient bills and placing them in window envelopes.

Procedure 47-2: Posting an NSF Check. The bank has returned Maria Ryan's check No. 938 for $10.00 marked NSF (not sufficient funds). Your bank charges $15.00 for each returned check. Using today's date, enter the returned check as an adjustment as well as the bank fee on the day sheet. Her old balance was zero.

Notes

JOURNAL OF DAILY CHARGES, PAYMENTS & DEPOSITS

PLACE
FIRST PEG
HERE

	DATE	PROFESSIONAL SERVICE	FEE	PAYMENT	ADJUST-MENT	NEW BALANCE	OLD BALANCE	PATIENT'S NAME	
1									1
2									2
3									3
4									4
5									5
6									6
7									7
8									8
9									9
10									10
11									11
12									12
13									13
14									14
15									15
16									16
17									17
18									18
19									19
20									20
21									21
22									22
23									23
24									24
25									25
26									26
27									27
28									28
29									29
30									30
31								TOTALS THIS PAGE	31
32								TOTALS PREVIOUS PAGE	32
33								TOTALS MONTH TO DATE	33

COLUMN A   COLUMN B   COLUMN C   COLUMN D   COLUMN E

MEMO _____

_____

_____

_____

DAILY-FROM LINE 31

ACCOUNTS RECEIVABLE PROOF	
Column E	
Plus Column A	
Sub-Total	
Minus Column B	
Sub-Total	
Minus Column C	
Equals Column D	

Box 1

MONTH-FROM LINE 31

ACCOUNTS RECEIVABLE PROOF	
Accts. Receivable Previous Day	$
Plus Column A	
Sub-Total	
Minus Column B	
Sub-Total	
Minus Column C	
Accts. Receivable End of Day	

Box 2

(From Hunt SA: *Saunders fundamentals of medical assisting student mastery manual,* St. Louis, 2007, Saunders.)

Notes

PLACE
FIRST PEG
HERE

JOURNAL OF DAILY CHARGES, PAYMENTS & DEPOSITS

		DATE	PROFESSIONAL SERVICE	FEE	PAYMENT	ADJUST-MENT	NEW BALANCE	OLD BALANCE	PATIENT'S NAME		
1											1
2	●										2
3											3
4											4
5											5
6	●										6
7											7
8											8
9											9
10	●										10
11											11
12											12
13											13
14	●										14
15											15
16											16
17											17
18	●										18
19											19
20											20
21											21
22	●										22
23											23
24											24
25											25
26	●										26
27											27
28											28
29											29
30	●										30
31										TOTALS THIS PAGE	31
32										TOTALS PREVIOUS PAGE	32
33										TOTALS MONTH TO DATE	33

COLUMN A   COLUMN B   COLUMN C   COLUMN D   COLUMN E

●

MEMO _____
_____
_____
_____

DAILY-FROM LINE 31	
ACCOUNTS RECEIVABLE PROOF	
Column E	
Plus Column A	
Sub-Total	
Minus Column B	
Sub-Total	
Minus Column C	
Equals Column D	

Box 1

MONTH-FROM LINE 31	
ACCOUNTS RECEIVABLE PROOF	
Accts. Receivable Previous Day	$
Plus Column A	
Sub-Total	
Minus Column B	
Sub-Total	
Minus Column C	
Accts. Receivable End of Day	

Box 2

(From Hunt SA: *Saunders fundamentals of medical assisting student mastery manual,* St. Louis, 2007, Saunders.)

Notes

Procedure 47-3: Posting an Overpayment. You receive check No. 332 in the amount of $70.00 from James Winston for payment of charges for an office visit one month ago. Using today's date, enter the payment on the day sheet used for Procedure 47-2. Mr. Winston's previous balance was $10.00. Remember to post negative amounts in parentheses.

Procedure 47-4: Processing a Refund. Prepare a refund for James Winston in order to bring the balance of his account to zero. Post the refund on the third line of the day sheet used for Procedure 47-2 as a credit adjustment. Write a check to James Winston for the refund amount using the first check form below. Leave the signature line blank, since you are not authorized to sign checks. The old balance of the checking account is $4,166.82. Complete the check stub. Prepare a letter to James Winston informing him that you are enclosing a check for the amount of his overpayment. His address is James Winston, 25 Magnolia Lane, Western, XY 44770. Inform him that he can call you at extension 24 if he has any questions. Assume that you will print the letter on office letterhead, and sign the letter using your own name and the title Medical Assistant on the next line. This means that a reference line is not necessary. Specify the check on the enclosure line. (Enc: Check #1837)

Notes

1837

DATE _____
TO _____
FOR _____

BALANCE BROUGHT FORWARD		
DEPOSITS		
BALANCE		
AMT THIS CK		
BALANCE CARRIED FORWARD		

BLACKBURN PRIMARY CARE ASSOCIATES, PC
1990 Turquiose Drive
Blackburn, WI 54937
608-459-8857

1837

94-72/1224

DATE _____

PAY TO THE
ORDER OF _____ $ _____

_____ DOLLARS

DERBYSHIRE SAVINGS
Member FDIC
P.O. BOX 8923
Blackburn, WI 54937

FOR _____

⑈055003⑈ 446782011⑈ 678800470

1838

DATE _____
TO _____
FOR _____

BALANCE BROUGHT FORWARD		
DEPOSITS		
BALANCE		
AMT THIS CK		
BALANCE CARRIED FORWARD		

BLACKBURN PRIMARY CARE ASSOCIATES, PC
1990 Turquiose Drive
Blackburn, WI 54937
608-459-8857

1838

94-72/1224

DATE _____

PAY TO THE
ORDER OF _____ $ _____

_____ DOLLARS

DERBYSHIRE SAVINGS
Member FDIC
P.O. BOX 8923
Blackburn, WI 54937

FOR _____

⑈055003⑈ 446782011⑈ 678800470

1839

DATE _____
TO _____
FOR _____

BALANCE BROUGHT FORWARD		
DEPOSITS		
BALANCE		
AMT THIS CK		
BALANCE CARRIED FORWARD		

BLACKBURN PRIMARY CARE ASSOCIATES, PC
1990 Turquiose Drive
Blackburn, WI 54937
608-459-8857

1839

94-72/1224

DATE _____

PAY TO THE
ORDER OF _____ $ _____

_____ DOLLARS

DERBYSHIRE SAVINGS
Member FDIC
P.O. BOX 8923
Blackburn, WI 54937

FOR _____

⑈055003⑈ 446782011⑈ 678800470

(From Hunt SA: *Saunders fundamentals of medical assisting student mastery manual,* St. Louis, 2007, Saunders.)

Notes

Procedure 47-5: Creating an Accounts Receivable Aging Record. Create a patient aging report based on information from the accounts of the following patients. Assume that you are creating the report on 11/30 for bills which were sent on the first day of the month after the service was provided: 8/1, 9/1, 10/1, or 11/1. Beside each account on the report, mark the action that should be taken according to Procedure 47-5.

Daryl P. Sanders
24 Lakeview Drive
Western, XY 44770

Date	Professional Service	Fee	Payment	Adjustment	New Balance
6/4/XX	99202, cash payment	55.00	20.00		35.00
6/28/XX	Ins. ck #219		20.00		15.00

Lloyd Hanson
10 High Street
Western, XY 44770

Date	Professional Service	Fee	Payment	Adjustment	New Balance
7/15/XX	99204, 93000, ck #664	150.00	15.00		135.00
7/28/XX	Ins ck #604 (for 6/15)		128.00	7.00	0.00
8/25/XX	99212	48.00	15.00		33.00

Maria Rivera Santos
160 Underwood Street
Western, XY 44770

Date	Professional Service	Fee	Payment	Adjustment	New Balance
9/28/XX	99204, ck #259	135.00	27.00		108.00

Thomas Maxwell
1100 Main Street
Western, XY 44770

Date	Professional Service	Fee	Payment	Adjustment	New Balance
9/1/XX	99213, 81002, 98000, ck #322	122.00	50.00		72.00
10/12/XX	99212, ck #602	48.00	15.00		105.00
10/15/XX	Ins ck #2298 (for 9/1)		56.00	16.00	33.00

Notes

Account Aging Report

Patient Name	Last Payment	Current 0 - 30	Past 31 - 60	Past 61 - 90	Past 91 - 120	Past 121+	Total Balance

(From Hunt SA: *Saunders fundamentals of medical assisting student mastery manual,* St. Louis, 2007, Saunders.)

Notes

Procedure 47-6: Writing a Collection Letter. Write a collection letter to each individual on the aging report above if you marked the account: "Payment is now overdue." Instruct the recipient to pay the bill or contact the office to make other arrangements. Use the date of 11/30/XX and assume that the letters will be printed on office letterhead. Sign any letter using your own name and use the title, Medical Assistant, on the next line.

Procedure 47-7: Posting a Collection Agency Payment. You received a payment from a collection agency of $50.00 (check No. 554) for the account of Helen McDonald. The current balance of her account is zero. Using line 4 on the day sheet, post a credit adjustment as a reverse collection. Using line 5, post the collection agency payment. Total all columns of the day sheet and balance the day sheet.

Notes

☑ EVALUATION OF COMPETENCY

Ⓓⓥⓓ Procedure 47-1: Processing Patient Bills

Name: _____   Date: _____

Evaluated By: _____   Date: _____

Performance Objective

Outcome:	Process patient bill.
Conditions:	Given the following: computer, patient accounts, paper or statement forms, window envelopes, and postage.
Standards:	Time: 10 minutes. Student completed procedure in ____ minutes.
	Accuracy: Satisfactory score on the Performance Evaluation Checklist.

Performance Evaluation Checklist

Trial 1	Trial 2	Point Value	Performance Standards
		•	Located patient accounts in the computer database.
		•	Selected accounts to be billed.
		•	Printed patient statements using paper forms or forms generated by the computer program.
		•	Verified that statements printed correctly.
		•	Folded statements so that patient name and address would be facing outward.
		•	Inserted statements in window envelopes.
		•	Verified that name and address were visible through the window.
		•	Placed postage on envelopes and set aside for mailing.
		∗	Prepared statements correctly for mailing.
		∗	Completed the procedure within 10 minutes.
			TOTALS

Evaluation of Student Performance

EVALUATION CRITERIA			COMMENTS
Symbol	Category	Point Value	
∗	Critical Step	16 points	
•	Essential Step	6 points	
▷	Theory Question	2 points	
Score calculation: 100 points			
– _____ points missed			
_____ Score			
Satisfactory score: 85 or above			

CAAHEP Competencies Achieved:

Psychomotor (Skills)
☑ VI. 2. b. Perform billing procedures.
☑ VI. 3. Use computerized office billing systems.

ABHES Competencies Achieved:
☑ 8. i. Perform billing and collection procedures.
☑ 8. w. Use manual or computerized bookkeeping systems.

EVALUATION OF COMPETENCY

Procedure 47-2: Posting an NSF Check

Name: _____   Date: _____

Evaluated By: _____   Date: _____

Performance Objective

Outcome:	Post an NSF check.
Conditions:	Given the following: computer, patient accounts, returned check, day sheet, pen, and calculator.
Standards:	Time: 10 minutes. Student completed procedure in ____ minutes.
	Accuracy: Satisfactory score on the Performance Evaluation Checklist.

Performance Evaluation Checklist

Trial 1	Trial 2	Point Value	*Performance Standards*
		●	Located the patient account for the patient whose check was returned.
		●	Wrote the patient's name and old balance on the first open line of the day sheet.
		●	Created a new transaction for the patient in the computer account, and posted the returned check using the code for "NSF check" or "adjustment charge" depending on office policy.
		●	Entered the returned check fee in the computer account using the code for "returned check fee," verifying that insurance would not be billed.
		●	Wrote "NSF check," the check number, and "returned check fee" in the *professional service* column of the day sheet.
		●	Placed the amount of the check in the adjustment column in parentheses.
		▷	Explained the difference between the notation for a credit adjustment and a debit adjustment.
		●	Entered the returned check fee on the day sheet in the *fee* column.
		●	Entered the sum of the NSF check, the returned check fee, and the old balance in the *new balance* column.
		✳	When totaling the adjustment column of the day sheet, subtracted the adjustment from the total of other adjustments.
		●	Notified the patient by telephone or letter that the check was returned and a fee was charged.
		●	Enclosed an updated patient statement with a letter.
		✳	Completed the procedure within 10 minutes.
			TOTALS

Evaluation of Student Performance

EVALUATION CRITERIA			COMMENTS
Symbol	Category	Point Value	
✱	Critical Step	16 points	
●	Essential Step	6 points	
▷	Theory Question	2 points	

Score calculation: 100 points

    – _____ points missed

    _____ Score

Satisfactory score: 85 or above

CAAHEP Competencies Achieved:

Psychomotor (Skills)

☑ VI. 2. g. Post non-sufficient fund (NSF) checks.

Affective (Behavior)

☑ VI. 1. Demonstrate sensitivity and professionalism in handling accounts receivable activities with patients.

ABHES Competencies Achieved:

☑ 8. p. Post non-sufficient funds (NSF).

EVALUATION OF COMPETENCY

Procedure 47-3: Posting an Overpayment

Name: _____ Date: _____

Evaluated By: _____ Date: _____

Performance Objective

Outcome:	Post an overpayment.
Conditions:	Given the following: computer, patient accounts, payment check(s), day sheet, pen, and calculator.
Standards:	Time: 5 minutes. Student completed procedure in ____ minutes.
	Accuracy: Satisfactory score on the Performance Evaluation Checklist.

Performance Evaluation Checklist

Trial 1	Trial 2	Point Value	Performance Standards
		●	Located the patient account for the patient with an overpayment.
		●	Created a new transaction for the patient in the computer account, and posted the payment using the correct code (patient check or insurance check) linked to the charges being paid.
		●	Noted that the balance due is a negative number.
		▷	Explained the meaning of a negative number as a balance in the accounts receivable.
		●	Entered the type of payment and check number in the *professional service* column of the day sheet.
		●	Entered the amount of the payment in the *payment* column of the day sheet.
		●	Entered the sum of the payment and the old balance in the *new balance* column in parentheses.
		✱	When totaling the adjustment column of the day sheet, subtracted the negative balance from the total.
		●	Arranged to clear the negative balance from the system according to office policy.
		✱	Completed the procedure within 5 minutes.
			TOTALS

Evaluation of Student Performance

EVALUATION CRITERIA			COMMENTS
Symbol	Category	Point Value	
∗	Critical Step	16 points	
●	Essential Step	6 points	
▷	Theory Question	2 points	

Score calculation: 100 points

　　　　　　－＿＿＿＿ points missed

　　　　　　＿＿＿＿ Score

Satisfactory score: 85 or above

CAAHEP Competencies Achieved:

Psychomotor (Skills)

☑ VI. 2. e. Process a credit balance.

Affective (Behavior)

☑ VI. 1. Demonstrate sensitivity and professionalism in handling accounts receivable activities with patients.

ABHES Competencies Achieved:

☑ 8. n. Process credit balances.

EVALUATION OF COMPETENCY

Procedure 47-4: Processing a Refund

Name: _____   Date: _____

Evaluated By: _____   Date: _____

Performance Objective

Outcome:	Process a refund.
Conditions:	Given the following: computer, patient accounts, payment check(s), day sheet, pen, calculator, and printer.
Standards:	Time: 10 minutes. Student completed procedure in _____ minutes.
	Accuracy: Satisfactory score on the Performance Evaluation Checklist.

Performance Evaluation Checklist

Trial 1	Trial 2	Point Value	*Performance Standards*
		●	Located the patient account in the computer.
		●	Entered the patient's name and old balance on the first open line of the day sheet.
		●	Calculated the amount to be refunded.
		●	Created a new transaction in the computer and entered the amount of the refund using the code for a refund.
		●	Verified that the patient's balance was zero after the transaction was entered.
		●	Wrote "Refund for Overpayment" in the *professional services* column of the day sheet.
		●	Entered the amount of the refund in the *adjustment* column.
		●	Subtracted the amount of the refund from the old balance, and entered zero in the *new balance* column.
		●	Wrote a check for the amount of the refund leaving the signature line blank.
		●	Recorded the check number, date, payee, and reason for the check on the check stub or in the check register.
		●	Subtracted the amount of the check from the checking account balance and entered the balance carried forward.
		●	Wrote a letter to the patient explaining the refund and prepared an envelope.
		●	Signed the letter and clipped the check to the letter and envelope.
		●	Left the check, letter, and envelope in the designated location to obtain a physician signature on the check.
		∗	Posted transaction correctly and prepared a letter without errors.
		∗	Completed the procedure within 10 minutes.
			TOTALS

Evaluation of Student Performance

EVALUATION CRITERIA			COMMENTS
Symbol	Category	Point Value	
∗	Critical Step	16 points	
●	Essential Step	6 points	
▷	Theory Question	2 points	

Score calculation: 100 points

−_____ points missed

_____ Score

Satisfactory score: 85 or above

CAAHEP Competencies Achieved:

Psychomotor (Skills)
☑ VI. 2. f. Process refunds.

Affective (Behavior)
☑ VI. 1. Demonstrate sensitivity and professionalism in handling accounts receivable activities with patients.

ABHES Competencies Achieved:

☑ 8. o. Process refunds.

EVALUATION OF COMPETENCY

Procedure 47-5: Creating an Accounts Receivable Aging Record

Name: _____   Date: _____

Evaluated By: _____   Date: _____

Performance Objective

Outcome:	Create an accounts receivable aging record.
Conditions:	Given the following: computer, patient accounts, accounts receivable aging record analysis form (optional), office policy or procedure manual, and pen.
Standards:	Time: 15 minutes. Student completed procedure in _____ minutes.
	Accuracy: Satisfactory score on the Performance Evaluation Checklist.

Performance Evaluation Checklist

Trial 1	Trial 2	Point Value	Performance Standards
		•	Used the reports function of the computer billing program to print an aging report for patients and insurance companies, or created the report manually from individual patient accounts.
		•	Reviewed the accounts on the report and marked the appropriate action for each account according to office policy.
		•	Marked all accounts less than 31 days old: "No action needed."
		•	Marked accounts with unpaid insurance claims older than 31 days: "Follow up with insurance."
		•	Marked accounts 31 to 60 days old with paid insurance claims according to office policy (e.g., "Attach first claim note to statement").
		•	Marked accounts 61 to 90 days old with paid insurance claims according to office policy (e.g., "Attach second claim note to statement").
		•	Marked accounts 91 to 120 days old with paid insurance claims according to office policy (e.g., "Telephone patient").
		•	Reviewed previous collection attempts for accounts over 120 days.
		•	Prepared a collection letter for each account over 120 days informing the patient of a specific deadline and intended action if payment is not received.
		•	Filed a copy of any collection letter in the patient's medical record.
		•	Recorded all action taken beside each account on the report.
		•	Documented any telephone calls and/or collection letter in the progress notes of the patient's medical record.

Trial 1	Trial 2	Point Value	*Performance Standards*
		∗	Analyzed outstanding accounts accurately, performed appropriate follow up, and documented correctly.
		∗	Completed the procedure within 15 minutes.
			TOTALS

CHART	
Date	

Evaluation of Student Performance

EVALUATION CRITERIA			COMMENTS
Symbol	Category	Point Value	
∗	Critical Step	16 points	
•	Essential Step	6 points	
▷	Theory Question	2 points	
Score calculation: 100 points			
−_____ points missed			
_____ Score			
Satisfactory score: 85 or above			

CAAHEP Competencies Achieved:

Psychomotor (Skills)
☑ VI. 2. c. Perform collection procedures.

ABHES Competencies Achieved:

☑ 8. i. Perform billing and collection procedures.

EVALUATION OF COMPETENCY

Procedure 47-6: Writing a Collection Letter

Name: _____   Date: _____

Evaluated By: _____   Date: _____

Performance Objective

Outcome: Write a collection letter.

Conditions: Given the following: accounts receivable aging report, computer, patient accounts, letterhead stationery, envelope, and printer.

Standards: Time: 10 minutes.   Student completed procedure in _____ minutes.

Accuracy: Satisfactory score on the Performance Evaluation Checklist.

Performance Evaluation Checklist

Trial 1	Trial 2	Point Value	*Performance Standards*
		•	Determined which accounts were over 120 days old from an accounts receivable aging report.
		•	Reviewed accounts over 120 days to be sure that there are no extenuating circumstances for which the patient might be given more time to pay.
		•	Set up a letter for the first account over 120 days using the format preferred by the office.
		•	Identified the patient's address from the patient information sheet or computer screen.
		•	Included the outstanding balance, the date charges were incurred, the service provided, and the amount paid by insurance in the letter.
		•	Described any previous telephone conversations and/or agreements in the letter.
		•	Stated the amount of the outstanding balance and the date by which it must be paid.
		•	Entered the typed signature of the individual designated by office policy to write collection letters. Used a reference line if another staff member will sign the letter.
		•	Signed the letter or placed it in the designated location to obtain a signature.
		•	Prepared an envelope.
		•	Copied the letter and filed the copy in the patient's medical record and/or a collection follow-up file.
		•	Placed a notation on the aging report and in the computer account that the letter was sent to the patient.
		•	Placed the letter in the envelope and mailed the letter.
		*	Created error-free letter and envelope.
		*	Completed the procedure within 10 minutes.
			TOTALS

Evaluation of Student Performance

EVALUATION CRITERIA			COMMENTS
Symbol	Category	Point Value	
*	Critical Step	16 points	
•	Essential Step	6 points	
▷	Theory Question	2 points	

Score calculation: 100 points

     – _____ points missed

     _____ Score

Satisfactory score: 85 or above

CAAHEP Competencies Achieved:

Psychomotor (Skills)
☑ IV. 10. Compose professional/business letters.
☑ VI. 2. c. Perform collection procedures.
☑ IX. 8. Apply local, state and federal health care legislation and regulation appropriate to the medical assisting practice setting.

Affective (Behavior)
☑ VI. 1. Demonstrate sensitivity and professionalism in handling accounts receivable activities with patients.
☑ IX. 3. Recognize the importance of local, state and federal legislation and regulations in the practice setting.

ABHES Competencies Achieved:

☑ 8. i. Perform billing and collection procedures.
☑ 8. dd. Serve as liaison between physician and others.
☑ 8. jj. Perform fundamental writing skills including correct grammar, spelling, and formatting techniques when writing prescriptions, documenting medical records, etc.

EVALUATION OF COMPETENCY

Procedure 47-7: Posting a Collection Agency Payment

Name: _____   Date: _____

Evaluated By: _____   Date: _____

Performance Objective

Outcome:	Post a collection agency payment.
Conditions:	Given the following: computer, patient account, payment check, day sheet, calculator, and pen.
Standards:	Time: 5 minutes. Student completed procedure in ____ minutes.
	Accuracy: Satisfactory score on the Performance Evaluation Checklist.

Performance Evaluation Checklist

Trial 1	Trial 2	Point Value	Performance Standards
		●	Located the account of the patient for whom a check has been received from the collection agency.
		●	Wrote the patient's name and old balance on the first open line of the day sheet.
		▷	Explained why the account balance was adjusted to zero when the account was sent for collection.
		●	Created a new transaction for the patient, selected the code for "Reverse collection," and entered the amount of the check.
		●	Verified that the computer showed a positive balance after this entry.
		●	Wrote "Reverse collection" in the professional service column of the day sheet.
		●	Entered the amount of the check in the adjustment column of the day sheet in parentheses as a debit adjustment.
		▷	Explained the difference between the notation for a credit adjustment and a debit adjustment.
		✳	When totaling the adjustment column of the day sheet, subtracted the debit adjustment from the total of the credit adjustments.
		●	Entered the amount of the check in the new balance column.
		●	In the computer, on a new line, selected the code for "Collection agency payment," and entered the amount of the check.
		●	Verified that the patient balance returned to zero.
		●	On the next line of the day sheet entered the patient's name again, and wrote the amount of the collection agency check as the old balance.
		●	Wrote "Collection agency payment" and the check number in the professional service column of the day sheet.
		●	Entered the amount of the check in the payment column.

Trial 1	Trial 2	Point Value	Performance Standards
		•	Entered zero in the new balance column.
		*	Completed the procedure within 5 minutes.
			TOTALS

Evaluation of Student Performance

EVALUATION CRITERIA			COMMENTS
Symbol	Category	Point Value	
*	Critical Step	16 points	
•	Essential Step	6 points	
▷	Theory Question	2 points	

Score calculation: 100 points

−_____ points missed

_____ Score

Satisfactory score: 85 or above

CAAHEP Competencies Achieved:

Psychomotor (Skills)
☑ VI. 2. h. Post collection agency payments.

ABHES Competencies Achieved:

☑ 8. q. Post collection agency payments.

48

The Medical Assistant as Office Manager

CHAPTER ASSIGNMENTS

√ After Completing	Date Due	Textbook Page(s)	TEXTBOOK ASSIGNMENTS	Possible Points	Points You Earned
		1109-1128	Read Chapter 48: The Medical Assistant as Office Manager		
		1113 1126	Read Case Study 1 Case Study 1 questions	5	
		1119 1126-1127	Read Case Study 2 Case Study 2 questions	5	
		1124 1127	Read Case Study 3 Case Study 3 questions	5	
			TOTAL POINTS		

√ After Completing	Date Due	Study Guide Page(s)	STUDY GUIDE ASSIGNMENTS (CTA: Critical Thinking Activity)	Possible Points	Points You Earned
		1241	Pretest	10	
		1242	Term Key Term Assessment	19	
		1243-1246	Evaluation of Learning questions	32	
		1246	CTA A: Fire Protection	10	
		1247	CTA B: Equipment Inventory List	10	
		1247	CTA C: Supply Inventory List	10	
		1247	CTA D: Patient Bill of Rights	10	
		1247-1248	CTA E: Evacuation Plan	10	
		1248	CTA F: Community Resources for Emergency Preparedness	10	
		1248	CTA G: Incident Report	10	

√ After Completing	Date Due	Study Guide Page(s)	STUDY GUIDE ASSIGNMENTS (CTA: Critical Thinking Activity)	Possible Points	Points You Earned
			CD Activity: Chapter 48 Establishing and Maintaining a Supply Inventory and Ordering System	10	
			CD Activity: Chapter 48 Processing an Employee Payroll	10	
			CD Activity: Chapter 48 Apply Your Knowledge questions (Record points earned)		
		1241	Posttest	10	
			ADDITIONAL ASSIGNMENTS		
			TOTAL POINTS		

√ When Assigned by Your Instructor	Study Guide Page(s)	Practices Required	LABORATORY ASSIGNMENTS (Procedure Number and Name)	*Score
	1249	2	**DVD Practice for Competency** 48-1: Performing Routine Maintenance of Equipment Textbook reference: pp. 1116-1117	
	1251-1252		**Evaluation of Competency** 48-1: Performing Routine Maintenance of Equipment	*
	1250	3	**DVD Practice for Competency** 48-2: Taking a Supply or Equipment Inventory Textbook reference: pp. 1119-1120	
	1253-1254		**Evaluation of Competency** 48-2: Taking a Supply or Equipment Inventory	*
	1250	3	**Practice for Competency** 48-3: Locating Community Resources Textbook reference: pp. 1124-1125	
	1255-1256		**Evaluation of Competency** 48-3: Locating Community Resources	*
			ADDITIONAL ASSIGNMENTS	

Notes

Name _____   Date _____

True or False

_____   1. Stationery, envelopes, and billing forms should be located in the administrative area of the medical office.

_____   2. Old telephone logs should be shredded when they are discarded.

_____   3. Rigid biohazard waste containers are usually stored under the sink in an examination room.

_____   4. The waiting room often has a sign requesting that patients pay copayments at the time of the visit.

_____   5. Falls are a common cause of workplace injury.

_____   6. Treatment rooms or special procedure rooms are usually kept a little warmer than examination rooms.

_____   7. The medical assistant is usually responsible for changing the plastic liners in biohazard waste containers.

_____   8. The doors to the laboratory and medical records shelves or area may have an additional lock.

_____   9. Fire doors can be propped open during the day but must be tightly closed at night or if a fire begins.

_____   10. An equipment inventory includes the date of purchase, cost, and serial number of each piece of equipment.

[?] **POSTTEST**

True or False

_____   1. Business operations may be performed at the front desk or separate area of the medical office.

_____   2. Each examination room should have a sink and wall-mounted paper towel dispenser.

_____   3. Biohazard waste containers with a plastic liner only need to be covered at night.

_____   4. The medical office may have a display rack with informational brochures in the waiting room.

_____   5. Tripping or slipping without falling may still cause workplace injuries.

_____   6. A good temperature for the office waiting room is 70°F to 72°F.

_____   7. All cleaning is done at night in the medical office by an outside cleaning company.

_____   8. Controlled substances should always be stored in an area with two locks and two separate keys.

_____   9. Smoke detectors that are wired into the office alarm system do not have batteries.

_____   10. A supply inventory is used to keep records for tax purposes.

✏Term KEY TERM ASSESSMENT

Directions: Match each medical term with its definition.

_____ 1. Back order

_____ 2. Depreciation

_____ 3. Gross pay

_____ 4. Inventory

_____ 5. Invoice

_____ 6. Minutes

_____ 7. Net pay

_____ 8. *Per diem*

_____ 9. Policy

_____ 10. Procedure

_____ 11. Purchase order (PO)

_____ 12. Reorder point

_____ 13. Risk management

_____ 14. Salary

_____ 15. Service contract

_____ 16. Social Security tax (FICA)

_____ 17. Vendor

_____ 18. Warranty

_____ 19. W-4 form

A. A written record of the proceedings of a meeting
B. The form used to claim allowances for federal income tax reporting
C. The total amount earned in a time period by an employee before any deductions
D. A guiding principle for the management of a medical office or business
E. A tax collected from employees to fund the Social Security program
F. A fixed amount of wages that does not depend on the number of hours worked
G. A detailed list of items in stock or in possession of an individual or business
H. A promise by the manufacturer to repair or replace defective parts in an item during a specific time period
I. A term used for items ordered that cannot be shipped immediately, usually because they are out of stock
J. A number on a supply inventory that indicates when a specific item should be reordered
K. A list of the steps to handle a certain situation or perform a certain task
L. The actual amount of money paid directly to an employee after taxes and other deductions
M. An agreement that provides for service for a piece of equipment after the warranty expires
N. The form used to order supplies as well as the order itself
O. An itemized bill for items that have not been prepaid
P. Employees who are scheduled by the day according to office needs
Q. Accounting methods to respond to the loss of value of a property or piece of equipment over time
R. The process of assessing risk and putting policies and procedures in place to minimize it
S. A company from whom supplies or equipment is purchased

EVALUATION OF LEARNING

Directions: Fill in each blank with the correct answer.

1. Write a general statement identifying the type of equipment and supplies needed in the administrative area of the medical office.

   a. Equipment: _____

   _____

   b. Supplies: _____

   _____

2. Write a general statement identifying the type of equipment and supplies needed for examination rooms and treatment rooms.

   a. Equipment: _____

   _____

   b. Supplies: _____

   _____

3. What are four common signs that might be found in a medical office waiting room?

   _____

   _____

4. List five activities that are considered part of routine maintenance.

   _____

   _____

   _____

5. Identify two important components for controlling the air in the medical office.

   _____

   _____

6. What parts of the medical office are MAs usually responsible for cleaning and/or tidying?

   _____

   _____

   _____

7. Describe briefly how to clean storage cabinets and drawers.

   _____

   _____

8. In addition to the general security system, which areas in the medical office should be kept locked?

_____

_____

_____

9. Identify four important fire protection measures used in medical offices.

_____

_____

_____

10. Identify two reasons why it is important to maintain an accurate inventory of equipment.

_____

_____

11. Describe how service contracts work. When do they go into effect?

_____

_____

12. What are some helpful things to do when a new piece of equipment is placed into service?

_____

_____

13. Name five types of information that should be included on a supply inventory list.

_____

_____

_____

14. What is the reorder point on a supply inventory list? How is it used?

_____

_____

15. What is the MA's responsibility for restocking administrative and clinical areas?

_____

_____

16. Why is a tracking number or purchase order number useful when ordering supplies?

_____

_____

17. Identify three steps the MA should take when supplies are delivered.

_____

_____

_____

18. How can staff meetings help create an environment for teamwork?

_____

_____

_____

19. Describe two methods to prepare meeting participants, keep a meeting running smoothly, and keep track of decisions made during the meeting.

_____

_____

20. What paperwork is required for a new employee?

_____

_____

21. What are five things that must be documented in an employee's payroll record?

_____

_____

_____

22. Identify three types of deductions that the employer must withhold from an employee paycheck.

_____

23. What is unemployment tax, and how is it paid?

_____

_____

24. When preparing payroll checks for employees, what five items of information must be recorded in the payroll record for each employee?

_____

_____

_____

25. What is the MA's responsibility in relation to the physician and office schedule?

_____

_____

_____

26. What are four tasks that the MA might need to perform when making travel arrangements for a physician or other staff member?

_____

_____

27. Differentiate between a policy and a procedure.

_____

28. Identify three reasons why it is valuable for organizations to have procedure manuals available.

_____

_____

29. Identify eight types of community resources to whom patients might be referred for information or services.

_____

_____

_____

_____

30. Describe when incident reports are completed and how they fit into the risk management plan of an organization.

_____

_____

31. Give four examples of damage or injury that should be covered by the medical office's general property and/or liability insurance.

_____

_____

32. What kind of protection is provided by professional liability insurance?

_____

_____

CRITICAL THINKING ACTIVITIES

A. FIRE PROTECTION

Make a list of fire protection equipment and supplies for the medical office shown in Chapter 1, Figure 1-4. Include items that might be part of the office building (such as a sprinkler system), as well as the location of fire extinguishers and other equipment.

_____

_____

_____

_____

_____

B. EQUIPMENT INVENTORY LIST

Create an inventory list of equipment in the clinical laboratory of your medical assisting program. Include the name of each piece of equipment, a description, and a serial number or school ID number. Set up your list with columns for at least three dates to check off items when you take inventory.

C. SUPPLY INVENTORY LIST

Working with at least one classmate, set up a supply inventory list for at least 15 supply items that might be used during the physical examination. The categories should include the following: item name, quantity in stock, reorder point, and quantity to reorder. For this assignment, a **supply** meets one or more of the following conditions:

- It is consumed in use
- It is expendable, and if it is damaged, it will be replaced rather than repaired
- It costs less than $250.00

Assume that your office wants to keep a 3-month supply of each item on hand. Assume that 100 patients are seen in the office each day, five days a week. Assume that there will be a 2-week delay between the time the order is placed and the time the order is received.

D. PATIENT BILL OF RIGHTS

Based on the national Consumer Bill of Rights and Responsibilities for Health Care of 1997, create a list of patient rights related to the care they will receive in your office and which might be included in a medical office policy. Use language that is simple and direct, assuming that this list might be given to patients. You can view a summary at the following website: http://www.hcqualitycommission.gov/cborr/exsumm.html.

_____
_____
_____
_____
_____
_____
_____
_____
_____
_____
_____
_____
_____
_____

E. EVACUATION PLAN

Create an evacuation plan for a specific room in the school where you are receiving your medical assisting training. You may choose a classroom or laboratory. Include each of the following elements:

1. Conditions under which an evacuation would be necessary: _____

_____

_____

2. Conditions under which it may be better to stay in place: _____

_____

_____

3. Individual authorized to order an evacuation and back-up individual: _____

_____

4. Specific route and exits to be used for evacuation: _____

_____

_____

5. Procedures for assisting disabled individuals to evacuate: _____

_____

_____

6. Means of determining that all individuals have left the area: _____

_____

_____

7. Means of accounting for employees after evacuation: _____

_____

_____

F. COMMUNITY RESOURCES FOR EMERGENCY PREPAREDNESS
Make a list of community resources for emergency preparedness in your community. Include names and contact information.

_____

_____

_____

_____

_____

_____

_____

_____

_____

_____

_____

G. INCIDENT REPORT
You are working in a medical office, and a patient slips and falls in the corridor when being taken back to an examination room. The physician is called, assists the patient to get up, and finds a bruise on the right hip but no other apparent injury. The physician instructs the patient to telephone if any problems arise later and documents the examination and findings in the patient's medical record. It is office policy to fill out an incident report for any fall that occurs in the office. Make a list of all information that you would have to include on the incident report.

_____

_____

_____

_____

_____

_____

_____

_____

_____

_____

_____

PRACTICE FOR COMPETENCY

Procedure 48-1: Performing Routine Maintenance of Equipment. Perform routine maintenance of both administrative and clinical equipment such as the autoclave, electrocardiograph, photocopier, and/or fax machine. Complete an equipment maintenance log for each item.

<table>
<tr><td colspan="3" align="center">Equipment Maintenance Log</td><td></td></tr>
<tr><td>Equipment description:</td><td colspan="3"></td></tr>
<tr><td>Serial Number:</td><td></td><td>Model Number:</td><td></td></tr>
<tr><td></td><td></td><td></td><td>Initials</td></tr>
<tr><td>Date:</td><td colspan="2">Action Taken/Comments:</td><td></td></tr>
<tr><td></td><td colspan="2"></td><td></td></tr>
<tr><td></td><td colspan="2"></td><td></td></tr>
<tr><td></td><td colspan="2"></td><td></td></tr>
<tr><td></td><td colspan="2"></td><td></td></tr>
<tr><td></td><td colspan="2"></td><td></td></tr>
</table>

<table>
<tr><td colspan="3" align="center">Equipment Maintenance Log</td><td></td></tr>
<tr><td>Equipment description:</td><td colspan="3"></td></tr>
<tr><td>Serial Number:</td><td></td><td>Model Number:</td><td></td></tr>
<tr><td></td><td></td><td></td><td>Initials</td></tr>
<tr><td>Date:</td><td colspan="2">Action Taken/Comments:</td><td></td></tr>
<tr><td></td><td colspan="2"></td><td></td></tr>
<tr><td></td><td colspan="2"></td><td></td></tr>
<tr><td></td><td colspan="2"></td><td></td></tr>
<tr><td></td><td colspan="2"></td><td></td></tr>
</table>

Procedure 48-2: Taking a Supply or Equipment Inventory. Take a supply and equipment inventory using the lists you prepared for Critical Thinking Activities B and C above. Prepare a list of supplies to be ordered.

Procedure 48-3: Locating Community Resources. Make a list of community resources to which patients may be referred including visiting nurse services, homemaker services, meal delivery, senior services, etc.

EVALUATION OF COMPETENCY

Procedure 48-1: Performing Routine Maintenance of Equipment

Name: _____   Date: _____

Evaluated By: _____   Date: _____

Performance Objective

Outcome:	Perform equipment maintenance and document on equipment maintenance log.
Conditions:	Given the following: piece of equipment to be maintained, cloth for dusting, maintenance log sheet, and supplies necessary for the piece or equipment (such as paper, batteries, toner, fluids, etc).
Standards:	Time: 10 minutes. Student completed procedure in ____ minutes.
	Accuracy: Satisfactory score on the Performance Evaluation Checklist.

Performance Evaluation Checklist

Trial 1	Trial 2	Point Value	Performance Standards
		•	Located the piece of equipment to be maintained.
		•	Checked all electrical cords to be sure there is no fraying or malfunction.
		•	Checked the piece of equipment for cracks, dents, or other damage, obvious impairment or malfunction.
		•	Checked any keyboard or keypad for cracks, faded numbers, or other impairment.
		▷	Explained what to do if the piece of equipment was damaged.
		•	Dusted or cleaned the outside or case of the piece of equipment according to manufacturer's directions.
		•	Checked leads and other wires, or other tubing.
		•	Checked or changed batteries, fluid, toner, or other essential components.
		•	Scheduled any required maintenance if appropriate.
		•	Filled out the equipment maintenance log correctly.
		✶	Completed the procedure within 10 minutes.
			TOTALS

Equipment Maintenance Log		
Equipment description:		
Serial Number:	**Model Number:**	

		Initials
Date:	**Action Taken/Comments:**	

Evaluation of Student Performance

EVALUATION CRITERIA			COMMENTS
Symbol	Category	Point Value	
∗	Critical Step	16 points	
•	Essential Step	6 points	
▷	Theory Question	2 points	

Score calculation: 100 points

− _____ points missed

_____ Score

Satisfactory score: 85 or above

CAAHEP Competencies Achieved:

Psychomotor (Skills)

☑ V. 9. Perform routine maintenance of office equipment with documentation.

ABHES Competencies Achieved:

☑ 8. y. Perform routine maintenance of administrative and clinical equipment.

EVALUATION OF COMPETENCY

Procedure 48-2: Taking a Supply or Equipment Inventory

Name: _____ Date: _____

Evaluated By: _____ Date: _____

Performance Objective

Outcome:	Take a supply and equipment inventory.
Conditions:	Given the following: inventory list, notebook or cards, items to inventory, and pen.
Standards:	Time: 15 minutes. Student completed procedure in _____ minutes.
	Accuracy: Satisfactory score on the Performance Evaluation Checklist.

Performance Evaluation Checklist

Trial 1	Trial 2	Point Value	*Performance Standards*
		●	Obtained list of items in inventory, inventory notebook, or box of inventory cards.
		●	Checked each item in the inventory record against items present in the area being inventoried.
		●	Validated serial numbers or equipment and checked the expiration date of supplies.
		●	Discarded any expired supplies and did not include in the inventory count.
		●	Documented any missing piece of equipment after making an effort to locate.
		●	Documented any item that needed repair.
		●	Flagged any supplies close to or below the reorder point as needing to be reordered.
		●	Checked that information on the inventory card or list was correct and complete.
		●	Made sure that the storage space was tidy and arranged so that items with the oldest expiration date were at the front of the storage area.
		●	Placed inventory cards, list, or book in the proper location for follow-up.
		✱	Completed the procedure within 15 minutes.
			TOTALS

Evaluation of Student Performance

EVALUATION CRITERIA			COMMENTS
Symbol	Category	Point Value	
∗	Critical Step	16 points	
•	Essential Step	6 points	
▷	Theory Question	2 points	

Score calculation: 100 points

−_____ points missed

_____ Score

Satisfactory score: 85 or above

CAAHEP Competencies Achieved:

Psychomotor (Skills)
☑ V. 10. Perform an office inventory.

ABHES Competencies Achieved:

☑ 8. z. Maintain inventory equipment and supplies.

EVALUATION OF COMPETENCY

Procedure 48-3: Locating Community Resources

Name: _____   Date: _____

Evaluated By: _____   Date: _____

Performance Objective

Outcome:	Locate community resources.
Conditions:	Given the following: local telephone book, office list of community resources, computer, local hospital newsletter(s), library access, local newspapers, pen, and notepad.
Standards:	Time: 15 minutes. Student completed procedure in _____ minutes.
	Accuracy: Satisfactory score on the Performance Evaluation Checklist.

Performance Evaluation Checklist

Trial 1	Trial 2	Point Value	Performance Standards
		•	Researched local sources to identify community agencies.
		•	As resources were identified, created a list.
		•	Included pertinent information such as name, services available, address, telephone number, web address, contact information, and other useful information.
		•	Transferred handwritten list to a computer document.
		•	Grouped resources by category and alphabetized within each group.
		•	Obtained physician approval of finished list.
		•	Updated the list when information changed, new resources were identified.
		•	Used a list of community resources for patients to make recommendations to patients and families.
		＊	Completed the procedure within 15 minutes.
			TOTALS

Evaluation of Student Performance

EVALUATION CRITERIA			COMMENTS
Symbol	Category	Point Value	
✳	Critical Step	16 points	
●	Essential Step	6 points	
▷	Theory Question	2 points	

Score calculation: 100 points

       − _____ points missed

       _____ Score

Satisfactory score: 85 or above

CAAHEP Competencies Achieved:

Psychomotor (Skills)

☑ XI. 12. Maintain a current list of community resources for emergency preparedness.

ABHES Competencies Achieved:

☑ 8. 3. Locate resources and information for patients and employers.

49

Obtaining Employment

CHAPTER ASSIGNMENTS

√ After Completing	Date Due	Textbook Page(s)	TEXTBOOK ASSIGNMENTS	Possible Points	Points You Earned
		1129-1144	Read Chapter 49: Obtaining Employment		
		1137 1143	Read Case Study 1 Case Study questions	5	
		1138 1143	Read Case Study 2 Case Study questions	5	
		1141 1144	Read Case Study 3 Case Study questions	5	
			TOTAL POINTS		

√ After Completing	Date Due	Study Guide Page(s)	STUDY GUIDE ASSIGNMENTS (CTA: Critical Thinking Activity)	Possible Points	Points You Earned
		1259	Pretest	10	
		1260	Key Term Assessment	5	
		1261-1263	Evaluation of Learning questions	24	
		1264-1267	CTA A: Preparing a Resumé	15	
		1267-1268	CTA B: Preparing a Cover Letter	10	
		1268	CTA C: References	10	
		1268-1269	CTA D: Interview Questions	10	
			CD Activity: Chapter 49 Apply Your Knowledge questions (Record points earned)		
		1259	Posttest	10	

√ After Completing	Date Due	Study Guide Page(s)	STUDY GUIDE ASSIGNMENTS (CTA: Critical Thinking Activity)	Possible Points	Points You Earned
			ADDITIONAL ASSIGNMENTS		
			TOTAL POINTS		

Name _____   Date _____

❓ PRETEST

True or False

_____ 1. Networking to find employment means applying for jobs using the Internet.

_____ 2. It is recommended to limit a resumé to one page.

_____ 3. Hobbies and other personal information are included in the last section of a resumé.

_____ 4. A functional resumé is recommended when an individual wants to change to a different type of work.

_____ 5. Begin a resumé with your name, address, telephone number, and e-mail address.

_____ 6. The medical assisting externship and volunteer work should not be included under *Work Experience*.

_____ 7. When describing job duties, use all past tense or all participle forms of verbs.

_____ 8. It is assumed that a medical assistant has a valid CPR certification, and it isn't necessary on the resumé.

_____ 9. The medical assistant should always ask permission before using a supervisor's name as a reference.

_____ 10. The medical assistant may ask about a salary range during the interview.

❓ POSTTEST

True or False

_____ 1. Using several methods to identify potential employers is an important step to find a job.

_____ 2. If a resumé is submitted to an employer, it is not necessary to complete a job application.

_____ 3. A resumé that categorizes experience according to skills is called a *chronological resumé*.

_____ 4. When including information about education, it should be listed with the most recent first.

_____ 5. The high school and date diploma was received should always be included on a resumé.

_____ 6. It is important not to leave gaps of time unaccounted for on a resumé.

_____ 7. Job duties may be summarized in bullet form on a resumé.

_____ 8. The names and addresses of three personal references should be listed on the resumé.

_____ 9. Resumés can be sent through the mail, attached to e-mail, by fax, or attached to an online application.

_____ 10. The interviewer should not ask about marital status or number of children during a job interview.

♪Term **KEY TERM ASSESSMENT**

Directions: Match each medical term with its definition.

1. Burnout

2. Continuing education unit (CEU)

3. Cover letter

4. Networking

5. Resumé

A. A summary of information about a person that describes education, work experience, and other information

B. A letter sent with one or more documents (such as a resumé) to provide an explanation

C. Contacting acquaintances and their contacts who may know of potential jobs

D. Disillusionment with work and physical or emotional exhaustion

E. A standard measure of 10 hours of qualified instruction or contact hours as defined by a specific profession

EVALUATION OF LEARNING

Directions: Fill in each blank with the correct answer.

1. What are the two parts of successful job hunting?

   _____

   _____

2. What are three questions the MA might ask himself or herself when setting goals for job hunting?

   _____

   _____

   _____

3. Identify three resources to identify potential employers other than newspaper or Internet advertisements.

   _____

   _____

   _____

4. Describe what a resumé is, and identify its function.

   _____

   _____

   _____

5. Should an MA include personal information on a resumé? Why or why not?

   _____

   _____

6. Describe three styles of resumés.

   _____

   _____

   _____

7. What information should be included on a resumé?

   _____

   _____

8. What specific information should be included in the education section of a resumé?

_____

_____

_____

9. Discuss two ways that previous experience can be presented, and give advantages and disadvantages of each.

_____

_____

_____

_____

10. In a previous job at a supermarket, the MA often helped put price tags on new items and arrange them in the store. Describe this using the past tense as she might include it on a resumé.

_____

_____

11. In a previous job at a retail store, the MA worked at the cash register. Describe this using the participle form of the verb as it would appear in a bulleted list.

_____

_____

12. What are three types of information that might be included in the "Special Skills" section of a resumé?

_____

_____

13. How should the MA prepare a list of references?

_____

_____

14. What format should be used for the final version of a resumé?

_____

_____

15. What is the purpose of a cover letter when sending out resumés?

_____

16. What are the advantages and disadvantages of faxing a resumé?

_____

_____

17. In addition to a resumé, what information should the MA bring when applying for a job?

_____

_____

18. Identify six specific ways that the MA can make a favorable impression during a job interview.

_____

_____

_____

_____

19. What kinds of questions might an MA ask during a job interview?

_____

_____

20. What kind of follow-up is appropriate after a job interview?

_____

_____

21. After obtaining employment, how can the MA keep his or her administrative and clinical skills current?

_____

_____

_____

22. Identify three specific actions an MA can take to avoid or respond to job burnout.

_____

_____

23. Identify four benefits for members of a national professional organization.

_____

_____

_____

24. Identify four routes that an MA may take to advance his or her career.

_____

_____

CRITICAL THINKING ACTIVITIES

A. PREPARING A RESUMÉ

Complete the following information as a basis for preparing your resumé.

1. Identify the kind of job(s) you are looking for:

First choice

_____

Second choice

_____

2. Summarize your education beginning with your most recent:

Name of school _____

City _____ State _____

Dates attended: _____/_____/_____ to _____/_____/_____

Degree: _____ Date: _____/_____/_____

Major (or courses completed if you did not graduate):

_____

_____

Awards, GPA (if higher than 3.0), Dean's list (dates):

_____

Previous education (beyond high school)

Name of school _____

City _____ State _____

Dates attended: _____/_____/_____ to _____/_____/_____

Degree: _____ Date: _____/_____/_____

Major (or courses completed if you did not graduate):

_____

_____

Awards, GPA (if higher than 3.0), Dean's list (dates):

_____

Provide information for other educational experience.

_____

_____

Other relevant training and dates of completion including first aid training, CPR training, and computer training.

_____

_____

_____

Other skills including foreign languages spoken and skills you have learned but never practiced in an externship or work setting.

_____

_____

_____

3. Summarize your experience in the health care field beginning with your most recent. Include your medical assisting externship.

Name of organization or physician: _____

City _____ State _____

Dates of experience: _____/_____/_____ to _____/_____/_____

Type of experience or job title: _____

Indicate if the following apply: Externship/Practicum _____ Volunteer _____ Part-time _____ Summer _____

Identify your duties and responsibilities, one per line. Use a consistent form (e.g., "prepared patients for examinations," "responsible for preparing patients for examinations").

_____

_____

_____

_____

_____

_____

Identify any special accomplishments, promotions, or other positive outcomes from this position.

_____

_____

Next most recent health-related experience:

Name of organization or physician: _____

City _____ State _____

Dates of experience: _____/_____/_____ to _____/_____/_____

Type of experience or job title: _____

Indicate if the following apply: Externship/Practicum _____ Volunteer _____ Part-time _____ Summer _____

Identify your duties and responsibilities, one per line. Use a consistent form (e.g., "prepared patients for examinations," or "responsible for preparing patients for examinations").

_____

_____

_____

_____

_____

_____

Identify any special accomplishments, promotions, or other positive outcomes from this position.

_____

_____

Next most recent health-related experience:

Name of organization or physician: _____

City _____ State _____

Dates of experience: _____/_____/_____ to _____/_____/_____

Type of experience or job title: _____

Indicate if the following apply: Externship/Practicum _____ Volunteer _____ Part-time _____ Summer _____

Identify your duties and responsibilities, one per line. Use a consistent form (e.g., "prepared patients for examinations," or "responsible for preparing patients for examinations").

_____

_____

_____

_____

_____

_____

Identify any special accomplishments, promotions, or other positive outcomes from this position.

_____

_____

Provide information for other experience in the health care field.

_____

_____

4. Identify work experience that is not related to health care. Include all full-time jobs, but if you have not been employed consistently, include part-time and/or summer employment, volunteer experience, or time spent as a homemaker.

Employer (or organization): _____

City _____ State _____

Dates of experience: _____/_____/_____ to _____/_____/_____

Type of experience or job title: _____

Indicate if the following apply: Externship/Practicum _____ Volunteer _____ Part-time _____ Summer _____

Identify your duties and responsibilities, one per line. Use a consistent form (e.g., "prepared patients for examinations," or "responsible for preparing patients for examinations").

_____

_____

_____

_____

_____

_____

Identify any special accomplishments, promotions, or other positive outcomes from this position.

_____

_____

Provide information for other work experience.

_____

_____

Next most recent experience:

Employer (or organization): _____

_____ State _____

f experience: _____/_____/_____ to _____/_____/_____

Type of experience or job title: _____

Indicate if the following apply: Externship/Practicum _____ Volunteer _____ Part-time _____ Summer _____

Identify your duties and responsibilities, one per line. Use a consistent form (e.g., "prepared patients for examinations," or "responsible for preparing patients for examinations").

_____

_____

_____

_____

_____

_____

Identify any special accomplishments, promotions, or other positive outcomes from this position.

_____

_____

Provide information for other work experience.

_____

_____

Next most recent experience:

Employer (or organization): _____

City _____ State _____

Dates of experience: _____/_____/_____ to _____/_____/_____

Type of experience or job title: _____

Indicate if the following apply: Externship/Practicum _____ Volunteer _____ Part-time _____ Summer _____

Identify your duties and responsibilities, one per line. Use a consistent form (e.g., "prepared patients for examinations," or "responsible for preparing patients for examinations").

_____

_____

_____

_____

_____

_____

Identify any special accomplishments, promotions, or other positive outcomes from this position.

_____

_____

Provide information for other work experience.

_____

_____

B. PREPARING A COVER LETTER
Complete the following information to help you prepare a cover letter to accompany your resumé when you look for a job.

1. Describe in one sentence the reason that you are currently seeking a job.

_____

_____

_____

2. Describe the type of position you seek (job title, full-time, and/or part-time) and when you will be available to begin working.

_____

_____

_____

3. Describe your personal qualifications in a few sentences focusing on your strengths as a person, as well as your skills.

_____

_____

_____

C. REFERENCES

Complete the following information to help you prepare a list of at least three references. If possible, include a supervisor from employment and/or externship and an instructor or coach from your educational program. Indicate if you have already obtained permission from the person to use him or her as a reference.

Name: _____ Permission Requested: _____

This person's relationship to you: _____

Contact information:

Employer: _____ Job Title: _____

Address: _____

_____

Telephone Number: _____

Name: _____ Permission Requested: _____

This person's relationship to you: _____

Contact information:

Employer: _____ Job Title: _____

Address: _____

_____

Telephone Number: _____

Name: _____ Permission Requested: _____

This person's relationship to you: _____

Contact information:

Employer: _____ Job Title: _____

Address: _____

_____

Telephone Number: _____

Provide information for two other references.

_____

_____

D. INTERVIEW QUESTIONS

Prepare a personalized and thoughtful response to each of the following questions you might be asked during a job interview.

1. Where do you see yourself in 5 years?

_____

_____

_____

_____

_____

2. Describe a difficult situation you have had at work and how you handled it.

_____

_____

_____

_____

_____

3. What could you contribute to our office?

_____

_____

_____

_____

_____

4. What are some of your weaknesses or areas you need to work on?

_____

_____

_____

_____

_____

5. What would your medical assisting instructor say about you if I were to call her for a reference?

_____

_____

_____

_____

_____

Notes

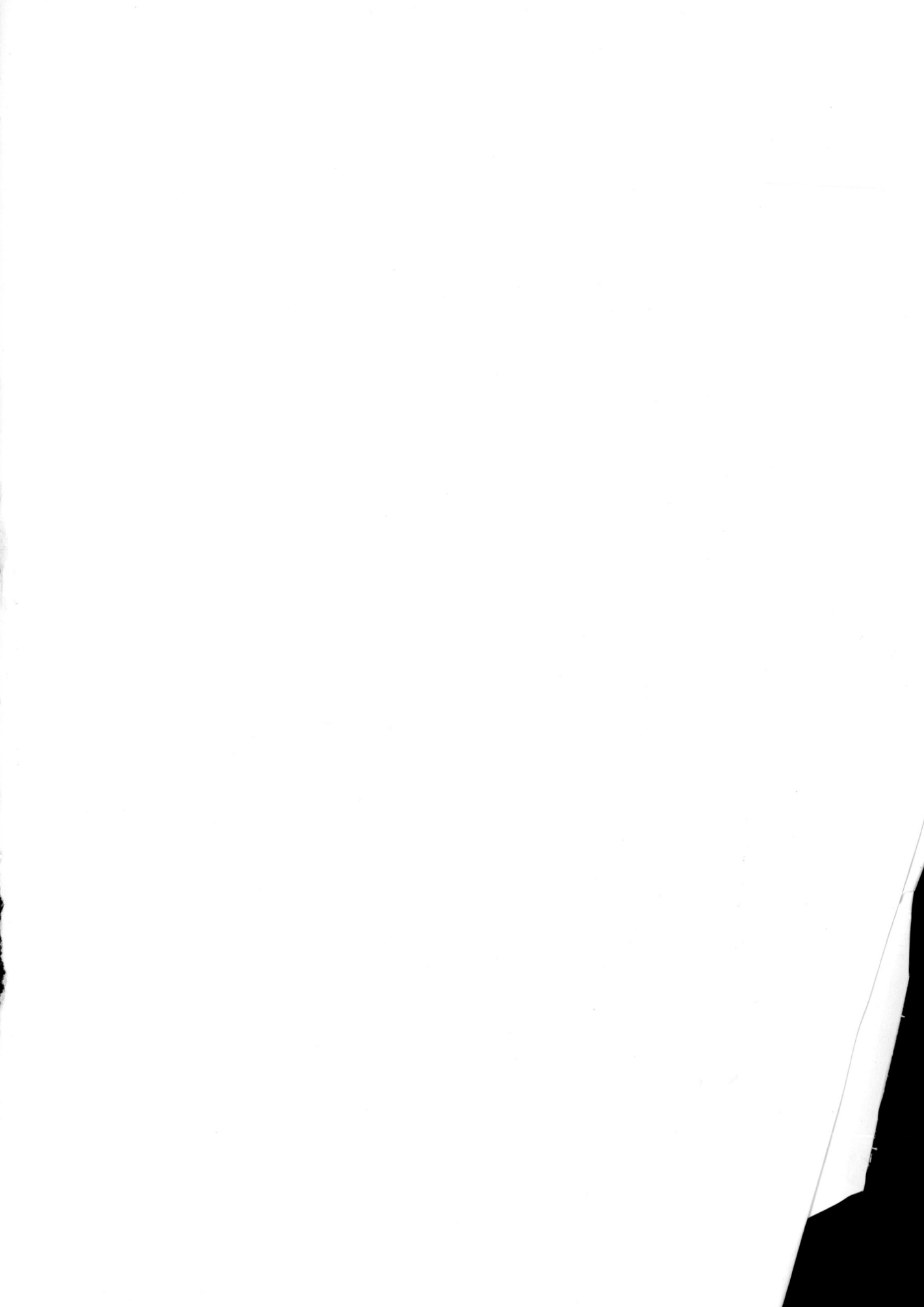